Psychotropic Medications and Developmental Disabilities: The International Consensus Handbook

Steven Reiss and Michael G. Aman

Nisonger Center
The Ohio State University

The Ohio State University Nisonger Center (Publisher)
Sponsored by the Arc of the United States
Distributed by the American Association on Mental Retardation

This book is dedicated to Maggi Reiss and Marsha Aman.

_____

ISBN 0-9658966-0-9

Published by The Ohio State University Nisonger Center. Distributed by the American Association on Mental Retardation. Sponsored by The Arc of the United States. Printed in the United States of America

Psychotropic Medication and Developmental Disabilities:
The International Consensus Handbook

Steven Reiss and Michael G. Aman (Editors)
The Ohio State University Nisonger Center

co-sponsored by The Arc of the United States

PREFACE

APPENDICIES

Preface

Since the 1970s, many concerns have been raised about the use of psychotropic medications for people with mental retardation and developmental disabilities (MR/DD). Policy makers concerned about frequent use have cited surveys showing that some 30% to 50% of the adults in U.S. institutions, and 25% to 40% of those in the community, take psychotropic medications on a daily basis. The drugs sometimes are prescribed indefinitely, with no specified endpoint to treatment. Many of the patients are nonverbal and cannot easily alert caregivers concerning possible adverse effects. Particularly in children, the drugs may interfere with learning, making acquisition of basic skills and knowledge even more difficult.

Another concern is the shortage of physicians trained to work with this population. Many physicians are trained in either mental retardation (pediatrics) or mental illness (psychiatry), but not in both. Because there is little interdisciplinary training, our medical schools produce few physicians trained to serve the needs of people who have a "dual diagnosis" (both mental retardation and mental illness). Consequently, many physicians are unfamiliar with the issues of dual diagnosis.

More research is needed on the safety and efficacy of psychotropic drugs when used with this population. Although data are limited, there are reasons to believe that these drugs sometimes interact with MR/DD or are effective at different dosages. Scientific research is needed to establish diagnostic conditions, identify effective dosage levels, and delineate adverse and interaction effects.

CONSENSUS PROCESS

These considerations suggest the need for an authoritative reference book on the use of psychotropic medicines with patients with MR/DD. In 1991 we sought to address this need by creating a consensus process. A significant number of influential medical, scientific, and public policy figures have supported this process. However, some people questioned the meaning of the word "consensus." Does "consensus" mean that everybody will reach agreement? What happens when this cannot be achieved? Who will participate in the process? Is it possible for the diverse elements of our field—physicians, scientists, and consumers—to reach a consensus? Since a consensus opinion can be invalid, some argued that it is better to establish knowledge solely through science.

Our Goals

Our consensus process was designed to identify the common observations of a large group of responsible scientists and practitioners and to integrate this information with that obtained from the relevant scientific literature. We did not seek to eliminate diversity of opinion; instead, our goal was to create a valid process in which competing ideas could be tested and improved. All too often, untested ideas have been propagated outside of peer-reviewed sources or presented at workshops; by creating a consensus process, we reduced the future influence of untested ideas and increased the likelihood of debate and discussion prior to practice. We sought to promote appropriate practices and to reduce extreme, risky, or abusive practices.

The Making of the Handbook

Our consensus process represents a coming together of various elements of the developmental disabilities field. There are many forces in our field that divide; in contrast, our process was intended to unite. The diverse groups participating in the process worked effectively together, producing this reference book and new guidelines for practice.

Our process was diverse and inclusive. It included seven professional disciplines (neurology, nursing, pharmacy, pediatrics, psychiatry, psychology, and special education) from 11 nations, as well as consumers and families. We invited participation from nearly everybody we could think of who actively published in the area or presented at national conferences (see Reiss and Aman, in press). We invited heads of University Affiliated Programs to nominate additional persons. We invited panel members to nominate additional persons. We organized an international conference to provide a forum for people in the field to comment on the work of the consensus committees.

This book represents the culmination of six years' effort. From our perspective, the three main activities were to organize the international consensus panel; to organize the international consensus conference held on June 15 and 16, 1995; and to edit the committee reports and draft chapters into a coherent volume. The last two of these activities represented an enormous amount of work. The effort is described in Reiss and Aman (in press).

Reiss' role was to organize the consensus panel; to plan and organize the international consensus conference; to edit content related to psychopathology and assessment; and to edit for clarity of expression. The initial idea for this project was Reiss'. Aman's role was to edit the drug chapters and co-edit the other chapters. This is a book on psychopharmacology; Aman was the primary editor for content related to psychopharmacology. Aman's ideas provided the basis for organizing the book and the chapters. Every sentence in the book was carefully considered by each editor, sometimes more than once. Many of the chapters were revised repeatedly in an effort to meet high standards of quality.

Here are some specific ways in which this book may be used.

1. Physicians may use the book to learn about the observations and opinions of the consensus panel and various committees that wrote the book.

2. Agencies may provide a copy of the book to consulting physicians as a means of strengthening the information on which decisions are made.

3. Teams and review panels may use the book to reflect on their roles, identify best practices, and strengthen methods for monitoring for adverse effects.

4. Consumers may use the book to help formulate questions to physicans and service providers.

5. Researchers may use the text as a reference volume to help set the stage for future research.

6. The book may be used to help identify extreme, idiosyncratic, inappropriate, or abusive practices.

Steven Reiss
Michael G. Aman
Columbus, Ohio

INTENDED USES

The content of this book represents the views of a large number of authorities. Although these views are not a "consensus" in the sense that all panel members agree with all statements, they are views endorsed generally by a number of authorities with diverse backgrounds. The book is intended to be comprehensive and authoritative.

Users should appreciate that consensus opinions are not necessarily valid opinions. The consensus opinions in this book represent a conservative statement of our best estimate of what is known at this point in time. Ultimately, only scientific research can establish validity. With future research, it is likely that some of the consensus opinions in this book will change, perhaps to a substantial degree. What we consider to be knowledge is not static or absolute; it is subject to change with new information and future experiences.

REFERENCE

Reiss, S., & Aman, M.G. (in press). The international consensus process on psychopharmacology and mental retardation. *Journal of Intellectual Disability Research.*

Diagnosis of Mental Disorders in People with Mental Retardation

Ludwik S. Szymanski[1], Bryan King[2], Benjamin Goldberg[3], Andrew H. Reid[4], Bruce J. Tonge[5], and Nancy Cain[6]

"Conduct may be founded on the hard rock or the wet marshes"

— F. Scott Fitzgerald,
The Great Gatsby

THE DIAGNOSIS OF MENTAL DISORDERS

Although there is no single definition of *mental disorder*, the concept is described as follows in the 1994 version of the American Psychiatric Association's (APA) *Diagnostic and Statistical Manual of Mental Disorders* (DSM-IV):

" a clinically significant behavioral or psychological syndrome or pattern that occurs in an individual and that is associated with present distress (e.g., a painful symptom) or disability (i.e., impairment in one or more important areas of functioning) or with a significantly increased risk of suffering death, pain, disability, or an important loss of freedom." (APA, 1994, p. xxi)

The term "diagnosis" is an application of a standardized name to a certain problem, and in general medicine, a recognition and naming of a disease. The *Random House Dictionary* (1987) gives the following definition: "a. The process of determining by examination the nature and circumstances of a diseased condition; b. the decision reached from such an examination." According to *Webster's International Dictionary* (3rd ed.), diagnosis means: "a. The art and act of identifying a disease from its signs and symptoms; b. a concise technical description of a taxonomic entity giving its distinguishing characters; c. investigation or analysis of the cause or nature of a condition, situation or problem" (p. 622). These definitions include naming the disease entity; describing its properties, circumstances, and causation; and making recommendations.

There are several levels of diagnoses. The pathoetiologic diagnosis describes the specific causation and the mechanism of the disorder (e.g., lobar pneumonia caused by *Streptococcus pneumoniae*). It is the most accurate type of diagnosis and most likely to lead to specific treatment, especially when it is confirmed by physical or laboratory findings. A syndromic diagnosis is based on the presence of a cluster (syndrome) of symptoms and signs (e.g., pneumonia may be indicated by fever, cough, breathing difficulties, and crepitation heard on auscultation of the chest.) This diagnosis is not specific because various agents may cause a syndrome. Diagnosis is even less specific when it is based on a single symptom, such as cough. The diagnosis of most mental disorders is either syndromic (e.g., at least 6 of 12 criteria have to be met for a diagnosis of autistic disorder) or monosymptomatic (e.g., sterotypic movement disorder with self-injurious behavior [SIB]).

Because the diagnosis of many mental disorders cannot be based on etiology, some authorities have stressed the importance of understanding individual psychopathology rather than fitting the patient into a rigid, diagnostic classification. This approach was supported by psychodynamic theorists, who focused on the pathology of personality development, unconscious conflicts, defenses, and other mental processes. However, formal psychiatric diagnosis made a comeback in the 1960s when progress in elucidating the roles of neurotransmitters brought mental disorders back into the realm of medicine. The growing use of psychoac-

1 Director of Psychiatry, Developmental Evaluation Center, Children's Hospital, Boston, MA
2 Assistant Professor of Psychiatry, University of California at Los Angeles, Los Angeles, CA
3 Emeritus Professor of Developmental Neuropsychiatry, University of Western Ontario, London, Ontario, Canada
4 Consultant Psychiatrist, Royal Dundee Liff Hospital, Dundee, Scotland
5 Professor of Developmental Psychiatry, Monash University, Clayton, Victoria, Australia
6 Clinical Assistant Professor of Psychiatry, University of Rochester School of Medicine and Dentistry, Rochester, NY

tive drugs also led to an increased need for standard diagnostic criteria. Today, formal diagnosis is critical for the controlled studies of drug effects, for replicability of possible results, and for comparisons across studies.

In this chapter, *diagnosis* refers to a comprehensive diagnostic understanding as well as a formal diagnostic label. Szymanski and Crocker (1989) used the term "expanded diagnosis" to encourage descriptions that include factors initiating and maintaining the symptoms, the person's strengths and functional level, and the need for intervention in various domains. A comprehensive assessment approach was further developed by the American Association on Mental Retardation's (AAMR) definition of mental retardation (AAMR, 1992), which requires that the assessment of people with mental retardation include the following four dimensions: intellectual and adaptive; psychological and emotional; physical, health, and etiological; and environmental. Thus, **there is general agreement that a diagnostic label alone is not sufficient in the assessment of a person with mental retardation.**

The importance of establishing diagnosis is well illustrated by recent research findings indicating that different cases of aggression can be associated with different mental disorders. Aggression is sometimes associated with depression (Reiss & Rojahn, 1993), paranoia (Reiss, 1992), psychosis, or personality disorder (Goldberg, Gitta, & Puddephatt, 1992). That is, some people are aggressive because they are unhappy and irritable, some because they are quick to perceive insult, some because they hear voices telling them to attack, and some because they are maladjusted and have turned to aggression as a habit for solving their problems. For many others, aggression may actually be an appropriate response to an inappropriate environmental situation. Psychiatric diagnoses help clinicians determine what type of aggression is present and how to respond in terms of treatment.

Frequently an aberrant behavior in a person with mental retardation is described as a behavior disorder, as opposed to a mental disorder. There is no official definition of the term *behavior disorder*, but it is commonly thought to refer to maladaptive, especially disruptive, behaviors, that are learned responses to environmental antecedents or consequences. The use of this concept sometimes overlooks two considerations (Szymanski, 1994). One consideration is that there are elements of learned behavior in the clinical presentation of every mental disorder. The other consideration is that the DSM-IV is atheoretical in that diagnosis is made mostly on the basis of observed behavioral manifestations

and not causation (unless causation is clear, such as "due to general medical condition"). Thus, there may not be a need to distinguish between behavioral and mental disorders; it may be more productive to determine which mental disorder syndrome is manifested by the behavior in question and then, the etiology, or factors initiating and maintaining the behavior. This strategy of course, assumes that the general criteria for mental disorder are met and that the individual has a persistent, aberrant, maladaptive behavioral pattern, rather than a minor, transitory, or situational behavior.

During the consensus process that resulted in the publication of this book, the opinion was voiced that it would not be appropriate to make a diagnosis of a mental disorder in every case of an aberrant behavior, and this is certainly true. Equally, the DSM-IV is not intended to be used to make a diagnosis of a mental disorder, for example, in every instance of a disobedient child. Thus, one should not make a diagnosis of intermittent explosive disorder for a person who exhibits aggressive behavior in a poorly staffed, sheltered workshop but behaves well in an adequately staffed residence.

THE EVOLUTION OF CLASSIFICATION SYSTEMS OF MENTAL DISORDERS

The modern classification systems were strongly influenced by Emil Kraepelin, who stressed objective and detailed description of the clinical features of mental disorders. He also noticed symptom overlap among various disorders.

The DSM has been the primary classification system for the diagnosis of mental disorders in the United States and is increasingly becoming the international model. There have been five versions. What is sometimes called a paradigm shift occurred in 1980 when the publication of DSM III signalled a change from a psychodynamic to a neuroscientific model.

The DSM I (APA, 1952) was based partially on the classification developed by the APA's Committee on Nomenclature and Statistics. It referred to disorders as "reactions" to psychological, social, and biological factors. DSM-I and the DSM-II (APA, 1968) gave general descriptions which reflected both psychobiological views and the psychodynamic model. The DSM-II was frequently criticized (Spitzer & Fleiss, 1974) for having unreliable diagnostic categories and for including few or no treatment implications.

The DSM-III (APA, 1980) represented a radical shift to a descriptive model, having its roots in the Kraepelinian focus on description of clinical observations. The disorders were grouped according to clinical presentation rather than presumed psychodynamic mechanism, and diagnostic categories were defined by specific, objective criteria describing clinical symptoms. The DSM-III specified that a minimal number of criteria had to be met before a diagnosis could be made. The DSM-III also introduced a multiaxial model, whereby diagnosis was made on five axes: (I), mental disorder; (II), developmental and personality disorders; (III), relevant physical disorders; (IV), psychosocial stressors; and (V), level of adaptive functioning. The DSM-III-R (APA, 1987) was an improved version of the DSM-III because it incorporated experience gathered in the clinical use of the DSM-III. In the DSM-IV (APA, 1994) developmental disorders are diagnosed on Axis I, whereas mental retardation and personality disorders are diagnosed on Axis II.

The DSM-I, DSM-II and, to a lesser degree, DSM-III were developed by individuals recognized as experts in the field, and represented the developers' efforts to achieve compromise between various views. The DSM-IV represents another step toward a research-based, neuroscience model of mental disorders. By international agreement, it was developed to be compatible with the ICD-10 (WHO, 1992). The DSM-IV is expected to include the same coding as the ICD-10.

The importance of a formal diagnostic system might be still denied by some mental health professionals. Behaviorists view maladaptive behaviors as expressions of learned responses rather than of diseases, and psychoanalysts believe that the underlying psychodynamics are not reflected in the formal diagnosis. Increasingly these are becoming minority views: The importance and usefulness of classification and diagnosis is generally accepted. Today, most of those who do research on the effectiveness of psychoactive drugs utilize DSM diagnostic categories as do virtually all of those who do influential cognitive research on psychopathology. The diagnostic system is essential in epidemiological research and formulation of public policy, and it is legally mandated by many state regulations and health insurance policies. Diagnostic understanding is necessary for designing a treatment program. For most patients and their families, a diagnosis will reduce confusion and uncertainty.

The following discussion of diagnosis is based, to the extent possible, on the DSM-IV (APA, 1994).

THREE QUESTIONS GUIDING PSYCHIATRIC DIAGNOSIS

One issue about which some disagreement continues concerns the terminology used to refer to the co-occurence of mental illness and mental retardation. The term *dual diagnosis*, introduced by Frank Menolascino, is widely used in this field. However, Szymanski and Grossman (1984) noted that this term is sometimes confusing. In the general mental health field, this term is commonly used for people who have both mental illness and substance abuse. Another concern is that a derivative term—*dually diagnosed*—has been used to classify people, rather than disorders, and in such cases the label can lead to discrimination. Although dissatisfaction with this term seems to be widespread, no substitute term has been widely adopted, although increasingly the writers of major texts refer to the comorbidity of mental disorder and mental retardation.

Discussions of psychiatric diagnosis and mental retardation generally have focused on the following three questions.

1. To what extent is it possible to establish a psychiatric diagnosis, according to standard diagnostic classification, for people who have both mental retardation and aberrant behaviors?

In the 1970s and 1980s a general consensus emerged that mental disorders can be diagnosed for people with mild mental retardation and reasonably good communicative skills, using standard diagnostic criteria. The diagnosis becomes more difficult for people with more severe mental retardation whose verbal skills are poor. Some people with severe mental retardation can be diagnosed using DSM-IV criteria that are modified to reflect their impairments and life circumstances, whereas others show patterns of symptoms and aberrant behaviors that cannot be easily fit into DSM-IV criteria for a specific mental disorder. However, the DSM-IV major diagnostic categories provide a subcategory of NOS (not otherwise specified), which can be used in such cases, to indicate at least that the person meets the general criteria for the diagnostic category but that a more specific diagnosis is not possible. The DSM-IV also includes several diagnoses based on a single symptom, such as stereotypic movement disorder and intermittent explosive disorder. Importantly, these diagnoses require that other, more specific disorders be excluded first. Thus, they should not be used in every case of a person with aggressive behavior.

Bregman (1991) reviewed the relevant literature and found at least several studies in which researchers utilized DSM-III criteria and were able to diagnose a broad spectrum of mental disorders among people who had mental retardation. Bouras, Brooks, and Drummond (1994) examined 356 people referred to a community psychiatric service in England over a period of 10 years. The sample included 57.6% with mild mental retardation, 27.4% with moderate mental retardation, and 15% with severe mental retardation. They were able to make a DSM-III-R diagnosis for 42.8% of the people they evaluated. In the remaining cases, behavioral problems were evident, but it was not possible to determine a specific psychiatric diagnosis.

2. What modifications of diagnostic criteria might be needed to diagnose mental disorders in people with mental retardation?

The clinical manifestations of mental disorders in people with mental retardation are modified by factors such as the cognitive and communication skill level; associated sensory, motor, and other disabilities that the person might have; life experiences; and learning opportunities. The most important influence is the language skills level, because many diagnostic criteria are based on an individual's communications. Some subjective symptoms, such as delusions, hallucinations, and thought disorder, cannot be ascertained if a person cannot communicate them. This problem occurs with young children and is not unique to mental retardation.

Although most psychopathology is manifested by essentially the same symptoms in people with mental retardation as in the general population (Philips, 1966), clinical presentation of some disorders may be significantly modified when the cognitive skills fall below certain levels. For example, a number of theorists have suggested that the very expression of psychopathology may change at low IQ levels (Aman, 1991; Reid, 1993; Reiss, 1994). If so, and if such "diagnostic metamorphoses" do occur, they still need to be demonstrated by research investigation. This is ultimately an empirical question for which an answer is not presently at hand.

A number of professionals have discussed criteria and methods for assessing and diagnosing psychiatric disorders for people with mental retardation (Reiss, 1994, pp. 102-103; Sovner, 1986; Szymanski, 1980). Sovner (1986) has described a phenomenon of psychosocial masking, in which specific psychiatric symptoms may be expressed in more simple or altered ways in people with mental retardation, and Reiss (1994) has stressed the importance of focusing on recognizable patterns of symptomatology that emerge as changes in typical functioning during periods

of regression. Modifications that have been suggested for specific disorders are discussed later in this chapter.

Researchers developed a number of psychometric instruments to aid in the assessment and diagnosis of mental disorders for this population. The more established instruments, such as the Aberrant Behavior Checklist (Aman, Singh, Stewart, & Field, 1985a) and the Reiss Screen for Maladaptive Behavior (Reiss, 1988; Reiss & Valenti-Hein, 1994), have research bases derived from well over 1,000 people and are widely used. The factor analytic research on these instruments has provided details on the specific ways in which mental disorders are expressed among people with mental retardation.

Researchers have discussed the relevance of developmental models for psychiatric diagnosis for people with mental retardation. In developmental models, aberrant behavior is diagnosed by comparing an individual with a group norm. This is how certain developmental disorders, such as mental retardation, are diagnosed. For many mental disorders, however, aberrant behavior is diagnosed by comparing an individual's current behavior to the same individual's premorbid behavior (Reiss, 1994, p. 42). In such cases, knowledge of normative development is not essential for a diagnosis, because the critical comparison is intra-individual.

3. To what extent does formal diagnosis aid in the selection of a specific treatment with psychoactive drugs?

Even though the causes of many mental disorders and symptoms are unknown, psychiatric diagnosis can help in the selection of appropriate medication and overall treatment plans, including non-pharmacological interventions. When a specific subcategory of a mental disorder cannot be diagnosed with confidence, which is not uncommon, treatment selection can be aided by identification of specific symptom clusters or precise specification of target behavior. However, symptomatic treatment is not definitive because a single symptom might be caused by a variety of disorders, each one requiring a different treatment.

There was once hope that for each diagnosis there would be a specific medication that alone would effect a cure. However, our experience with psychopharmacology to date indicates that reality is not this simple. For example, although a stimulant medication may reduce hyperactivity and impulsivity and increase attention span, behavioral and educational approaches are necessary to teach the socially appropriate communication of frustration. Similarly, in general medicine, not every case of essential hypertension responds to the same medication, and, even if there is a response, additional measures such as dietary or lifestyle changes and stress management are needed for a person to recover and maintain health.

Schatzberg and Cole (1991) offered the following three reasons to explain why matching a psychopharmacological treatment with a specific diagnosis is successful in only some cases: The disorder is not easily classified in many people; some people with a classic diagnosis do not respond to the traditional treatment for that disorder; and many drugs have wider actions than traditionally thought. For example, selective serotonin reuptake inhibitors are used for treatment of obsessive-compulsive disorders and depressive diseases, whereas tricyclic antidepressants are used for treatment of depression, enuresis, hyperactivity, and panic disorder.

Although a removal of a target symptom is important, the real goal should be to achieve a maximally feasible quality of life. For example, a person whose aggressive outbursts were ameliorated by the use of propranolol, but who developed the side effect of depression, should not be considered as a therapeutic success. Obviously, this person has not achieved an acceptable quality of life.

COMPONENTS OF A DIAGNOSTIC CLINICAL EXAMINATION

The initial diagnostic evaluation should be comprehensive. Quick medication reviews lasting a few minutes and leading to a prescription to control the behavior in question, regardless of the broader clinical presentation, are inappropriate.

The basic principles of psychiatric assessment apply to people who have mental retardation, but diagnostic techniques have to be adapted to the person's developmental level, especially the person's communication skills. A detailed discussion of the psychiatric clinical examination of persons with mental retardation is outside the scope of this chapter and can be found in standard textbooks (Reiss, 1994; Szymanski & Wilska, 1996). Here the three basic components are described: obtaining a detailed history, conducting a direct interview, and making a diagnostic formulation.

A *detailed history* should be obtained from all sources and caregivers, because many people with mental retardation may be unable to provide one themselves. Because the behavior leading to the referral might be a result of the person having to adapt to an abnormal environment, the history has to include a description of the person's environment, quality of life, and reason for referral. It is important to identify situations in which the presenting problems do and do not occur. For example, an aggressive behavior in a workshop only, but not in living situation, calls for investigation of the workshop environment and not for an immediate prescription. Not only the presenting complaints but also the general behavior, adaptation, and emotional functioning should be assessed. A detailed history of prior use of psychotropic drugs should include their indication, positive and negative effects, range of doses administered, and duration of treatment. The past assessment of the etiology of the mental retardation should be reviewed and updated as needed. Objective behavioral data should be obtained and analyzed and be used to form a baseline for measuring treatment effects. Appropriate behavioral rating scales are very helpful for this purpose.

A *direct interview* with the referred person is essential. Lack of verbal language is a reason for a longer, not shorter, interview which may also include observing the person in work and living situations.

Diagnostic formulation should follow an assessment of the total information and should include consideration of the person's life experience, learning, understanding, and communication level.

APPLYING DIAGNOSTIC CATEGORIES TO PEOPLE WITH MENTAL RETARDATION

Pervasive Developmental Disorders

The basic feature of pervasive developmental disorders (PDD) is a disturbance in multiple areas of development. PDD category is subdivided into autistic disorder, Asperger's disorder, Rhett syndrome, childhood disintegrative disorder, and PDD NOS (including atypical autism). Mental retardation is present in up to 80% of the people with PDD. An exception is Asperger's disorder; by definition, there is no delay in language and cognitive development in this disorder.

A diagnosis of autistic disorder requires that at least 6 of 12 criteria be met, including at least two of the first subgroup (qualitative impairment in social interaction), at least one of the second subgroup (qualitative impairment in interpersonal communication), and at least one of the third subgroup (restricted, repetitive, and stereotyped patterns of behavior, interests, and activities). Impairments in social interactions are central to the diagnosis of autism; these impairments are not the same as shyness or avoiding others. In addition to the required six criteria, the child must display delays or abnormal functioning, with onset before age of three years, in at least one of the following areas: social interaction, language (in social communication), and symbolic or imaginative play. Considerable clinical experience and often several interviews are required to recognize when symptoms are inherent in the individual rather than reactions to the immediate situation.

A common mistake has been to diagnose a PDD in people with mental retardation who present with a speech delay and self-stimulatory behavior. Such individuals are usually able to engage in interpersonal, reciprocal interaction and in interpersonal communication, appropriate to their developmental level, which rules out a PDD. The DSM-IV underwent extensive field testing in an effort to reduce the high rate of false positives (Volkmar et al., 1994). A frequent false-positive diagnosis is of PDD NOS. This diagnosis might be made only if the basic features of PDD are present, including impairment in social interaction, but the required number of criteria are not met or they are subthreshold.

Diagnosis of an autistic disorder in children with mental retardation is usually not difficult. A more difficult diagnostic challenge is posed by adults with autistic disorder who have developed some ability to relate to familiar people. A detailed developmental history is helpful in such cases.

Attention-Deficit Hyperactivity Disorder

According to the DSM-IV, attention-deficit hyperactivity disorder (ADHD) is a unitary phenomenon, with subtypes that are differentiated by the predominance of the symptom pattern (inattention and hyperactivity-impulsivity). Most of the diagnostic criteria reflect observable behaviors so that the presence of verbal language is usually not necessary in order to make the diagnosis. The diagnosis in people with mental retardation may be problematic because of a lack of normative data on attention span at various developmental levels and ages. Another problem, irrespective of mental retardation, occurs when a person is described as "hyper" in one setting (typically school or work

place) and as "calm" in another setting. This suggests that the problem might be situational; for example, a person may behave differently when faced with boring, difficult, or anxiety-provoking tasks. In such instances, behavior management, rather than psychotropic drugs, is usually indicated.

Conduct Disorder

The essential feature of conduct disorder is "a repetitive and persistent pattern of behavior in which the basic rights of others, or major age-appropriate societal norms or rules are violated" (APA, 1994, p. 85). This pattern includes aggression, property damage, deceitfulness, theft, and rule violation. In making this diagnosis, consideration needs to be given to the individual's personal circumstances. Mitigating factors include cognitive level and the person's ability to understand required social rules such as the concept of ownership of property, behaviors prevalent in a particular setting (such as an institution), and whether or not the behavior is manifested in only one setting.

Oppositional Defiant Disorder

This disorder is characterized by behavior toward authority figures that is "negativistic, defiant, disobedient, and hostile" (APA, 1994, p. 91). It requires that individuals have the ability to understand what is expected of them. Additionally, the behavior has to be markedly greater than would be anticipated in people of comparable developmental level. This diagnosis is not equivalent to the term *noncompliance* commonly used by caregivers for people who do not follow orders. In fact, in some cases noncompliance may reflect good judgment and adaptation. It might be the only way a nonverbal person can express an opinion that differs from that of the caregiver.

Pica and Rumination Disorder

These behaviors, which are seen with some frequency among people with significant mental retardation, also are formal DSM-IV diagnoses. It should be kept in mind that concurrent mood or anxiety disorders might be reflected in an increase in pica behavior. As with other disorders, these diagnoses are made only if the behaviors are inappropriate for the developmental level and severe enough to require attention.

Tourette and Other Tic Disorders

These disorders, according to DSM-IV, are characterized by motor movements and vocalizations that are rapid, sudden, not rhythmic, recurrent, and usually frequent. People with these disorders may feel that their urges to move or vocalize are irresistible, but usually they can suppress them for certain lengths of time. Swearing (coprolalia) is commonly thought of as typical of Tourette disorder, but it occurs infrequently and certainly not in nonverbal people. The diagnosis of these disorders is difficult, because many people with mental retardation engage in self-stimulatory behaviors that may include stereotypic movements (see next section). The latter are often more complex and intentional, although ascertaining intentionality may be difficult with nonverbal people.

Stereotypic Movement Disorder

This disorder can occur with or without SIB. The diagnosis is indicated if stereotypic behavior leads to significant functional impairment requiring treatment. The DSM-IV introduced the specifier "with self-injurious behavior," which is used if there is physical damage requiring medical treatment, as happens in certain cases of head-banging, self-biting, self-hitting, and picking at skin and bodily orifices.

SIB occurs in about 2% to 3% of people with mental retardation known to state service programs (Borthwick-Duffy & Eyman, 1990; Rojahn, 1986). It is more common among people residing in institutions. Predisposing factors for SIB include presence of severe or profound mental retardation, Lesch-Nyhan syndrome, PDD, Cornelia de Lange syndrome, and sometimes fragile X syndrome.

Psychological motivational factors for SIB have been divided into three groups: self-stimulatory, attention-seeking, and avoidance of task demands (e.g., Carr, 1977; review by Reiss, 1994). These have formed the basis of two psychological approaches, called functional analysis (Iwata, Dorsey, Slifer, Bauman, & Richman, 1982) and communication theory (Carr & Durand, 1985). Each of these approaches enjoys widespread support within the field. However, Reiss (1994) has suggested that the data supporting communication theory are subject to alternative explanations.

Researchers also have suggested that disorders of the endogenous opioid and serotonin systems may play a role in the genesis or maintenance of SIB (King, 1993;

Sandman, 1990). Although this view seems to be gaining influence, there is still widespread disagreement about the causes of self-injury, and additional research is needed (Aman & Singh, 1991; Gualtieri, 1989). Because the presence of the SIB is not a discriminating factor among psychiatric diagnoses, a comprehensive differential diagnostic assessment is necessary (Gualtieri, 1989).

Schizophrenia and Other Psychotic Disorders

Definitions of psychosis vary, from a narrow one, which includes delusions and hallucinations, to a broader one, which also includes disordered thought processes and behavior. Schizophenia is the most common example of psychotic disorder. It affects about 1% of the population and appears to be about as common in people with and without mental retardation (Reiss, 1994). The symptoms of schizophrenia may be positive or negative. The positive symptoms include hallucinations (false sensory experiences, such as hearing voices), delusions (firmly held false beliefs), and grossly disorganized speech and behavior. The negative symptoms include loss of normal functions, such as apathy, blunting, or incongruity of emotional responses and poverty of thought and speech. The diagnostic criteria also include regression (significant deterioration in functioning from pre-illness levels) and major disturbance in the person's adaptive functioning. A certain level of language is necessary to ascertain the presence of DSM-IV symptoms of schizophrenia, such as delusions, hallucinations, and disorganized speech. Technically at least, schizophrenia might be also diagnosed if there is grossly disorganized behavior and negative symptoms. The condition is sometimes associated with agitation, bizarre behavior, aggression, and anxiety.

The DSM-IV distinguishes among the following psychotic disorders: schizophrenia, schizophreniform disorder, schizoaffective disorder, delusional disorder, brief psychotic disorder, shared psychotic disorder, psychotic disorder due to general medical condition, substance-induced psychosis, and psychotic disorder NOS. Schizophrenia is subtyped as paranoid, disorganized, catatonic, undifferentiated, and residual. Schizophrenia is coded according to different patterns of course, that may be continuous, episodic with progressive deficit, episodic with stable deficit, episodic and remittent, or with incomplete or complete remission. Psychotic symptoms may occur also in mood disorders.

The interest in the relationship between mental retardation and psychosis is longstanding. Kraepelin (1896) took the view that approximately 7% of cases of schizophrenia or "dementia praecox" arose on the basis of mental retardation. He also suggested that certain forms of retardation with developmental mannerisms and stereotypies might be early cases of schizophrenia, and he proposed the term "propfschizophrenia" for this condition. Although he later modified his views and agreed that the rhythmic movements seen in some people with severe mental retardation did not, in fact, signify schizophrenia, he continued to believe that dementia praecox beginning in the first decade of life could produce "states of weakness ... regarded as imbecility or idiocy." This suggestion stimulated a debate as to whether schizophrenia in people with mental retardation was a clinically distinct condition, in which a schizophrenic psychosis of particularly early onset could bring about a state of severe learning disability, or whether the complex hand and finger movements and stereotypies seen in some such people with mental retardation were "a form of schizophrenia played out upon the psychomotor level rather than the symbolic" (Earl, 1934). By the late 1930s, however, the term *propfschizophrenia* had come to mean so many things to so many investigators that it ceased to be of clinical use and gradually withered away.

Hayman (1939) maintained that people with the most severe mental retardation showed "an undifferentiated psychosis," with a constitutional periodicity in some cases. Herskovitz and Plesset (1941) suggested that schizophrenia could not be diagnosed on clinical grounds for patients with an IQ much below 50. The present view is that the diagnosis of schizophrenia is clinical and firmly rooted in language-based phenomenology (Reid, 1993). As a result, this diagnosis, and particularly more specific diagnosis of the subtype of schizophrenia, cannot be made with confidence for people with an IQ much below around 45. Meadows et al. (1991) maintained that it should be possible to substantiate this diagnosis using standardized diagnostic instruments, such as the Schedule for Affective Disorders and Schizophrenia (Endicott & Spitzer, 1978). Clarke (in press), Meadows et al. (1991) and Reiss (1994), however, have advanced alternative views affirming the possibility of diagnosing schizophrenia in people with severe mental retardation.

Mood Disorders

The primary problem in mood disorders is an aberrant occurrence of mood states, which may be depressed (commonly called low) or elevated (high, manic).

Major depressive episode and manic episode are building blocks of specific diagnoses. In hypomanic episode, the presentation is similar to manic episode, but the symptoms are milder and do not result in major functional impairment.

There are several subcategories of mood disorders. For the diagnosis of major depressive disorder, at least five of nine clearly defined symptom categories have to be met for at least two weeks. Seven of the nine can be satisfied for people without language skills. The major symptoms are severely depressed mood, anhedonia (loss of interest in formerly pleasurable activities), and disturbance of sleep, appetite, energy level, and activity level. The essential criteria for a major depression are listed in Table 1-1, and comparable symptoms that may occur in the context of mental retardation are noted. Similarly, Table 1-2 shows a comparison of criteria and symptoms for manic episode.

Bipolar I disorder is indicated by at least one occurrence of a manic or mixed episode. In bipolar II disorder, an individual has a history of cyclical moods that include major depressive episodes, and of hypomanic or subthreshold manic episodes instead of classic mania. In cyclothymic disorder, an individual's cyclical mood swings do not reach the point of mania or depression but nevertheless cause clinically significant distress or impairment in social or occupational function. When four or more episodes occur in a given year, the term *rapid cycling mood disorder* is used. In dysthymic disorder, a chronic mild to moderate depressed mood lasts for at least one year in the case of adolescents and for at least two years in the case of adults.

The comorbidity of mood disorders and mental retardation was not fully recognized until the early 1970s. Reid (1972) published influential case studies. Sovner and Hurley (1983) summarized the evidence in the literature for this diagnosis. Szymanski and Biederman (1984) reported results of a study of people with Down syndrome, in whom depression and anorexia nervosa were diagnosed and treated. Reiss and Trenn (1984) and Reiss and Benson (1985) reported on outpatients with dysthymia. Matson, Kazdin, and Senatore (1984) reported the first rating instrument for depression, and Reiss (1988) reported the first sets of normative and demographic data with combined sample sizes exceeding 1,000 people. Today, a consensus has been reached that people with mental retardation are vulnerable to mood disorders. Overall prevalence rates might be about as high as in the general population (Reiss, 1994, p. 82). However, depressed mood is more common among school children with mental retardation than among

Table 1-1. Criteria for Major Depressive Episode

DSM IV Criterion	Example in Mental Retardation
1. Depressed mood most of the day, as indicated by either subjective report or observation made by others. In children and adolescents, it can be irritable mood.	Description by caregivers of a change from being happy and smiling or laughing or of having a sense of humor to an absence of these characteristics. Tearfulness, increase in somatic complaints, irritability.
2. Markedly diminished interest or pleasure in all, or almost all, activities most of the day, nearly every day.	Loss of interest in friends, apathy, inability to enjoy activities enjoyed in the past, refusal to participate in previously favored activities.
3. Significant weight loss when not dieting or weight gain, or decrease or increase in appetite nearly every day.	Refusal to go to the dining table or refusal to eat once there. This may be reported by caregivers only as noncompliance and should be asked about specifically. Food stealing, hoarding.
4. Insomnia or hypersomnia nearly every day.	Behavioral disturbances in the evening might overshadow underlying sleep disturbances.
5. Psychomotor agitation or retardation nearly every day.	Agitation may be manifested by pacing, by the inability to sit still, or as general restlessness. Agitation may also be manifested by the appearance of, or an increase in, self-injurious behavior, stereotypy, running away, aggression, or other behavior. Decreased speech, trouble completing activities of daily living.
6. Fatigue or loss of energy nearly every day.	Decrease in productivity or a regression in skills.
7. Feelings of worthlessness or excessive or inappropriate guilt (which may be delusional) nearly every day.	Comments such as "nobody likes me" or "I can't do this job."
8. Diminished ability to think or concentrate, or indecisiveness, nearly every day.	Decreased productivity or regression of skills. An individual may begin a task but not follow through. Decreased attention to the task may also occur. "Noncompliance."
9. Recurrent thoughts of death (not just fear of dying), recurrent suicidal ideation without a specific plan, or a suicide attempt or a specific plan for committing suicide.	Deliberate, potentially lethal acts. Self-injurious behavior. Offering self up to peers who are known to aggress.

school children with no mental retardation (Schloss, Epstein, & Cullinan, 1988). Aggressive behavior may also be associated with clinically significant levels of depressed mood (Reiss & Rojahn, 1993). And, as with people who do not have mental retardation, depression in people with mental retardation is strongly associated with low levels of social support and with poor social skills (Reiss & Benson, 1985).

Anxiety Disorders

Anxiety disorders are manifested in severe disruptions in everyday functioning caused by significant anxiety or avoidance. The DSM-IV lists 11 subtypes of anxiety disorder. Panic disorder is relatively uncommon and has only recently been reported for people with mental retardation. Posttraumatic stress disorder (PTSD) is indicated by a

Table 1-2. Criteria for Manic Episode

DSM IV Criterion	Example in Mental Retardation
A. A distinct period of abnormally and persistently elevated, expansive, or irritable mood, lasting at least 1 week (or any duration if hospitalization is necessary) must be present.	Shouting, yelling and screaming, refusal to do what others ask, such as expected chores or goal-related activities. Aggression or property destruction. Silliness, teasing, singing, and dancing may be indications of expansive mood. Behavior may be labeled "manipulative" rather than recognized as evidence of elevated or expansive mood.
B. During the period of mood disturbance, three (or more) of the following symptoms have persisted (four if the mood is only irritable) and have been present to a significant degree:	
1. Inflated self-esteem or grandiosity.	Individuals may have unrealistic goals, perhaps related to a belief that they do not have mental retardation. Inflated self-esteem may be hard to identify and easy to overlook.
2. Decreased need for sleep (e.g., feels rested after only 3 hours of sleep).	An individual is up all or much of the night, displays a great deal of energy, and does not attempt to nap throughout the day. Increase in maladaptive behavior at night.
3. More talkative than usual or pressure to keep talking.	Non-stop talking or constant vocalization may be the way pressured speech presents.
4. Flight of ideas or subjective experience that thoughts are racing.	Rapid shifts in conversation from one topic to another.
5. Distractibility (i.e. attention too easily drawn to unimportant or irrelevant external stimuli).	Distractibility, "non-compliance," loss of productivity at work or at school.
6. Increase in goal-directed activity (either socially, at work or school, or sexually) or psychomotor agitation.	Intrusiveness, public masturbation, or notable increase in same. Aggression, assault, disruption, increased eating, self-stimulatory behavior, change in frequency or intensity of rituals.
7. Excessive involvement in pleasurable activities that have a high potential for painful consequences (e.g. engaging in unrestrained buying sprees, sexual indiscretions, or foolish business investments).	Increased sexual preoccupation and sexual activity, increased or frequent masturbation.

persistent tendency to reexperience a traumatic event in several ways. The past requirement that the event be so extreme that it is outside of normal human experience has been deleted, and the focus is now on the person's intense reaction to that event. Reports of PTSD in people with mental retardation have focused on victims of phys-

ical and sexual abuse. McNally (1993) has found a negative correlation between the severity of PTSD symptoms over time and the IQ of combat soldiers. Apparently, the soldiers with higher IQs were better able to resolve their traumatic experiences so that symptom severity decreased over time. If this correlation holds for people with mental retardation, it would suggest that increased vulnerability to PTSD exists in this population.

Obsessive-compulsive disorder (OCD) is characterized by the presence of intrusive thoughts and repetitive behaviors that are performed to neutralize the fear and worry associated with obsessions. Reports of OCD in people with mental retardation have included classic cases of people who check and hoard (Matson, 1982). Although the DSM-IV allows for "poor insight" as a qualifier, whereby individuals may for the most part not recognize the excessive or unreasonable nature of their behaviors, it can often be a challenge to distinguish between a stereotypic movement and a true compulsion in a nonverbal person. By definition, compulsions should generally cause some distress, as distinct from the neutral feeling or even pleasure that one may witness when observing a person with severe mental retardation repetitively flip a light switch off and on, or flush toilets, or twirl a string.

Researchers have considered the extent to which certain cases of SIB can be considered examples of OCD (King, 1993; Vitiello, Spreat, & Behard, 1989). OCD and SIB are similar in that both entail the occurrence of ritualistic behavior. Dissimilarities include the fact that OCD is positively correlated with IQ, whereas SIB is negatively correlated with IQ. OCD can be treated by psychological fear-exposure techniques, whereas SIB cannot be treated in this manner (Reiss, 1994, p. 79). In order to demonstrate that SIB is a form of OCD, it must be shown that the SIB is performed to reduce anxiety (by definition, OCD is an anxiety disorder) rather than for self-stimulation, attention, or some other motivation.

Anxiety disorders also include phobias. Specific phobias are intense fears and avoidance of specific objects or situations, whereas social phobia is an intense fear of being humiliated. People with mental retardation are vulnerable to the full range of phobias.

Generalized anxiety disorder is indicated by significant levels of anxiety and worry for at least six months. Although anxiety lasting long periods of time is seen in some people with mental retardation, it is sometimes unclear whether or not awareness and worry are present.

Overall prevalence rates for anxiety disorders appear to be at least as common as those seen in the general population. Phobia is the most common type of anxiety disorder seen in people with mental retardation.

Personality Disorders

As is indicated in the DSM-IV, personality traits can be defined by patterns of individual emotional and motivational responses that develop over the course of the individual's life. The term *personality disorders* is used when these patterns are inflexible, result in maladaptive behavior and dysfunction, are evident across a broad range of personal and social situations, and markedly differ from the expectations of the individual's culture. Their onset is in early adolescence or adulthood, they are stable over time, and they lead to distress or impairment.

The most common maladaptive personality traits among people with mental retardation are conduct problems, distrust and suspiciousness, excessive attention-seeking, dependency, social avoidance, and nonassertiveness.

Eaton and Menolascino (1982) observed an occurrence of personality disorders in 27.1% of a clinic-based population of people with mental retardation. Reid and Ballinger (1987) reported that 56 percent of a sample of institutionalized adults with mild or moderate mental retardation showed abnormal personality features, and in 22% the presence of a personality disorder was suggested. Reiss (1992) found abnormal personality traits in up to 40% of a random sample of people with mental retardation living in a metropolitan area. Zigler and Burack (1989) have suggested that psychopathology is more common in people with mental retardation because of a high rate of occurrence of maladaptive personality traits.

In the DSM-IV, 10 personality disorders are listed that can be grouped into three clusters based on descriptive similarities. Cluster A may be indicated by behavior that is odd or eccentric, such as paranoia (pervasive distrust and suspiciousness; quick to perceive insult), acute discomfort in close relationships, and display of cognitive or perceptual distortions. Cluster B may be indicated by dramatic, emotional, or erratic behavior, including antisocial behavior, instability in personal relationships, excessive attention-seeking, excessive need for admiration, and a lack of empathy. Cluster C may be indicated by feelings of inadequacy, hypersensitivity to negative evaluation, excessive submissiveness, dependency, preoccupation with orderliness or control, and perfectionism.

Clinicians sometimes confuse personality disorders with other mental disorders. For example, psychotic disorders are commonly confused with Cluster A personality disorders, mood or psychotic disorders with Cluster B personality disorders, and anxiety disorders with Cluster C personality disorders. To avoid this confusion, clinicians should pay careful attention to exact DSM-IV diagnostic criteria and text descriptions and keep in mind that in personality disorders the behavioral patterns must be pervasive, enduring, and be present at least since adolescence.

The most influential research on personality in individuals with mental retardation has been reported by Zigler (1971) and his colleagues, who have documented experiments with "outerdirectness" and other personality characteristics. Zigler and Burack (1989) have suggested that the high rate of psychopathology seen in people with mental retardation is related to maladaptive personality traits resulting from negative social experiences. Goldberg et al. (1992) has reported some preliminary data on possible associations between clusters of personality disorders and the severity of mental retardation.

Paraphilias

Reiss (1990) found that 3 persons (1.5%) in a representative community sample of 205 had a significant problem with sexual behavior. Among the behaviors reported by other clinical researchers were public masturbation (Barmann & Murray, 1981), pedophilia (Polvinale & Lutzker, 1980), transvestism, frotteurism, and zoophilic exhibitionism. Prior to making a diagnosis of paraphilia, other mental disorders should be considered, including mania, schizophrenia, borderline personality disorders, and encephalopathy.

Sexual offense is a major reason for imprisonment of people with mental retardation. At any given moment, about 1% of people with mental retardation are in prison (Day, 1993). Over the course of the life span, fewer than 3% of people with mental retardation are imprisoned (Dyggve & Kodahl, 1979). Comparing offenders with and without mental retardation, Day (1993) found that sexual offenses accounted for a disproportionately high percentage of the criminal convictions of offenders with mental retardation.

MENTAL DISORDERS DUE TO A GENERAL MEDICAL CONDITION

The DSM-IV has eliminated organic mental disorder as a separate category. The phrase, "due to a general medical condition," is used instead. The DSM-IV requires that this phrase should be used only when there is evidence that the mental disorder is the direct physiological consequence of a medical condition. The specific diagnosis of that conditon should be separate-

ly noted on Axis III. The general medical conditions may be as varied as hypothyroidism, amphetamine intoxication, brain tumor, vascular disorders, and physical trauma.

These changes in the DSM-IV should end the past practice of using the organic diagnosis for any maladaptive behavior of people with mental retardation. The rationale was that if mental retardation due to biological etiology was present, any accompanying psychopathology could be ascribed to the same causation. In DSM-IV, the diagnosis, "due to a general medical condition," is used only when there is evidence of *both* organic pathology *and* its primary causative relationship to the behavioral symptomatology. In some situations such a relationship is implied by the chronology—for example, behavioral symptoms appearing at the time of onset of seizure disorder. It should be noted, however, that usually psychosocial or environmental factors contribute to the clinical presentation as well. These factors may maintain the problem rather than initiate it.

The DSM-IV lists these disorders in several sections:

- *General disorder categories.* If both the specific criteria for a disorder (e.g., mood disorder) *and* general criteria for the disorder due to a general medical condition are met, then the appropriate diagnosis might be: mood disorder due to ... (The general medical condition to be specified).

- *Mental disorders due to a general medical condition not elsewhere classified* includes catatonic disorder, personality change, and mental disorder NOS.

- *Delirium, dementia, and amnestic and other cognitive disorders* form a separate section.

- *Substance-related disorders,* which previously were listed with organic mental disorders, are now in a separate section.

Dementia

Although age of onset prior to 18 years is one of the diagnostic criteria for mental retardation, there is no age criterion for a diagnosis of dementia. Some clinicians have a misconception that in every case when the IQ declines after age 18, the diagnosis of dementia should be made. However, the DSM-IV criteria for dementia also include poor adaptive skills, memory impairment, and at least one other cognitive disturbance. These features must represent a decline from the premorbid level. Determination of these impairments

Table 1-3. Suggested Medications Based on Psychiatric Diagnosis in MR/DD[7]

Diagnosis	Medications
Adjustment Disorder	1. anxiolytics
aggression (chronic & organic)	1. beta blockers 2. buspirone 3. anticonvulsants
akathisia (neuroleptic induced)	1. beta blockers (propranolol)
Attention-Deficit Hyperactivity	1. stimulants 2. tricyclic antidepressants
Autism	1. neuroleptics
Depressive Disorders	1. antidepressants
enuresis	1. tricyclic antidepressants
Generalized Anxiety Disorder	1. anxiolytics 2. antidepressants
Hyperactivity	1. clonidine
Mania	1. lithium 2. valproate, carbamazepine 3. benzodiazepines
Obsessive-Compulsive Disorder	1. clomipramine, fluoxetine, paroxetine
Panic Disorder	1. antidepressants 2. benzodiazepines
pica (zinc deficiency)	1. zinc supplement
Schizophrenia	1. neuroleptics
Self-Injurious Behavior	1. naltrexone 2. neuroleptics 3. antidepressants 4. beta-blockers
sleep problems (no psychiatric disorder)	1. melatonin 2. benzodiazepines 3. clonidine
Tourrette syndrome (also tics)	1. neuroleptics 2. anxiolytics 3. clonidine

7 See appropriate chapters is this book for details.

may be difficult if not impossible in very young children, and for that reason the DSM-IV allows that making a diagnosis of dementia might not be appropriate before ages 4-6 years and is not necessary if the condition is sufficiently characterized by the diagnosis of mental retardation alone.

CONCLUSION

The recent versions of the DSM (III, III-R, and IV) have become widely used throughout much of the world. Part of their appeal is based on the provision of well-defined symptoms needed to establish a given diagnosis. This chapter addresses the applicability of the DSM for people with mental retardation, the modifications need-ed to facilitate valid diagnoses in this group, and how formal diagnoses aid in choosing appropriate psychotropic medications. As this chapter illustrates, it is possible to establish valid and reliable diagnoses for the majority of people with both mental retardation and behavioral or emotional symptoms. Brief descriptions are also provided of the major DSM categories and of modifications that may prove helpful in assessing people with mental retardation. Knowledge of valid diagnostic categories and the identification of suitable treatments is an evolving process that will probably continue to grow at an accelerating rate.

Table 1-3 summarizes the major indications for psychopharmacological agents, as concluded in this book based on the results of the consensus process. The relationship between psychiatric diagnosis and psychopharmacological agent is shown in this table.

REFERENCES

Aman, M. G. (1991). *Assessing psychopathology and behavior problems in persons with mental retardation: A review of available instruments* (DHHS Publication No. ADM 91–1712). Rockville, MD: U.S. Department of Health and Human Services.

Aman, M.G., & Singh, N.N. (1991). Pharmacological intervention. In J.L. Matson & J.A. Mulick (Eds.), *Handbook of Mental Retardation* (2nd ed., pp. 347–372). Elmsford, New York: Pergamon Press.

Aman, M.G., Singh, N.N., Stewart, A.W., & Field, C.J. (1985). The Aberrant Behavior Checklist: A behavior rating scale for the assessment of treatment effects. *American Journal of Mental Deficiency, 89,* 485–491.

American Association on Mental Retardation (AAMR). (1992). *Mental retardation: Definition, classification, and systems of supports.* Washington, DC: Author.

American Psychiatric Association. (1952). *Diagnostic and statistical manual of mental disorders* (1st ed.). Washington, DC: Author.

American Psychiatric Association. (1968). *Diagnostic and statistical manual of mental disorders* (2nd ed.). Washington, DC: Author.

American Psychiatric Association. (1980). *Diagnostic and statistical manual of mental disorders* (3rd ed.). Washington, DC: Author.

American Psychiatric Association. (1987). *Diagnostic and statistical manual of mental disorders* (3rd ed. revised). Washington, DC: Author.

American Psychiatric Association. (1994). *Diagnostic and statistical manual of mental disorders* (4th ed.). Washington, DC: Author.

Barmann, B.C., & Murray, W.J. (1981). Suppression of inappropriate sexual behavior by facial screening. *Behavior Therapy, 12,* 730–735.

Borthwick-Duffy, S.A., & Eyman, R.K. (1990). Who are the dually diagnosed? *American Journal on Mental Retardation, 94,* 586–595.

Bouras, N., Brooks, D., & Drummond, K. (1994). Community psychiatric services for people with mental retardation. In N. Bouras (Ed.), *Mental health in mental retardation* (pp. 293–299). New York: Cambridge University Press.

Bregman, J. (1991). Current developments in the understanding of mental retardation: Part II. Psychopathology. *Journal of the American Academy of Child and Adolescent Psychiatry, 30,* 861–872.

Carr, E.G. (1977). The motivation of self-injurious behavior: A review of some hypotheses. *Psychological Bulletin, 84,* 800–816.

Carr, E.G., & Durand, V.M. (1985). The social-communicative basis of severe behavior problems in children. In S. Reiss & R.R. Bootzin (Eds.), *Theoretical issues in behavior therapy* (pp. 219–254). New York: Academic Press.

Clarke, D.J. (in press). Prader-Willi syndrome and psychoses: Three case reports. *British Journal of Psychiatry.*

Day, K. (1993). Crime and mental retardation: A review. In C.R. Hollin & K. Howells (Eds.), *Clinical approaches to the mentally disordered offender* (pp. 111–144). New York: Wiley.

Dyggve, H., & Kodahl, T. (1979). Disease patterns among 942 mentally retarded persons in a Danish county. *Acta Psychiatrica Scandinavica, 5,* 381–394.

Earl, C.J.C. (1934). The primitive catatonic psychosis of idiocy. *British Journal of Medical Psychology, 14,* 231–253.

Eaton, L.E., & Menolascino, F.J. (1982). Psychiatric disorders in the mentally retarded: Types, problems and challenges. *American Journal of Psychiatry, 139,* 1297–1303.

Endicott, J., & Spitzer, R.L. (1978). A diagnostic interview: The Schedule for Affective Disorders and Schizophrenia. *Archives of General Psychiatry, 35,* 837–844.

Goldberg, B., Gitta, M.Z., & Puddephatt, A. (1992). *Personality and trait disturbances in an adult mental retardation population: Significance for psychiatric management.* Presented at the International Association for the Scientific Study of Mental Deficiency, Gold Coast, Australia.

Gualtieri, C.T. (1989). The differential diagnosis of self-injurious behavior in mentally retarded people. *Psychopharmacology Bulletin, 25,* 358–363.

Hayman, M. (1939). The interrelations of mental defect and mental disorder. *Journal of Mental Science, 85,* 1183–1193.

Herskovitz, H.H., & Plesset, M.R. (1941). Psychoses in adult mental defectives. *Psychiatric Quarterly, 15,* 574–588.

Iwata, B.A., Dorsey, M.F., Slifer, K.J., Bauman, K.E., & Richman, G.S. (1982). Toward a functional analysis of self-injury. *Analysis and Intervention in Developmental Disabilities, 2,* 3–20.

King, B.H. (1993). Self-injury by people with mental retardation: A compulsive behavior hypothesis. *American Journal on Mental Retardation, 98,* 93–112.

Kraepelin, E. (1896). *Dementia: Praecox and*

paraphrenia. (R.M. Barclay, Trans.). Edinburgh, Scotland: Livingstone.

Matson, J.L. (1982). Treating obsessive-compulsive behavior in mentally retarded adults. *Behavior Modification, 6,* 551–567.

Matson, J.L., Kazdin, A.E., & Senatore, V. (1984). Psychometric properties of the Psychopathology Inventory for Mentally Retarded Adults. *Applied Research in Mental Retardation, 5,* 881–889.

McNally, R.J. (1993). Stressors that produce posttraumatic stress disorder in children. *Journal of Consulting and Clinical Psychology, 3,* 531–537.

Meadows, G., Turner, T., Campbell, L., Lewis, S.W., Reveley, M.A., & Murray, R.M. (1991). Assessing schizophrenia in adults with mental retardation. *British Journal of Psychiatry, 158,* 103–105.

Philips, I. (1966). Children, mental retardation and emotional disorder. In I. Philips (Ed.), *Prevention and treatment of mental retardation* (pp. 111–122). New York: Basic Books.

Polvinale, R.A., & Lutzker, J.R. (1980). Elimination of assaultive and inappropriate sexual behavior by reinforcement and social restitution. *Mental Retardation, 18,* 27–30.

Reid, A.H.(1972). Psychoses in adult mental defectives: II. Schizophrenic and paranoid psychoses. *British Journal of Psychiatry, 12,* 213–218.

Reid, A.H. (1993). Schizophrenic and paranoid syndromes in persons with mental retardation: Assessment and diagnosis. In R.J. Fletcher & A. Dosen (Eds.), *Mental health aspects of mental retardation.* New York: Lexington Books.

Reid A.H., & Ballinger, B.R. (1987). Personality disorder in mental handicap. *Psychological Medicine, 17,* 983–987.

Reiss, S. (1988). *The Reiss Screen for Maladaptive Behavior.* Worthington, OH: IDS Publishing Corporation.

Reiss, S. (1990). Prevalence of dual-diagnosis in community-based day programs in the Chicago metropolitan area. *American Journal on Mental Retardation, 94,* 578–585.

Reiss, S. (1992). Assessment of a man with dual diagnosis. *Mental Retardation, 30,* 1–6.

Reiss, S. (1994). *Handbook of challenging behavior: Mental health aspects of mental retardation.* Worthington, OH: IDS Publishing Corporation.

Reiss, S., & Benson, B.A. (1985). Psychosocial correlates of depression in mentally retarded adults: Minimal social support and stigmatization. *American Journal of Mental Deficiency, 89,* 331–337.

Reiss, S., & Rojahn, J. (1993). Joint occurrence of depression and aggression in children and adults with mental retardation. *Journal of Intellectual Disability, 37,* 287–294.

Reiss, S., & Trenn, E. (1984). Consumer demand for outpatient mental health services for mentally retarded people. *Mental Retardation, 22,* 112–115.

Reiss, S., & Valenti-Hein, D.(1994). Development of a psychopathology rating scale for children with mental retardation. *Journal of Consulting and Clinical Psychology, 62,* 28–33.

Rojahn, J. (1986). Self-injurious and stereotypic behavior of noninstitutionalized mentally retarded people: Prevalence and classification. *American Journal of Mental Deficiency, 91,* 268–276.

Sandman, C.A. (1990). The opiate hypothesis in autism and self injury. *Journal of Child and Adolescent Psychopharmacology, 1,* 237–248.

Schatzberg, A.F., & Cole, J.O. (1991). *Manual of clinical psychopharmacology* (2nd ed.). Washington, DC: American Psychiatric Press.

Schloss, P.J., Epstein, M.H., & Cullinan, D. (1988). Depression characteristics among mildly handicapped students. *Journal of the Multihandicapped Person, 1,* 293–302.

Sovner, R. (1986). Limiting factors in the use of DSM-III criteria with mentally ill/mentally retarded persons. *Psychopharmacology Bulletin, 22,* 1055–1059.

Sovner, R., & Hurley, A.D. (1983). Do the mentally retarded suffer from affective illness? *Archives of General Psychiatry, 40,* 61–62.

Spitzer, R.L., & Fleiss, J.L. (1974). A reanalysis of the reliability of psychiatric diagnosis. *British Journal of Psychiatry, 125,* 341–347.

Szymanski, L.S. (1980). Psychiatric diagnosis of retarded persons. In L.S. Szymanski & P.E. Tanguay (Eds.), *Emotional disorders of mentally retarded persons* (pp 61–81). Baltimore: University Park Press.

Szymanski, L.S. (1994). Mental retardation and mental health: Concepts, aetiology and incidence. In N. Bouras (Ed.), *Mental health in mental retardation: Recent advances and practices* (pp. 19–33). Cambridge, England: Cambridge University Press.

Szymanski, L.S., & Biederman, J. (1984). Depression and anorexia nervosa of persons with Down's syndrome. *American Journal of Mental Deficiency, 89,* 246–251.

Szymanski, L.S., & Crocker, A.C. (1989). Mental retardation. In H.I. Kaplan & B.J. Sadock (Eds.), *Comprehensive textbook of psychiatry* (Vol. 5). (pp. 1728–1771) Baltimore: Williams & Wilkins.

Szymanski, L.S., & Grossman, H. (1984). Dual implications of dual diagnosis. *Mental Retardation, 22,* 155–156.

Szymanski, L.S., & Wilska, M. (1996). Mental retardation. In A.Tasman, J. Kay, & J.A. Lieberman (Eds.), *Psychiatry (pp. 605–635).* Philadelphia: Saunders.

Vitiello, B., Spreat, S., & Behard, D. (1989). Obsessive-compulsive disorder in mentally retarded patients. *Journal of Nervous and Mental Diseases, 177,* 233–235.

Volkmar, F.R. et al. (1994). Field trial for autistic disorder in DSM-IV. *American Journal of Psychiatry, 151,* 1361–1367.

World Health Organization (WHO) (1992). *International classification of diseases* (10th ed.). Geneva, Switzerland: Author.

Zigler, E. (1971). The retarded child as a whole person. In H.E. Adams & W.K. Boardman (Eds.), *Advances in experimental clinical psychology* (pp. 47–121). Elmsford, NY: Pergamon Press.

Zigler, E., & Burack, J. (1989). Personality development and the dually diagnosed person. *Research in Developmental Disabilities, 10,* 225–240.

Past Research on Psychopharmacology of People with Mental Retardation and Developmental Disabilities[1]

Stephen R. Schroeder[2], Nick Bouras[3], Cynthia R. Ellis[4],
Andrew H. Reid[5], Curt Sandman[6], John S. Werry[7], Henry Wisniewski[8]

The history of psychopharmacology for treating people with mental retardation and developmental disabilities is similar to that for treating mental illness (Ayd, 1991). Although the literature on history is limited, some relevant information was published in 1991 in the anniversary issues of the *Journal of the Experimental Analysis of Behavior* and 1990 in the anniversary issue of *Journal of Psychopharmacology*. There also are some published first-hand accounts from pioneers in the field. For example, a particularly stimulating account was given by Heinz Lehman (1993) of McGill University as a special lecture at the 30th annual meeting of the American College of Neuropsychopharmacology, entitled "Before They Called it Psychopharmacology." In this lecture, he portrayed the historical milestones in terms of a chronology of important discoveries and their historical significance (see Figure 2-1, top two panels). We adapted Lehman's schema and drew a similar one for the history of psychopharmacology in the field of mental retardation and developmental disabilities (see Figure 1, bottom panel).

Lehman distinguished between psychopharmacotherapy, the clinical discipline based on empirical observations, and psychopharmacology, the scientific discipline based on systematic research programs. He observed that these two disciplines do not always function in close coordination. When collaboration between scientists and clinicians is inadequate, serious mistakes are likely. For instance, prescription of neuroleptics for behavior control of people with mental retardation and developmental disabilities in the 1950s and 1960s was based mostly on flawed clinical research that lacked proper methodology and a theoretical base (Sprague & Werry, 1971). The trial-and-error use of neuroleptics for these patients without a proper psychiatric diagnosis is no longer considered accepted practice. If the clinical practice had been coordinated more with scientific knowledge, more rigorous evaluations would have been conducted and far fewer neuopleptics would have been given. In the next section, we survey chronologically drugs that were not originally developed for use with people with mental retardation and developmental disabilities but later came to be used with this population.

DEVELOPMENT OF PSYCHOTHERAPEUTIC DRUGS, 1857-1949

Bromides

Introduced by Locock in 1857, bromides are the oldest anticonvulsants. Locock thought bromides acted by lowering sex drive; since at that time excessive masturbation was thought to be the cause of epilepsy, bromides

1 The preparation of the manuscript was supported by NICHD grants #02528, #26927, and #23042 to Stephen R. Schroeder.
2 Director of Schiefelbusch Institute for Life Span Studies, University of Kansas, Lawrence, KS
3 Senior Lecturer in Psychiatry, Guy's Hospital-London Bridge, London, England, United Kingdom
4 Assistant Professor of Pediatrics and Psychiatry, Medical College of Virginia, Richmond, VA
5 Consultant Psychiatrist, Royal Dundee Liff Hospital, Dundee, Scotland (UK)
6 Professor-in-Residence, University of California at Irvine
7 Emeritus Professor of Psychiatry, University of Auckland, Auckland, NZ
8 Professor and Director, NYS Institute for Basic Research in Developmental Disabilities, Staten Island, NY

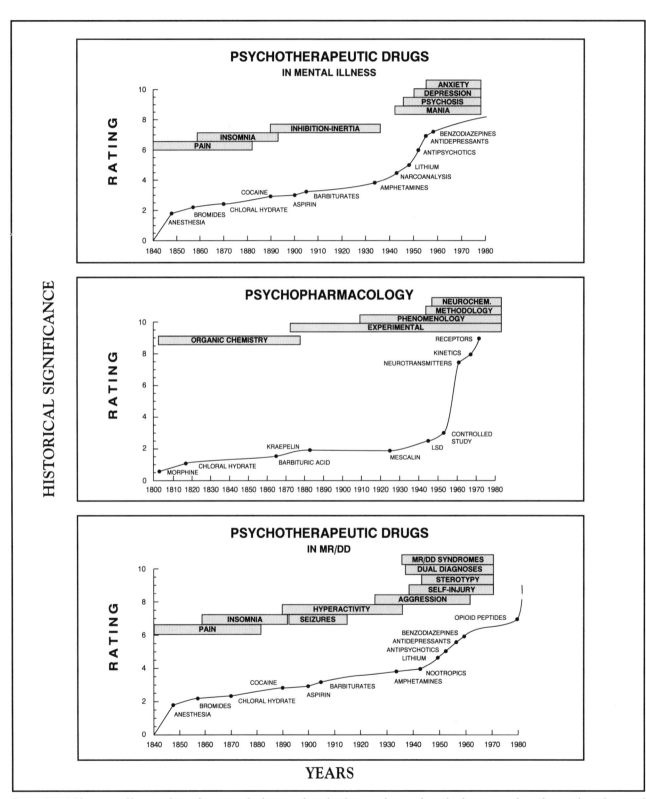

Figure 2-1. Milestones of historical significance in the history of psychopharmacology and psychotherapeutic drugs for people with mental illness and mental retardation and developmental disabilities. Ratings on the ordinate of the top two panels are from Lehman (1993). Ratings in the bottom panel are from the present authors. (From Kugelmass, 1956).

were used to treat this condition. Later bromides were used for insomnia and anxiety in addition to their continued use as anticonvulsants.

Barbiturates

The barbiturates, synthesized by Fischer and Von Mering in 1903, were introduced in 1912 as a hypnotic for insomnia. They also were used in the past as the primary medications for seizure control for people with developmental disabilities. In the 1950s and 1960s, newer anticonvulsants largely replaced the barbiturates, which have toxic and addictive potential. The barbiturates' labile psychotropic effects are familiar to clinicians (Gualtieri, 1991). The psychotropic effects of anticonvulsants (carbamazepine, valproic acid, and the benzodiazepines) have only recently been studied.

Amphetamines

Amphetamines were originally introduced by Prinzmetal and Bloomberg in 1935 as a potential cure for inertia and depression. However, the discovery by both Bradley (1937) and Molitch and Eccles (1937) that amphetamines reduce disruptive behavior and hyperactivity and improve academic performance in school children is often marked as the beginning of psychopharmacology for children. This finding was also important for people with mental retardation and developmental disabilities because it focused attention on a syndrome involving brain damage that required medication. Still (1902) and Tredgold (1908) were the first to describe hyperactivity as we know it today.

Hyperactivity was believed to be related to deficits in inhibitory volition, moral control, and sustained attention caused by early mild, undetected brain damage. These concepts of impaired attention, impaired regulation of activity, and impaired impulse control that were "paradoxically" reduced by stimulants have occupied researchers to the present day (Barkley, 1991). The fact that stimulants are used mostly among people with mild to moderate mental retardation, as opposed to those with more severe mental retardation, is probably related to this early concept of minimal brain dysfunction (Cutler, Little, & Strauss, 1940). It is also related to the finding that there were fewer responders among those with more severe ranges of retardation (Aman, Marks, Turbott, Wilsher, & Merry, 1991a, 1991b) and those with autism (Campbell, Fish, Shapiro, & Floyd, 1972).

Lithium

In Australia Cade (1949) introduced the use of lithium salts to quiet agitated manic states. However, it took 20 years before a technology was developed to manage lithium's toxicity. Once this happened, lithium became the primary long-term treatment for agitated manic episodes. Lithium was first used for people with mental retardation and developmental disabilities to treat aggression (Dostal & Zvolsky, 1970) and later self-injurious behavior ([SIB]; Cooper & Fowlie, 1973).

DEVELOPMENT OF PSYCHOTHERAPEUTIC DRUGS, 1950-1960

Antipsychotics

Charpontier synthesized chlorpromazine from promethazine in 1950 at the Rhone Poulene Laboratories in France. He was interested in its sedative properties for anesthesiology. Delay, Deniker, and Harl (1952) tried the new sedative with 38 patients with acute psychoses and discovered an antipsychotic effect. They reported that "manic excitation and more generally psychotic agitation, aggressiveness, and delusiveness conditions of schizophrenia improved, but deficiency symptoms did not change markedly (p. 274)." Before long psychiatrists in the United States were performing their own trials (Bair & Herold, 1955), and the revolution of biological psychiatry had begun. It is still dominating that field. In order to convey the drama of the discovery of neuroleptics, it is best to use the words of one of its pioneers (Lehman, 1993).

At the brink of World War II, I parachuted from Europe into the new world of North American psychiatry. Let me sketch for you the picture of psychiatry in the early 1940s. We had Kraepelin's and Bleuler's guides to the diagnosis of the major psychoses, manic depressive disorder, and schizophrenia. We had only two theories to explain the rest of the psychiatric illnesses, the neuroses and personality disorders: Freud's psychoanalysis and Pavlov's and Skinner's theories and findings on conditioning and learning.

Our two major therapies were insulin-induced hypoglycemic coma and electroconvulsive shock therapies (ECTs) for schizophrenia and affective disorders; and we had psychoanalysis and some derivative psychotherapy for the treatment of the neuroses. Paraldehyde and the barbiturates were about our only means to quell agitation and violence in addition to physical restraint and seclusion. In the 1940s mental illness was generally viewed as a hopeless stigma to be treated in hospitals with a variety of unspecific shock treatments. The scientific paradigm surrounding schizophrenia was hypoxia of the brain, and possibly the whole organism, as expressed succinctly by Freeman in 1931, "a generalized inherent tendency to ...deficient oxidative process" (Freeman, 1931). I remember a group of students making hospital rounds with me in 1952 in Montreal. We were looking at two young schizophrenic patients gesturing excitedly toward the ceiling from where they were hearing frightening voices. One of the students asked afterwards, "Will we ever get a pill to help these people?" I smiled patronizingly and replied that, unfortunately, it would never be as simple as "just a pill."

Not more than a year later I read one Sunday morning some medical literature that a pharmaceutical detail man had left with my secretary, saying: "This is about some new drug that is so good that these papers will sell it." I immediately set up a clinical trial of chlorpromazine with some psychotic patients, most of them schizophrenic. Within days, some of the patients had stopped hallucinating and within two weeks a few were in remission and ready to leave the hospital. I assumed we were seeing a series of flukes, and perhaps resulting from an extremely strange chance selection in the sample. It seemed almost as improbable as winning one million dollars twice in a lottery.

Much as I wanted to believe what I was seeing, I didn't for a long time. Even in my correspondence with other clinicians in the United States working with the phenothiazines neither I, nor they, dared to attribute specific antipsychotic effects to these drugs. We thought it might be a new modification of some sedating and inhibiting action, but we did not label the drugs antipsychotic. In 1956, when I was addressing the Canadian Medical Association, I introduced the term "antipsychotic" apologetically, and more as a metaphor than a designation.

It did not cross our minds that the new drugs might help the chronic back-ward patients, those who had not responded to insulin coma and ECT. However, we put a number of these "hopeless" patients on chlorpromazine for its symptomatic sedative effect and to our amazement, some of them actually went into remission. Again, it took us at least two years to accept the fact that at least some chronic schizophrenia patients were improving, even remitting, with phenothiazines.

Epistemologically speaking, psychiatry now had the cart before the horse. For the first time in history, we had drugs that suppressed hallucinations and delusions, drugs that could bring some chronic psychotic patients back to remission, drugs that could prevent psychotic relapses and, in addition to these quasimiracles, drugs that could produce parkinsonian symptoms. Could all this be explained by the simple paradigm of deficient oxidative processes in the brain? No way. The action mechanism of the new drugs were a mystery in the early 1950s. (pp. 294-302)

A plausible explanation for a mechanism of action of antipsychotic drugs in terms of blockade of dopamine neurons was proposed only a decade later by Carlsson and Lindquist (1963).

Reserpine was in vogue about the same time as chlorpromazine was, although its tranquilizing properties were known in India since 1755. It was rediscovered by Swiss scientists in the 1950s. Reserpine was important because it led to interest in 5-hydroxytryptophan and serotonergic theories of schizophrenia and depression. Reserpine also came to be widely used among people with mental retardation.

Given the hype accorded these new miracle drugs, they were soon adopted for use with people with mental retardation and developmental disabilities. An abstract by Davies (1954) appeared in *Lancet* on the effectiveness of chlorpromazine on mental deficiency. Bair and Herold (1955) followed up with the first full report of chlorpromazine for hyperactivity. The use of antipsychotics spread rapidly, so that, by 1956, the pharmacopoeia for aments looked something like the table recommended by Kugelmass (1956) in Figure 2-2. Antipsychotics were prescribed for a wide variety of problems.

By 1970, the prevalence of psychotropic drug use in U.S. residential facilities for people with mental retardation and developmental disabilities was more than 50 percent (Lipman, 1970). Neuroleptics were by far the most frequently prescribed psychotropic medication. In their classic review of psychotropic drugs, Sprague and Werry (1971) cited more than 100 studies in which antipsychotics were used; many of these studies were methodologically inadequate. Subsequent reviewers (Aman, 1983; Baumeister et al., 1993) have come to

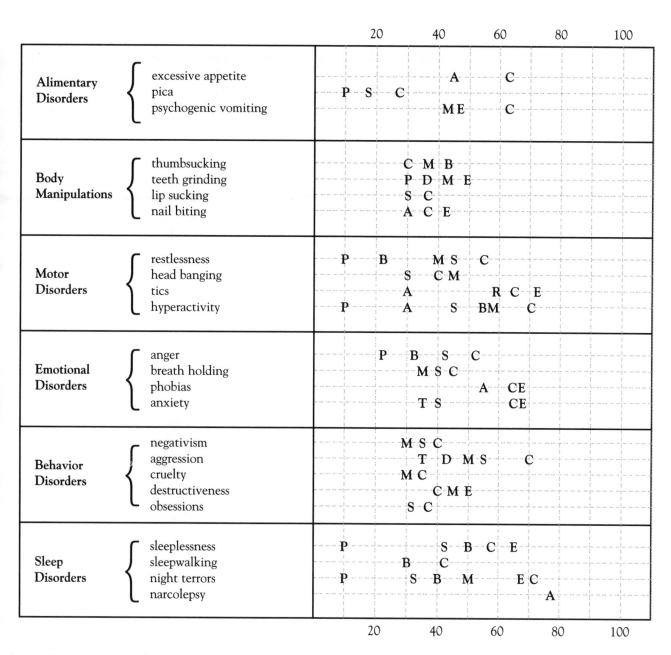

Figure 2-2. Comparative effectiveness of psychochemotherapeutic agents in amentia symptomatology of children. Code A = amphetamine; B = Benadryl (diphenhydramine hydrochloride); C = chlorpromazine; D = Dilantin (phenytoin); E = Equanil (meprobamate); M = Miltown (meprobamate); P = phenobarbital; R = Ritalin (methylphenidate); S = Serpasil (reserpine); T = Tolserol (mephenesin). From Kugelmass, 1956.

similar conclusions. With the increasing concerns for extrapyramidal side effects, especially tardive dyskinesia, the use of neuroleptics for people with mental retardation and developmental disabilities has decreased. Other less toxic drugs have been used in recent years; however, the use of neuroleptics is still widespread.

Antidepressants

The discovery of antidepressants followed shortly after the discovery of antipsychotics. Kuhn's paper on imipramine (1957) stimulated interest in tricyclic antidepressants; in 1957 Crane discovered, by accident, another category of antidepressants, called monoamine oxidase inhibitors (MAOIs). Although antidepressants have been used extensively with people with depressive disorders, they have been used less frequently for people with mental retardation and developmental disabilities. Early reports by Carter (1960) and Bender and Faretra (1961) proved overly optimistic. Sprague and Baxley (1979) summarized the results of these early studies by showing that those reporting negative results were methodologically more sound than those showing positive results. MAOIs currently are infrequently prescribed for people with mental retardation and developmental disabilities because of their side effects, which may result in hypertension.

Serotonin-related disorders include more than just affective disorders. Serotonin-modulating antidepressants were used successfully to treat panic disorders by Klein (1964). Other disorders that may respond to serotonin-modulating drugs are aggression and severe behavior disorders in persons with mental retardation and developmental disabilities. For example, researchers have found that these conditions are associated with affective disorders in this population (Reiss & Rojahn, 1993; Sovner & Hurley, 1983). Other considerations relevant to the use of antidepressants for people with aggression and severe behavior problems are as follows: (a) possible effects of 5-hydroxytryptophan on SIB in Lesch-Nyhan syndrome (Mizuno & Yugari, 1974, 1975; Nyhan, Johnson, Kaufman, & Jones, 1980); (b) elevated serotonin levels in some children with autism (Ritvo et al., 1970); (c) possible effects of fenfluramine on their clinical symptoms (Geller, Ritvo, Freeman, & Yuwiler, 1982); and (d) possible effectiveness of serotonin reuptake inhibitors on aggression and SIB associated with mood disorders in people with mental retardation or developmental disabilities (Thompson, Hackenberg, & Schaal, 1991).

Benzodiazepines

Benzodiazepines are the most commonly prescribed class of drugs for anxiety. They were introduced into the clinical literature by Harris in 1960. They are sometimes called selective CNS depressants because they are GABA receptor agonists. Early research also indicated positive effects on hostility and aggression (Boyle & Tobin, 1961; Feldman, 1962). Chlordiazepoxide (LaVeck & Buckley, 1961) and diazepam (Galambos, 1965) were also shown to have positive effects on subjects with

mental retardation. There is a small but growing variety of other anxiolytic drugs that are used to treat behavior disorders, probably because of their relatively benign side effects. However, the nature of their selective effects are still somewhat unclear.

THE ROOTS OF PSYCHOPHARMACOLOGY

The middle panel of Figure 2-1 shows the course of the scientific discipline of psychopharmacology for the general population.

Early in the 19th century there was considerable debate as to whether or not the effects of hashish, alcohol, or opiates might reveal anything about the mind. Although these drugs were considered to be poisons for the body, Cartesian mind-body dualism was still in vogue so that people could wonder if the drugs might have beneficial effects on the mind (Healy, 1993). A major force in opposition to this view was Wilhelm Wundt, the chairman of philosophy at the University of Leipzig, who formed the first psychology laboratory in 1879. He studied subjective experience by introspection.

Wundt is generally considered the father of modern psychology. One of his first students in 1883 was Emil Kraepelin, the father of modern psychiatry. His goal was "to study the effects of poisons on intellectual processes" (Healy, 1993). He named this discipline pharmacopsychology to emphasize its phenomenology. Kraepelin was the first to conduct controlled experiments on the psychological effects of mind-altering compounds. In this manner, the interdisciplinary partnership between psychiatry and psychology was evident in Kraepelin's work; today, interdisciplinary partnership in psychopharmacology research includes a broad range of disciplines. Although the biological basis of psychopharmacology has grown so enormously that it may seem predominant, the psychological element remains central, because there is as yet no other way to measure the targeted neurochemical effects.

The ideas of placebo controls, group designs, blind evaluations, statistical tests, and informed consent were often resisted by many clinicians in psychopharmacology, even into the 1950s. Clinical savvy was thought to be enough. Medical ethics was not yet an important discipline. Several disasters—for example, the effects of thalidomide on fetal development—forced governmental regulation of clinical drug trials. A rationale for stages of trials (open, single-blind, double-blind) was promoted by the U.S. Food and Drug Administration. As a result, the research improved dramatically. This increase in experimental rigor was also seen in the psychopharmacology research on effects with people with mental retardation and developmental disabilities, although it arrived later in the 1970s. Aman (1991) has performed an excellent review of instruments for measuring psychopathology in mental retardation.

An important contributor to experimental rigor not shown in Figure 2-1 is the field of behavior pharmacology. Although the effects of drugs on conditioning can be traced to Skinner and Heron (1937) and Pavlov (1927), modern behavior pharmacology usually is traced to two papers by Dews (1955a, 1955b) in which he showed that different doses of pentobarbital, methamphetamine, and scopolamine had very different effects on fixed interval versus fixed ratio schedules of reinforcement (Laties, 1986). Since then, an enormous amount of work has been done showing a variety of drug-environment interactions with the behavioral repertoire. Brady (1959) summarized the utility of these methods.

> First, a relatively broad spectrum of behavioral response patterns can be quantitatively and operationally identified and defined. Simple and complex discriminative capacities are assessable within the limits of an experimental situation which also provides a reliable estimate of general activity level, motor functioning, and sensory decrements. Second, specific aspects of an organism's behavioral repertoire can be selectively evaluated and dependably separated within a response pattern. Emotional or affective reactions can be independently assessed without complicated and equivocal interpretive problems involving nonspecific behavioral and motor disturbances, debilitation, and the like. And finally, it is now quite clear that such operant conditioning techniques are sensitive to a wide variety of experimental operations, including central nervous system damage, electrical stimulation, and pharmacologic agents. Specific aspects of a behavioral repertoire can be altered differentially with experimental controls inherently present within the remainder of the response pattern. (p. 55)

Behavior pharmacology and its companion discipline of applied behavior analysis have been very important for people with mental retardation and developmental disabilities. Precision in measurement, single-subject designs, and a host of conditioning techniques developed over the last 40 years have revolutionized how we

view the learning capacities of people with mental retardation as well as the prognosis for treating the behavior disorders they sometimes display. A particular contribution of behavior pharmacology in this arena is to show fine-grained measurements of the relative efficacy of a particular drug dose both on a behavior disorder and on learning and performance (Williams & Saunders, 1997). This is very important, because the sedative effects of many of the drugs used may interfere with learning and cognition, which are the central concerns in mental retardation.

Animal models have played a significant role in the study of mental illness in humans because they allow researchers to (a) experimentally produce analogous disorders caused by similar etiological factors, (b) mimic homologous human symptoms, (c) test pharmacological responsiveness to putative therapeutic drugs, and (d) test the underlying neurobiological substrates of a disorder. Animal models have also been very important for the psychopharmacology of mental retardation and developmental disorders, by aiding our understanding of hyperactivity (Robbins & Sahakian, 1979), stereotyped behavior (Lewis & Baumeister, 1982), SIB (Breese et al., 1984a), and aggression (Tessel, Schroeder, Stodgell, & Loupe, 1975), and of the drugs that may selectively affect them.

DEVELOPMENT OF PSYCHOPHARMACOTHERAPY

The bottom panel of Figure 2-1 shows some of the major milestones in the history of the use of psychotherapeutic drugs for people with mental retardation and developmental disabilities. The early history, with the exception of that of nootropic (knowledge enhancing) drugs, is patterned very much after the history of psychotherapeutic drugs for mental disorders. Psychopharmacotherapy for people with mental retardation and developmental disabilities came of age in the 1970s and 1980s, and most of its major milestones have occurred since that time. In this section we address the advent of nootropics, systems for dual diagnosis, and three specific neurochemical models for SIB and aggression.

Nootropic Drugs

Nootropic drugs are substances that are believed to enhance cognition by facilitating learning; improving memory; and reducing impairments produced by hypoxia, aging, head trauma, ethanol, and a long list of other threats to CNS integrity (Freeman, 1966). Sarter (1991) reviewed a list of 47 of these cognition enhancers, 22 of which have been tested in humans. Only a few of them, such as piracetam, have shown any promise.

Attempts to raise the IQ of people with mental retardation date back to the introduction of glutamic acid in 1943. A supra normal diet of glutamic acid was reported not only to improve seizure control, but also to raise scores on IQ tests (Albert, Hoch, & Waelsch, 1946). Contemporary reviewers, such as Austin and Ross (1960), all concurred that the more carefully designed studies were negative almost without exception, and interest in the glutamic acid diet faded. The story is not over, however: Glutamic acid derivatives are major neuroexcitatory substances. Modern studies of glutamate's role in memory function may reopen the question of cognitive enhancement.

During the 1950s and 1960s, other substances were tried for cognitive enhancement, including stimulants, vitamin B, vitamin E, thyroid hormone, chronic gonadotrophin hormone, and low doses of neuroleptics. None of these substances showed promise (Louttit, 1965). Today, there is still some research interest in raising intelligence levels by treating a vitamin deficiency state, by giving supplements of normal amounts of vitamin B6 and B12, and by megavitamin therapy (Benton & Cook, 1991; Rimland, Calloway, & Dreyfus, 1978). Comprehensive reviews of these recent studies (Aman & Singh, 1988; Conners, 1993) yielded the same conclusion as did previous reviews: There is little support for these treatments. Well-controlled studies of diet for people with mental retardation and developmental disabilities are very difficult to do.

Systems of Dual Diagnosis

Menolascino coined the term *dual diagnosis* (Steven Reiss, personal communication). The increasing prominence of this concept in the 1970s and 1980s has had a major impact on attempts to classify people with mental retardation or developmental disabilities who also have a mental disorder. An effort is often made to ascertain whether a person has a dual diagnosis, so that an appropriate medication specific to the psychiatric condition can be prescribed. An important milestone was the publication of the DSM-III (American Psychiatric Association [APA], 1980), which set the stage for dual diagnosis. It introduced explicit diagnostic criteria, a multiaxial system, and a descriptive approach that represented a paradigm shift from a psychodynamic to a biological model of psychiatry. This approach promoted empirical research on psychopharmacology as a mode of treatment of mental disorders. Two early important descriptions of dual diagnosis were provided by Eaton and Menolascino (1982) and by Sovner and Hurley (1983). The phenomenon of "diagnostic overshadowing," introduced by Reiss, Levitan, and Szyszko (1982) is also a seminal finding that has been replicated.

NEUROCHEMICAL HYPOTHESES FOR SELF-INJURY (SIB) AND AGGRESSION

The discovery of Lesch-Nyhan syndrome in 1964 (Lesch & Nyhan, 1964) was a major milestone in the psychopharmacology of developmental disabilities. Unlike many other milestones, this one did not have its roots in the study of mental illness. The Lesch-Nyhan syndrome was the first genetic disorder for which a high frequency of a distinctive behavioral phenotype (i.e., self-biting) existed in its population. For years, Lesch-Nyhan syndrome has served as a neurobiological window for studying neurotransmitter functions and pharmacotherapy for SIB. Early hypotheses concerning serotonin dysfunction led to clinical trials with 5-hydroxytryptophan, but it showed only a temporary improvement (Mizuno & Yugari, 1974, 1975; Nyhan et al., 1980). Lloyd et al.'s 1981 important postmortem study of three Lesch-Nyhan cases revealed a 60% to 90% depletion of dopamine and elevation of serotonin in striatal neurons. This finding led Breese, an animal neuropharmacologist, to propose a rat model of neonatal 6-hydroxydopamine lesions as a second hypothesis to account for self-biting in Lesch-Nyhan syndrome (Breese et al., 1984a, 1984b). This rat model has many far-reaching implications for the behavioral and pharmacological treatment and prevention of SIB.

Sandman et al. (1983) proposed the opioid peptide hypotheses for explaining SIB. These hypotheses, which are compatible with those related to serotonin dysfunction, were based on the observation that some people with SIB seem to be insensitive to pain. Perhaps their endorphin system was malfunctioning and could be modulated by endorphin blockers such as naloxone. The first clinical trials of naloxone by Sandman et al. (1983) showed a dose-response effect. This result has been replicated with its orally administered counterpart, naltrexone, in some studies but not others (see Chapter 17). Sandman et al.'s neurochemical hypotheses for SIB have started a new generation of models and theories that have much more specificity in persons with mental retardation and developmental disabilities than was the case for previous theories. Such work, which requires interdisciplinary collaboration to do well, seems to represent a significant contribution to the study of psychopharmacology for people with mental retardation and developmental disabilities.

NEED FOR RESEARCH

Historically, research on psychopharmacology for people with mental retardation and developmental disabilities has been limited by over-regulation and inadequate funding. The former has made it difficult in the United States to obtain the permissions needed to conduct clinical psychopharmacological research with this population (Sprague, 1990). In some past cases, up to 14 levels of prior approval were needed before research could begin. Although the population is fragile and needs to be protected, 14 required approvals are too many. Many authorities are concerned that individuals are being denied the advantages of newly discovered drugs. A second major obstacle is inadequate funding for training and research. Research funding in this area is less than 1% of the federal funds allocated to other areas of mental health or mental retardation. In some years, the National Institutes of Health (NIH) funded only a few relevant research projects in the entire country.

CONCLUSION

Progress has been made since psychopharmacology was begun more than 150 years ago when the rise of organic chemistry permitted the synthesis of myriad new compounds. Until 1950 most of these drugs had only general effects, such as sedation. However, astute clinicians in 1952 observed new and specific psychotropic effects. The search for psychiatric drugs included the use of animal models for testing clinical effects and for elucidating the biological sources of such effects. In the last decade, hypotheses about alterations in brain chemistry and their behavioral effects have led to the search for drugs with specific actions. Although conceived in clinical empiricism and nourished by serendipity, psychopharmacology at the close of the 20th century is increasingly becoming a laboratory science. The future of psychopharmacology in the field of mental retardation and developmental disabilities looks even brighter in the 21st century, with the advent of new neurochemical hypotheses, new drugs, and new methodologies to study them. Some obstacles continue to remain, however.

ACKNOWLEDGMENTS

Research and preparation of this chapter were supported by NICHD Grants 02528, 26927, and 23042 to Stephen R. Schroeder.

REFERENCES

Albert, K., Hoch, P., & Waelsch, H. (1946). Preliminary report on the effect of glutamic acid in mentally retarded subjects. *Journal of Nervous and Mental Diseases, 104*, 263–274.

Aman, M.G. (1983). Psychoactive drugs in mental retardation. In J.L. Matson & F. Andrasik (Eds.), *Treatment and innovations in mental retardation* (pp. 455–513). New York: Plenum Press.

Aman, M.G. (1991). *Assessing psychopathology and behavior in persons with mental retardation: A review of available instruments.* Rockville, MD: U.S. Department of Health and Human Services.

Aman, M.G., Marks, R.E., Turbott, S.H.,

Wilsher, C.P., & Merry, S.N. (1991a). Clinical effects of methylphenidate and thioridazine in intellectually subaverage children. *Journal of the American Academy of Child and Adolescent Psychiatry, 30*, 246–256.

Aman, M.G., Marks, R.E., Turbott, S.H., Wilsher, C.P., & Merry, S.N. (1991b). Methylphenidate and thioridazine in the treatment of intellectually subaverage children: Effects on cognitive-motor performance. *Journal of the American Academy of Child and Adolescent Psychiatry, 30*, 816–824.

Aman, M.G., & Singh, N.N. (Eds.). (1988). *Psychopharmacology of the developmental disabilities.* New York: Springer-Verlag.

American Psychiatric Association. (1980).

Diagnostic and statistical manual of mental disorders (3rd ed.). Washington, D.C.: American Psychiatric Press.

American Psychiatric Association. (1994). *Diagnostic and statistical manual of mental disorders* (4th ed.). Washington, D.C.: American Psychiatric Press.

Austin, A.W., & Ross, S. (1960). Glutamic acid and human intelligence. *Psychological Bulletin, 57*, 429–434.

Ayd, F.J. (1991). The early history of modern psychopharmacology. *Neurophsychopharmacology, 5*, 71–84.

Bair, H.V., & Herold, W. (1955). Efficacy of chlorpromazine in hyperactive mentally retarded children. *Archives of Neurology and Psychiatry, 74*, 363–364.

Barkley, R.A. (1991). *Attention deficit hyper-*

activity disorder. New York: Guilford Press.

Bender, L., & Faretra, G. (1961). Organic therapy in pediatric psychiatry. *Diseases of the Nervous System, 22* (Suppl. 4), 110–111.

Benton, D., & Cook, R. (1991). Vitamin and mineral supplements improve the intelligence scores and concentration of six-year-old children. *Personality and Individual Differences, 12,* 1151–1158.

Boyle, D., & Tobin, J.M. (1961). Pharmaceutical management of behavior disorders: Chlordiazepoxide in covert and overt expressions of aggression. *Journal of the Medical Society, 58,* 427–429.

Bradley, C. (1937). The behavior of children receiving benzedrine. *American Journal of Psychiatry, 94,* 577–585.

Brady, J.V. (1959). Comparative psychopharmacology: Animal experimental studies on the effects of drugs on behavior. In J.D. Cole & R.W. Gerard (Eds.), *Psychopharmacology: Problems in evaluation* (NRC Publication No. 583, pp. 47–53). Washington, D.C.: National Academy of Sciences, National Research Council.

Breese, G.R., Baumeister, A.A., McGowan, T.J., Emerick, S., Frye, G.D., Crotty, K., & Mueller, R.A. (1984a). Behavioral differences between neonatal- and adult-6-hydroxydopamine-treated rats to dopamine agonists: Relevance to neurological symptoms in clinical syndromes with reduced brain dopamine. *Journal of Pharmacology and Experimental Therapeutics, 231,* 343–354.

Breese, G.R., Baumeister, A.A., McGowan, T.J., Emerick, S., Frye, C.D., & Mueller, R.A. (1984b). Neonatal-6-hydroxydopamine treatment: Model of susceptibility for self-mutilation in the Lesch-Nyhan syndrome. *Pharmacology, Biochemistry and Behavior, 21,* 459–461.

Cade, J.F.J. (1949). Lithium salts in the treatment of psychotic excitement. *Medical Journal of Australia, 36,* 349–352.

Campbell, M., Fish, B., Shapiro, T., & Floyd, A. (1972). Acute responses of schizophrenic children to a sedative and "stimulating" neuroleptic: A pharmacological yard stick. *Current Therapeutic Research, 14,* 759–766.

Carlsson, A., & Lindquist, M. (1963). Effect of chlorpromazine or haloperidol on formation of 3-methoxytyramine and normetanephrine in mouse brain. *Acta Pharmacologica, 20,* 140–144.

Carter, C. H. (1960). Isocarboxazid in the institutionalized mentally retarded. *Diseases of the Nervous System, 21,* 568–570.

Conners, C.K. (1993). Nootropics and food. In M.G. Aman & J.S. Werry (Eds.), *Practitioner's guide to psychoactive drugs for children and adolescents* (pp. 373–389). New York: Plenum Medical Books.

Cooper, A.F., & Fowlie, H.C. (1973). Control of gross self-mutilation with lithium carbonate. *British Journal of Psychiatry,* 122, 370–371.

Crane, G.E. (1957). Iproniazid phosphate (Marsilid): A therapeutic agent for mental disorders and debilitating diseases. *Psychiatric Research Reports, 8,* 142–152.

Cutler, M., Little, J.W., & Strauss, A.A. (1940). Effect of benzedrine on mentally deficient children. *American Journal of Mental Deficiency, 45,* 59–65.

Davies, T.S. (1954). Chlorpromazine in mental deficiency. *Lancet, ii,* 819.

Delay, J., Deniker, P., & Harl, J.M. (1952). The treatment of excitement and agitation states by a method of medication derived from hibernotherapy. *Annals Medico-psychologiques, 110,* 267–273.

Dews, P. B. (1955a). Studies on behavior: I. Differential sensitivity to pentobarbital of pecking performance in pigeons depending on the schedule of reward. *Journal of Pharmacology and Experimental Therapeutics, 113,* 393–401.

Dews, P.B. (1955b). Studies on behavior: II. The effects of pentobarbital, methamphetamine and scopolamine on performances in pigeons involving discriminations. *Journal of Pharmacology and Experimental Therapeutics, 113,* 380–389.

Dostal, T., & Zvolsky, P. (1970). Antiaggressive effect of lithium salts in severe mentally retarded adolescents. *International Pharmacopsychiatry, 5,* 203–207.

Eaton, L., & Menolascino, F. (1982). Psychiatric disorders in the mentally retarded: Types, problems, and challenges. *American Journal of Psychiatry, 139,* 218–230.

Feldman, P.E. (1962). Analysis of the efficacy of diazepam. *Journal of Neuropsychiatry, 3,* 62–67.

Freeman, R.D. (1966). Drug effects on learning in children: A selective review of the past thirty years. *Journal of Special Education, 1,* 17–44.

Freeman, W. (1931). Psychochemistry: Some physico-chemical factors in mental disorders. *Journal of the American Medical Association, 93,* 293–296.

Galambos, M. (1965). Long-term clinical trial with diazepam on adult mentally retarded persons. *Diseases of the Nervous System, 26,* 305–309.

Geller, E., Ritvo, E.R., Freeman, B.J., & Yuwiler, A. (1982). Preliminary observations on the effects of fenfluramine on blood serotonin and symptoms in three autistic boys. *New England Journal of Medicine, 307,* 165–169.

Gualtieri, C.T. (1991). *Neuropsychiatry and behavioral pharmacology.* New York: Springer-Verlag.

Harris, T.H. (1960). Methaminodiazepoxide. *Journal of the American Medical Association, 172,* 128–129.

Healy, D. (1993). 100 years of psychopharmacology. *Journal of Psychopharmacology, 7,* 207–214.

Journal of the Experimental Analysis of Behavior. (1991), 56 (2), 167–415.

Journal of Psychopharmacology. (1990), 4 (3).

Klein, D.F. (1964). Delineation of two drug-responsive anxiety syndromes. *Psychopharmacologia, 5,* 397–408.

Kugelmass, I.N. (1956). Psychochemotherapy of mental deficiency in children. *International Record of Medicine and General Practice Clinics, 169,* 323–338.

Kuhn, R. (1957). The treatment of depressive states with an iminodibenzyl derivative (G22355). *Schweizerische Medizinische Wochenschrift, 87,* 1135–1140.

Laties, V.G. (1986). Lessons from the history of behavior pharmacology. In N.A. Krasnegor, D.B. Gray, & T. Thompson (Eds.), *Advances in behavior pharmacology: Vol. 5. Developmental behavioral pharmacology* (pp. 21–39). Hillsdale, NJ: Erlbaum.

LaVeck, G.D., & Buckley, P. (1961). The use of psychopharmacological agents in retarded children with behavior disorders. *Journal of Chronic Diseases, 13,* 174–183.

Lehman, H.E. (1993). Before they called it psychopharmacology. *Neuropsychopharmacology, 8,* 291–303.

Lesch, M., & Nyhan, W.L. (1964). A familial disorder of uric acid metabolism and central nervous system 22 function. *American Journal of Medicine, 36,* 561–570.

Lewis, M.H., & Baumeister, A.A. (1982). Stereotyped mannerisms in mentally retarded persons: Animal models and theoretical analyses. In N.R. Ellis (Ed.), *International review of research in mental retardation* (Vol. 12, pp. 123–161). New York: Academic Press.

Lipman, R.S. (1970). The use of psychopharmacological agents in residential facilities for the retarded. In F.J. Menolascino (Ed.), *Psychiatric approaches to mental retardation* (pp. 387–398). New York: Basic Books.

Lloyd, K.C., Hornykiewicz, O., Davidson, L., Shannak, K., Farley, I., Goldstein, M., Shibuya, M., Kelley, W., & Fox, I.H. (1981). Biochemical evidence of dysfunction of brain neurotransmitters in the Lesch-Nyhan syndrome. *The New England Journal of Medicine, 305,* 1106–1111.

Louttit, R.T. (1965). Chemical facilitation of intelligence among the mentally retarded. *American Journal of Mental Deficiency, 69,* 495–501.

Mizuno, T., & Yugari, Y. (1974). Self-mutilation in Lesch-Nyhan syndrome. *Lancet, 1,* 761.

Mizuno, T., & Yugari, Y. (1975). Prophylactic effects of L-5-hydroxytryptophan on self-mutilation in the Lesch-Nyhan syndrome. *Neuropediatrie, 6,* 13–23.

Molitch, M., & Eccles, A.K. (1937). The effect of benzedrine sulfate on the intelligence scores of children. *American Journal of Psychiatry, 94,* 587–590.

Nyhan, W.L., Johnson, H.G., Kaufman, I.A., & Jones, K.L. (1980). Serotonergic approaches to the modification of behavior in the Lesch-Nyhan syndrome. *Applied Research in Mental Retardation, 1*, 25–40.

Pavlov, I.P. (1927). *Conditioned reflexes* (V. Anrep, Trans.). London: Oxford University Press.

Reiss, S., Levitan, G.W., & Szyszko, J. (1982). Emotional disturbance and mental retardation: Diagnostic overshadowing. *American Journal of Mental Deficiency, 86*, 567–574.

Reiss, S., & Rojahn, J. (1993). Joint occurrence of depression and aggression in children and adults with mental retardation. *Journal of Intellectual Disability Research, 37*, 287–294.

Rimland, B., Calloway, E., & Dreyfus, P. (1978). The effect of high doses of vitamin B6 on autistic children: A double-blind crossover study. *American Journal of Psychiatry, 135*, 472–475.

Ritvo, E.R., Yuwiler, A., Geller, E., Ornitz, E.M., Saeger, K., & Plotkin, S. (1970). Increased blood serotonin and platelets in infantile autism. *Archives of General Psychiatry, 23*, 566–572.

Robbins, T.W., & Sahakian, B.J. (1979). "Paradoxical" effects of psychomotor stimulant drugs in hyperactive children from the standpoint of behaviour pharmacology. *Neuropharmacology, 18*, 931–950.

Sandman, C.A., Datta, P.C., Barron, J., Hoehler, F.K., Williams, C., & Swanson, J.M. (1983). Naloxone attenuates self-abusive behavior in developmentally disabled clients. *Applied Research in Mental Retardation, 4*, 5–11.

Sarter, M. (1991). Taking stock of cognition enhancers. *Trends in Psychopharmacology Reviews, 12*, 456–461.

Skinner, B.F., & Heron, W.T. (1937). Effects of caffeine and benzedrine upon conditioning and extinction. *Psychological Record, 1*, 340–346.

Sovner, R., & Hurley, A.D. (1983). Do the mentally retarded suffer from affective illness? *Archives of General Psychiatry, 40*, 61–67.

Sprague, R. L. (1990). Obstacles to including the mentally retarded in psychopharmacology research. In R.L. Sprague & D.J. Luchins (Chairs), *Obstacles to including the mentally retarded in psychopharmacology research*, Symposium conducted at the meeting of the American College of Neuropsychopharmacology, San Juan, PR.

Sprague, R.L., & Baxley, G.B. (1979). Drugs used for the management of behavior in mental retardation. In J. Wortis (Ed.), *Mental retardation* (Vol. 11, pp. 1–24). New York: Grune & Stratton.

Sprague, R.L., & Werry, J.S. (1971).

Methodology of psychopharmacological studies with the retarded. In N.R. Ellis (Ed.), *International review of research in mental retardation* (Vol. 5, pp. 148–220). San Diego, CA: Academic Press.

Still, G.F. (1902). Some abnormal psychical conditions in children. *Lancet, i*, 1008–1012, 1077–1082, 1163–1168.

Tessel, R.E., Schroeder, S.R., Stodgell, C.J., Loupe, P.S. (1995). Rodent models of mental retardation: Self-injury, aberrant behavior and stress. *Mental Retardation and Developmental Disabilities Reviews, 1*, 99–103.

Thompson, T., Hackenberg, T., & Schaal, D. (1991). *Pharmacological treatments for behavior problems in developmental disabilities* (NIH Publication No. 91-3410). Paper presented at the Consensus Development Conference on Destructive Behavior, National Institutes on Health, Bethesda, MD.

Tredgold, A.F. (1908). *Mental deficiency (amentia)*. New York: W. Wood.

Williams, D.C., & Saunders, K.J. (1997). Methodological issues in the study of drug effects on cognitive skills in mental retardation. In N. Bray (Ed.), *The international review of research in mental retardation*, (Vol. 21, pp.147–156). San Diego, CA: Academic Press.

Epidemiology and Psychoactive Medication

Christine Rinck, Ph.D.[1,2]

EPIDEMIOLOGY AND PSYCHOACTIVE MEDICATION

Psychoactive drugs are substances that produce behavioral, emotional, or cognitive changes (e.g., Aman & Singh, 1988), such as antipsychotic agents, antidepressants, and anti-anxiety agents that are usually thought of as psychiatric medications. Also included are a number of drugs that are not usually thought of as psychiatric medications. For example, anticonvulsant drugs that are used to control epileptic seizures often are not thought of as psychiatric medications; however, most (perhaps all) anticonvulsant drugs have psychoactive effects in addition to their effects in controlling seizures. The anticonvulsant drugs carbamazepine (Tegretol), valproate (Depakote and Epilim), and clonazepam (Klonopin), among others, have significant effects on behavior and emotion, especially in managing the psychiatric disorder known as mania.[3]

In 1970 Lipman published the first prevalence study on the use of psychoactive medications with people with mental retardation. He reported high rates, with some institutions prescribing psychoactive medications for as many as 80% or more of the residents. Similar rates soon were reported by other researchers. For example, Tu (1979) found that 42% of his sample were receiving psychoactive medication, whereas DiMascio (1975) reported a rate of 53%.

The results of the early prevalence studies raised concerns among many advocates and policymakers regarding possible inappropriate uses of psychoactive medications (Wolfensberger, 1984). It was thought that too many people were being given these medications and that sometimes the medications were used to sedate people rather than to treat a specific disorder or aberrant behavior. Too many people experienced *polypharmacy*, in which multiple psychoactive medications are given to manage the same symptoms in the same person. Some of the medications can have serious side effects; therefore, use requires a risk/reward analysis and careful monitoring.

With increased concerns came additional research designed to specify more precisely how many people with mental retardation receive one or more psychoactive medications. Researchers also studied various subpopulations of people with mental retardation. They have studied how rates of drug use may vary depending on psychiatric and behavioral conditions, and they have examined various standards of practice that may be associated with increases or decreases in the use of psychoactive medications.

The literature on the prevalence of psychoactive drug use among people with mental retardation is summarized and reviewed in this chapter. Although this literature permits some general conclusions, making comparisons of findings across studies is complicated by the following two considerations. First, because mental retardation is a dynamic field in which professional practices regarding psychoactive medications can change considerably over a period of only a few years, some results of prevalence studies may become outdated within a few years after they are obtained. New drugs are introduced every year, and preferences for various drug categories change with advances in research and changes in clinical thinking.

The second consideration involves methodology. Different investigators have included different medications under the rubric of psychoactive medication. For example, certain anticonvulsant medications can be

1 Director of Research, Institute for Human Development, University of Missouri at Kansas City, Kansas City, MO
2 Other committee members: Martin Agran, Ph.D., Associate Professor of Special Education, Utah State University; B. I. Sacks, M.D., University of London, United Kingdom
3 Many researchers distinguish between the terms *psychoactive* and *psychotropic* drugs (Aman & Singh, 1988). Psychoactive drugs are those that produce behavioral, emotional, or cognitive effects, whereas psychotropic drugs are agents prescribed specifically for the purposes of altering the client's behavior or emotions (Aman & Singh, 1988). Psychotropic drugs do not include certain agents that may have behavioral or emotional effects (e.g., certain drugs used to treat asthma and most anticonvulsants). In this chapter, the expression "psychoactive medication" will be used to refer to medications that have behavioral, emotional, or cognitive effects, unless a more specific meaning is stated; for example, where the original author distinguished between psychoactive and psychotropic drugs, we have endeavored to do likewise here.

prescribed either for epilepsy or for psychiatric conditions. One researcher might include all anticonvulsant medications as examples of psychoactive medications, another might include anticonvulsant medications only when they are given for psychiatric conditions, and a third might not include anticonvulsant medications at all. These differences in methods can produce significant differences in outcome, producing apparent discrepancies in findings across studies on the prevalence of psychoactive drug use. Naturally, researchers who include all uses of anticonvulsant medications typically obtain higher overall prevalence estimates than do those who subtract out the number of people given these medications for epilepsy and other nonpsychiatric conditions.

PREVALENCE OF PSYCHO-ACTIVE MEDICATION USE

Comprehensive lists of outcomes and prevalence studies are presented in Tables 3-1 and 3-2. In this section, findings regarding the use of psychoactive medications are summarized by major clinical category.

Antipsychotics

Antipsychotic medications constitute a large group of psychoactive agents that includes seven different classes: phenothiazines, butyrophenones, thioxanthenes, dihydroindolones, dibenzoxazepines, diphenylbutylpiperidines, and tricyclic dibenzodiazepines (Campbell, Gonzalez, Ernst, Silva, & Werry, 1993). These drugs also have been called *neuroleptics*, because they are capable of causing profound motor effects (e.g., dystonias) that, in the early days, were thought to mimic a neurologic disorder. As will be seen later in this chapter, unfortunately this eventually proved to be the case, as is exemplified by the side effect known as tardive dyskinesia. These agents were also called major tranquilizers, because they induce calm and tend to diminish arousal. The drugs are prescribed to treat thought disorder, especially when these symptoms are associated with diagnoses of schizophrenia, bipolar disorder with psychosis, major depressive disorder with psychosis, Tourette syndrome, autism, hyperactivity, aggressiveness, and conduct disorder (Campbell et al., 1993).

Antipsychotic agents are the most frequently prescribed category of psychoactive medication with people with mental retardation, especially in institutions (Hill, Balow, & Bruininks, 1985; Intagliata & Rinck, 1985; Spreat,

Serafin, Behan, & Leiman, 1993). Recent studies have indicated widely varying prevalence rates for different samples of people in community-based facilities. For example, Lepler, Hodas, and Cotter-Mack (1993) reported a rate of 5%, whereas Pary (1993) reported a rate of 42%.

The drugs thioridazine and chlorpromazine (especially thioridazine) are among the most commonly prescribed antipsychotic agents in clients with mental retardation (Aman, Sarphare, & Burrow, 1995). In recent years, haloperidol also has been widely prescribed (e.g., Briggs, 1989; Buck & Sprague, 1989). The drugs thioridazine and haloperidol are also frequently prescribed for people with autism (Aman, Van Bourgondien, Wolford, & Sarphare, 1995).

The long-term use of antipsychotic medications is associated with a number of side effects, especially various tremors and movement disorders such as pseudo-Parkinsonism, dystonia, akathisia, akinesia, and tardive dyskinesia. These adverse reactions to treatment can interfere with the performance of daily activities. Such side effects are commonly treated with anticholinergic agents, such as benztropine (Cogentin) and amantadine (Symmetrel). Researchers have found that anticholinergic agents have been prescribed at rates ranging from around 3% to as high as 22% for the various samples surveyed (see Table 3-2). According to one study, the anticholinergic agents were used for a higher percentage of older versus younger people (Pary, 1993).

There is evidence that the use of antipsychotic agents among people with mental retardation is declining. A number of factors account for this decrease in use. Some researchers have expressed concern about the potentially damaging side effects of antipsychotic agents. Another factor has been the growing trend among psychiatrists to diagnose mood disorders for many cases in which the past practice was to diagnose schizophrenia (Reid, 1993a). In recent years a number of influential psychiatrists have advocated the use of antidepressants instead of antipsychotics, especially for people with more severe forms of mental retardation (Reid, 1993b). Another influence has been the growing use of multidisciplinary review teams to assess the appropriateness of drug regimens (see Chapter 5). This has often led to a decrease in the use of psychoactive agents, including antipsychotic agents (Findholt & Emmett, 1990; Hancock, Weber, Kaza, & Hou, 1991).

Antidepressants

Antidepressant medications include several groups of agents: monoamine oxidase inhibitors, tricyclic antidepressants, heterocyclic antidepressants, and the newest group—the selective serotonin reuptake inhibitors like fluoxetine (Prozac). The drugs are prescribed to treat depressed mood, irritability, and associated conduct problems, especially when these symptoms are associated with diagnoses of mood disorder or anxiety disorder.

The rates of use of antidepressant medications in prevalence studies have varied from almost none (Briggs, 1989) to approximately 8% (Pary, 1993). In the only survey to be conducted for clients with autism, a rate of 6% was found (Aman, Van Bourgondien, Wolford, & Sarphare, 1995). The use of antidepressants has been found to be higher in community settings than in institutional settings. According to one study, older people were prescribed antidepressants more frequently than were younger people (Pary, 1993).

The use of antidepressants may be increasing. As was noted previously, a number of influential psychiatrists have suggested that in the past some mood disorders were misdiagnosed as psychotic disorders. The trend toward greater diagnosis of mood disorder is probably leading to increased use of antidepressant medications.

Anxiolytics and Hypnotics

Anxiolytics are anti-anxiety agents. They are used to treat nervousness, fears, panic attacks, and related behavioral conditions. Anxiolytic drugs, diazepam (Valium) and clonazepam (Klonopin), are sometimes used to treat people with epilepsy. Hypnotic agents are used to induce sleep. The most common hypnotics are flurazepam (Dalmane), diazepam, temazepam (Restoril), and triazolam (Halcion). Chloral hydrate (Noctec) and meprobamate (Miltown) once were widely prescribed as hypnotics, but their use has given way to the more specific and safer benzodiazepine group, of which diazepam is the prototype. The anxiolytics and hypnotics also include antihistamines such as diphenhydramine (Benadryl), barbiturates such as secobarbital (Seconal), and buspirone (BuSpar), a new anxiolytic that is unique in that it does not have hypnotic properties. All agents from this group except buspirone have both anti-anxiety and hypnotic properties.

The choice of drug (for anxiolytic versus hypnotic purposes) often hinges on absorption and elimination characteristics and sometimes on drug company promotion. Drugs with rapid absorption and relatively short half-lives (e.g., 4 to 8 hours) are often preferred as hypnotics, whereas agents producing longer-lasting and more even drug concentrations over the day are often preferred as anxiolytic drugs. Poindexter (1989) found that anxiolytic

medications were prescribed for 1.3% of a sample of 474 people residing in an Intermediate Care Facility/Mental Retardation (ICF/MR). Most of those in the sample were adults, and the majority had severe or profound mental retardation. In contrast, White (1983) found that these medications were prescribed for 20.4% of a sample of 435 residents (both adolescents and adults) living in a developmental center. However, this figure included drugs that were used as anticonvulsants (e.g., diazepam, clonazepam) and PRN (taken as needed only) prescriptions.

Stimulants

Stimulant medications include methylphenidate (Ritalin) and dextroamphetamine (Dexedrine), which are prescribed widely for the treatment of attention-deficit hyperactivity disorder (ADHD) in children. These drugs are given to improve attention, impulse control, task-relevant behavior, and compliance with rules (Barkley, DuPaul, & Costello, 1993). In a 1981 review of drug surveys, Gadow found rates of stimulant use at about 1% to 2% of elementary school students enrolled in classes for students with mild mental retardation. More recently researchers have obtained rates of 6% to about 7% (Safer & Krager, 1988). Gadow (1985) suggested that 7.5% of students with mild mental retardation are being treated with a stimulant medication at any given point in time. Use of stimulants has been found to be a little bit higher in institutions versus community-based facilities (Hill et al., 1985; Intagliata & Rinck, 1985). In the only survey done among subjects with autism, Aman, Van Bourgondien, Wolford, and Sarphare (1995) found that 12% of children aged 7 to 13 years were taking stimulant drugs. This is not surprising, as the stimulants are helpful for managing hyperactivity and ADHD, and hyperactivity has long been regarded as a common symptom in autism.

Antimanic Agents

Lithium is perhaps the most commonly used psychoactive medication for the treatment of manic behavior and bipolar disorder. Pary (1993) found that lithium was prescribed for 6% of a sample of 369 adults and older adults in the catchment area of Allegheny County in Pennsylvania. The subjects in this study came from a multitude of settings including independent, family-supervised, supervised community, and institutional. Lepler et al. (1993) obtained rates of 9.5% and 5.8% for 42 and 52 adults surveyed in

1987 and 1989, respectively, in a community-based agency that operated day, residential, and support programs.

Anticonvulsants

Jacobson (1982) found that about 25% of the people with mental retardation receiving services in New York State had epilepsy. Not surprisingly, there is widespread use of anticonvulsants among people with mental retardation because the rate of epilepsy tends to increase with functional impairment. Most agents used to treat epilepsy also have psychoactive effects. Some commonly used anticonvulsant drugs include phenobarbital and other barbiturates, phenytoin (Dilantin), carbamazepine (Tegretol), valproic acid (Depakene, Epilim), and ethosuximide (Zarontin). Some new, recently developed anticonvulsant drugs include felbamate (Felbatol) and gabapentin (Neurontin). Three anticonvulsant agents are also used for their effects in managing psychiatric disorders. Carbamazepine, valproate, and clonazepam are all effective in managing manic disorder. Two groups of researchers evaluated the extent of use of anticonvulsants for behavioral control. Lepler et al. (1993) found an initial rate of 7.3%, which decreased over a three-year period to 5.8%. Aman, Sarphare, and Burrow (1995) surveyed 1,101 adults in group homes and found that 5.4% of subjects were receiving anticonvulsants for psychiatric or behavioral problems. The most common target behaviors listed for these drugs were pica, destructive behavior, psychosis, and aggression.

FACTORS ASSOCIATED WITH USE OF PSYCHOACTIVE AGENTS

Level of Mental Retardation

Research studies on the prevalence of psychopathology and behavioral problems in people with mild as compared with severe mental retardation have yielded inconsistent results (Reiss, 1994, pp. 18-19). The results of some studies suggest greater psychopathology among persons with mild mental retardation (e.g., Borthwick-Duffy, 1994; Jacobson, 1982; Reiss & Valenti-Hein, 1994), whereas other researchers reported lower rates for people with mild mental retardation (Lund, 1985; Philips & Williams, 1975; Reiss, 1988). Reiss (1994) concluded that there may be little or no difference in overall prevalence rates of psychopathology

for adults with mild versus severe mental retardation, but that rates may be significantly higher for children with mild as compared with severe mental retardation.

Researchers have obtained inconsistent results regarding the use of psychoactive agents as a function of severity of mental retardation. Some researchers found that psychoactive agents were used more often with people with severe disabilities (Aman, Sarphare, & Burrow, 1995; Hancock et al., 1991; Hill et al., 1985; Jacobson, 1988), whereas others found no correlation (Anderson & Polister, 1993; Buck & Sprague, 1989; Burd et al., 1991). Others still have found evidence of more medication use among people with mild disabilities (Aman, Sarphare, & Burrow, 1995; Martin & Agran, 1985; Stone, Alvarez, Ellman, Hom, & White, 1989). Aman, Van Bourgondien, Wolford, and Sarphare (1995), who surveyed subjects with autism in North Carolina, found a greater use of antipsychotics and anticonvulsants in subjects with more severe mental retardation.

Gender

Generally, gender has not been an important variable in prevalence studies of dual diagnosis. For example, only small differences have been obtained in mean scores for male versus female subjects on standardized dual diagnosis instruments (e.g., Reiss, 1988; Reiss & Valenti-Hein, 1990, 1994). When gender effects have been obtained for people with mental retardation, moreover, they correspond to similar effects reported for the general population. For example, depression is more commonly seen in women with mental retardation, whereas aggression is more common in men (Reiss & Trenn, 1984).

Most researchers have found that men and women with mental retardation are equally likely to be given psychoactive medications (Aman, Sarphare, & Burrow, 1995; Buck & Sprague, 1989; Burd et al., 1991; Harper, Wadsworth, & Michael, 1989; Intagliata & Rinck, 1985; Jacobson, 1988; Martin & Agran, 1985). Hancock et al. (1991) and Tu and Smith (1979) both found that a greater proportion of women were receiving psychoactive medications. It is not clear why these two studies showed different patterns. In their survey of drug use by subjects with autism, Aman, Van Bourgondien, Wolford, and Sarphare (1995) observed no gender-related medication patterns.

Psychiatric Diagnosis

Very few studies have focused on psychiatric diagnosis

and the use of psychoactive agents in people with mental retardation. One noteworthy finding, however, is that a diagnosis of psychosis is particularly likely to be associated with drug therapy (Aman, Sarphare, & Burrow, 1995; Jacobson, 1988; Pary, 1993; Tu & Smith, 1983). Psychoactive agents, especially antipsychotic medications, also have been widely prescribed for people with challenging behavior (Hill et al., 1985; Intagliata & Rinck, 1985; Jacobson, 1988). Individuals with aggressive or violent behavior are very likely to be given drug therapy (Aman, Sarphare, & Burrow, 1995; Rinck & Calkins, 1989; Stone et al., 1989; Tu & Smith, 1983). Medication also is commonly used to treat self-injurious behavior and hyperactivity (Briggs, 1989; Lepler et al., 1993).

Many people who receive psychotropic agents have no psychiatric diagnosis in their case files (Jacobson, 1988; Rinck & Rinck, 1991). In some of these cases, the individual is under treatment for a well specified behavioral condition, such as self-injury or stereotypic behavior. In other cases, however, the medications are prescribed without any specific target symptom or diagnosis.

Residential Setting

The use of psychoactive medications for people with mental retardation in institutional settings may be declining. Findings from the 1980s and earlier showed that these medications were used more often in institutions than in community settings (e.g., Intagliata & Rinck, 1985). Even for people in community placements, an institutional history was highly related to current psychotropic drug use (Martin & Agran, 1985). Recent studies, however, suggest comparable rates for institutions and the community (Anderson & Polister, 1993; Pary, 1993): The number of people with a dual diagnosis who still live in institutions is still proportionately higher. However, bizarre behaviors may be more readily tolerated in institutions, and institutions may be more likely to create active interdisciplinary review boards that have been found to decrease the use of psychoactive medications.

Rinck and Calkins (1989) surveyed 3,744 people with mental retardation in community placements in Missouri. They found a higher prevalence of psychotropic medication among older subjects (those aged 55 years and older) in medically oriented facilities than among those in group homes. In a national survey of older people with mental retardation, Anderson and Polister

(1993) found that large private facilities had the highest prevalence of psychotropic drugs. Only one study has been reported on the use of psychoactive medications in rural versus urban settings. Rinck and Calkins (1989) found that forty-three percent of older subjects (less than or equal to 55 years) in rural areas (less than 20,000 inhabitants) received antipsychotic drugs, as compared with 28% in small towns (population 20,000 to 250,000), and 7% in urban areas (population less than 250,000). Rinck and Calkins also reported that 5.3% of subjects in rural areas used anti-anxiety drugs, compared with less than 1% in small towns and 7.3% in urban areas.

Age

Researchers have found that the highest rates of treatment of dual diagnosis occur for people in late adolescence and early adulthood (e.g., Reiss, 1994, pp. 16-18; Reiss & Trenn, 1984). Rates of dual diagnosis are much lower for children aged ten or less than for any other age group (Reiss & Valenti-Hein, 1994; Rojahn, Borthwick-Duffy, & Jacobson, 1993). Researchers have found little or no correlation between age and prevalence of dual diagnosis for people between the ages of about 30 and about 55. Some researchers have found high rates for elderly people (Coyle, 1988; Davidson et al., 1992; Harper & Wadsworth, 1990), but others have observed no differences in rates for elderly compared with nonelderly people (Jacobson & Harper, 1989).

A number of researchers have found that older people use more psychoactive medications (Anderson, 1992; Errickson, Bock, Young, & Silverstein, 1981; Hill et al., 1985; James, 1986), whereas others have found no relationship (Buck & Sprague, 1989; Hancock et al., 1991; Harper et al., 1989; Linaker, 1990; Pary, 1993; Tu & Smith, 1979). Jacobson (1988) found a curvilinear relationship, with the highest prevalence among the youngest and the oldest people. The reasons for use of psychoactive medications may differ for older versus younger people. Younger people may be more likely to receive drug treatment for aggression. Rinck and Calkins (1989) found that psychoactive medications were more commonly used for those people aged 65 or older who resided in a rural area or in a medically oriented facility.

A number of factors need to be considered in interpreting studies on the relationship between psychoactive medication use and age. For example, older people with mental retardation may experience more medication because more of them have a diagnosis of dementia (Zigman, Seltzer, & Silverman, 1994). Older people are also more likely to reside in medically oriented facilities, which in general are more likely than many other types of settings to rely on psychoactive medication (Avon, Dreyer, Connelly, & Soumerai, 1989).

APPROPRIATE USE OF PSYCHOACTIVE MEDICATION

The appropriateness of psychoactive medication use was examined by Bates, Smeltzer, and Arnoczky (1986), who compared the type of medication with the individual's psychiatric diagnosis. This information was extracted from the medical files of residents in state developmental centers. They found appropriate use for 45%, and probable inappropriate use for 39% of residents; they were uncertain about the remaining 16%. Because the study is more than a decade old, the degree to which the findings are still relevant needs to be determined by additional research.

A number of researchers have examined the issue of appropriateness of use by discontinuing medications in questionable cases or as part of planned periods known as drug holidays. Heistad, Zimmermann, and Doebler (1982) evaluated the effects of a drug-free holiday that was ordered by a court of law. The participants were residents in a developmental center in Minnesota. The researchers found that between 37% and 56% of the people were probably or definitely better off on the medication in terms of overall behavioral adjustment, quality of life, and job performance. However, as many as 44% of the people did not seem to have been benefiting from the previous medicine(s) they were taking. The findings suggested a significant rate of inappropriate use of psychoactive medications among people with mental retardation. However, these findings are more than 15 years old and may not be relevant to today's practices.

Efforts to ensure appropriate uses of medications have included the establishment of interdisciplinary team reviews. Virtually all states require interdisciplinary teams to monitor psychoactive medications for people with mental retardation. These teams usually comprise some combination of administrators, direct care providers, mental retardation technicians, nurses, pharmacists, psychologists, and social workers (Glaser & Morreau, 1986). The reviews typically include a determination of the reason for the drug prescription in terms of a psychiatric diagnosis or specification of a target

behavior. The team also may specify methods for evaluating effectiveness and dates for reassessment.

Especially in institutions, the implementation of the interdisciplinary team process has decreased both the numbers of people receiving medications and dosage levels. Findholt and Emmett (1990) found that implementation of an interdisciplinary review process had a major impact on a state developmental center housing between 436 and 509 residents. Initially, 41% of the residents were receiving antipsychotic medications, 14% antidepressants, 16% anxiolytics, and 10% polypharmacy. Eight years after the review process was begun, 12% received antipsychotics, 3% anxiolytics, and less than 1% polypharmacy. Similar findings were reported by Briggs, Hamad, Garrard, and Willis (1984) and by Briggs (1989). Lepler et al. (1993) reported that the use of psychotropic drugs decreased from a 20% prevalence rate to 17% over a 10-year period and that dosage levels were reduced by 75% for those still prescribed medications. Spreat et al. (1993) reported a 6% decrease in active prescriptions and a 46.5% decrease in dosage.

CONCLUSION

The use of psychoactive medications with people with mental retardation has been examined in numerous research studies conducted over the last 25 years. Between 12% and 43% of the people in the research samples were receiving at least one psychoactive medication. The most commonly used class of medication is the antipsychotics (neuroleptics), although the use of antidepressants is increasing and the prevalence of anticonvulsants has always been high. More selective use of anticonvulsants for specific psychiatric applications (e.g., treating manic disorder) is increasing. Although in the past psychoactive medications were used more often in institutions than in community settings, today's rates may be approximately equal for the various settings. Few consistent relationships have been reported regarding the impact of age and severity of mental retardation on psychoactive drug use. More research is needed to focus on the relationship of psychoactive drugs to other factors (e.g., setting or the subject's characteristics). Inappropriate uses of psychoactive medication may be declining, but too few methodologically sound studies have been reported from which to draw a firm conclusion. Most researchers have found that the practice of using interdisciplinary team reviews resulted in significant reductions in the use of psychoactive medication.

Table 3-1. Major Drug Prevalence Surveys (1970-1996)
% Receiving Medication

Author, publication date, and subgroups	Number of persons surveyed	Psychotropics	Anticonvulsants	Total %	Drugs most commonly prescribed
Public residential facilities studies					
Lipman (1970)	institutional[a]	51[b]	NR[c]	NR	thioridazine, chlorpromazine, trifluoperazine, diazepam, chlordiazepoxide
Spencer (1974)	585	22+	24	51+	phenobarbital, haloperidol, chlorpromazine, phenytoin, thioridazine
Bullmore, cited in Kirman (1975)	617	NR	26	60	NR
DiMascio (1975)					phenobarbital, phenytoin,
facility 1	1,232	26	21	NR	thioridazine, chlorpromazine,
facility 2	785	53	90	NR	primidone, diazepam
Sewell & Werry (1976)	254	40	NR	NR	thioridazine, chlorpromazine, methotrimeprazine, nitrazepam
Cohen & Sprague (1977)	1,924	51	36	66	thioridazine, phenytoin, phenobarbital, diazepam, primidone, mesoridazine
Hughes (1977)	219	NR	NR	68	phenobarbital, phenytoin, diazepam, chlorpromazine, thioridazine, haloperidol
Pulman, Pook, & Singh (1979)	435	47	34	60	phenytoin, diazepam, carbamazepine, trimeprazine, haloperidol, phenobarbital
Silva (1979)	260	NR	24	66	phenytoin, phenobarbital, thioridazine, hydroxyzine, primidone
Tu (1979)	2,238	42	27	58	thioridazine, chlorpromazine, mesoridazine, diazepam, thiothixene
Craig & Behar (1980)					piperidine, aliphatic, piperazine,
1970 sample	161	83	NR	83+	neuroleptics, tricyclic
1977 sample	92	86	NR	86+	antidepressants
Jonas (1980)	596	NR	NR	70	chloral hydrate, carbamazepine, thioridazine, diazepam, haloperidol
LaMendola, Zaharia, & Carver (1980)					
1974 sample	NR	27	NR	34	NR
1978 sample	NR	20	NR	21	NR

Author, publication date, and subgroups	Number of persons surveyed	Psychotropics	Anticonvulsants	Total %	Drugs most commonly prescribed
Errickson, Bock, Young, & Silverstein (1981)					
public resid. group	2,808	30	NR	NR	NR
ICF/MR group	3,004	23	NR	NR	NR
Inoue (1982)					
prestudy group	445	33.5	NR	NR	NR
poststudy group	415	36.9	NR	NR	NR
White (1983)	415	19	36	51	carbamazepine, thioridazine, phenytoin, sodium valproate, haloperidol
Radinsky (1984)					phenytoin, phenobarbital, thioridazine, carbamazepine chlorpromazine, haloperidol
public resid. group	1,687	27+	48	51	
ICF/MR group	388	23+	56	67	
Hill, Balow, & Bruininks (1985)	992	30	36	51+	anticonvulsants (unspecified), phenothiazines, hypnotics
Intagliata & Rinck (1985)	171	54	42	76	phenytoin, phenobarbital, thioridazine, diazepam, chlorpromazine
Aman, Richmond, Stewart, Bell, & Kissel (1987)					
U.S. sample	531	37+	41	58	NR
New Zealand	937	39+	28	60	NR
Briggs (1989)					thioridazine, haloperidol, chlorpromazine
1984 group	730	18.7	NR	NR	
1987 group	695	18.7	31.3	44.2	
Buck & Sprague (1989)	5,766	28.9	NR	NR	haloperidol, chlorpromazine
Stone, Alvarez, Ellman, Hom, & White (1989)	6,450	35.0	NR	NR	NR
Burd et al. (1991)	809	17.8	20.4	37.0	NR
Hancock, Weber, Kaza, & Hou (1991)					
1979 sample	139	30	NR	NR	NR
1983 sample	139	24	NR	NR	NR
1988 sample	139	12	NR	NR	NR
Community-based studies					
Hansen & Keogh (1971)	229[c,d]	31	NR	NR	CNS sedatives/tranquilizers, CNS stimulants, antihistamines

Author, publication date, and subgroups	Number of persons surveyed	Psychotropics	Anticonvulsants	Total %	Drugs most commonly prescribed
Gadow (1981)					
sibling group	435	24	23	24	
group home	461	29	34	32	
special home	385	46	43	43	lithobid
Gadow & Kalachnik (1981)	3,306[c,e]	7	12	18	phenytoin, phenobarbital, methylphenidate, primidone, thioridazine, diazepam
Radinsky (1984)	575[c,f]	36	33	36	thioridazine, phenytoin, phenobarbital, haloperidol, carbamazepine
Martin & Agran (1985)	178[c,g]	32+	24	48	phenytoin, thioridazine, phenobarbital, haloperidol, chlorpromazine
Aman, Field, & Bridgman (1985)					
preschool group	126	2	31	33	carbamazepine, phenytoin,
spec. ed. group	356	3	17	21	thioridazine, sodium valproate,
adult ctr. group	530	14	18	29	phenobarbital, haloperidol
Hill, Balow, Bruininks (1985)	962[c,f]	26	22	40+	anticonvulsants (unspecified), phenothiazines, benzodiazepines
Intagliata & Rinck (1985)	295[c,f]	36	21	48	thioridazine, phenytoin, phenobarbital, primidone, chlorpromazine
Schalock, Foley, Toulouse, & Stark (1985)					
1981 group	41	30.5	NR	NR	NR
1983 group	41	20.0	NR	NR	NR
Gowdey, Zarfas, & Phipps (1987)	1,389[c,h]	20	23	40	phenytoin, phenobarbital, carbamazepine, thioridazine, chlorpromazine
Poindexter (1989)	1,282	18.6	21.8	34.6	thioridazine, tofranil, lithobid,
1978 group	474	32.1	NR	NR	xanax, cogentin, phenytoin
1983 group	474	27.4	NR	NR	
1987 group	474	12.2	NR	NR	
Zaharia & Struxness (1991)	1,282	18.6	21.8	34.6	
Lepler, Hodus, & Cotter-Mack (1993)					
1986 group	42	21	7.1[a]	NR	NR
1989 group	52	19	5.8[a]	NR	NR
Pary (1993)					
20-39 yrs.	208	NR	23	50	NR
40-54 yrs.	90	NR	31	63	NR
55+	71	NR	20	66	NR

Author, publication date, and subgroups	Number of persons surveyed	Psychotropics	Anticonvulsants	Total %	Drugs most commonly prescribed
Gualtieri & Schroeder (1985)	1,467 CAS[c,i]	17	6	NR	antipsychotics (unspecified), antiepileptics, antidepressants
Spreat, Serafin, Behan, & Leiman (1993)					
1990 group		45.0	NR	NR	NR
1991 group		42.6	NR	NR	NR
Aman, Sarphare, & Burrow (1995)	1,101	25.7	5.4	27.0	haloperidol, chlorpromazine, carbamazepine, sodium valproate, phenobarbital, lithium carbonate
Studies of other settings					
Gadow (1976)	2,559[c,k]	8	7	14	methylphenidate, phenytoin, phenobarbital, primidone, thioridazine
Krager, Safer, & Earhart (1979)	3,867	15+	NR	NR	NR
Ahsanuddin, Ivey, Schlotzhauer, Hall, & Prosen (1983)	100[l]	66	NR	NR	thioridazine, chlorpromazine, others unspecified
Aman, Van Bourgondien, Wolford, & Sarphare, 1995	838[m]	22.1	13.2	38.9	thioridazine, haloperidol, chlorpromazine

a   Residents of 109 institutions.
b   This figure may be an overestimate, as the survey asked how many residents had been, or were currently being, treated with psychotropic medication.
c   Medication prescribed only for behavioral or psychiatric conditions.
d   Pupils with educational handicap.
e   Pupils with trainable handicap.
f   Community residential facility.
g   Community residential agency.
h   Group home.
i   Children included in a class action suit in North Carolina.
j   Only antipsychotics surveyed.
k   Early childhood special education program (Illinois) for children, 3-5 years, with developmental handicaps.
l   Child psychiatric facilities.
m Members with autism in the Autism Society of North Carolina.
NR = Not reported.

Note: Table has been adapted and extended, by permission, from Aman and Singh (1988).

Table 3-2. Prevalance Presented by Drug Group (1970-1996)
% Receiving Medication

Author, publication data, and subgroups	Anti-psychotic	Anxiolytic/ hypnotic	Anti-depressant	Anti-manic	Stimulant	Anti-Parkinson	Anti-hypertensive
Studies of institutional facilities							
Lipman (1970)	39.0	8.0	4.0	NR	NR	NR	NR
Pulman, Pook, & Singh (1979)	26.4	20.5[a,i]	.23	NR	.9	6.2	NR
Silva (1979)	21.2	12.7[j]	NR	NR	NR	3.5	NR
Inoue (1982)	40.7	15.1[b]	4.9	.4	NR	NR	NR
White (1983)	14.0	6.3[b]	1.7	NR	NR	2.4	NR
Hill, Balow, & Bruininks (1985)	29.9	12.7[b]	1.1	.6	.4	3.3	NR
Intagliata & Rinck (1985)	45.0	16.9	1.2	.6	1.2	NR	NR
James (1986)[c]	36.0	20.0	16.0	.6	NR	NR	NR
Briggs (1989)							
1984 group	16.6	.5	.7	1.2	.1	NR	NR
1987 group	14.5	3.2	2.0	2.3	0	NR	NR
Buck & Sprague (1989)[d]	25.0	5.2	5.0	1.2	.2	6.0	NR
Poindexter (1989)							
1978 group	30.1	2.6	0.2	NR	.8	NR	NR
1983 group	21.3	2.8	0.6	1.5	.6	NR	NR
1987 group	9.5	2.1	0.4	2.7	NR	NR	NR
Findholt & Emmett (1990)							
1979 group	40.8	13.0[e]	10.5[e]	2.0	NR	NR	NR
1987 group	11.9	3.0[e]	1.14[e]	1.0	NR	NR	NR
Hancock, Weber, Kaza & Hou (1991)							
1979 group	30.0	1.4	NR	0	NR	3.6	NR
1983 group	24.0	2.9	.7	1.4	NR	NR	NR
1988 group	12.0	5.0	NR	0	NR	NR	NR
Spreat, Serafin, Behan & Leiman (1993)							
in 1990	45.0	NR	NR	NR	NR	NR	NR
in 1991	42.6	NR	NR	NR	NR	NR	NR
Studies of community facilities							
Gadow & Kalachnik (1981)[f]	1.3	.2	.18	NR	1.8	NR	NR
Martin & Agran (1985)	29.7	3.0	5.0	0	NR	23.0	NR
Hill, Balow, & Bruininks (1985)	20.5	7.7[b]	1.2	.2	.4	4.2	NR
Intagliata & Rinck (1985)							
public resid. group	28.8	9.8	3.4	NR	.3	NR	NR
community group	45.0	26.3	1.2	.6	1.2	NR	NR
Aman, Field, & Bridgman (1985)							
preschool group	0	.8	0	NR	NR	NR	NR
special schools group	2.0	1.0	.8	NR	NR	NR	NR
adult ctrs. group	11.0	2.8	2.0	NR	NR	NR	NR

Author, publication data, and subgroups	Anti-psychotic	Anxiolytic/ hypnotic	Anti-depressant	Anti-manic	Stimulant	Anti-Parkinson	Anti-hypertensive
Schalock, Foley, Toulouse, & Stark (1985)							
1977 group	15.8	NR	NR	NR	NR	NR	NR
1981 group	30.5	NR	NR	NR	NR	NR	NR
1983 group	20.0	NR	NR	NR	NR	NR	NR
Gowdey, Zarfas, & Phipps (1987)	13.6	4.5	3.1	.9	NR	3.3	NR
Rinck & Calkins (1989)							
21 yrs. & under group	NR	2.0	NR	NR	NR	NR	NR
25-54 yrs. group	25.1	4.8	NR	NR	NR	NR	NR
55-64 yrs. group	35.6	6.8	NR	NR	NR	NR	NR
65-74 yrs. group	35.9	4.8	NR	NR	NR	NR	NR
75 & older group	30.9	20.0	NR	NR	NR	NR	NR
Burd et al. (1991)	10.0	3.1	3.2[g]	1.9	0.3	NR	2.3
Lepler, Hodas, & Cotter-Mack (1993)							
1987 group	14.3	4.0	4.8	9.5	0	9.5	7.1
1989 group	9.1	5.8	5.8	5.8	0	5.8	1.9
Pary (1993)							
20-39 age group	26	13	7	5	NR	8	NR
40-54 age group	37	16	8	6	NR	8	NR
55 & older group	42	8	10	7	NR	18	NR
Aman, Sarphare, & Burrow (1995)	21.2	4.2[b]	4.0	10.6	.1	5.1	1.8
Aman, Van Bourgondien, Wolford, & Sarphare (1995)[j]	12.2	6.3[b]	6.1	13.2	6.6	NR	4.4

a   Includes PRN (as needed) medication.
b   May be an overestimate, because the rating does not correct for possible use of multiple drugs by same person. This is total of anxiolytic and sedative medication, reported separately.
c   Elderly population monitored over a 20-year period.
d   Determined from billing slips of Medicaid recipients in nursing homes.
e   Approximately half of the subjects were taking anticonvulsants, for which ratings are not included. It is possible that some anticonvulsants were given as anxiolytics or antimanic drugs.
f   School-age children and adolescents.
g   Does not include mood stabilizers that also are classed as anticonvulsants (e.g., sodium valproate, carbamazepine).
h   Sample comprised subjects with autism.
i   This figure includes benzodiazepines only. A further 14.7% of residents were taking trimeprazine for sleep. Because both benzodiazepines and trimeprazine were given on a PRN basis and any overlap is not reported, trimeprazine use is not reported here.
j   Does not include agents that were likely being used as anticonvulsants (e.g., phenobarbital).
NR = Not reported.

REFERENCES

Ahsanuddin, K.M., Ivey, J.A., Schlotzhauer, D., Hall, K., & Prosen, H. (1983). Psychotropic medication prescription patterns in 100 hospitalized children and adolescents. *Journal of the American Academy of Child Psychiatry, 22,* 361–364.

Aman, M.G., Field, C.J., & Bridgman, G.D. (1985). City-wide survey of drug patterns among non-institutionalized retarded persons. *Applied Research in Mental Retardation, 5,* 159–171.

Aman, M G., Richmond, G., Stewart, A.W.,

Bell, J.C., & Kissel, R C. (1987). The Aberrant Behavior Checklist: Factor structure and the effect of subject variables in American and New Zealand facilities. *American Journal of Mental Deficiency, 91,* 570–578.

Aman, M.G., Sarphare, G., & Burrow, W.H.

(1995). Psychotropic drugs in group homes: Prevalence and relationship to demographic/psychiatric variables. *American Journal on Mental Retardation, 99,* 500–509.

Aman, M.G., & Singh, N.N. (1988). Patterns of drug use, methodological considerations, measurement techniques, and future trends. In M.G. Aman & N.N. Singh (Eds.), *Psychopharmacology of the developmental disabilities* (pp. 1–28). New York: Springer Verlag.

Aman, M.G., Van Bourgondien, M.E., Wolford, P.C., & Sarphare, G. (1995). Psychotropic and anticonvulsant drugs in subjects with autism: Prevalence and patterns of use. *Journal of the American Academy of Child and Adolescent Psychiatry, 34,* 1672–1681.

Anderson, D. (1992). Healthy and institutionalized: Health and related conditions among older institutionalized persons with developmental disabilities. *Journal of Applied Gerontology, 8,* 228–241.

Anderson, D., & Polister, B. (1993). Psychotropic medications use among older adults with mental retardation. In E. Sutton, A. Factor, B. Hawkins, T. Heller, & G. Seltzer (Eds.), *Older adults with developmental disabilities: Optimizing choice and change* (pp. 61–75). Baltimore: Sage.

Avon, J., Dreyer, P., Connelly, K., & Soumerai, S. (1989). Use of psychoactive medications and the quality of care in rest homes. *New England Journal of Medicine, 327,* 227–232.

Barkley, R.A., DuPaul, G.J., & Costello, A. (1993). Stimulants. In J.S. Werry & M.G. Aman (Eds.), *Practitioner's guide to psychoactive drugs for children and adolescents* (pp. 205–237). New York: Plenum Medical.

Bates, W.J., Smeltzer, D.J., & Arnoczky, S. (1986). Appropriate and inappropriate use of psychotherapeutic medications for institutionalized mentally retarded persons. *American Journal of Mental Deficiency, 90,* 363–370.

Borthwick-Duffy, S.A. (1994). Epidemiology and prevalence of psychopathology in people with mental retardation. *Journal of Consulting and Clinical Psychology, 62,* 17–27.

Briggs, R. (1989). Monitoring and evaluating psychotropic drugs for persons with mental retardation: A follow-up report. *American Journal on Mental Retardation, 93,* 633–639.

Briggs, R., Hamad, C., Garrard, S., & Willis, F. (1984). A model for evaluating psychoactive medication use with the mentally retarded. In J. Mulick & B. Mallory (Eds.), *Transitions in mental retardation: Advocacy, technology, and science* (pp. 229–248). Norwood, NJ: Ablex.

Buck, J.A., & Sprague, R.L. (1989). Psychotropic medication of mentally retarded residents in community long-term care facilities. *American Journal on Mental Retardation, 93,* 618–623.

Burd, L., Fisher, W., Veseley, B.N., Williams, M., Kerbeshian, J., & Leech, C. (1991). Prevalence of psychoactive drug use among North Dakota group home residents. *American Journal on Mental Retardation, 96,* 119–126.

Campbell, M., Gonzalez, N.M., Ernst, M., Silva, R.R., & Werry, J.S. (1993). Antipsychotics (neuroleptics). In J.S. Werry & M.G. Aman (Eds.), *Practitioner's guide to psychoanalytic drugs for children and adolescents* (pp. 269–296). New York: Plenum Medical.

Cohen, M.N., & Sprague, R.L. (1977, March). *Survey of drug usage in two midwestern institutions for the retarded.* Paper presented at the Gatlinburg Conference on Research in Mental Retardation, Galtinburg, TN.

Coyle, J.T. (1988). Psychiatry, neuroscience, and the double disabilities. In J.A. Stark, F.J. Menolascino, M.H. Albarelli, & V.C. Gray (Eds.), *Mental retardation and mental health: Classification, diagnosis, and treatment services* (pp. 81–89). New York: Springer Verlag.

Craig, T. J., & Behar, R. (1980). Trends in the prescription of psychotropic drugs (1970–1977) in a state hospital. *Comprehensive Psychiatry, 21,* 336–345.

Davidson, P.W., Cain, N.N., Sloan-Keeves, J.E., Kramer, B., Quinjano, L.E., Van Heyningen, J., & Giesow, V.E. (1992). *Aging effects on severe behavior disorders in community-based clients with mental retardation.* Paper presented at the meeting of the Gerontological Society of America. Washington, D.C.

DiMascio, A. (1975, May). *Psychotropic drug usage in the mentally retarded: A review of 2000 cases.* Paper presented at the workshop on Psychotropic Drugs and the Mentally Retarded, Portland, OR.

Errickson, E., Bock, W., Young, R.C., & Silverstein, B.J. (1981). Psychotropic drug use in Title XIX (ICF-MR) facilities for the mentally retarded in Minnesota. In R. Young & J. Kroll (Eds.), *The use of medications in controlling the behavior of the mentally retarded: Proceedings* (pp. 82–88). Minneapolis: University of Minnesota.

Findholt, N.E., & Emmett, C.G. (1990). Impact of interdisciplinary team review on psychotropic drug use with persons who have mental retardation. *Mental Retardation, 28,* 41–46.

Gadow, K.D. (1976, April). *Psychotropic and anticonvulsant drug usage in early childhood special education program I. Phase one: A preliminary report: Prevalence, attitude, training, and problems.* Paper presented at the meeting of the Council for Exceptional Children, Chicago, Illinois.

Gadow, K.D. (1981). Prevalence of drug treatment for hyperactivity and other childhood behavior disorders. In K.D. Gadow & J. Loney (Eds.), *Psychosocial aspects of drug treatment for hyperactivity* (pp. 13–76). Boulder, CO: Westview Press.

Gadow, K.D. (1985). Prevalence and efficacy of stimulant drug use with mentally retarded children and youth. *Psychopharmacology Bulletin, 21,* 291–303.

Gadow, K.D., & Kalachnik, J. (1981). Prevalence and pattern of drug treatment for behavior and seizure disorders of TMR students. *American Journal of Mental Deficiency, 85,* 588–595.

Glaser, B.A., & Morreau, L.E. (1986). Effects of interdisciplinary team review on the use of antipsychotic agents with severely and profoundly mentally retarded persons. *American Journal of Mental Deficiency, 90,* 371–379.

Gowdey, C.W., Zarfas, D.E., & Phipps, S. (1987). Audit of psychoactive drug prescription in group homes. *Mental Retardation, 25,* 331–334.

Gualtieri, C.T., & Schroeder, S.R. (1985). Unpublished data on children in a class action suit (North Carolina) for children with behavioral, developmental, and neurological handicaps. Chapel Hill, N.C.: University of North Carolina.

Hancock, R.D., Weber, S. L., Kaza, R., & Hou, K. S. (1991). Changes in psychotropic drug use in long-term residents of an ICF/MR facility.

Hansen, P., & Keogh, B.K. (1971). Medical characteristics of children with educational handicaps: Implications for the pediatrician. *Clinical Pediatrician, 10,* 726–730.

Harper, D.C., & Wadsworth, J.S. (1990). Dementia and depression in elders with mental retardation: A pilot study. *Research in Developmental Disabilities, 11,* 177–198.

Harper, D.C., Wadsworth, J.S., & Michael, A.L. (1989). Psychotropic drug use in older developmentally disabled with behavior difficulties. *Research in Developmental Disabilities, 10,* 53–60.

Heistad, G.T., Zimmermann, R.L., & Doebler, M.J. (1982). Long-term usefulness of thioridazine for institutionalized mentally retarded patients. *American Journal of Mental Deficiency, 87,* 243–251.

Hill, B. K., Balow, E. A., & Bruininks, R. H. (1985). A national study of prescribed drugs in institutions and community residential facilities for mentally retarded people. *Psychopharmacology Bulletin, 21,* 279–284.

Hughes, P.S. (1977). Survey of medication in a subnormality hospital. *British Journal of Mental Subnormality, 23,* 88–94.

Inoue, F. (1982). A clinical pharmacy service to reduce psychotropic medication use in an institution for mentally handicapped persons. *Mental Retardation, 20,* 70–74.

Intagliata, J., & Rinck, C. (1985). Psychoactive drug use in public and community residential facilities for mentally retarded persons. *Psychopharmacology Bulletin, 21,* 268–278.

Jacobson, J.W. (1982). Problem behavior and

psychiatric impairment within a developmentally disabled population: I. Behavior frequency. *Applied Research in Mental Retardation, 3,* 121–139.

Jacobson, J.W. (1988). Problem behavior and psychiatric impairment within a developmentally disabled population: III. Psychotropic medication. *Research in Developmental Disabilities, 9,* 23–38.

Jacobson, J.W., & Harper, M.S. (1989). Mental health status of older persons with mental retardation in residential care settings. *Australia and New Zealand Journal of Developmental Disabilities, 15,* 301–309.

James, D.H. (1986). Psychiatric and behavioral disorders amongst older severely mentally handicapped inpatients. *Journal of Mental Deficiency Research, 30,* 341–345.

Jonas, O. (1980). Patterns of drug prescribing in a residential centre for the intellectually handicapped. *Australian Journal of Developmental Disabilities, 6,* 25–30.

Kirman, S.B. (1975). Drug therapy in mental handicap. *British Journal of Psychiatry, 127,* 545–549.

Krager, J.M., Safer, D., & Earhart, J. (1979). Type and prevalence of medication used to treat hyperactive school children: Follow-up survey results. *Journal of School Health, 49,* 317–321.

LaMendola, W., Zaharia, E.S., & Carver, M. (1980). Reducing psychotropic drug use in an institution for the retarded. *Hospital and Community, 31,* 271–272.

Lepler, S., Hodas, A., & Cotter-Mack, A. (1993). Implementation of an interdisciplinary psychotropic drug review process for community-based facilities. *Mental Retardation, 31,* 307–315.

Linaker, O.M. (1990). Frequency and determinants for psychotropic drug use in an institution for the mentally retarded. *British Journal of Psychiatry, 156,* 525–530.

Lipman, R.S. (1970). The use of psychopharmacological agents in residential facilities for the retarded. In F.J. Menolascino (Ed.), *Psychiatric approaches to mental retardation* (pp. 387–389). New York: Basic Books.

Lund, J. (1985). The prevalence of psychiatric morbidity in mentally retarded adults. *Acta Psychiatrica Scandinavica, 72,* 563–570.

Martin, J.E., & Agran, M. (1985). Psychotropic and anticonvulsant drug use by mentally retarded adults across community residential and vocational placements. *Applied Research in Mental Retardation, 6,* 33–49.

Pary, R. (1993). Psychoactive drugs used with adults and elderly adults who have mental retardation. *American Journal on Mental Retardation, 98,* 121–127.

Philips, I., & Williams, N. (1975). Psychopathology and mental retardation: A study of 100   mentally retarded children: I. Psychopathology. *American Journal of Psychiatry, 132,* 1265–1271.

Poindexter, A.R. (1989). Psychotropic drug patterns in a large ICF/MR facility: A ten-year experience. *American Journal on Mental Retardation, 93,* 624–626.

Pulman, R.M., Pook, R.B., & Singh, N.N. (1979). Prevalence of drug therapy for institutionalized mentally retarded children. *Australian Journal of Mental Retardation, 5,* 212–214.

Radinsky, A.M. (1984). *A descriptive study of psychotropic and anti-epileptic medication use with mentally retarded persons in three residential environments.* Unpublished doctoral dissertation, University of Pittsburgh.

Reid, A.H. (1993a). Schizophrenia and paranoid syndromes in persons with mental retardation: Assessment and diagnosis. In R. Fletcher & A. Dosen (Eds.), *Mental health aspects of mental retardation—Progress in assessment and treatment* (pp. 98–110). New York: Lexington Books.

Reid, A.H. (1993b). Schizophrenia and paranoid syndromes in persons with mental retardation: Treatment and assessment. In R. Fletcher & A. Dosen (Eds.), *Mental health aspects of mental retardation—Progress in assessment and treatment.* New York: Lexington Books.

Reiss, S. (1988). The development of a screening measure for psychopathology in people with mental retardation. In E. Dibble & D.B. Gray (Eds.), *Assessment of behavior problems in persons with mental retardation living in the community* (DHHS Publication No. [ADM] 90–1642). Washington, D.C.: National Institute of Health.

Reiss, S. (1994). *Handbook of challenging behavior: Mental health aspects of mental retardation.* Worthington, OH: IDS Publishing Corporation.

Reiss, S., & Valenti-Hein, D. (1990). *Reiss Scales for Children's Dual Diagnosis: Test manual.* Worthington, OH: IDS Publishing Corporation.

Reiss, S., & Valenti-Hein, D. (1994). Development of a psychopathology rating scale for children with mental retardation. *Journal of Consulting and Clinical Psychology, 62,* 28–33.

Reiss, S., & Trenn, E. (1984). Consumer demand for outpatient mental health services for mentally retarded people. *Mental Retardation, 22,* 112–115.

Rinck, C., & Calkins, C. (1989). Patterns of psychotropic medication use among older persons with developmental disabilities. *Journal of Applied Gerontology, 8,* 216–228.

Rinck, C., & Rinck, W. (1991, May). *Tardive dyskinesia and older persons with developmental disabilities.* Paper presented at the meeting of the American Association on Mental Retardation, Crystal City, MD.

Rojahn, J., Borthwick-Duffy, S.A., & Jacobson, J.W. (1993). The association between psychiatric diagnoses and severe

behavior problems in mental retardation. *Annals of Clinical Psychiatry, 5,* 163–170.

Safer, D.J., & Krager, J.M. (1988). A survey of medication treatment for hyperactive-inattentive students. *Journal of the American Medical Association, 260,* 2256–2270.

Schalock, R., Foley, J., Toulouse, A., & Stark, J. (1985). Medication and programming in controlling the behavior of mentally retarded individuals in community settings. *American Journal on Mental Retardation, 89,* 503–509.

Sewell, J., & Werry, J. S. (1976). Some studies in an institution for the mentally retarded. *New Zealand Medical Journal, 84,* 317–319.

Silva, D.A. (1979). The use of medication in a residential institution for mentally retarded persons. *Mental Retardation, 17,* 285–288.

Spencer, D.A. (1974). A survey of the medication in a hospital for the mentally handicapped. *British Journal of Psychiatry, 124,* 507–508.

Spreat, S., Serafin, C., Behan, D., & Leiman, S. (1993). Tranquilizer reduction trials in a residential program for persons with mental retardation. *Hospital and Community Psychiatry, 44,* 1100–1102.

Stone, R. K., Alvarez, W. F., Ellman, G., Hom, A. C., & White, J. F. (1989). Prevalence and prediction of psychotropic drug use in California developmental centers. *American Journal on Mental Retardation, 93,* 627–632.

Tu, J.B. (1979). A survey of psychotropic medication in mental retardation facilities. *Journal of Clinical Psychiatry, 40,* 125–128.

Tu, J.B., & Smith, J T. (1979). Factors associated with psychotropic medication in mental retardation facilities. *Comprehensive Psychiatry, 20,* 289–295.

Tu, J.B., & Smith, J T. (1983). The Eastern Ontario Survey: A study of drug-treated psychiatric problems in the mentally handicapped. *Canadian Journal of Psychiatry, 28,* 270–276.

White, A.J.R. (1983). Changing patterns of psychoactive drug use with the mentally retarded. *New Zealand Medical Journal, 96,* 686–688.

Wolfensberger, W. (1984). *Voluntary association on behalf of societally devalued and/or handicapped people.* Downsview, Ontario: National Institute on Mental Retardation.

Zaharia, E.S., & Struxness, L. (1991). Comparative survey of drug use in a community service system. *Mental Retardation, 29,* 191–194.

Zigman, W. B., Seltzer, G. B., & Silverman, W. P. (1994). Behavioral and mental health changes associated with aging in adults with mental retardation. In M. Seltzer, M. Krauss, & M. Janicki (Eds.), *Life course perspectives on adulthood and old age* (pp. 67–91). Washington, DC: American Association on Mental Retardation.

Guidelines for the Use of Psychotropic Medication

John E. Kalachnik[1], Bennett L. Leventhal[2], David H. James[3], Robert Sovner[4],
Theodore A. Kastner[5], Kevin Walsh[6], Steven A. Weisblatt[7], Margaret G. Klitzke[8,9]

INTRODUCTION

The use of psychotropic medication for individuals with developmental disabilities has been the focus of considerable controversy and legal activity (Beyer, 1988; Singh, Guernsey, & Ellis, 1992; Sprague, 1982). In addition to the involvement of a vulnerable population and a pattern of historical misuse, the underlying issues revolve around whether the right people are treated and whether psychotropic medication is properly monitored and managed (Aman, 1983; Gadow & Poling, 1988; Keppel & Gualtieri, 1989; Scheerenberger, 1983, 1987; Thompson, Hackenberg, & Schaal, 1989). Over the period of 1970-1995, a set of basic guidelines has evolved from a variety of sources such as regulatory authorities, accreditation organizations, professional groups, legal decisions, and published research. In this chapter, we review the historical development of psychotropic medication guidelines, describe the biopsychosocial model, and list specific psychotropic medication guidelines along with comments and relevant resources.

It is important to note that this chapter is not designed to be a legal or regulatory document. Appropriate laws, regulations, or state codes should be consulted. Additionally, nomenclature may not be uniform across countries, and the reader is urged to substitute wording appropriate for his or her culture. Some examples of interchangeable terms are "patient," "client," "resident," "consumer," or "individual"; "guardian," "proxy," or "legally authorized representative"; "hospital" or "public residential facility"; and "unlicensed drug indication" or "unlabelled drug indication." Furthermore, readers outside the United States may need to substitute ICD-10 for DSM-IV and an authoritative body for the U. S. Food and Drug Administration (FDA).

DEFINITION OF GUIDELINES

We intentionally selected the term "guidelines" instead of "standards" in part because we were interested in promoting education and application rather than legal standards. A guideline is defined as "an indication or outline of future policy or conduct" in Webster's International Dictionary (p. 1009), whereas a standard is "something that is set up and established by authority as a rule..." (p. 2223). Thus, the term "guidelines" has less of a legal or mandatory connotation than the term "standard."

As used by Eddy (1992), the terms standards, guidelines, and options permit different degrees of flexibility on the part of practitioners. A practice policy is considered a standard if the health and economic consequences of an intervention are sufficiently well known to permit decisions and if there is virtual unanimity among practitioners about the desirability and proper use of the intervention. Standards permit the least degree of flexibility in their application; exceptions to a standard are unusual and require significant justification. A practice policy is considered a guideline if the outcomes of an intervention are well enough understood to permit decisions about its proper use and if it is preferred by an appreciable majority of people. Guidelines are not necessarily endorsed by all authorities; they should be followed in most cases, but depending on the patient, the setting, and other factors, they can be tailored to fit specific indi-

1 Co-Chair, Minnesota Department of Human Services, St. Paul, MN
2 Co-Chair, Professor of Psychiatry and Pediatrics, University of Chicago, Chicago, IL
3 Consultant in Psychiatry of Developmental Disabilities, Budock Hospital, Toro, (UK)
4 Associate Professor of Psychiatry, Tufts University, Boston, MA
5 Associate Professor of Clinical Pediatrics, Columbia University, and DDC Medical Director, Morristown Memorial Hospital, Morristown, NJ
6 Director of Research, Center for Human Development, Morristown Memorial Hospital, Morristown, NJ
7 Assistant Professor of Clinical Psychiatry, Albert Einstein College of Medicine, Bronx, NY
8 Associate Medical Director for DD Unit, Emma Pendleton Bradley Hospital, E. Providence, RI
9 The other committee members were Nancy Cain, M.D., Edwin Cook, M.D., Max Friedrich, M.D., Benjamin Goldberg, M.D., Ruth Hamilton, Ph.D., James Hillard, M.D., Richard Kern, M.D., James Mulick, Ph.D., Allan Reiss, M.D., Steven Ruedrich, M.D., B.I. Sacks, M.D., Luis Salvador, Ph.D., Akihiko Takahashi, M.D., James Wilson, Pharm.D., Harold Woodward, Ed.D.

viduals and situations. Guidelines permit a moderate amount of flexibility in their application. A practice policy is a treatment option if treatment outcomes are not known, if outcomes are known but patients' preferences are not known, if outcomes are known but patients are indifferent, or if patients' preferences are evenly divided. Options have the highest degree of flexibility.

Eddy also described the difference between pathway and boundary guidelines. Pathway guidelines (also referred to as protocols or algorithms) direct practitioners along a preferred management path. Boundary guidelines (also referred to as criteria or parameters) define the limits of proper practice. In effect, pathway guidelines draw a path through a field and say, "Stay on this path," whereas boundary guidelines place fences in a field and say, "Take any path you want, but stay within these fences."

A similar schema was described by the Agency for Health Care Policy and Research (1993). "Clinical practice guidelines" were defined as systematically developed statements to assist practitioners and patients in making decisions about appropriate health care for specific clinical circumstances. "Standards of quality" were defined as authoritative statements of minimal levels of acceptable performance or results, excellent levels of performance or results, or the range of acceptable performance or results. The guidelines in this chapter are best described as boundary guidelines and systematically developed statements to assist practitioners and patients in making decisions about appropriate care.

HISTORICAL REVIEW OF PSYCHOTROPIC MEDICATION GUIDELINES

It is critical to remember that psychotropic medication guidelines were influenced by social forces, attitudes, and alternative interventions. Although the discovery of chlorpromazine (Thorazine) in 1952 is heralded as the beginning of modern psychopharmacology, a number of significant events occurred prior to this date, including the discovery or use of chloral hydrate in 1869, paraldehyde in 1882, barbiturates in 1903, rauwolfia serpentina in 1931, amphetamine in 1937, phenytoin in 1940, and lithium in 1949. Indeed, attempts to alter behavior go back to antiquity, and history and folklore provide accounts of stupor, sedation, or hypnosis induced through the use of alcohol, laudanum (preparations containing opium or a solution of opium in alcohol),

and herbs (Ayd, 1991; Baldessarini, 1980; Gadow & Poling, 1988; Harvey, 1980; Kaplan & Sadock, 1988).

In relation to individuals with developmental disabilities, few published reports existed until the 1940s. Paraldehyde and hypnotic drugs such as chloral hydrate were the primary drugs used to manage behavior prior to the 1950s. Like the modern era of psychopharmacology in general, the modern era of psychopharmacology for individuals with developmental disabilities began with reports of chlorpromazine use in 1954 and 1955 (Gadow & Poling, 1988; Scheerenberger, 1983; Thompson et al., 1989).

Concerns about the misuse of psychotropic medication began to appear as early as 1958. Greiner (1958) commented that "...in the years to come, the retarded may claim an all-time record, of having the greatest variety and the largest tonnage of chemical agents shoveled into them" and "If your aim is helping the retarded, I urge you to avoid the casual clinical trial of drugs. Make them good trials, or don't make them at all" (cited in Gadow & Poling, 1988, p. 144). Two sentinel studies established a scientific basis for the concerns surrounding the use of psychotropic medication. In 1967 Lipman presented a survey suggesting that more than 50% of individuals with developmental disabilities in institutions were prescribed psychotropic medication and that neuroleptic medication, especially thioridazine and chlorpromazine, accounted for the majority of use (Lipman, 1967, 1970). In 1971 Sprague and Werry reviewed more than 180 published psychotropic drug studies that were undertaken with individuals with developmental disabilities in terms of scientific methodology and concluded that:

> ...very few empirically verified generalizations can be made about psychotropic drugs with the mentally retarded, yet it is just as clear that this series of methodologically weak, experimentally poor, and statistically inept studies have not provided a fair, sensitive measure of the behavioral effects of the drugs, effects which are routinely assumed to be present considering the widespread use of these drugs. (p. 168)

These concerns went largely unheeded and set the stage for literally dozens of individual and class-action lawsuits.

Development of Standards

The year 1952 is usually considered the beginning of standards within the field of mental retardation because that is when the American Association on Mental Deficiency (AAMR) published a committee report on standards for institutions. With support from the National Institute of Mental Health, AAMR then initiated a major standards development project in 1959 which was published in 1964. With support from the Mental Retardation Branch of the U.S. Public Health Service, an evaluation instrument was developed in 1965, and 134 state institutions were surveyed from 1966 to 1969.

AAMR formed the National Planning Committee on Accreditation of Residential Centers for the Retarded in 1966 because of interest from other organizations that recognized the advantages of establishing a single standards-setting and survey agency. In 1969, this group established the structure for what is now known as the Accreditation Council on Services for People with Disabilities (ACD) and accepted an invitation to join what is now known as the Joint Commission on Accreditation of Healthcare Organizations (JCAHO). JCAHO was established in 1951 to continue the hospital accreditation program founded by the American College of Surgeons in 1918. ACD published standards for residential facilities in 1971 and for community agencies in 1973. These were combined into one set of standards in 1977. ACD formed its own accreditation program when JCAHO reorganized in 1979 (Accreditation Council for Facilities for the Mentally Retarded [ACMR], 1971, 1973; Accreditation Council for Services for Mentally Retarded and Other Developmentally Disabled Persons [ACMRDD], 1977, 1983; Accreditation Council on Services for People with Developmental Disabilities [ACDD], 1987, 1990; ACD, 1993, 1995; American Association on Mental Deficiency Project on Technical Planning in Mental Retardation, 1964; JCAHO, 1995a, 1995b; Sparr & Smith, 1990).

State governments traditionally financed institutions, but the Intermediate Care Facilities for the Mentally Retarded (ICFMR) benefit was enacted by law in 1971 as an optional, federally-funded, state Medicaid program. The U.S. Department of Health, Education, and Welfare, now known as the U.S. Department of Health and Human Services, was directed to develop federal regulations, which appeared for the first time in 1974. These essentially incorporated 1971 ACD standards. Responsibility was transferred to the Health Care Financing Agency (HCFA) in 1977, which made slight modifications in 1978 and major revisions in 1988 (Department of Health, Education, and Welfare [DHEW], 1974; HCFA, 1978, 1988; Sparr & Smith, 1990).

By 1970, some professionals had published general guidelines for the use of psychotropic medication for individuals with developmental disabilities (Freeman, 1970). Honigfeld and Howard (1973) wrote an influential set of early psychotropic medication guidelines, *"Evaluating Your Medical Colleagues,"* that were applicable across populations, and Mason and Granacher (1980) wrote guidelines for antipsychotic medication use. Professional task forces became involved by the mid-1970s on issues such as behavior therapy in psychiatry and tardive dyskinesia (TD). Task forces continued to work through the 1980s and 1990s, issuing reports on topics ranging from the role of psychiatry in developmental disabilities to the use of antipsychotic medication at high doses (American Psychiatric Association [APA], 1974, 1979, 1989, 1990, 1992; APA Committee on Research on Psychiatric Treatments, 1992; Arnold, 1993; Royal College of Psychiatrists' Consensus Panel, 1994; Sovner, 1986; World Health Organization Heads of Centres Collaborating in WHO Co-ordinated Studies on Biological Aspects of Mental Illness [WHO], 1990).

Formal standards of care specific to psychotropic medication appeared for the first time on May 5, 1971, in ACMR standards for institutions:

> Chemical restraint shall not be used excessively, as punishment, for the convenience of staff, as a substitute for program, or in quantities that interfere with a resident's habilitation program (ACMR, 1971, p. 22).

United States District Court Judge Frank Johnson expanded this concept through a 1972 *Wyatt v. Stickney* order:

> Residents shall have a right to be free from unnecessary or excessive medication. The resident's records shall state the effects of psychoactive medication on the resident. When dosages of such are changed or other psychoactive medications are prescribed, a notation shall be made in the resident's record concerning the effect of the new medication or new dosages and the behavior changes, if any, which occur.

> Medication shall not be used as punishment, for the convenience of staff, as a substitute for a habilitative program, or in quantities that interfere with the resident's habilitation program (cited in Sprague, 1982, pp. 380-381).

In 1973, ACMR applied its 1971 chemical restraint statement for institutions to community facilities and altered *chemical restraint* to *medication* (p. 46). The only mention of psychotropic medication in the original 1974 federal regulations was the exact 1971 ACMR chemical restraint statement (DHEW, 1974). In 1974 the Mental Health Law Project petitioned the U.S. Food and Drug Administration (FDA) to stop the unapproved use of phenothiazine medication with individuals with developmental disabilities. A 12-member FDA Advisory Panel was formed, and recommendations were made that ultimately resulted in package insert material that describes how properly to use these medications. These recommendations included little support for daily doses greater than 500 mg of chlorpromazine or 400 mg of thioridazine, little evidence of efficacy beyond six months, potential interference with learning performance, and periodic reductions to ascertain the need for continued use (Beyer, 1988; Lehr, Gilbert, Tatel, Foer, & Kahan, 1975; Lipman, DiMascio, Reatig, & Kirson, 1978; Rinck, Guidry, & Calkins, 1989; Singh et al., 1992; Sprague, 1975, 1982).

United States District Court Judge Earl Larson expanded the depth and breadth of psychotropic medication standards through orders resulting from *Welsch v. Likins* (1976) and *Welsch v. Dirkswager* (1977) (see Sprague, 1982). These orders limited the use of antipsychotic medication in the treatment of severe behavior disorders in persons with mental retardation and developmental disabilities. They also required a specific description of the behavior to be changed by the medication, a baseline period of at least one month unless the justification for a shorter period was provided, the use of recognized data collection methods such as time sample and frequency counts to measure target behaviors, the use of data to evaluate medication efficacy after initiation or dose or drug type change, and periodic drug holidays to determine whether major tranquilizers continued to be necessary. These orders were the legal source of the widely used term *drug holiday*, although the order itself only required that a plan be developed, said nothing about the rate of reduction, and allowed use of antipsychotics inconsistent with the order provided the clinical justification was recorded.

In 1977 ACMRDD expanded the original 1971 chemical restraint statement and classified psychotropic medication as a behavior management method. Psychotropic medication was to represent the least restrictive alternative, lead to a less restrictive way of managing the behavior, reflect a decision by the interdisciplinary team, and be incorporated into the individual's program plan. Target behavior definitions and data methods to judge medication efficacy were incorporated, but the definition of drug holiday was modified to allow for gradual dosage reductions. Four additional standards were incorporated. First, an evaluation had to document whether psychotropic medication benefits outweighed the harmful effects of the behavior. Second, psychotropic medication was to be reviewed and approved by an agency's behavior management and human rights committees prior to implementation. Third, written informed consent was required from the appropriate individual. And fourth, less restrictive methods were to be systematically attempted and shown to be ineffective before a psychotropic medication could be used for maladaptive or problem behavior.

Federal regulation revision in 1978 did not alter the 1974 regulations concerning chemical restraint; however, resident rights allowed the resident to refuse treatment, participate in planning his or her own care, and receive full information about his or her health and medical conditions. Informed consent was required from the individual's parent or legal guardian if chemical restraint was used during a behavior modification session. A new standard limited the use of chemical restraint to an emergency, which was defined as injury to self (HCFA, 1978).

United States District Court Judge Edward Gigonux applied the previously described antipsychotic standards to all psychotropic medications in the 1978 *Wuori v. Zitnay* consent decree (see Sprague, 1982). This decree further required a method to assess side effects and the person's progress or response to treatment including monitoring and recording, appropriate laboratory tests and analysis of results, and carefully considered and monitored withdrawal of psychotropic medication at least annually in order to determine the need for the medication or dose level. The decree also required an annual review by a psychopharmacology consultant if any of the following occurred: the concurrent use of more than one antipsychotic medication; the concurrent use of an antipsychotic medication with an antianxiety, antidepressant, or antimania medication; the use of anticonvulsant medication in the absence of seizures; the use of anti-Parkinsonian medication in the absence of extrapyramidal side effects; the use of antipsychotic medication in the event of serious side effects including, but not limited to, TD; or submission of a written statement of concern by any staff member.

In the 1980 *Clites v. Iowa* case, Iowa District Court Judge Harold Martin awarded more than $750,000, upheld on appeal, to an individual with developmental disabilities who developed TD after long-term antipsychotic medication use (see Sprague, 1982). This was the first TD case tried to verdict with an extensive and widely distributed written opinion (Gualtieri, Sprague, & Cole, 1986). The case required close monitoring of antipsychotic medication for TD and other harmful effects, antipsychotic medication reduction and discontinuation if TD occurred unless evidence of effectiveness was present, and TD education as part of the informed consent process. This case also concluded that standards were not met because active treatment for the underlying problem behavior did not occur, and because informed consent was not obtained.

ACDD revisions in 1987 gave emphasis to the use of functional analysis, limited emergency psychotropic medication intervention to three times within six months before a written plan is needed, and required monthly psychotropic medication reviews to consider possible reduction and elimination. The revision of federal regulations in 1988 incorporated most of the standards developed over the previous decade. Several, however, were modified. Quarterly rather than monthly psychotropic medication reviews were to occur unless the individual was not progressing toward objectives, in which case the review was to be as often as necessary. Gradual psychotropic medication withdrawal was to occur at least annually and be coordinated with the interdisciplinary team unless clinical evidence contraindicated a reduction. By this time, 28 states had regulations for institutional facility psychotropic medication use, and 23 states had regulations for community facility psychotropic medication use (Rinck et al., 1989).

Resentment about regulation of psychotropic medication increased in the early 1990s. Sources of resentment included narrow interpretation by surveyors, excessive paperwork to document compliance, excessive anti-medication views of some interdisciplinary teams, and limitations in effecting genuine staff change. The message conveyed was one of frustration with micromanagement and creative interference. Although the *Osheroff v. Chestnut Lodge* case (see Klerman, 1990) was settled out of court, it touched on the issue of an individual's right to effective treatment with psychotropic medication when providers persisted in the non-use of antidepressant medication despite clinical evidence to support its use (Brown, 1990; Holburn, 1990, 1992; Jacobson, 1990; Jacobson & Otis, 1992; Klerman, 1990).

In 1993 ACD shifted from specific standards toward outcome-based performance measures. This appeared to be a response to the aforementioned concerns and the need to alter an ACD model that had evolved to categorize all psychotropic medication use as highly restrictive. Another important factor prompting the shift was an increasing acknowledgment of mental illness in a significant number of individuals with developmental disabilities (Crews, Bonaventura, & Rowe, 1994;

Menolascino, 1989; Reiss, 1990; Sovner & Hurley, 1989). Interest in this population was sparked in 1980 by a major diagnostic advance, the DSM-III (APA, 1980), which was further refined with the DSM-III-R (APA, 1987) and the current DSM-IV (APA, 1994).

Psychotropic medication standards appear to have come full circle while advancing one turn of the wheel. The 1974 petition to the FDA to stop the unapproved use of antipsychotic drugs did not include a request for complete elimination of these drugs for individuals with psychosis; it called for terminating use for the control of behavior or mental retardation (Lehr et al., 1975). Lipman (1967) and Sprague and Werry (1971) were concerned not with the appropriate use of antipsychotic medication for individuals with psychosis, but with the extensive use of these drugs for people without an indicated condition. Federal regulators were concerned with client protection and the inability of professionals and organizations to put their own houses in order (Sparr & Smith, 1990). Concerns about accreditation, legal, and professional issues forced the development of informed consent and the extension of empirical monitoring for all psychotropic medication whether such medication was used for behavior change or mental illness. Some standards or their interpretation became so micromanaged that they conveyed an anti-medication position. Consequently, to ensure proper psychotropic medication use while simultaneously avoiding restriction and micromanagement, some standards have come to focus more on quality of life outcomes.

THE BIOPSYCHOSOCIAL MODEL

If there is one unifying concept underlying contemporary psychotropic medication use on the applied clinical level, it is the biopsychosocial model. This model was developed in 1977 by the physician George Engel (Engel, 1977, 1980). Engel contended that traditional biomedicine was in crisis because of its adherence to a model of disease that was no longer adequate for the scientific tasks and social responsibilities of either medicine or psychiatry. According to Engel, the biomedical model was based on these outmoded concepts: a reductionistic premise that complex phenomena are only derived from molecular biology, which can ultimately explain all biological events; mind-body dualism, or the doctrine that the mental is separate from the physical; and exclusionism, or the omission of whatever cannot be explained by the underlying molecular biology concept. Such a model, Engel contended, resulted in unfortunate attitudes toward patients as well as expensive practices such as unnecessary hospitalization, overuse of drugs, excessive surgery, and inappropriate use of diagnostic tests.

In contrast, the biopsychosocial model is based on a general systems theory that incorporates natural hierarchical systems ranging from the minute—molecules, cells, and tissues—to the complex—the person and his or her experiences, other people, family, community, and the surrounding culture. The basic premise is that the systems are interdependent so that an event at one level potentially affects systems at other levels. In order to provide optimal patient care, biological, psychological, and sociological aspects of care must be acknowledged and addressed.

The biopsychosocial model is not without its critics. Although they endorse the model, Sadler and Hulgas (1992) note three reasons why it has not had great success in changing physicians' behavior in actual clinical problem solving. First, within day-to-day problem solving the systems' hierarchy provides no functional priority of one level over another. Second, methodological limits are placed on the scope of medical inquiry. And third, economics plays a role in decision making, a reality in the care of individuals with developmental disabilities as well (Meinhold & Mulick, 1990, 1992; Meinhold, Mulick, & Teodoro, 1994). In order to encourage greater practicing of the biopsychosocial model on the day-to-day clinical level, they proposed the "three faces model." The three faces, or aspects, and the questions they posed are as follows: (1) *the epistemic aspect*—what is the problem? (2) *the pragmatic aspect*—what actions need to be taken and what will be their consequences? and (3) *the ethical aspect*—what value implications do my actions have?

The value of the biopsychosocial model and the three faces model is that problems are addressed from a variety of integrated treatment modalities. This is critical in the care of individuals with developmental disabilities, for whom active treatment has been a driving force for change.

PSYCHOTROPIC MEDICATION GUIDELINES

It is not possible to develop psychotropic medication guidelines to address every conceivable procedural or clinical situation. Regulatory and reimbursement agency review, legal system due process, and professional actions unique to specific psychotropic medications or individual case profiles will affect the application of any guideline. Within this context, it is perhaps valuable to reiterate the overriding guideline for the use of psychotropic medication, "There is no substitute for thoughtful, careful, systematic, individualized management in the psychopharmacotherapy of patients with MR/DD" (Arnold, 1993, p. 196). In reviewing the guidelines, the reader should begin with the chart which is accompanied by a series of "what it means" and "what it does not mean" statements. These statements and the comments are intended to assist in the application of the guideline.

Guideline 1 Comment. One must ascertain the purpose of a prescription in order to evaluate whether or not the use of a medication should be considered psychotropic. The term "psychotropic medication" cannot be defined solely in terms of chemical compositon; this is because medications typically classified as psychotropic usually have nonpsychotropic applications, whereas those approved for nonpsychotropic purposes may later be shown to have psychotropic applications for some individuals. Moreover, new medications are continually being developed so that efforts to develop a comprehensive listing of psychotropic medications may become outdated within several months.

The phrase "stabilize or improve" was chosen in order to avoid words such as *control, modify,* or *normalize.* Psychotropic medication is not intended to control, modify, or normalize an individual who, outside of legal due process, is the locus of control and the ultimate decision maker. The purpose of psychotropic medication is to improve or stabilize a condition which is interfering with a person's quality of life.

References. Aman, 1983; APA Committee, 1992; Freeman, 1970; HCFA, 1992.

Guideline 2 Comment. This is an epiphany in the field consisting of the original May 5, 1971 psychotropic medication statement and subsequent court cases. The emergency initiation of psychotropic medication for general sedation properties is not necessarily inappropriate, but it is considered extreme and requires a number of controls (e.g., generally limited to 12 hours with renewal up to 72 hours before legal due process is required for further use). The emergency initiation of psychotropic medication is limited to situations in which (a) the individual presents an imminent and substantial risk of physical danger to self or others, (b) the medication is neces-

Guideline 1: Psychotropic Medication Definition

Guideline	What It Means	What It Does Not Mean
A psychotropic medication is any drug prescribed to stabilize or improve mood, mental status, or behavior.	This includes medications typically classified as antipsychotic, antianxiety, antidepressant, antimania, stimulant, or sedative-hypnotic.	This definition does not include situations when medications typically classified as psychotropic are prescribed for other conditions or diagnoses (e.g., diazepam can be prescribed for spasticity, and haloperidol can be prescribed for Huntington's Chorea).
	This includes other medications not typically classified as psychotropic when such medication is prescribed to improve or stabilize mood, mental status, or behavior (e.g., carbamazepine is generally classified as an antiepileptic medication but can be prescribed for affective disorders).	This definition does not include situations when medications not typically classified as psychotropic are prescribed for other conditions or diagnoses (e.g., if carbamazepine is prescribed for epilepsy, it is not a psychotropic medication).
	This includes herbal or nutritional substances when such substances are used to stabilize or improve mood, mental status, or behavior.	This definition does not include situations such as giving someone a glass of warm milk when he cannot sleep or a multi-vitamin tablet in the morning.

sary to ensure the physical safety of the individual or others, and (c) less restrictive alternatives are first attempted and shown to have failed or are considered and rejected as being inappropriate for the situation. The individual's guardian must be promptly notified of any emergency initiation or admission to an acute care facility.

References. ACDD, 1987, 1990; ACMR, 1971; Crabbe, 1989; HCFA, 1978, 1988; Hickman, Resnick, & Olson, 1982; Howe, 1984; Sovner & Hurley, 1987; see Sprague, 1982, for a review of *Wyatt v. Stickney* (1972), *Welsch v. Dirkswager* (1977), and *Wuori v. Zitnay* (1978).

Guideline 3 Comment. A coordinated multidisciplinary care plan is important to address the interactive nature of biochemical, psychological, and sociological aspects of care. In some cases, index behavior or symptoms may not be eliminated or only return to prior levels, meaning that the behavior or condition will still have to be addressed by the individual or others. Behaviors or symptoms may worsen as well as improve and may do so in different settings. Although the stage is often set for learning or a return to normal activity, psychotropic medication in and of itself does not teach new skills or necessary cognitive strategies.

Multidisciplinary team members, including the prescriber, do not approve the use of psychotropic medication within a multidisciplinary care plan. The individual, if competent, or his or her guardian does. Numerous problems can be avoided if the physician does not unilaterally prescribe psychotropic medication in a nonemergency situation (a) outside a coordinated multidisciplinary care plan approved by the individual or guardian, and (b) without a full psychiatric and functional assessment. Similarly, numerous problems can be avoided if other multidisciplinary team members (a) communicate relevant and organized information to the prescriber so the best decision regarding psychotropic medication can be made, and (b) do not interfere with psychotropic medication decisions within the parameters of the multidisciplinary care plan approved by the individual or guardian. Disagreements between multidisciplinary members regarding the use of psychotropic medication should be presented to the individual or guardian for a decision. If the individual is incompetent and no guardian exists, disagreements should be referred to appropriate peer or external review bodies.

Common shortcomings in care plans are a lack of specified parameters for psychotropic medication use and a lack of planned alternatives in the event of nonresponse or side effects. These potentially lead to reactive

Guideline 2: Inappropriate Use

Guideline	What It Means	What It Does Not Mean
Psychotropic medication shall not be used excessively, as punishment, for staff convenience, as a substitute for meaningful psychosocial services, or in quantities that interfere with an individual's quality of life.	When this guideline is not followed, psychotropic medication becomes chemical restraint or is not being used in the best interest of the individual.	This is not intended to curtail the legitimate use of psychotropic medication to treat psychiatric disorders that are known to be medication responsive. This does not mean short-term chemical restraint should not be used for extreme situations when other procedures fail or are not appropriate for the situation.
	Excessive includes inappropriately high doses or inappropriately long periods of time relative to the diagnosis or condition of concern. Punishment includes the use of psychotropic medication in response to an individual who is (1) exercising his or her legal rights or (2) appropriately responding to inappropriate staff or peer behavior (e.g., striking out at a staff member who is improperly confiscating the individual's possessions or fighting with a peer who is attempting to assault the individual). Staff convenience includes the use of psychotropic medication to compensate for poorly trained staff, staff shortages, poor environmental conditions, or nonaddressed medical or health concerns. Substitute for meaningful psychosocial services includes the use of psychotropic medication to replace more appropriate or necessary therapeutic, behavioral, or educational interventions. Interference with quality of life means that while a specific behavior or condition may be improved, a decline in functional status or learning ability compromises the individual to a greater degree than does the behavior or condition.	This does not mean maintenance medication cannot be used for psychiatric conditions if (1) a valid diagnosis is established and (2) there is evidence that the medication is needed.

instead of proactive planning, wasteful use of time, poor coordination among care team members, violations of existing informed consent, frustration with delays while further assessments and informed consent are obtained, and erosion of the therapeutic alliance. Numerous problems can be avoided by specifying variables such as psychotropic medication dose levels and ranges, titration plans, response timelines, actions in the event of side

Guideline 3: Multidisciplinary Care Plan

Guideline	What It Means	What It Does Not Mean
Psychotropic medication must be used within a coordinated multidisciplinary care plan designed to improve the individual's quality of life.	Psychotropic medication alone is not a care plan. A number of professionals and responsible parties may be involved in an overall plan to teach skills, monitor intervention, alter environmental stressors, provide other therapy, and provide patient and family education.	The individuals involved in a care plan may not be the same for every case. The prescriber may not be responsible for coordinating the overall care plan. If he or she is not, the responsible party, such as a case manager or family member, should be identified.
	Psychotropic medication parameters must be clearly established. These include titration plans, dosage range, response timelines, expected duration, other medication in the event of nonresponse, actions in the event of side effects or other adverse events, outcome indicators, and review points.	Every possible option does not have to be identified. Parameters can be altered as events develop as long as they are communicated and relevant informed consent updated.
	Multidisciplinary care members must not work in isolation. Psychotropic medication changes must be communicated to other multidisciplinary team members and coordinated with changes in life activity or therapy. Similarly, life activity or other therapy changes must be communicated to the prescriber and coordinated with psychotropic medication decisions.	Prescribers or other team members do not have to attend every decision or conference. Communication may occur via telephone, e-mail, fax, or interactive TV. This does not mean emergency actions cannot be taken. Serious events or prodromal signs may also require noncoordinated changes. This does not mean all minor changes must be coordinated.
	This guideline applies to PRN orders.	This does not include stat orders that by definition constitute emergency intervention.

effects, alternative psychotropic medication in the event of nonresponse, outcome indicators, expected duration of use, and a timeline for periodic review of the person's progress. Outcome indicators provide a means for reviewing progress. These should specify a change in index behavior baseline level and quality of life activity. Specific timelines to evaluate a psychotropic medication may help minimize the possibility of premature conclusions of ineffectiveness or continuing a noneffective medication. Four to eight weeks (in some cases, longer) are required for many psychotropic medications to have their full effect.

This is a critical guideline, and its message should not be overlooked within any debate about the role of vari-ous multidisciplinary team members in regard to psychotropic medication. The treatment team must work together not only to conduct assessments and establish intervention strategies, but also to monitor systematically the strategies selected.

References. ACD, 1993; ACDD, 1990; ACMRDD, 1977; Arnold, 1993; Bishop, 1992; Crabbe, 1989; Engel, 1977, 1980; Fahs, 1988; HCFA, 1988, 1992; Kaplan & Sadock, 1988; Mason & Granacher, 1980; Schooler, 1993; Sovner & Hurley, 1987; Werry, 1993.

Guideline 4 Comment. The psychiatric diagnosis and behavioral-pharmacologic hypothesis models both view maladaptive behavior as a final common pathway reflect-

Guideline 4: Diagnostic And Functional Assessment

Guideline	What It Means	What It Does Not Mean
The use of psychotropic medication must be based on a psychiatric diagnosis or a specific behavioral-pharmacological hypothesis resulting from a full diagnostic and functional assessment.	A diagnostic and functional assessment addresses (1) organic and medical pathology; (2) psychosocial and environmental conditions; (3) health status; (4) current medications; (5) the presence of a psychiatric condition; (6) history, previous intervention, and results; and (7) a functional analysis of behavior.	This guideline does not mean a psychotropic medication cannot be changed provided the psychiatric and functional assessment is still valid, the possible change has been outlined or updated in the multidisciplinary care plan, and the existing informed consent allows for such change.
	A functional analysis of behavior addresses (1) what, if any, antecedents or consequences affect or control a behavior; (2) whether behavior represents a deficit or excess, or is situationally inappropriate; (3) whether different patterns occur in different situations; and (4) possible schedule of reinforcement effects.	Findings from a functional analysis of behavior are not intended to curtail the legitimate use of psychotropic medication to treat psychiatric disorders known to be medication responsive.
	A psychiatric diagnosis is based on DSM-IV criteria. A behavioral-pharmacological hypothesis is based on the function of the behavior and a medication's known psychopharmacology (e.g., antecedent aversive stimuli such as taunts lead to aggression; a serotonin agonist may increase the reactivity threshold and thereby lowers the possibility of aggression; appropriate skills to handle taunts are taught).	Neither a psychiatric diagnosis nor a behavioral-pharmacological hypothesis is intended to convey the appropriateness of initially instituting (1) a psychotropic medication, (2) a non-psychotropic intervention, or (3) both. Such a decision will depend on the severity of and circumstances surrounding an individual case.

ing an individual's response to environmental demands, physical discomfort, or disturbances in neurochemical and physiological function. The goal of each is to see past nonspecific maladaptive behavior, determine the function or source, and determine whether an underlying environmental-responsive behavior disorder explains the presenting problem. Both models stress the interactive effects among behavior, environment, and neurochemistry and recognize that more complex variables must be considered. For example, a contemporary psychiatric formulation considers the functional significance of a person's behavior in multiple settings based on an objective assessment. A contemporary functional assessment considers that in some cases a person's behavior may have no functional significance because the problem may originate neurochemically. The sequencing of pharmacologic and non-

pharmacologic interventions will depend on the individual and whether a drug-responsive condition is present.

Whichever model is used, it is important to avoid the following errors when conducting assessments for purposes of formulating a diagnosis or reasonable hypothesis from which to develop a care plan: (a) failing to recognize the contribution of the environment, (b) failing to recognize the presence of a psychiatric condition, (c) overdiagnosing psychosis and schizophrenia, (d) using behavioral norms more appropriate for persons without developmental disabilities, (e) assigning a psychiatric diagnosis to justify more easily a pharmacologic intervention, and (f) viewing drugs and psychosocial interventions as either/or choices rather than a flexible combination in a constantly evolving relationship specific to the individual.

References. ACMRDD, 1977, 1983; ACDD, 1987,

Guideline 5: Informed Consent

Guideline	What It Means	What It Does Not Mean
Written informed consent must be obtained from the individual, if competent, or the individual's guardian before the use of any psychotropic medication and must be periodically renewed.	If not competent, the individual must be included to the degree possible.	Informed consent does not have to be obtained before the emergency use of psychotropic medication.
	Information must be presented orally, in writing, in layperson's terms, in an educational manner, and in a manner ensuring communication (e.g., sign language for an individual with a hearing impairment).	As long as the guardian has provided written informed consent, the appropriate use of psychotropic medication should not be affected by a guardian who will not return telephone calls or attend properly announced reviews.
	The time interval for renewing informed consent depends on the individual and treatment phase (e.g., first time use may indicate renewal 3 to 6 months later) but is at least once per year.	The recommended time period for renewal of informed consent applies only if the risk:benefit ratio for continued treatment has not changed.
	Information includes at least (1) the diagnosis or hypothesis, the specific signs or symptoms to be changed, and how they will be monitored; (2) a description of the proposed treatment, the expected benefits, the probability of success, how long it will take for benefits to occur, and the expected duration of use; (3) the feasible alternatives including the prognosis if the proposed treatment is not undertaken; (4) expected and unexpected risks and adverse effects including incidence, severity, and significance; (5) specific information about the proposed psychotropic medication including dose, appropriate dosage range for the individual, route of administration, plans if the medication is unsuccessful, and drug, alcohol, and food interactions; (6) an explanation of the right to refuse the treatment or to change one's mind, and that consent is time-limited and must be periodically renewed; and (7) the identity of the professionals involved and how to contact them.	

1990; Bishop, 1992; Crabbe, 1989; Gardner & Cole, 1987; Gualtieri & Keppel, 1985; Rogoff, 1984; Schaal & Hackenberg, 1994; Schroeder, 1990; Sovner, 1986, 1994; Sovner & Hurley, 1985, 1989; Thompson, Egli, Symons, & Delaney, 1994.

Guideline 5 Comment. Books and monographs have been written about informed consent and related concepts such as the right to refuse treatment. Contemporary models view informed consent as part of a greater ethical duty to establish a therapeutic alliance

Guideline 6: Index Behaviors And Empirical Measurement

Guideline	What It Means	What It Does Not Mean
Specific index behaviors and quality of life outcomes must be objectively defined, quantified, and tracked using recognized empirical measurement methods in order to monitor psychotropic medication efficacy.	Index behaviors are also referred to as target behaviors, signs (observable evidence), or symptoms (subjective sensations reported by the patient).	This guideline is not intended to suggest that other factors are not important (e.g., prodromal signs of relapse, life event changes or stress suggesting relapse, side effects, or changes in non-psychotropic therapy).
	Recognized empirical measurement methods include frequency count, duration recording, time sample, interval recording, permanent products, and rating scales.	Other information and the subjective observations of an individual who has the ability to provide such information can also be used to assess treatment. This guideline does not preclude the use of other methods such as laboratory learning tasks.
	A baseline quantification must occur before the nonemergency initiation or addition of any psychotropic medication. Although a baseline period will vary depending on the severity of the situation, a reasonable period is 2 to 4 weeks.	This does not mean an existing medication must be discontinued in order to obtain a baseline. A baseline is a period of time accepting existing interventions against which subsequent change is compared.
	Measurement must occur on an ongoing and consistent basis after the initiation of any psychotropic medication, especially before and after any dose or drug change.	This does not mean daily measurement must occur in every case. Measurement may vary depending on diagnosis, condition, severity, living situation, treatment phase, actual or planned intervention change, or subjective reports suggesting more intense measurement.

with the individual. Involving the individual in all decisions related to his or her care is a central tenet of this concept. Succinctly, in a nonemergency situation, if a competent individual or his/her guardian refuses consent for a psychotropic medication and the prescriber still considers the medication necessary, appropriate procedural and legal due process must be followed before the medication can be prescribed.

No credible authority advocates the use of psychotropic medication in a nonemergency situation without informed consent. Concern, however, has been expressed about the use of written informed consent, but with most individuals with developmental disabilities, it is the guardian and not the individual who provides informed consent. Written informed consent provides a

structure to the process and is useful given the understanding that an informed consent form (a) is an adjunct to oral explanation and educating the patient, (b) is not a substitute for "process informed consent" or the continual communication and contact between multidisciplinary professionals and the individual or guardian on all issues, (c) can be misdesigned to be excessively vague or complex, (d) does not provide legal protection if patients or guardians do not understand the information or what they are signing, and (e) does not ensure that a professional will obtain informed consent or quality informed consent. Educational material written in layperson's language for patients is critical within this process, because such material is associated with increased efforts to educate patients, is "paradoxically reassuring" to the patient should side effects occur, and is respectful of the lay individual and the learning process involved.

This guideline provides for each multidisciplinary care group to determine the best mechanism for obtaining formal written informed consent. In some situations a prescriber may obtain informed consent. In others, a nurse may obtain informed consent. In still others, a social worker may coordinate informed consent. Any procedure must adhere to the following observation by Kaplan and Sadock (1988): "Respect for persons incorporates and goes beyond informed consent. It is unfortunate that so much emphasis has been placed on informed consent—its rituals, documentation, and difficulties—at the expense of the higher ethical standard of respect for persons" (p. 121).

References: ACMRDD, 1977; American Bar Association Commission on the Mentally Disabled, 1986; APA, 1979, 1992; Applebaum, Lidz & Meisel, 1987; Bernstein, 1988; HCFA, 1978, 1988, 1992; Howe, 1984; JCAHO, 1995a; Kaplan & Sadock, 1988; Kennedy & Sanborn, 1992; McElroy, Keck, & Friedman, 1995; Simon, 1987; Singh et al., 1992; Sovner & Hurley, 1985; Sprague & Galliher, 1988; Werry & Aman, 1993.

Guideline 6 Comment. Behavior and mental state are much more difficult to assess than are other medical conditions such as hypertension. Specific index behaviors and quality of life outcomes assist the physician, other multidisciplinary care team members, and the patient or guardian to evaluate progress over a drug trial. The term *index behavior* is used instead of *target behavior* in order to reinforce Guideline 4, which emphasizes psychotropic medication use based on a psychiatric diagnosis or specific behavioral-pharmacologic hypothesis. The behavior per se is not being treated.

Quality of life outcome is an important measure because index behavior improvement usually leads to an improved quality of life by removing an obstacle to the rehabilitation process. Quality of life serves as a check against potential functional status decline despite specific index behavior improvement. Index behaviors are not entirely omitted in favor of quality of life measures because quality of life is a molar rather than molecular concept and may not change for a period of time despite index behavior improvement. As an analogy, blood pressure readings are not omitted in favor of quality of life when medication for hypertension is prescribed.

Although subjective information provided by very verbal individuals during face to face interviews should not be minimized or overlooked, a number of authorities have suggested the importance of objective behavioral indicators of clinical status. Sovner and Hurley (1987) noted, "In our opinion, behavioral monitoring of treatment provides the most effective way of making decisions regarding the response of mentally retarded persons treated with psychotropic medication" (p. 48). Crabbe (1989) stressed the need for specific target symptoms and observed, "Psychiatrists are adjusting to clinical data collecting from behavioral observations and reports rather than traditional interviewing which has limitations in nonverbal clients" (pp. 19–20). Index behavior measurement is a critical concept within the integration of psychiatric and behavioral schools of thought because the best approach to behavioral pharmacological management is to obtain good data. Other multidisciplinary care team members must remember that the prescriber needs empirical data in a succinct, usable, and longitudinal format such as a graphic representation.

A baseline period will vary according to the individual case. Generally, a 2- to 4-week period is sufficient. At least one court case, *Welsch v. Likins* (see Sprague, 1982), required a 1-month period, and some DSM-IV psychiatric diagnoses such as that for depression require at least two consecutive weeks of symptoms. Such a period provides a more accurate measure of the behavior or condition and helps prevent overreaction to a bad week or normal variation. In some instances, 2 to 4 weeks may not provide sufficient time for a valid baseline. For example, if an index behavior rate is improving over several weeks prior to treatment, it is difficult to determine whether continued improvement after medication intervention would have occurred in the absence of treatment. As a result, treatment may be erroneously continued.

Index behavior data do not automatically mandate clinical decisions. Empirical data are part of a first pass review and must be examined in the context of diagnosis and other life events. For example, if an index behavior has increased, suggesting current treatment is ineffective, recognizing that the individual is experiencing acute stress would mandate no medication changes in order to allow for reassessment once the stressor has been "psychologically processed."

Crabbe observed that the length of psychiatric treatment varies; that is, treatment may ensue for 3 weeks, 6 weeks, 12 months, 3 years, or indefinitely. The situation is dynamic and not static, and acute, chronic, and maintenance treatment phases change as do the environment and the individual. It is not always possible or necessary to collect index behavior data every day for

Guideline 7: Side Effects Monitoring

Guideline	What It Means	What It Does Not Mean
The individual must be monitored for side effects on a regular and systematic basis using an accepted methodology which includes a standardized assessment instrument.	A standardized assessment instrument is used in addition to any recommended physiological and laboratory assessments.	This does not mean side effects cannot occur at other times and that staff or other personnel should not be trained to recognize side effects. This does not mean client reports or other information from caregivers cannot be used.
	Standardized assessment instruments mean (1) a published or recognized scale or (2) a checklist constructed from standard pharmaceutical or medical references (e.g., *United States Pharmacopeia* or *Facts and Comparisons*). Standardized instruments do not diagnose side effects. They provide information for further inquiry or follow-up by professionals.	
	A direct examination should accompany the use of the assessment instrument.	The prescriber does not have to conduct every assessment. Other parties such as nurses may report the information to the physician for review.
	Monitored on a regular basis means every person receiving drug therapy must be assessed at least once (1) every 3 to 6 months and (2) after the initiation of a new psychotropic medication or a dose increase. Systematic basis means some coordinated procedure to conduct, review, record, and act on assessment information.	The frequency of assessments will depend on individual circumstances (e.g., high risk clients may require weekly assessments, whereas stabilized maintenance clients living independently may only make appointments once per year).

every individual. This especially applies to individuals in home health care or semi-independent living situations or to individuals with certain psychiatric conditions such as refractory bipolar disorder or schizophrenia requiring maintenance medication. However, some form of ongoing, consistent, and periodic data collection is necessary to track and review status. If data are collected periodically, more frequent data collection should occur during acute treatment phases and when drug or dose changes are considered.

References. ACD, 1993; ACMRDD, 1977; Aman, Hammer, & Rojahn, 1993; APA, 1974; Arnold, 1993; see Beyer, 1988, for a review of *Halderman v. Pennhurst* (1977); Bishop, 1992; Crabbe, 1989; Hall, 1971; Handen, 1993; HCFA, 1988, 1992; Kaplan & Sadock, 1988; Mason & Granacher, 1980; Rojahn & Schroeder, 1983; Schroeder, 1990; Sovner, 1986, 1994; Sovner & Hurley, 1985, 1987; see Sprague, 1982, for a discussion of *Doe v. Hudspeth* (1977), *Welsch v. Likins* (1976), *Welsch v. Dirkswager* (1977), and *Wuori v.*

Guideline 8: Tardive Dyskinesia Monitoring

Guideline	What It Means	What It Does Not Mean
If antipsychotic medication or other dopamine-blocking drugs are prescribed, the individual must be monitored for tardive dyskinesia on a regular and systematic basis using a standardized assessment instrument.	Other dopamine-blocking drugs include amoxapine and metoclopramide.	
	A standardized assessment instrument means the use of a published or recognized scale such as AIMS, DISCUS, TDRS, or TRIMS.	This guideline does not preclude the use of specialized methods (e.g., electromyography, accelerometers, or ultrasound).
	Monitoring on a regular basis means at least once every 6 months.	This guideline does not preclude assessments being carried out on a more frequent basis for some individuals (e.g., those in a high-risk group, with signs of developing TD, or needing treatment intervention for severe TD).
	If a TD-causing drug is discontinued, assessments should occur 1 and 2 months after discontinuation to check for withdrawal TD.	If a medication known to cause TD is prescribed for a short period of time (e.g., less than 90 days), 1 and 2 month assessments do not have to occur unless high-risk factors are involved. Assessments do not have to be conducted at every medication reduction, especially when done on a gradual basis.
	If persistent TD has been diagnosed and an antipsychotic medication or other dopamine-blocking drug is no longer prescribed, assessments should continue to occur every 6 to 12 months. Systematic basis mean some coordinated procedure to conduct, review, record, and act on assessment information.	This guideline does not mean assessments must continue for remitted TD unrelated to ongoing medication or other therapy used to treat the TD.

Zitnay (1978); Steingard, Allen, & Schooler, 1994; Thompson et al., 1989.

Guideline 7 Comment. The monitoring of side effects is critical because side effects may be harmful to the person's health. Side effects may be behavioral in nature and may intensify underlying behavior problems. They are associated with numerous hospital admissions per year as well as litigation. Even when health consequences are minor, side effects may cause discomfort such that patient noncompliance or impaired quality of life occurs.

Side effects with mild to moderate severity are more likely to be detected when standardized questionnaires and assessment methods are used. Despite the value of lab tests, side effects occur within normal blood ranges, and most functional side effects (e.g., tremor, ataxia, dysarthria, drooling, irritabilty, etc.) do not have lab tests. As Zametkin and Yamada (1993) noted, "Although such rating scales are probably not commonly used in practice for the assessment of side effects, their use is to be encouraged since they may elicit medication-induced symptoms that the patient or family might not have reported" (p. 88). Standardized side effect scales such as the Stimulant Drug Side Effects Rating Scale (Barkley, DuPaul, & Costello, 1993) have been developed for some medication classes or can be constructed from standard medical or pharmaceutical references such as the *United States Pharmacopeia* (United States Pharmacopeial Convention, 1995), *Facts and Comparisons* (1995), or *American Hospital Formulary Service Drug Information* (American Society of Hospital Pharmacists, 1995). Standardized side effect scales such as the Simpson-Angus Scale (Simpson & Angus, 1970) or the Barnes Akathisia Scale (Barnes, 1989) have been developed for specific side effects such as extrapyramidal side effects. The Adverse Drug Reaction Scale (Corso, Pucino, DeLeo, Calis, & Gallelli, 1992) was developed for all medication classes, whereas the Systematic Assessment for Treatment Emergent Effects (SAFTEE) (Levine & Schooler, 1986), the Dosage Record and Treatment Emergent Symptom Scale (DOTES) (National Institute of Mental Health, 1985), and the Monitoring of Side Effects Scale (MOSES) (Kalachnik, 1985) were for psychotropic medication classes.

The frequency with which side effects rating scales should be administered varies depending on factors such as the individual person, treatment phase, and specific medications. On the one hand, a person who is prescribed a psychotropic for the first time or undergoing numerous medication changes may need to be assessed weekly or more often for a period of time. On the other hand, an independent outpatient who is stabilized on low-dose maintenance medication for an established long-term condition may need to be assessed only once every 6 to 12 months. A general rule of thumb is to check systematically every 3 to 6 months as part of regular medication reviews and within a reasonable amount of time after the initiation of any new psychotropic medication or a dose increase.

Prescribers do not necessarily have to conduct every side effect assessment. Trained personnel such as nurses should conduct the majority of assessments. Scales can also be adapted into a self-report format for individuals capable of participating in such an activity. However, the prescriber should review assessments and directly examine the client periodically. Supplemental reports from parents and teachers and questioning of the interdisciplinary team are also valuable. The overall concept behind this guideline is to expect side effects and to look for them actively and systematically.

References. American Academy of Pediatrics Committee on Drugs, 1985; Beardsley, Freeman, & Appel, 1983; Bennett & Lipman, 1977; Crabbe, 1989; Gitlin, Cochran, & Jamison, 1989; see Grandquist, 1990, for HCFA Interpretive Guidelines; Grohmann et al., 1993; Hanzel, Kalachnik, & Harder, 1992; Herranz, Arteaga, & Armijo, 1982; JCAHO, 1995a; Marder et al., 1993; McElroy, Keck, & Friedman, 1995; Rabin, Markowitz, Ocepek-Welikson, & Wagner, 1992; Reiter & Kutcher, 1991; Scandinavian Society of Psychopharmacology, 1987; Simon, 1987; Singh et al., 1992; Sleator, Ullmann, & von Neumann, 1982; Sovner & Hurley, 1985; see Sprague, 1982, for a review of *Wuori v. Zitnay* (1978); Zametkin & Yamada, 1993; Zbinden, 1963.

Guideline 8 Comment. Tardive dyskinesia (TD) is a side effect of antipsychotic medication, amoxapine, and metoclopramide. The early detection (secondary prevention) of TD is critical to maximize the chances for reversal and to minimize its impact for individuals for whom long-term antipsychotic medication continues to be necessary. The APA (1992) has noted, "Systematic and reliable assessment of tardive dyskinesia is essential in both research and clinical settings" (p. 52). Jeste and Caligiuri (1993) further stated:

> The use of standardized rating scales is beneficial in the initial assessment of TD, but their follow-up value is also important. When administered at regular intervals, these scales can assist clinicians in judging the progression of symptoms in a diagnosed patient, in detecting sudden changes in the severity of symptoms, and in assessing response to treatments. We should point out, however, that the rating scales are not diagnostic instruments. (p. 308)

The four major TD scales are the Abnormal Involuntary Movement Scale (AIMS) (Guy, 1976), the Dyskinesia Identification System Condensed User Scale (DISCUS) (Sprague & Kalachnik, 1991), the Tardive Dyskinesia Rating Scale (TDRS) (Simpson, Lee, Zoubok, & Gardos, 1979), and the Texas Research Institute of Mental Sciences Dyskinesia Scale (TRIMS) (Smith, Allen, Gordon, & Wolff, 1983).

References. APA, 1979, 1992; APA Committee, 1992; Brown & Funk, 1986; Crabbe, 1989; Gardos & Cole, 1986; Jeste & Caligiuri, 1993; Kaplan & Sadock, 1988; Munetz & Schulz, 1986; Pi & Simpson, 1986;

Guideline 9: Regular And Systematic Review

Guideline	What It Means	What It Does Not Mean
Psychotropic medication must be reviewed on a regular and systematic basis.	The review schedule should be outlined in the care plan.	This guideline does not mean other reviews cannot occur or that the schedule cannot be changed.
	Systematic review means a coordinated procedure between all parties to (1) share, review, document, and act on information such as index behavior, quality of life, and side effects data, and (2) communicate drug, dose, and non-pharmacological changes.	
	Regular means at least once every 3 months and within 1 month of drug or dose changes.	More frequent reviews should occur when certain factors are present (e.g., high-risk profile).
9a. Clinical reviews must be conducted on a regular and systematic basis by the prescriber.	The prescriber must see the individual at each clinical review.	The frequency of clinical reviews may vary (e.g., acute cases may require weekly to monthly reviews, whereas stabilized maintenance cases may require 6 to 12 month reviews).
9b. Data reviews must be conducted on a regular and systematic basis by appropriate members of the multidisciplinary team.	Appropriate team members may vary depending on factors such as the setting, case, and type of review (e.g., an annual review or change in care plan may involve all members, whereas a 3-month review may only involve the individual or guardian, prescriber, nurse, and case manager).	All members do not have to be physically present at a review (e.g., reports may be provided for the prescriber or others to review, or telephone or interactive TV may be used). This does not mean the prescriber must carry out a complete physical examination or order a laboratory evaluation at every data review.
	A pharmacist must periodically review the individual drug regimen (e.g., every 3 to 12 months depending on factors such as a high-risk profile, the specific regimen, new medications, or significant dose changes).	

Simon, 1987; Sovner & Hurley, 1985; see Sprague, 1982, for a review of *Clites v. Iowa* (1980).

Guideline 9 Comment. Periodic reviews of data and clinical status are necessary to assess the risk:benefit ratio of continued psychotropic medication use. Whereas the manner of examination or observation of the individual by the prescriber is dictated by the individual's condition and the treatment, the data should be reviewed at least quarterly if dose is stabilized, and no more than one month after a drug or dose change unless unique situations present themselves. Unique situations may range from less frequent data reviews for successful independently living individuals on maintenance medication with few medication or dose changes to more frequent data reviews for individuals with severe conditions, a greater number of changes, or instability of data. Rules of thumb for considering more frequent reviews and

Guideline 10: Lowest Optimal Effective Dose

Guideline	What It Means	What It Does Not Mean
Psychotropic medication must be reviewed on a periodic and systematic basis to determine whether it is still necessary or, if it is, whether the lowest optimal effective dose is prescribed.	Lowest optimal effective dose (OED) means the least amount of medication required to improve or stabilize the problem.	This guideline does not mean that higher dose levels are necessarily inappropriate for some individuals as evidenced by improved outcome.
	If several psychotropic medications are prescribed, it may be possible to reduce the number of drugs, although a medication-free status is not possible.	This guideline does not mean that several psychotropic medications are always inappropriate (e.g., for treatment resistant cases showing improved outcome).
	Periodic means every medication review with in-depth risk:benefit analysis provided at least once per year.	This guideline does not preclude the use of more frequent in-depth risk:benefit analyses for some individuals (e.g., for those with a high-risk profile, first time use, etc.).
	Any reduction to determine the lowest OED must be gradual in nature including (1) the dose amount and (2) the length of time at a dose level.	This guideline does not mean that gradual reductions can or should occur in every situation (e.g., no lower dose forms are manufactured, short-term use, pharmacokinetics such as rapid excretion for lithium, etc.).
	Systematic means a review of variables such as the (1) views of the individual or guardian; (2) pattern of index behavior and quality of life data; (3) results of previous properly conducted reductions; (4) comparison of current drugs and dose levels to norms appropriate for the age group, population, diagnosis, and treatment phase; (5) new variables since drug initiation or the last reduction attempt; and (6) current drugs and dose levels compared to previous levels.	Drug holidays are not required every year. Nor do gradual reductions necessarily have to occur each year for established long-term drug-responsive conditions, provided proper variables are reviewed and the current drug and dose regimen is the lowest OED.

prescriber appointments are that individuals show regression or loss of skills already gained or failure to progress toward identified index behavior levels and quality of life outcomes.

There are a number of ways to structure psychotropic medication reviews depending on the setting. It is not necessary that all multidisciplinary team members be physically present for full participation at each review. In some situations, some members may conduct a preliminary review and forward recommendations and reports to the prescriber for review. In other situations,

a person such as a case manager may coordinate independent reviews at different times by different professionals. In some settings, only immediate health care professionals and the individual or guardian may be involved. In other settings, such as residential facilities with prescribers on staff, all members may attend all reviews. In still other settings all members may attend only an annual update meeting or provide reports if unable to attend.

It is helpful if the care plan specifies the degree of change in index behavior or quality of life activity that

Guideline 11: Frequent Changes

Guideline	What It Means	What It Does Not Mean
Frequent drug and dose changes should be avoided.	Medications can take varying times to work. Variables such as drug pharmacokinetics and recognized treatment times should be reviewed so as to minimize the number of changes.	This guideline does not mean that frequent changes cannot occur or are necessarily inappropriate (e.g., as part of an upward or downward titration plan or as a result of side effects).
	Drugs and doses should not be changed in a reactive manner to index behavior fluctuation, without consideration of the disorder being treated, or simply for change's sake.	This guideline does not mean drugs and doses cannot be changed if there is a valid reason for the change (e.g., prodromal signs of relapse emerge such that an existing medication's dose is altered and an additional medication is initiated).

prompt in-depth review, discussion, or appointment with the prescriber. For example, alerting the prescriber for in-depth discussion or appointment may be prompted by established prodromal signs of relapse, environmental stresses, and life events that increase the likelihood of relapse specific to the individual or diagnosis. If aggression typically varies between two and five times per month, a "red flag" level prompting in-depth prescriber medication review or appointment may be defined as "more than five aggressions per month for two consecutive months." Conversely, an indicator level prompting in-depth prescriber review for possible dose reduction may be defined as "less than two aggressions per month for six consecutive months."

Overall, if the following three concepts are followed, a psychotropic medication review mechanism as determined by the involved parties is probably acceptable. First, changes beyond those permitted in the established care plan should not be made without diagnostic and functional assessments and the informed consent of the individual or guardian (Guidelines 3-5). Second, a communication channel must be established for the individual, guardian, and other multidisciplinary care members to convey data or concerns to health care professionals. And third, a communication channel must be established for health care professionals to promptly communicate changes to the individual, guardian, and other multidisciplinary care members, even when these changes are within the parameters of the established care plan.

References: ACDD, 1987; APA Committee, 1992; Bishop, 1992; HCFA, 1988, Honigfeld & Howard, 1973; Mason & Granacher, 1980; Singh et al., 1992; Sovner & Hurley, 1985.

Guideline 10 Comment. There are four reasons for periodic consideration of gradual psychotropic medication reduction: (1) a complete remission may have been achieved in the person's clinical status, (2) an observed improvement in clinical status may not have been a result of the prescribed medication, (3) determining the lowest effective dosage may reduce the risk of long-term side effects, and (4) a medication or dose level may no longer be necessary. Although this guideline encourages review and reduction to determine continued need, it does not mandate an annual "drug holiday." It only requires that the possibility of a gradual dose reduction be considered. Possible contraindications include (a) the necessity of maintenance dose levels for certain disorders such as schizophrenia or bipolar disorder, (b) marked relapse during previous gradual reduction, (c) the current dose is already at the lower end of an established dose range for the individual, and (d) the individual has a long history of treatment failure and shows dramatically improved quality of life activity ("best he/she has ever been") with the current psychotropic medication regimen. The presence of contraindications at one point in time, however, does not mean that the individual should be omitted from future periodic review because circumstances change. For example, a new job or termination of a restrictive procedure may contraindicate lowest optimal effective dose (OED) reduction procedures for several months but not longer.

Kaplan and Sadock noted, "The brain is not a group of on-and-off neurochemical switches; rather it is an interactive network of neurons in a complex homeostasis. Thus the abrupt discontinuation of virtually any psychoactive drug is likely to disrupt further the brain's

Guideline 12: Polypharmacy

Guideline	What It Means	What It Does Not Mean
Keep psychotropic medication regimens as simple as possible in order to enhance compliance and minimize side effects.	Intraclass polypharmacy (i.e., the use of two psychotropic medications from the same therapeutic class at the same time) is rarely justified.	This guideline does not mean that short periods of using two medications from the same class cannot occur during crossover periods when one medication is initiated and increased as the other is reduced and discontinued. This guideline does not mean that intraclass polypharmacy is inappropriate for a unique case as is evidenced by improved index behavior and quality of life compared to each single agent.
	Interclass polypharmacy (i.e., the use of two or more psychotropic medications from different therapeutic classes at the same time) should be minimized.	This guideline does not mean that two or more drugs cannot be prescribed for an individual or that such medications are necessarily inappropriate for that individual (e.g., co-morbid conditions, acute situations requiring additional medication, refractory cases, cases not responding to single agents, diagnostic indicators, etc.).

functioning" (1988, p. 495). There are two reasons why gradual withdrawal is preferred over abrupt withdrawal. First, abrupt reduction increases the potential for withdrawal syndromes. These have been reported for many medications including tricyclic antidepressants, benzodiazepine antianxiety agents, antipsychotic medication, beta-blockers such as propranolol, and sedative-hypnotic medication. Second, abrupt discontinuation or large dose decreases may result in relapse and a return to original dose levels when, in fact, a lower maintenance dose may have been possible if gradual methodology was employed.

The definition of gradual reduction varies depending on the medication and the goal of the reduction. Is the goal to remove an ineffectual psychotropic medication or to determine the lowest dose? If the goal is to terminate ineffectual medication, gradual reduction is based upon avoidance of withdrawal effects. If the goal is to achieve the lowest OED, sufficient time is needed at each dose level to allow for meaningful data comparison. For example, propranolol is usually discontinued over at least two weeks to avoid withdrawal effects. However, if the goal is to determine whether a lower dose of propranolol is as effective as a higher dose in treating a condition, at least two to four weeks per dose level should be

considered in order to ensure that any changes are not an artifact of normal variability.

Many chronically administered psychotropic medications have long half-lives and are highly lipophilic (have an affinity for fatty tissue storage). Reduction schedules, therefore, are generally expected to be quite long with changes not more frequent than once per week and often over longer periods of time, sometimes up to two to three months. In some cases of schizophrenia with long-term exposure to antipsychotic medication, reductions may take place over periods as long as six months or more. Conditions that may warrant exceptions to gradual reductions include the following: (a) the medication has been prescribed for a short period of time, (b) a low dose is prescribed and no lower dose form is available, (c) a side effect such as neuroleptic malignant syndrome is present, (d) a medical or surgical situation is present, (e) a change is planned from one psychotropic medication to another within the same class, (f) the person is being treated in an inpatient acute care unit where limited time is allowed but a higher degree of expertise and monitoring is available, and (g) the pharmacokinetics of specific medications such as lithium or methylphenidate allow more rapid reductions.

Guideline 13: Practices To Minimize

Guideline	What It Means	What It Does Not Mean
Minimize the following practices to the degree possible:	These practices require evidence of need and positive outcome data.	This does not mean the practice may not help a specific individual.
13a. Long-term use of PRN (as needed) orders.	Long-term is more than a few weeks.	
13b. Long-term use of benzodiazepine antianxiety medications such as diazepam.	Long-term is more than 3 months.	Some benzodiazepines (e.g., clonazepam) may be used to treat affective or other conditions (e.g., TD).
13c. Use of long-acting sedative-hypnotic medications such as chloral hydrate.		
13d. Long-term use of shorter-acting sedative-hypnotics such as temazepam.	Long-term is more than 14 days.	This does not mean longer use may not be necessary in some cases.
13e. Anticholinergic use such as benztropine without signs of EPSE.		Prophylactic use may be necessary in some cases (e.g., high potency antipsychotic at a higher dose).
13f. Long-term use of anticholinergic medication.	Long-term is more than 3 to 6 months.	Long-term use may be necessary in some cases (see above example).
13g. Use of antipsychotic medication at high doses.	This is above (1) 500 mg chlorpromazine or (2) 10 to 15 mg haloperidol.	This does not mean some individuals may not respond to higher doses.
13h. Use of phenytoin, phenobarbital, and primidone as psychotropic medications.		This does not mean these medications are inappropriate for the treatment of: (1) some types of epilepsy, or (2) some resistant psychiatric disorders as evidenced by index behavior and quality of life improvement compared to other agents.

References. Arnold & Aman, 1991; Bishop, 1992; Cantopher, Olivieri, Cleave, & Edwards, 1990; Casey & Gerlach, 1984; Coulter, 1988; Crabbe, 1989; Fielding, Murphy, Reagan, & Peterson, 1980; Fischbacher, 1982; Gardos & Cole, 1986; Garner, Kelly, & Thompson, 1993; HCFA, 1988, 1992; Kales, Bixler, Tan, Scharf, & Kales, 1974; Kaplan & Sadock, 1988; Marder et al., 1993; Noyes, Garvey, Cook, & Perry, 1988; Pi & Simpson, 1986; Schooler, 1993; Schwinghammer, 1982; Sovner & Hurley, 1984, 1985; see Sprague, 1982, for a review of *Doe v. Hudspeth* (1977), *Welsch v. Likins* (1976), *Welsch v. Dirkswager* (1977), and *Wuori v. Zitnay* (1978).

Guideline 11 Comment. Most psychotropic medications require an extended time for effectiveness. Preestablished timelines within the care plan (see Guideline 3) help prevent overreaction to day-to-day fluctuations in the frequency or severity of index behaviors. Werry observed, "It takes a sure knowledge of psychopharmacology and of psychiatry to resist fiddling, while drugs and/or disorders operate to a different drummer" (1993, p. 18).

References. Crabbe, 1989; Sovner & Hurley, 1985, 1987; Werry, 1993.

Guideline 12 Comment. Polypharmacy increases the risk

Guideline 14: Peer Or External Review

Guideline	What It Means	What It Does Not Mean
Establish a system of peer or external review of psychotropic medication prescribing that incorporates a mechanism of flagging cases of greatest concern.	A continuous quality improvement (CQI) or quality improvement model should be used.	This guideline does not mean that a committee must review and approve every instance of psychotropic medication use.

---

of drug interactions, adverse reactions, cost, and noncompliance. Without a clear diagnostic indication, polypharmacy is usually unnecessary for individuals with developmental disabilities. This guideline is not intended to discourage the use of two or more psychotropic medications given appropriate therapeutic indications. Rather, it is intended as a reminder that inappropriate polypharmacy can insidiously manifest itself when medications are added to treat a condition that may not necessarily be fully correctable or responsive to medication. The routine addition of a psychotropic medication to the treatment regimen without consideration of discontinuation of a prior psychotropic medication should be avoided.

References. Aman, 1985; Aman, Hammer, & Rojahn, 1993; Crabbe, 1989; Kaplan & Sadock, 1988; Rogoff, 1984; Sovner, 1994; Sovner & Hurley, 1985; see Sprague, 1982, for a discussion of *Doe v. Hudspeth* (1977); Werry, 1993.

Guideline 13 Comment. This guideline provides a series of professional recommendations regarding minimizing the use of specific practices or medications. The practices listed should be avoided whenever possible.

Long-term use of PRNs (Guideline 13a). PRNs are standing orders that physicians leave for nurses, directing them to medicate a person if a certain behavior or event occurs. Recent studies suggest a powerful placebo effect. Regular use of a PRN beyond a few weeks indicates a need to consider an environmental cause or to review the treatment plan. PRN orders should be reserved for behavior that occurs sporadically or unpredictably and does not abate quickly. If a PRN order is used, it must be part of a multidisciplinary care plan (see Guideline 3; Druckenbrod, Rosen, & Cluxton, 1993; Sovner & Hurley, 1985; Vitiello et al., 1991).

Use of benzodiazepine antianxiety and sedative-hypnotic medication (Guidelines 13b, 13c, and 13d). The long-term use of these medications may lead to diminishing effectiveness, tolerance, and pronounced withdrawal reactions. The benzodiazepine antianxiety medications are

associated with behavioral disinhibition in some individuals. Long-acting sedative-hypnotic medications such as chloral hydrate are associated with behavioral disinhibition in individuals with developmental disabilities. Although shorter-acting sedative hypnotics are preferred over longer-acting sedative hypnotics, it is generally recommended to avoid the long-term use of any sedative-hypnotic medication if possible (American Society of Hospital Pharmacists, 1995; APA Committee, 1992; Barron & Sandman, 1985; Thompson et al., 1989).

Use of anticholinergic medication (Guidelines 13e and 13f). Anticholinergic medication is associated with unpleasant autonomic side effects such as dry mouth, constipation, blurred vision, and urinary retention; memory loss; and other disadvantages such as cognitive disturbance. Most authorities do not recommend anticholinergic medication use without signs of extrapyramidal side effects, especially when a low-dose therapy is initiated. Additionally, anticholinergic medication may no longer be required as the body adapts to extrapyramidal side effects or when lower antipsychotic medication maintenance levels are reached (APA Committee, 1992; Casey & Gerlach, 1984; Mason & Granacher, 1980; Marder et al., 1993; Royal College, 1994; see Sprague, 1982, for a discussion of *Doe v. Hudspeth* (1977); WHO, 1990).

Use of high doses of antipsychotic medication (Guideline 13g). There is little evidence for the effectiveness of antipsychotic medication for individuals with developmental disabilities with dosages above 500 mg of chlorpromazine (Thorazine) or 400 mg of thioridazine (Mellaril). In most cases of schizophrenia, there is little clinical effect beyond 10 to 20 mg of haloperidol (Haldol) and fluphenazine (Prolixin). Individuals who require high-dose therapy should not be undermedicated, but close review of such cases should occur because high doses are generally not required on a long-term basis and increase the risk of serious side effects (APA Committee, 1992; American Society of Hospital Pharmacists, 1995; Kane & Marder, 1993; Lipman et al.,

Table 4–1. Psychotropic Medication Guideline Summary
The 10–4 Principle

Do's

1. Treat any substance prescribed to improve or stabilize mood, mental status, or behavior as a psychotropic medication (Guideline 1).

2. Use psychotropic medication within a coordinated multidisciplinary care plan (Guideline 3).

3. Use psychotropic medication based on a psychiatric diagnosis or a specific behavioral-pharmacologic hypothesis and only after conducting complete diagnostic and functional assessments (Guideline 4).

4. Obtain written informed consent from the individual or guardian and establish a therapeutic alliance involving all decision-makers (Guideline 5).

5. Track treatment efficacy by defining objective index behaviors and quality of life outcomes and measure them using empirical methods (Guideline 6).

6. Monitor for side effects using standardized assessment instruments (Guideline 7).

7. Monitor for tardive dyskinesia using standardized assessment instruments if antipsychotic or other dopamine blocking medications are prescribed (Guideline 8).

8. Conduct clinical and data reviews on a regular and systematic basis (Guideline 9).

9. Strive to use the lowest optimal effective dose (Guideline 10).

10. Evaluate drug and monitoring practices through a peer or team quality review or improvement group (Guideline 14).

Don'ts

1. Don't use psychotropic drugs excessively, for convenience, as a substitute for meaningful psychosocial services, or in quantities that interfere with quality of life activity (Guideline 2).

2. Avoid frequent drug and dose changes (Guideline 11).

3. Avoid intraclass polypharmacy and minimize interclass polypharmacy to the degree possible in order to decrease the likelihood of patient noncompliance and side effects (Guideline 12).

4. Minimize to the degree possible (Guideline 13):

    Long-term PRN orders

    Use of long-acting sedative-hypnotics (e.g., chloral hydrate)

    Long-term use of short-acting sedative hypnotics (e.g., temazepam)

    Long-term use of benzodiazepine antianxiety medications (e.g., diazepam)

    High antipsychotic medication doses

    Long-term use of anticholinergic medication (e.g., benztropine)

1978; Mason & Granacher, 1980; Royal College, 1994; Sovner & Hurley, 1985).

Use of phenobarbital, phenytoin, and primidone (Guideline 13h). There is little recent evidence for using these antiepileptic drugs (AEDs) as psychotropic medications for individuals with developmental disabilities. Even when used for epilepsy, they are associated with a number of side effects. If psychotropic medication, especially antipsychotic medication, and barbiturate AEDs such as

phenobarbital or primidone are prescribed, the possibility of AED barbiturate exacerbation of index behaviors and the inadvertent use of psychotropic medication should be reviewed (Aman, 1983, 1985; Gadow & Poling, 1988; Singh et al., 1992; Thompson et al., 1989; United States Pharmacopeial Convention, 1995).

Guideline 14 Comment. External or peer review has major public health implications and generally results in cost savings and favorable outcome. It is especially important for community residential or public residential facilities, managed health care agencies, and organizations contracting to coordinate overall living care (e.g., organizations contracting to provide case management services to oversee semi-independent living).

Peer review teams should include not only qualified people who have experience or training in contemporary psychotropic medication practices (e.g., psychiatrists, pharmacists, and nurses), but also other representatives such as consumers or guardians, psychologists, and social workers who may have other valid insights. The goal of the committee is not to eliminate psychotropic medication, but to review psychotropic medication use from a quality improvement model. Although every case does not necessarily have to be reviewed, a system should be developed for identifying cases of greatest concern (e.g., intraclass polypharmacy, acute dose levels for extended periods of time, long-term benzodiazepine antianxiety use, etc.). Random sampling of records should also occur to ascertain appropriate use, evaluation, and monitoring in terms of assessments of clinical status, quality of life, side effects monitoring, and renewal of informed consent.

References. ACDD, 1990; APA Committee, 1992; Beyer, 1988; Findholt & Emmett, 1990; HCFA, 1988; Mason & Granacher, 1980.

SUMMARY

Over the past 25 years, a set of basic psychotropic medication guidelines has emerged through a combination of accreditation, professional, legal, and regulatory sources. Taken as a whole, they provide a framework from which to lay the abuses of the past to rest, retain the lessons learned in order to prevent reoccurrence, and incorporate new knowledge. The 14 guidelines that this framework comprises are summarized in Table 4-1, in which the guidelines are divided into 10 do's and 4 don'ts. If practitioners, consumers, and organizations can respond to the "10–4 principle" and implement these guidelines, most psychotropic medication controversies can be avoided.

In the early to mid-1970s, guidelines were driven by concepts such as active treatment, multidisciplinary teams, and informed consent. From the late 1970s to the late 1980s, guidelines were driven by the need to develop a methodology to monitor index behaviors and side effects and to establish the lowest maintenance dose. Since that time, guidelines have been driven by the biopsychosocial model, the integration of behavioral psychology and clinical psychiatry, and quality of life outcome based performance measures.

The guidelines discussed herein are intended to be applied to the care of all individuals with developmental disabilities. Most individuals are cared for in the community, and the misuse of psychotropic medication can no longer be attributed to state institutional care. Psychotropic medication guidelines are especially critical because increasing economic constraints suggest that the concerns surrounding psychotropic medication in the past are not likely to dissipate in the future. The guidelines presented herein merge rational (controlling principles and underlying reason) and empirical (capable of being verified or disproved by observation) views.

REFERENCES

Accreditation Council for Facilities for the Mentally Retarded (ACMR). (1971). *Standards for residential facilities for the mentally retarded.* Chicago: Joint Commission on Accreditation of Hospitals.

Accreditation Council for Facilities for the Mentally Retarded (ACMR). (1973). *Standards for community agencies serving persons with mental retardation and other developmental disabilities.* Chicago: Joint Commission on Accreditation of Hospitals.

Accreditation Council for Services for Mentally Retarded and Other Developmentally Disabled Persons (ACMRDD). (1977). *Standards for services for developmentally disabled individuals.* Chicago: Joint Commission on Accreditation of Hospitals.

Accreditation Council for Services for Mentally Retarded and Other Developmentally Disabled Persons (ACMRDD). (1983). *Standards for services for developmentally disabled individuals.* Washington, DC: Author.

Accreditation Council on Services for People with Developmental Disabilities (ACDD). (1987). *Standards for services for people with developmental disabilities.* Boston: Author.

Accreditation Council on Services for People with Developmental Disabilities (ACDD). (1990). *Standards and interpretive guidelines for services to people with developmental disabilities.* Landover, MD: Author.

Accreditation Council on Services for People with Disabilities (ACD). (1993). *Outcome-based performance measures.* Towson, MD: Author.

Accreditation Council on Services for People with Disabilities (ACD). (1995). *Information and orientation packet.* Towson, MD: Author.

Agency for Health Care Policy and Research. (1993). *Clinical practice guideline development* (AHCPR Pub. No. 93–0023). Rockville, MD: U.S. Department of Health and Human Services, Public Health Service.

Aman, M.G. (1983). Psychoactive drugs in mental retardation. In J.L. Matson & F. Andrasik (Eds.), *Treatment issues and innovations in mental retardation* (pp. 455–513). New York: Plenum Press.

Aman, M.G. (1985). Drugs in mental retardation: Treatment or tragedy? *Australia and New Zealand Journal of Developmental Disabilities, 10,* 215–226.

Aman, M.G., Hammer, D., & Rojahn, J. (1993). Mental retardation. In T.H. Ollendick & M. Hersen (Eds.), *Handbook of child and adolescent assessment* (pp.

321–345). Needham Heights, MA: Allyn & Bacon.

American Academy of Pediatrics Committee on Drugs. (1985). Behavioral and cognitive effects of anticonvulsant therapy. *Pediatrics, 76,* 644–647.

American Association on Mental Deficiency Project on Technical Planning in Mental Retardation. (1964). Standards for state residential institutions for the mentally retarded [entire issue no. 21]. *American Journal of Mental Deficiency, 68.*

American Bar Association Commission on the Mentally Disabled. (1986). *The right to refuse psychotropic medication.* Washington, DC: American Bar Association.

American Psychiatric Association. (1974). *Behavior therapy in psychiatry: A report of the American Psychiatric Association task force on behavior therapy.* New York: Jason Aronson.

American Psychiatric Association. (1979). *Task force report 18: Tardive dyskinesia.* Washington, DC: American Psychiatric Press.

American Psychiatric Association. (1980). *Diagnostic and statistical manual of mental disorders* (3rd ed.). Washington, DC: American Psychiatric Press.

American Psychiatric Association. (1987). *Diagnostic and statistical manual of mental disorders* (3rd ed. revised). Washington, DC: American Psychiatric Press.

American Psychiatric Association. (1989). *Treatments of psychiatric disorders: A task force report of the American Psychiatric Association.* Washington, DC: American Psychiatric Press.

American Psychiatric Association. (1990). *Psychiatric services to adult mentally retarded and developmentally disabled persons: Task force report 30.* Washington, DC: American Psychiatric Press.

American Psychiatric Association. (1992). *Tardive dyskinesia: A task force report of the American Psychiatric Association.* Washington, DC: American Psychiatric Press.

American Psychiatric Association. (1994). *Diagnostic and statistical manual of mental disorders* (4th ed.) Washington, DC: American Psychiatric Press.

American Psychiatric Association Committee on Research on Psychiatric Treatments. (1992). Psychopharmacological screening criteria. *Journal of Clinical Psychiatry, 53,* 184–196.

American Society of Hospital Pharmacists. (1995). *American hospital formulary service drug information.* Bethesda, MD: Author.

Applebaum, P.S., Lidz, C.W., & Meisel, A. (1987). *Informed consent: Legal theory and clinical practice.* New York: Oxford.

Arnold, L.E. (1993). Clinical pharmacological issues in treating psychiatric disorders of patients with mental retardation. *Annals of Clinical Psychiatry, 5,* 189–197.

Arnold, L.E., & Aman, M.G. (1991). Beta blockers in mental retardation and developmental disorders. *Journal of Child and Adolescent Psychopharmacology, 1,* 361–373.

Ayd, F.J. (1991). The early history of modern psychopharmacology. *Neuropsychopharmacology, 5,* 71–84.

Baldessarini, R.J. (1980). Drugs and the treatment of psychiatric disorders. In L.S. Goodman & A. Gilman (Eds.), *The pharmacological basis of therapeutics* (6th ed., pp. 391–447). New York: Macmillan.

Barkley, R.A., DuPaul, G.J., & Costello, A. (1993). Stimulants. In J.S. Werry & M.G. Aman (Eds.), *Practitioner's guide to psychoactive drugs for children and adolescents* (pp. 205–237). New York: Plenum Press.

Barnes, T.R.E. (1989). A rating scale for drug-induced akathisia. *British Journal of Psychiatry, 154,* 672–676.

Barron, J., & Sandman, C.A. (1985). Paradoxical excitement to sedative-hypnotics in mentally retarded clients. *American Journal of Mental Deficiency, 90,* 124–129.

Beardsley, R.R., Freeman, J.M., & Appel, F.A. (1983). Anticonvulsant serum levels are useful only if the physician appropriately uses them: An assessment of the impact of providing serum level data to physicians. *Epilepsia, 24,* 330–335.

Bennett, B.S., & Lipman, A.G. (1977). Comparative study of prospective and voluntary reporting in determining the incidence of adverse drug reactions. *American Journal of Hospital Pharmacy, 34,* 931–936.

Bernstein, J.G. (1988). *Handbook of drug therapy in psychiatry* (2nd ed.). Littleton, MA: PSG.

Beyer, H.A. (1988). Litigation and use of psychoactive drugs in developmental disabilities. In M.G. Aman & N.N. Singh (Eds.), *Psychopharmacology of the developmental disabilities* (pp.29–57). New York: Springer-Verlag.

Bishop, A.C. (1992). Empirical approach to psychopharmacology for institutionalized individuals with severe or profound mental retardation. *Mental Retardation, 30,* 283–288.

Brown, G.W. (1990). Rule-making and justice: A cautionary tale. *Mental Retardation, 28,* 83–87.

Brown, P., & Funk, S.C. (1986). Tardive dyskinesia: Barriers to the professional recognition of an iatrogenic disease. *Journal of Health and Social Behavior, 27,* 116–132.

Cantopher, T., Olivieri, S., Cleave, N., & Edwards, J.G. (1990). Chronic benzodiazepine dependence: A comparative study of abrupt withdrawal under propranolol cover versus gradual withdrawal. *British Journal of Psychiatry, 156,* 406–411.

Casey, D.E., & Gerlach, J. (1984). Tardive dyskinesia: Management and new treatment. In H.C. Stancer, P.E. Garfinkel, &

V.M. Rafoff (Eds.), *Guidelines for the use of psychotropic medication: A clinical handbook* (pp. 183–203). Jamaica, NY: Spectrum.

Corso, D.M., Pucino, F., DeLeo, J.M., Calis, K.A., & Gallelli, J.F. (1992). Development of a questionnaire for detecting potential adverse drug reactions. *Annals of Pharmacotherapy, 26,* 890–896.

Coulter, D.L. (1988). Withdrawal of sedative anticonvulsant drugs from mentally retarded persons: Development of guidelines. *Journal of Epilepsy, 1,* 67–70.

Crabbe, H.F. (1989). *A guidebook for the use of psychotropic medication in persons with mental illness and mental retardation.* East Hartford, CT: Connecticut Department of Mental Retardation.

Crews, W.D., Bonaventura, S., & Rowe, F. (1994). Dual diagnosis: Prevalence of psychiatric disorders in a large state residential facility for individuals with mental retardation. *American Journal on Mental Retardation, 98,* 688–731.

Department of Health, Education, and Welfare. (1974, January 17). Medical assistance program. Intermediate care facility services. *Federal Register, 39,* 2220–2235.

Druckenbrod, R.W., Rosen, J., & Cluxton, R.J. (1993). As-needed dosing of antipsychotic drugs: Limitations and guidelines for use in the elderly agitated patient. *Annals of Pharmacotherapy, 27,* 645–648.

Eddy, D.M. (1992). *A manual for assessing health practices and designing practice policies: The explicit approach.* Philadelphia: American College of Physicians.

Engel, G.L. (1977). The need for a new medical model: A challenge for biomedicine. *Science, 196,* 129–136.

Engel, G.L. (1980). The clinical application of the biopsychosocial model. *American Journal of Psychiatry, 137,* 535–544.

Facts and comparisons. (1995). St. Louis: Author.

Fahs, J.J. (1988). Multidisciplinary psychiatric consultation in mental retardation. *Newsletter of the National Association for the Dually Diagnosed, 5* (2), 1–4.

Fielding, L.T., Murphy, R.J., Reagan, M.W., & Peterson, T.L. (1980). An assessment program to reduce drug use with the mentally retarded. *Hospital and Community Psychiatry, 31,* 771–773.

Findholt, N.E., & Emmett, C.G. (1990). Impact of interdisciplinary team review on psychotropic drug use with persons who have mental retardation. *Mental Retardation, 28,* 41–46.

Fischbacher, E. (1982). Effect of reduction of anticonvulsants on well-being. *British Medical Journal, 285,* 423–424.

Freeman, R.D. (1970). Use of psychoactive drugs for intellectually handicapped children. In N.R. Bernstein (Ed.), *Diminished people: Problems and care of the mentally retarded* (pp. 277–304). Boston: Little, Brown.

Gadow, K.D., & Poling, A.G. (1988). *Pharmacology and mental retardation*. Boston: College-Hill.

Gardner, W.I., & Cole, C.L. (1987). Managing aggressive behavior: A behavioral diagnostic approach. *Psychiatric Aspects of Mental Retardation Reviews, 6*, 21–25.

Gardos, G., & Cole, J.O. (1986). How to minimize tardive dyskinesia. *Hospital Therapy, 11*, 33–42.

Garner, E.M., Kelly, M.W., & Thompson, D.F. (1993). Tricyclic antidepressant withdrawal syndrome. *The Annals of Pharmacotherapy, 27*, 1068–1071.

Gitlin, M.J., Cochran, S.D., & Jamison, K.R. (1989). Maintenance lithium treatment: Side effects and compliance. *Journal of Clinical Psychiatry, 50*, 127–131.

Grandquist, L.G. (1990, October 9). *Legal and ethical issues arising from drug treatment of persons with developmental disabilities*. Minneapolis, MN: Legal Advocacy for Persons with Developmental Disabilities.

Greiner, T. (1958). Problems of methodology in research with drugs. *American Journal of Mental Deficiency, 64*, 346–352.

Grohmann, R., Strobel, C., Ruther, E., Dirschedl, P., Helmchen, H., Hippius, H., & Miller-Oerlinghausen, B. (1993). Adverse psychic reactions to psychotropic drugs: A report from the AMUP study. *Pharmacopsychiatry, 26*, 84–93.

Gualtieri, C.T., & Keppel, J.M. (1985). Psychopharmacology in the mentally retarded and a few related issues. *Psychopharmacology Bulletin, 21*, 304–309.

Gualtieri, C.T., Sprague, R.L., & Cole, J.O. (1986). Tardive dyskinesia litigation and the dilemmas of neuroleptic treatment. *Journal of Psychiatry & Law, 14*, 187–216.

Guy, W. (1976). *ECDEU assessment manual for psychopharmacology* (rev. ed.). Washington, DC: U.S. Government Printing Office.

Hall, R.V. (1971). *Behavior modification: The measurement of behavior*. Lawrence, KS: H & H Enterprises.

Handen, B.L. (1993). Pharmacotherapy in mental retardation and autism. *School Psychology Review, 22*, 162–183.

Hanzel, T.E., Kalachnik, J.E., & Harder, S.R. (1992). A case report of phenobarbital exacerbation of a preexisting maladaptive behavior partially suppressed by chlorpromazine and misinterpreted as chlorpromazine efficacy. *Research in Developmental Disabilities, 13*, 381–392.

Harvey, S.C. (1980). Hypnotics and sedatives. In L.S. Goodman & A. Gilman (Eds.), *The pharmacological basis of therapeutics* (6th ed., pp. 339–375). New York: Macmillan.

Health Care Financing Administration (HCFA). (1978, September 29). Standards for intermediate care facilities for the mentally retarded. *Federal Register, 43*, 45241–45253.

Health Care Financing Administration. (1988, June 3). Medicaid program: Conditions for intermediate care facilities for the mentally retarded. *Federal Register, 53*, 20448–20505.

Health Care Financing Administration. (1992, February 5). Medicare and medicaid programs; Omnibus nursing home requirements. Proposed rule: *Federal Register, 57*, 4516–4534.

Herranz, J.L., Arteaga, R., & Armijo, J.A. (1982). Side effects of sodium valproate in monotherapy controlled by plasma levels: A study in 88 pediatric patients. *Epilepsia, 23*, 203–214.

Hickman, F.J., Resnick, P.J., & Olson, K.B. (1982). Right to refuse psychotropic medication: An interdisciplinary proposal. *Mental Disability Law Review, 6*, 122–130.

Holburn, C.S. (1990). Rules: The new institutions. *Mental Retardation, 28*, 89–94.

Holburn, C.S. (1992). Rhetoric and realities in today's ICF/MR: Control out of control. *Mental Retardation, 30*, 133–141.

Honigfeld, G., & Howard, A. (1973). *Psychiatric drugs: A desk reference*. New York: Academic Press.

Howe, E.G. (1984). Legal aspects of psychopharmacology. *Psychiatric Clinics of North America, 7*, 887–900.

Jacobson, J.W. (1990). Regulations: Can they control staff compliance in human services systems? *Mental Retardation, 28*, 77–82.

Jacobson, J.W., & Otis, J.P. (1992). Limitations of regulations as a means of social control reform in developmental services. *Mental Retardation, 30*, 163–171.

Jeste, D.V., & Caligiuri, M.P. (1993). Tardive dyskinesia. *Schizophrenia Bulletin, 19*, 303–315.

Joint Commission on Accreditation of Healthcare Organizations (JCAHO). (1995a). *Accreditation manual for mental health, chemical dependency, and mental retardation developmental disabilities services*. Oakbrook Terrace, IL: Author.

Joint Commission on Accreditation of Healthcare Organizations (JCAHO). (1995b). *Comprehensive accreditation manual for hospitals*. Oakbrook Terrace, IL: Author.

Kalachnik, J.E. (1985). Medication monitoring procedures: Thou shall, here's how. In K.D. Gadow & A.G. Poling (Eds.), *Pharmacotherapy and mental retardation* (pp. 231–268). Boston: College-Hill.

Kales, A., Bixler, E.O., Tan, T., Scharf, M.B., & Kales, J.D. (1974). Chronic hypnotic-drug use: Ineffectiveness, drug-withdrawal insomnia, and dependence. *Journal of the American Medical Association, 227*, 513–517.

Kane, J.M., & Marder, S.R. (1993). Psychopharmacologic treatment of schizophrenia. *Schizophrenia Bulletin, 19*, 287–302.

Kaplan, H.I., & Sadock, B.J. (1988). *Synopsis of psychiatry. Behavior sciences. Clinical psychiatry* (5th ed.). Baltimore: Williams & Wilkins.

Kennedy, N.J., & Sanborn, J.S. (1992). Disclosure of tardive dyskinesia: Effect of written policy on risk disclosure. *Psychopharmacology Bulletin, 28*, 93–100.

Keppel, J.M., & Gualtieri, C.T. (1989). Monitoring psychopharmacology in programs for the retarded. In *Treatments of psychiatric disorders: A task force report of the American Psychiatric Association* (pp. 68–71). Washington, DC: American Psychiatric Press.

Klerman, G.L. (1990). The psychiatric patient's right to effective treatment: Implications of *Osheroff v. Chestnut Lodge. American Journal of Psychiatry, 147*, 409–418.

Lehr, D.J., Gilbert, G.E., Tatel, D.S., Foer, A.A., & Kahan, J.S. (1975). Legal restrictions on the use of phenothiazines in institutions for the mentally retarded. In *Workshop on psychotropic drugs and the mentally retarded* (Contract No. MF 282-75-0417PM, pp. 150–204). Rockville, MD: National Institute of Mental Health.

Levine, J., & Schooler, N.R. (1986). SAFTEE: A technique for the systematic assessment of side effects in clinical trials. *Psychopharmacology Bulletin, 22*, 343–381.

Lipman, R.S. (1967, May). *Results of a survey on psychotropic usage in institutions for the mentally retarded*. Paper presented at the meeting of the American Association on Mental Deficiency, Denver, CO.

Lipman, R.S. (1970). The use of psychopharmacological agents in residential facilities for the retarded. In F.J. Menolascino (Ed.), *Psychiatric approaches to mental retardation* (pp. 387–398). New York: Basic Books.

Lipman, R.S., DiMascio, A., Reatig, N., & Kirson, T. (1978). Psychotropic drugs and mentally retarded children. In M.A. Lipton, A. DiMascio, & K.F. Killam (Eds.), *Psychopharmacology: A generation of progress* (pp. 1437–1447). New York: Raven Press.

Marder, S.R., Ames, D., Wirshing, W.C., & Van Putten, T. (1993). Schizophrenia. *Psychiatric Clinics of North America, 16*, 567–587.

Mason, A.S., & Granacher, R.P. (1980). *Clinical handbook of antipsychotic drug therapy*. New York: Brunner/Mazel.

McElroy, S.L., Keck, P.E., & Friedman, L.M. (1995). Minimizing and managing antidepressant side effects. *Journal of Clinical Psychiatry, 56* (Suppl. 2), 49–55.

Meinhold, P.M., & Mulick, J.A. (1990). Risks, choices, and behavioral treatment. *Behavioral Residential Treatment, 5*, 29–44.

Meinhold, P.M., & Mulick, J.A. (1992). Social policy and science in the treatment of severe behavioral disorders: Defining and securing a healthy relationship. *Clinical Psychology Review, 12*, 585–603.

Meinhold, P.M., Mulick, J.A., & Teodoro,

J.M. (1994). Risks and SISIS-treatment litigation: Focus on the family. *Journal of Child and Family Studies, 3,* 403–415.

Menolascino, F.J. (1989). Model services for treatment/management of the mentally retarded-mentally ill. *Community Mental Health Journal, 25,* 145–155.

Munetz, M.R., & Schulz, S.C. (1986). Minimization and overreaction to tardive dyskinesia. *Schizophrenia Bulletin, 12,* 168–172.

National Institute of Mental Health. (1985). DOTES (Dosage record and treatment emergent symptom scale). *Psychopharmacology Bulletin, 22,* 347–381.

Noyes, R., Garvey, M.J., Cook, B.L., & Perry, P.J. (1988). Benzodiazepine withdrawal: A review of the evidence. *Journal of Clinical Psychiatry, 49,* 382–389.

Pi, E.H., & Simpson, G.M. (1986). Prevention of tardive dyskinesia. In N.S. Shah & A.G. Donald (Eds.), *Movement disorders* (pp. 181–193). New York: Plenum Press.

Rabin, J.G., Markowitz, J.S., Ocepek-Welikson, K., & Wagner, S.S. (1992). General versus systematic inquiry about emergent clinical events with SAFTEE: Implications for clinical research. *Journal of Clinical Psychopharmacology, 12,* 3–10.

Reiter, S., & Kutcher, S.P. (1991). Disinhibition and anger outbursts in adolescents treated with clonazepam. *Journal of Clinical Psychopharmacology, 11,* 268.

Reiss, S. (1990). Prevalence of dual diagnosis in community-based day programs in the Chicago metropolitan area. *American Journal on Mental Retardation, 94,* 578–585.

Rinck, C., Guidry, J., & Calkins, C.F. (1989). Review of states' practices on the use of psychotropic medication. *American Journal of Mental Deficiency, 93,* 657–668.

Rogoff, Mai-Lan (1984). Psychotropic medications and mentally retarded patients. In J.G. Bernstein (Ed.), *Clinical psychopharmacology* (2nd ed., pp. 211–231). Littleton, MA: John Wright.

Rojahn, J., & Schroeder, S.R. (1983). Behavioral assessment. In J.L. Matson & J.A. Mulick (Eds.), *Handbook of mental retardation* (pp. 227–243).

Royal College of Psychiatrists' Consensus Panel. (1994). The use of high-dose antipsychotic medication: Consensus statement. *British Journal of Psychiatry, 164,* 448–458.

Sadler, J.Z., & Hulgas, Y.F. (1992). Clinical problem solving and the biopsychosocial model. *American Journal of Psychiatry, 149,* 1315–1323.

Scandinavian Society of Psychopharmacology Committee of Clinical Investigations (UKU). (1987). The UKU side effects rating scale [entire issue]. *Acta Psychiatrica Scandinavica, 76* (Suppl. 334).

Schaal, D.W., & Hackenberg, T. (1994). Toward a functional analysis of drug treatment for behavior problems of people with developmental disabilities. *American Journal on Mental Retardation, 99,* 123–140.

Scheerenberger, R.C. (1983). *A history of mental retardation.* Baltimore: Paul H. Brookes.

Scheerenberger, R.C. (1987). *A history of mental retardation: A quarter century of promise.* Baltimore: Paul H. Brookes.

Schooler, N.R. (1993). Reducing dosage in maintenance treatment of schizophrenia. *British Journal of Psychiatry, 163* (Suppl. 22), 58–65.

Schroeder, S. R. (1990). Neuroleptic medications for persons with developmental disabilities. In M.G. Aman & N.N. Singh (Eds.), *Psychopharmacology of the developmental disabilities* (pp. 82–100). New York: Springer-Verlag.

Schwinghammer, T. (1982). Drug withdrawal syndromes. *U.S. Pharmacist, 7,* 35–48.

Simon, R.I. (1987). *Clinical psychiatry and the law.* Washington, DC: American Psychiatric Press.

Simpson, G.M., & Angus, J.W.S. (1970). A rating scale for extrapyramidal side effects. *Acta Psychiatrica Scandinavica, 212* (Suppl. 44), 11–19.

Simpson, G.M., Lee, J.H., Zoubok, B., & Gardos, G. (1979). A rating scale for tardive dyskinesia. *Psychopharmacology, 64,* 171–179.

Singh, N.N., Guernsey, T.F., & Ellis, C.R. (1992). Drug therapy for persons with developmental disabilities: Legislation and litigation. *Clinical Psychology Review, 12,* 665–679.

Sleator, E.K., Ullmann, R.K., & von Neumann, A. (1982). How do hyperactive children feel about taking stimulants and will they tell the doctor? *Clinical Pediatrics, 21,* 474–479.

Smith, R.C., Allen, R., Gordon, J., & Wolff, J. (1983). A rating scale for tardive dyskinesia and parkinsonian symptoms. *Psychopharmacology Bulletin, 19,* 266–276.

Sovner, R. (1986). Assessing the quality of a psychotropic drug regimen. In D. Rapoport & J. Parry (Eds.), *The right to refuse antipsychotic medication* (pp. 48–57). Washington, DC: American Bar Association.

Sovner, R. (1994). *Instructional guidelines for the appropriate use of psychotropic drug therapy with persons who have developmental disabilities.* Brookline, MA: Author.

Sovner, R., & Hurley, A.D. (1984). Discontinuing psychotropic drug therapy: Rationale, guidelines, and side effects. *Psychiatric Aspects of Mental Retardation Reviews, 3,* 41–44.

Sovner, R., & Hurley, A.D. (1985). Assessing the quality of psychotropic drug regimens prescribed for mentally retarded persons. *Psychiatric Aspects of Mental Retardation Reviews, 8/9,* 31–38.

Sovner, R., & Hurley, A.D. (1987). Objective behavioral monitoring of psychotropic drug therapy. *Psychiatric Aspects of Mental Retardation Reviews, 6,* 48–51.

Sovner, R., & Hurley, A.D. (1989). Ten diagnostic principles for recognizing psychiatric disorders in mentally retarded persons. *Psychiatric Aspects of Mental Retardation Reviews, 8,* 9–14.

Sparr, M.P., & Smith, W. (1990). Regulating professional services in ICFs/MR: Remembering the past and looking to the future. *Mental Retardation, 28,* 95–99.

Sprague, R.L. (1975). Research findings and their impact upon the FDA pediatric advisory panel. In *Workshop on psychotropic drugs and the mentally retarded* (Contract No. MF 282-75-0417PM, pp. 111–132). Rockville, MD: National Institute of Mental Health.

Sprague, R.L. (1982). Litigation, legislation, and regulations. In S.E. Bruening & A.D. Poling (Eds.), *Drugs and mental retardation* (pp. 377–413). Springfield, IL: Charles C Thomas.

Sprague, R.L., & Galliher, L. (1988). Litigation about psychotropic medication. In K.D. Gadow & A.G. Poling (Eds.), *Pharmacotherapy and mental retardation* (pp. 297–312). Boston: College-Hill.

Sprague, R.L., & Kalachnik, J.E. (1991). Reliability, validity, and a total score cutoff for the Dyskinesia Identification System: Condensed User Scale (DISCUS) with mentally ill and mentally retarded populations. *Psychopharmacology Bulletin, 27,* 51–58.

Sprague, R.L., & Werry, J.S. (1971). Methodology of psychopharmacological studies with the retarded. In N.R. Ellis (Ed.), *International review of research in mental retardation* (Vol. 5, pp. 147–219). New York: Academic Press.

Steingard, S., Allen, M., & Schooler, N.R. (1994). A study of the pharmacologic treatment of medication-compliant schizophrenics who relapse. *Journal of Clinical Psychiatry, 55,* 470–472.

Thompson, T., Egli, M., Symons, F., & Delaney, D. (1994). Neurobehavioral mechanisms of drug action in developmental disabilities. In T. Thompson & D.B. Gray (Eds.), *Destructive behavior in developmental disabilities: Diagnosis and treatment* (pp. 133–180). Thousand Oaks, CA: Sage.

Thompson, T., Hackenberg, T.D., & Schaal, D.W. (1989). Pharmacological treatments for behavior problems in developmental disabilities. In *Treatment of destructive behaviors in persons with developmental disabilities* (NIH Publication No. 91-2410, pp. 343–510). Rockville, MD: National Institutes of Health.

United States Pharmacopeial Convention. (1995). *United States pharmacopeia.* Rockville, MD: Author.

Vitiello, B., Hill, J.L., Elia, J., Cunningham,

E., McLeer, S.V., & Behar, D. (1991). P.R.N. medications in child psychiatric patients: A pilot placebo-controlled study. *Journal of Clinical Psychiatry, 52,* 499–501.

Werry, J.S. (1993). Introduction: A guide for practitioners, professionals, and public. In J. S. Werry & M.G. Aman (Eds.), *Practitioner's guide to psychoactive drugs for children and adolescents* (pp. 3–21). New York: Plenum Press.

Werry, J.S., & Aman, M.G. (Eds.). (1993). *Practitioner's guide to psychoactive drugs for children and adolescents.* New York: Plenum Press.

World Health Organization Heads of Centres Collaborating in WHO Co-ordinated Studies on Biological Aspects of Mental Illness. (1990). Prophylactic use of anti-cholinergics in patients on long-term neuroleptic treatment. *British Journal of Psychiatry, 156,* 412.

Zametkin, A.J., & Yamada, E.M. (1993). Monitoring and measuring drug effects: I. Physical effects. In J.S. Werry & M.G. Aman (Eds.), *Practitioner's guide to psychoactive drugs for children and adolescents* (pp. 75–97). New York: Plenum Press.

Zbinden, G. (1963). Experimental and clinical aspects of drug toxicity. In S. Garattini & P.A. Shore (Eds.), *Advances in Pharmacology* (Vol. 2, pp. 1–112). New York: Academic Press.

Interdisciplinary Teams[1]

Sharon Davis[2], Michael L. Wehmeyer[3], John P. Board, Jr.[4],
Sherman Fox[5], Fran Maher[6], and Beverly Roberts[7]

INTRODUCTION

In 1980 the Accreditation Council for Services for Mentally Retarded and Other Developmentally Disabled Persons recommended that psychoactive medications be used only as an integral part of an individualized program plan designed by an interdisciplinary team. Since that time, interdisciplinary teams have become much more involved in the decision-making and monitoring process for such medications (Lepler, Hodas, & Cotter-Mack, 1993). In this chapter, issues surrounding the use of interdisciplinary teams are summarized. What is their efficacy? What are the practical considerations in their implementation? What should be the scope of their authority?

Throughout this chapter, the term *team* will be used to mean *interdisciplinary team* or *review panel*. A team is a group of people from differing professions such as medicine, psychology, education, rehabilitation, counseling, and case management, as well as consumers (people with mental retardation) and their friends, family, and advocates. Because of the diversity of teams, it is difficult to draw conclusions that apply to them all. Some teams regulate medication use, whereas others serve as part of the treatment process. Some are in congregate care settings, whereas others are in the community. Some are intended to reduce overall reliance on psychoactive medications, whereas others are intended only to reduce inappropriate uses of such medications. Teams also differ in terms of both the disciplines represented and whether or not consumers are included.

PURPOSES OF TEAMS

Teams emerged as a response to the overuse of psychoactive drugs with people with mental retardation (Sprague, 1977; Sprague & Baxley, 1978). The concern about this situation was heightened by the fact that the medications were developed for use with adults with average cognitive ability, not for children and adults with mental retardation. There is a lack of scientifically sound studies on safety and efficacy with people with mental retardation and developmental disabilities (Sprague & Werry, 1971). Psychoactive medications may interfere with learning and other cognitive processes, a special concern with people with mental retardation (Aman & Singh, 1986; LaMendola, Zaharia, & Carver, 1980; Sprague & Werry, 1971).

Teams do more than reduce inappropriate uses of psychoactive medications. They often improve the quality of the clinical information used to diagnose behavior disorders and to prescribe medications. Without teams, physicians may not always have the time to complete a thorough review of all information about the consumer's behavior. A team approach using a broad range of input from all stakeholders—including the consumer, family, and staff—can provide a reliable, comprehensive, and data-oriented summary of the consumer's behavior (Kastner & Walsh, 1994; Lepler, Hodas, & Cotter-Mack, 1994).

The use of teams received impetus from a change in treatment philosophy. Today, service agencies prefer multimodal treatments that include behavior modification, environmental interventions, and psychoactive medications to treatment approaches based solely on psychoactive medications (Bishop, 1992). Generally, teams favor this multimodal approach and review a comprehensive range of treatment options.

Teams can help coordinate care for people living in community-based programs. In the last two decades, the

---

1 Additional consenting committee members: Martin Agran, Ph.D., Associate Professor, Department of Special Education, Utah State University; Benjamin Goldberg, M.D., Professor of Developmental Neuropsychiatry, University of Western Ontario, Canada

2 Director, Department of Research and Program Services, The Arc of the United States, Arlington, TX

3 Assistant Director, Department of Research and Program Services, The Arc of the United States, Arlington, TX

4 Chief of Medical Services, Michigan Department of Mental Health, Lansing, MI

5 Adjunct Professor of Psychiatry, Dartmouth College Medical School, Hanover, NH

6 The Arc of New Jersey, North Brunswick, NJ

7 Project Director, The Arc of New Jersey, North Brunswick, NJ

field of disability services has moved from centralized, congregate programs to community-based services and supports (Nirje, 1972; Taylor, Bogdan, & Racino, 1991; Wolfensberger, 1972). Although some people who reside in smaller, community-based residences need psychoactive medications (Burd et al., 1991; Gowdey, Zarfas, & Phipps, 1987; Rinck, Guidry, & Calkins, 1989), they have difficulty finding community-based health care providers who are familiar with mental retardation and developmental disabilities. In these cases, teams can help individuals find appropriate diagnostic and treatment services (Agran & Martin, 1982; Lepler et al., 1994).

Teams can help agencies promote self-determination and outcome-based evaluation (Ficker-Terrill & Rowitz, 1991; Gardner & Chapman, 1993; Luckasson et al., 1992; Perske, 1989). These trends place the individual and his or her family in a more visible and responsible role for decision making. Teams can be constituted to provide a vehicle for enhancing consumer choices and participation with regard to treatment issues.

Teams can help agencies monitor compliance with laws and regulations governing the use of psychoactive medications. The regulations are important in holding accountable the agencies and professionals serving people with mental retardation. Various standards, regulations, and legal decisions require agencies to create teams. Teams are mandated by the 1980 standards of the Accreditation Council for Services for Mentally Retarded and Other Developmentally Disabled Persons (1980) and the federal guidelines for intermediate care facilities for people with mental retardation. Legal decisions mandating the use of teams include *New York State Association for Retarded Citizens v. Rockefeller* (1975) and *Wyatt v. Stickney* (1972).

REDUCTION OF MEDICATION USE

Although the use of teams is still controversial among some professional groups, teams have been used to reduce reliance on psychoactive medications in the treatment of severe behavior problems. A number of researchers found that the introduction of teams in fact can reduce the use of psychoactive medications. In one of the better known studies, LaMendola et al. (1980) described a team's functioning in an institution. The team evaluated all residents and new admissions, held drug holidays to determine continued need for medica-

tions, conducted quarterly team reviews, discussed their findings with the residents' physicians, and set a predetermined time period within which the program had to be reevaluated. The percentage of residents receiving psychoactive medications declined from 34% to 21% between July 1974 and January 1978.

Schalock, Foley, Toulouse, and Stark (1985) described the functioning of a community-based team that decreased reliance on psychoactive medications. The team approved all new treatment plans and monitored the frequency and severity of changes in behavior. They favored the use of psychoactive medications only when behavioral programming alone was insufficient. Behavior programs were implemented for consumers with behavior problems. The effects of the programs were evaluated after 30 days. The programs were continued when the index behaviors decreased at least 5% in terms of their frequency or severity; the programs were either modified or continued when the index behaviors changed less than 5%; psychoactive medications were considered when the index behaviors changed more than 5%. If medications were attempted, the team required careful records of dates of introduction and changes in dosages. After 30 days of medication, the physicians continued or reduced the dosages when there was a 5% or greater decrease in index behaviors; and the physicians increased the dosages when there was a 5% or greater increase in problematic behaviors. Although physicians had the final authority to prescribe or change medications, the team could discontinue all treatment if a physician did not comply with their recommendations to reduce medications.

A nonequivalent between-groups design was used to evaluate the effect of the team on overall use of psychoactive medication. All participants exhibited stereotyped or noncompliant behavior. One group of residents was taking Thorazine at the time of referral to the program, whereas the other was not. Two years after the implementation of the team's program, the percentage of people on psychoactive medication declined from 30.5% to 20%.

Glaser and Morreau (1986) compared rates of use of antipsychotic medications in a public institution during a period when the medications were reviewed by a small medical group versus a larger team. In the first six months of the study, a medical group consisting of an attending physician, a clinical nurse, and a pharmacist reviewed each person's medications. During the second six-month period, a psychologist, a social worker, a primary caregiver, and a facility administrator were added to the team. The larger team established whether or not a valid psychiatric diagnosis had been made. In cases with no psychiatric diagnosis, the team determined an index behavior, discussed existing behavioral interventions, and examined data related to changes in the index behavior and the physical health of the individual. Finally, the team made revisions to the behavior plan and medications.

Glaser and Morreau found that 38 residents of one unit in the institution were receiving antipsychotic medication during the study period. Ten were identified by the larger team as receiving medications to treat symptoms of specifically diagnosed psychiatric disorders rather than specific index behaviors. These 10 persons were excluded from the study, leaving 28 participants. The researchers found a 6.5% overall decrease in medication use during the medical review versus a 28.5% decrease during the larger team review. There was a 19.5% decrease between the last medical review session and the first interdisciplinary team review meeting. Of the 28 participants, 5 were no longer receiving medication by the end of the study. Statistical analysis indicated that there were no significant differences in approximate oral equivalent doses between the start and end of the medical review phase of the study, but significant decreases occurred between the end of the medical phase and the start of the team phase, as well as between the start and end of the team phase. The reduction in medication use did not produce a statistically significant increase in accidents, but it was associated with a significant increase in the numbers of assaults and falls.

Briggs (1989) found that the introduction of a team decreased overall use of psychoactive medications at a large institution. At monthly meetings, the team examined the outcomes of behavioral and medication treatments, reviewed side effects, and applied previously agreed upon data-based criteria to recommend changes in dosage. Starting in 1979 and then annually from 1981 to 1987, the institution collected data on residents' use of psychoactive medications. Of 225 residents who were prescribed psychoactive medications during the eight-year period, 130 (58%) had the medication discontinued at some point in time. Of these, 90 (40% of the total group) were no longer taking medication at the time the study was completed. The team process was credited with maintaining an overall rate of 20% use of psychoactive medications, which is considered low for an institution, and ensuring dosage-reduction attempts in 91% of the cases.

Findholt and Emmett (1990) studied the impact of a team at a large state institution. Responding to the 1972

Wyatt v. Stickney decision, the facility formed a team in 1977. Each resident's medications were reviewed at least semi-annually. The team looked at all aspects of the person's functioning and then made a recommendation to the physician. The physician had the final authority for prescribing and changing medications. The investigators found a significant decrease in the use of psychotropic medications. From 1979 to 1987, the percentages of the institution's residents on psychoactive medication decreased from 41% to 12% for antipsychotics, from 14% to 2% for antidepressants, and from 13% to 3% for anxiolytics.

Lepler et al. (1993) described a team effort at a community-based agency. The team, which was coordinated by a nurse-practitioner, was composed of a behavioral specialist, staff members, and family. They met semi-annually as a group, although some individual team members met with each other more frequently. They identified existing or emerging psychiatric concerns and then discussed their findings with a community-based psychiatrist in regularly scheduled meetings. Between the start of the program in 1986 and April 1990 (or discharge date), 9 of the 12 individuals who had received psychoactive medications had experienced reductions in medication rates. Lepler et al. (1993) concluded that the use of the team contributed to decreased reliance on medications; however, Kastner and Walsh (1994) argued that the team had no effect. The mean number of medications per client remained about the same, 2.5 versus 2.8, as did the percentages of consumers receiving such medications, 18% versus 17%.

In conclusion, most researchers found that the formation of a team was associated with a reduction in the use of psychoactive medications. In some instances, however, the reduction in use in medication may have resulted from factors that were confounded with the introduction of teams. For example, Poindexter (1989) observed the use of psychoactive medications at a large Intermediate Care Facility for the Mentally Retarded and suggested that the reduced use in medications over a ten-year period might have been attributable to a number of factors. In addition to the team, the factors that might have been responsible for reduced reliance on medications included the increased age of the cohort, improved behavior modification techniques, increased input from all members of the interdisciplinary team, increased physician awareness of neurologic side effects, and increased precision in diagnosis of psychiatric disorders. Other possible factors were a change in treatment philosophy favoring behavioral interventions and federal and state regulations that restricted the use of psychoactive medications.

ISSUES ASSOCIATED WITH THE FORMATION OF TEAMS

The following is a discussion of some of the issues commonly encountered when teams are created.

Relationship Between Team and Physician

Given the responsibility physicians have for patients under their care, teams must be careful not to practice medicine (Kastner & Walsh, 1994). However, there is considerable concern on the part of physicians and other health professionals that they will lose ultimate authority for medical decision making to teams (Kastner & Walsh, 1994) due to inflexible, regulatory requirements. This issue was eloquently illustrated by Brown (1990) who published a "cautionary tale" concerning the fictional trial of a physician for not adequately treating a person with mental retardation who, as a result of his depression, had committed suicide, and the concurrent trial of the person's group home staff (team members) for practicing medicine without a license.

The prescription of medication requires detailed, technical knowledge. Physicians are justifiably concerned when the primary responsibility for making medication decisions is placed in the hands of laypeople or spread equally among team members. Teams must discuss their authority with physicians and develop a workable arrangement that respects all applicable laws and regulations governing the practice of medicine.

Recruiting Community-Based Psychiatrists

Today, residential services are moving from medically oriented, congregate settings to community-based, individualized services and supports. Although psychiatrists might be available for team meetings when they work for an institution, few community-based physicians have time to attend team meetings. The problem is complicated further by the fact that many people with mental retardation rely on Medicaid, which has a reimbursement rate so low that many physicians would be unwilling to accept it if they had to spend time at lengthy team meetings. Kastner and Walsh (1994) have argued that mandating the use of teams in the community could have unintended consequences, such as limiting access to psychiatric and neurological care. Team and other regulatory requirements increase the physician's administrative time and costs.

Apart from the issues of time and expense, it is difficult to find community-based physicians who have expertise in the use of psychoactive medications for people with mental retardation and developmental disabilities. Physicians are usually trained either in mental retardation (pediatrics) or in mental illness (psychiatry), but not in both. There is little cross-fertilization between these disciplines. Consequently, there is a severe shortage of trained physicians to work with people who have both mental retardation and mental illness.

Working with Multiple Physicians

Another issue community teams must address is how to work with multiple physicians. It is unlikely that all of the community-based physicians treating a consumer will be able to attend team meetings. Problems can occur when consumers are treated by group practices, where they see different physicians at different times. Additionally, Schalock et al. (1985) found that some consumers living in the community were taking multiple medications that had been prescribed by different physicians who were each unaware of the other's prescriptions. Teams need to identify procedures to ensure coordinated care when multiple physicians are involved.

Defining Excessive Use of Medication

The goal of reducing excessive reliance on psychoactive medications must be carefully defined so as not to eliminate medications that consumers actually need. Teams should seek to eliminate unnecessary uses of psychoactive medications, not all uses. Sometimes psychoactive medications offer the best treatment for an individual's condition. As Kastner and Walsh (1994, p. 244) put it, "lower rates of psychotropic drug use are not necessarily associated with improvements in health status" for people with mental retardation and developmental disabilities.

Kastner and Walsh (1994) have called for caution in mandating the use of teams. They argued that, "as health care reform moves forward, the cost, quality and effectiveness of new programs must be carefully studied before being presented as models for replication" (p. 244). This warning seems particularly prudent when discussing the use and misuse of psychoactive medications with people with mental retardation. Teams need to consider carefully procedures that ensure that they do not remove effective medications that actually are helping consumers.

OTHER METHODS FOR IMPROVING PRACTICE

Teams represent only one method to improve standards of practice. The following additional ideas have been suggested.

Psychiatric Diagnosis

One way to increase appropriate uses of psychoactive medication is to make psychiatric diagnoses whenever possible. Inappropriate medications are most likely when index behaviors are treated without consideration of psychiatric diagnosis. For example, aggression may be symptomatic of depression (Reiss & Rojahn, 1993), paranoia (Reiss, 1992), psychosis, personality disorder (Reiss, 1994), or some other psychiatric disorder. Because different medications are used to treat depression and psychosis, the diagnosis of psychiatric conditions associated with aggression aids the selection of appropriate medications. Therefore, some have argued that the main goal for systemic change should be to ensure that individuals with mental retardation receive a complete psychiatric evaluation from a mental health professional who is knowledgeable about people who have a dual diagnosis.

However, opinions on the importance of psychiatric diagnosis vary. For a variety of reasons, it is not always possible to determine a valid psychiatric diagnosis (Arnold, 1993; Sovner, 1986). The psychiatric nomenclature used for people with mental retardation is still evolving because some individuals have symptoms that do not match known psychiatric diagnoses (Fawcett, 1995). Others have symptoms that are masked and difficult to identify. In an effort to study these problems, Havercamp (1996) found that the reliability of psychiatric rating scales break down at about IQ 25. In many cases, it may be impossible to establish a psychiatric diagnosis below IQ 25. In a related study, Bouras, Brooks, and Drummond (1993) found that a psychiatric diagnosis could be made for only 42.8% of the consumers evaluated at a community psychiatric service in England.

Because of the special difficulties of diagnosing psychiatric disorders in people with mental retardation, virtually all authorities urge careful evaluation of a comprehensive array of information (King, DeAntonio, McCracken, Forness, & Ackerland, 1994; Levitas & Gilson, 1990; Reiss, 1994; Szymanski & Tanguy, 1980). The following sources of information are considered by the diagnostic teams of the Division of Prevention and Treatment of Developmental Disorders in the Department of Psychiatry at University of Medicine and Dentistry of New Jersey:

- a clear presenting complaint
- a complete history of the present illness
- past medical and psychological history
- a patient interview, with a mental status examination appropriate to cognitive capacity
- a summary and formulation
- a diagnosis according to criteria set forth in the DSM IV (1994), modified as necessary, along with recommendations keyed to the diagnosis

Many programs also use standardized assessment instruments.

When a psychiatric diagnosis cannot be established, consideration should be given to objective indices, such as the frequency and severity of maladaptive behavior. Especially troublesome is the use of psychiatric medications based on vague impressions of behavior. For example, Chadsey-Rusch and Sprague (1989) found that decisions to maintain consumers' neuroleptic drugs were linked more closely to the staff members' perceptions than to objective data such as frequency counts.

Training

Education is crucial to improving standards of practice. For example, Avorn et al. (1992) evaluated the impact of a comprehensive outreach program that provided physicians with an opportunity to attend workshops on psychoactive medications. A pre-post, matched-sample control group design was used with nearly 400 consumers in each group. Consumers whose physicians were involved in the educational program experienced a significant decrease in psychoactive medication use compared with those in the control group. The results suggest that education is effective in the promotion of appropriate use of psychoactive medications. When health care professionals have the knowledge they need to be more effective, the role of teams may change from regulation to service coordination.

CONSTITUTION AND OPERATION OF TEAMS

Various aspects of creating and operating teams have been discussed in the literature. Some of these are summarized here.

Composition of Teams

Teams usually have a wide range of participants. Who comprises a team depends on both the purposes of the team and whether the team is located in the community or in an institution. The following are some specific examples of team variations.

- Findholt and Emmett (1990) constituted a team that included an attending physician, a registered nurse, a registered pharmacist, a doctoral-level psychologist, the agency's supervisor of education, a director of residential living, and direct-care staff members. They suggested that optional participants might include the family and other interested people.
- Briggs (1989) suggested that a team in an institution might include a primary care physician, a psychiatrist, a nurse-practitioner, a nurse, a psychologist, a social worker, and direct-care staff members.
- A team constituted by Glaser and Morreau (1986) consisted of an attending physician, a clinical nurse, a pharmacist, a psychologist, a social worker, and the agency's direct-care staff and administrator.
- In one of the few reports of a community-based team, Lepler et al. (1993) described a team that included a nurse-practitioner as the chair, a behavior specialist or a psychologist, direct-care staff members, family members or an advocate, and the consumer. Although the community-based psychiatrists were unable to attend team meetings, the team's recommendations were discussed with them at the consumers' regularly scheduled appointments.
- Teams described by Schalock et al. (1985) included agency staff such as psychologists, social workers, administrators, and others. These teams forwarded their recommendations to the community-based psychiatrist, who considered their suggestions. The psychiatrist remained the final decision maker regarding the prescription of medication, but the team had the authority to discontinue the treatment if the psychiatrist did not implement their recommendations.

Generally, these examples concern teams that were constituted primarily for the purpose of reviewing psychoactive medication (see Findholt & Emmet, 1990; Lepler et al., 1993). At many community agencies, however, the teams that monitor medications have been constituted for some other purpose, such as monitoring residential, educational, employment, or habilitation services (Glaser & Morreau, 1986). When teams are constituted to monitor a variety of services in addition to psychoactive medication, their composition will be dictated by their specific functions and duties.

Consumers

Unfortunately, many teams may be operated at the convenience of their professional members in a manner that discourages consumer and family participation. For example, meetings may be scheduled more at the convenience of the professional members, without adequate consideration of the schedule of consumers and their families. Too few teams have considered consumers and family members to be equal partners in the decision-making process. A notable exception, however, was the community-based team reported by Lepler et al. (1993). This team recognized consumers and families as full partners, demonstrating that a partnership can be accomplished in a practical and effective manner. In agencies where teams only review psychoactive medications, issues of consumer rights may be handled by human rights committees. In many other agencies, however, teams are charged with enforcing the rights of patients and consumers regarding psychoactive medications.

Teams need to consider a number of issues regarding informed consent. They need to ensure that consent is truly informed. The consent should be based on the consumer's receiving adequate information about treatments, risks, and benefits. The information should be presented in an understandable, nontechnical manner. Where needed, alternative formats should be provided, such as translations, audiotapes, and braille. Teams should not assume automatically that people with mental retardation are incapable of giving consent. Although many people with mental retardation have difficulty providing fully informed consent, several studies indicate that when consumers are given training and support, they can provide some degree of informed consent (Lindsey, 1994; Lindsey & Luckasson, 1991; Morris, Niederbuhl, & Mahr, 1993). Teams should ensure that such training is available.

Teams should make every effort to ensure that consumers either accept or reject treatment. When a person is unable to provide consent, and there is no family member or guardian available, teams should work with a human rights committee. They can identify a proxy consent-provider—such as a human rights officer, the agency's chief operating officer, or a representative of an advocacy agency—to act in the best interest of the individual.

Teams need to pay much more attention to consumers, families, and guardians. In particular, they need to provide timely notifications of meetings, which they often do not do. Consumers and families should have meaningful choices in treatment options. Teams should discuss ways to provide consumers and families with decision-making authority. The published literature on teams provides few discussions of the role of consumers and families, suggesting that this topic has not received adequate attention.

Authority of Teams

Agencies need to define the authority of teams, especially regarding the roles of consumers and physicians on issues of medication. In our view, patients should have the final authority to accept or to reject treatment. When patients are not competent, the authority should rest with the family or guardian.

Who is ultimately responsible, the team or the physician? The various published articles on teams do not address the issue of ultimate responsibility. The issue is important, however, and it is frequently raised by attending physicians. As far as we could determine from the literature, there is no precedent for the removal of either legal or ethical responsibility from the physician regarding the course of a patient's medical treatment. We could find no reported instances in which the final responsibility for medical decisions was taken away from physicians and given to a team.

Emergencies

Special rules may be needed for emergency situations. In emergencies, physicians need to be able to act without having to consult first with a team because teams may not be able to meet on very short notice. Emergency plans should permit physicians to act as required by a situation. The plans also should specify how quickly a team must subsequently convene.

Team Functions

Teams may be constituted for a variety of purposes, including monitoring medications, strengthening the process of treatment decision making, and implement-

ing a particular philosophy of treatment. For example, the team described by Schalock et al. (1985) implemented the agency's philosophy that, whenever possible, behavioral programming should be instituted instead of psychoactive medication. This team recommended psychoactive medications only after a systematic behavioral program had failed to eliminate a maladaptive behavior. The final decisions about medication, however, were made by physicians, not the team.

Lepler et al. (1993) identified the following goals for their team: (a) ensuring proper communication between personnel from day and residential settings with regard to medication monitoring and decision making; (b) establishing a system in which medication decisions are based on observations of specific index behaviors; (c) using the most positive, least restrictive types of interventions that have a chance of improving an individual's functioning and quality of life; (d) coordinating interventions and proceeding in a systematic manner in the evaluation of each treatment variable and its effect on an individual's performance; and (e) incorporating the expertise of professionals, direct-services staff, and, when possible, the consumer in the decision-making process. The team's primary functions were to: (a) differentiate among psychiatric, medical, or behavioral reasons for maladaptive behavior; (b) monitor changes in an individual's status using objective behavioral measurements; and (c) recommend appropriate adjustments of medication or behavior interventions.

Briggs (1989) described a team that met monthly to review drug and behavioral programming. This team monitored the effects of treatment on specified, measurable index behaviors. The team reviewed side effects and determined future drug use according to criteria previously agreed upon. The attending physician was part of the team.

Glaser and Morreau (1986) described a team that regulated and monitored the prescription of antipsychotic agents. This team addressed the specific concern, widely shared among both consumer advocates and leading psychiatrists, that antipsychotic medications are overused with people with mental retardation. The team also assessed the effects of medication changes on the number and types of injuries reported.

Additionally, teams can have important educative functions. They can help busy physicians keep up with the latest research results. They can help psychologists and social workers learn about specific medications. They can teach direct-care staff to recognize side effects and to use behavior programs. Training also should be provided to family members, school professionals, and others providing services to the consumer.

Medications Subject to Review

There is no consensus on precisely which medications should be subject to review from a team. Some authorities hold that teams should review medications only when they are given in the absence of a psychiatric diagnosis. The more widely held view, however, is that all psychoactive medications should be reviewed, even when psychiatric diagnoses have been made. Several states have policies defining a psychoactive medication as any drug administered for the management and treatment of behavior. Under these policies, the purpose for which the drug is prescribed, not its pharmacological characteristics, determines its classification as a psychoactive drug.

Sources of Information

Teams participating in treatment planning should take into account reports of the following information.

1. The team should have a psychiatric report in which either a diagnosis of mental illness is made or a discussion is presented indicating why a diagnosis is not possible. The report should be based on information concerning sleep patterns, appetite, activity level, mood, presence or absence of hallucinations, delusional thinking, suicidal or homicidal ideation, confusion, regression, and other possible psychiatric symptoms. Standardized dual diagnosis instruments may be helpful. The team also should review behavioral data, such as the frequency, duration, and severity of the maladaptive behavior. The team should evaluate the responses of staff or others to the behavior and try to identify antecedent stimulus conditions that affect the occurrence of the behavior.
2. The team should have a report from a recent physical examination, made by a physician who is knowledgeable about developmental disabilities. The team should consider the possibility that behavior problems are caused by a physical problem such as a seizure disorder, fatigue, or an abscessed tooth. The medical data reviewed by the team should include the person's seizure history and previous medication history.
3. The team should have reports indicating the consumer's psychological functioning and social history.
4. The team should look in the records for a signed, informed consent from either the consumer or the consumer's family, guardian, or both.
5. The team should review previous behavior management or treatment plans, examine facts about how well those plans worked, and consider less restrictive procedures. Behavior management or treatment programs should include guidelines on accelerative and decelerative interventions to run concurrently with psychoactive medication administration.
6. The team should know the individual's current medications and have information about their interactions.
7. The team should consider alternative explanations for behavioral changes. For example, did a favorite staff person recently leave the agency? Did a friend or family member become ill?
8. The team should determine whether potential adverse reactions and side effects are documented for each medication. Procedures to evaluate the emergence of such reactions should be in place, such as regularly scheduled evaluations by nursing staff.
9. The team should consider whether the dosage levels are appropriate.
10. The team should compare the individual's current behavior with baseline information to evaluate medication dosages and the possibility that changes are needed. Staff should gather behavioral data in a reliable, systematic manner during baseline and treatment periods.
11. If drug holidays are safe for the individual, the team should ensure that they are used to evaluate the continued need for medications.
12. The team should consider the possibility that aberrant behavior is related to gender- or age-specific health issues, such as premenstrual syndrome, menopausal symptoms, or arthritis.
13. The team should know how long the individual has received medications.
14. The team should have evaluations of the effects of all treatments on the individual's behavioral, social, communicative, and cognitive functioning.

Teams should talk with people who are familiar with the circumstances, the consumer, and the family. These sources can corroborate or contradict the written documentation. They may provide details not available in written records.

Training of Team Members

Team members who assist with treatment decisions should receive training about psychoactive medications and indications in people with mental retardation and developmental disabilities. This should include training regarding the various types of psychoactive medications, indicated uses, common misuses, common side effects, and possible adverse reactions. Team members need reference information about specific medications, dosages, and potential side effects. Additionally, team members should have training in basic decelerative and accelerative behavioral procedures and in data collection procedures.

The amount of training needed varies depending on what the team is supposed to do. Teams that are constituted exclusively in an oversight and monitoring role need training in the diagnosis of psychiatric illness and in the administration of psychoactive medications.

Community-Based Teams

Researchers have focused mostly on facility-based teams that are charged with reviewing psychoactive medications. Because the number of people living in congregate residential settings is declining, more attention needs to be paid to the functions of teams in community settings, such as in group homes and supported living arrangements.

CONCLUSIONS

We have reached agreement on the following points.

1. Agencies can justify constituting teams that have clearly defined goals and objectives.

(a) Teams reduce inappropriate uses of psychoactive medications. In the past, medications have been overused in enough situations to warrant oversight. The potentially deleterious side effects from many of these medications make overuse a particular concern.

(b) A number of factors contribute to inappropriate uses of psychoactive medications. These include inadequate oversight; the absence of research on safety and efficacy specific to people with mental retardation and developmental disabilities; inadequate attention to psychiatric diagnosis; inadequate attention to dosage levels; inadequate

monitoring of treatment and side effects; lack of relevant blood tests; the prescription of medication for indefinite time periods, with no identified endpoint of treatment; inadequate consideration of possible health factors causing irritation, pain, fatigue, or frustration; inadequate consideration of environmental changes in the consumer's life; and inadequate consideration of alternatives to psychoactive medications.

(c) Teams gather information in ways that aid treatment planning. They provide physicians with broad, relatively reliable summaries of the consumer's behavior and psychological functioning. They can balance the subjective and incomplete reports physicians sometimes obtain when they talk with only a few informants about the consumer's behavior.

(d) Teams help agencies meet regulations and other legal responsibilities regarding due process and the use of psychopharmacological agents. They also help document outcomes.

2. The field of disability services has moved from congregate settings where professionals are the primary, if not sole, decision makers, to services that focus on community integration and involve consumers and their families at all levels of decision making. Teams should operate in a manner consistent with this trend.

3. People with mental retardation need access to mental health care providers who can conduct a comprehensive psychiatric review and make recommendations regarding treatment and the use of psychoactive medications.

4. Teams represent only one of a number of strategies to improve standards of practice regarding the use of psychoactive medications by people with mental retardation. Other strategies include greater use of psychiatric diagnosis and continuing education programs.

5. Practitioners have some justifiable concerns when teams are mandated. Teams are best created in a voluntary manner based on a careful consideration of specific circumstances.

6. Additional research is needed to evaluate the effects and costs of teams under various circumstances. The traditional facility-based model may not be relevant to community settings, where different models may be needed. The standard against which models of service delivery should be judged is how well they address the unique needs of the individual.

7. Teams should include the consumer, his or her family or guardian, and representatives from the medical, social, psychological, educational, and service delivery areas.

8. The attending physician is crucial to the team. If he or she cannot attend team meetings, as will be the case in many community-based programs, procedures must specify how the team's discussion and information will be relayed in a reliable manner.

(a) Each member's role must be decided. Particular attention needs to be given to the responsibilities of the physician and the team in the prescription and monitoring of medication and in the overall treatment process. The unique role of the physician warrants further discussions among consumers, family members, physicians, and other potential team members.

(b) It is unlikely, although desirable, that the consumer's physician attend every meeting. When this is not possible, the team may designate an alternative health practitioner, such as a nurse or nurse-practitioner, as the panel's liaison to accompany the individual and his or her family member to the physician's office to discuss issues raised at the full panel meeting.

9. There is an urgent need for increased training of psychiatrists, physicians, and other health care providers who serve people with mental retardation and developmental disabilities. These professionals need information on the use, abuse, and misuse of psychoactive medications.

10. People with mental retardation and their families must play a meaningful role in decision making regarding treatment and services.

(a) The team and others have a responsibility to ensure that consumers and their families are actively involved in the decision-making process.

(b) There needs to be a discussion among all concerned regarding the role of the consumer and his or her family in the decision-making process. Consumers should have the right to refuse treatment and seek both alternative options and second opinions. Normally, the consumer, in conjunction with his or her family or guardian, should have the final word about taking medications.

11. Teams should not be created solely for the purpose of reducing reliance on psychoactive medication. Instead, the goal should be to reduce only inappropriate uses of such medications.

12. Team members should receive training in the use, abuse, risks, and benefits of psychoactive medications; components of a psychiatric evaluation; basic accelerative and decelerative behavior management techniques; and data collection procedures.

13. Teams that are part of treatment decision making should perform the following tasks:

(a) provide reliable information to the physician;

(b) ensure that a current psychiatric evaluation is available;

(c) ensure that a current psychological evaluation is available;

(d) monitor behavior and health;

(e) respond to emergency situations;

(f) ensure that the treatment regimen is being carried out; and

(g) coordinate interventions, including medications, behavior programming, and other health-related areas such as diet.

14. Teams participating in treatment decision making should consider information from a variety of sources, including the consumer and the family; medical, social, and psychological histories; diagnostic and previous intervention results; and direct-care staff members.

15. Teams should ensure that their agencies are in compliance with applicable regulations.

16. Teams should work with human rights and other committees to ensure informed consent, adequate notification, and the participation of consumers, families, and guardians in the decision-making process.

REFERENCES

Accreditation Council for Services for Mentally Retarded and Other Developmentally Disabled Persons (1980). *Standards for services for developmentally disabled individuals*. Washington, DC: Author.

Agran, M., & Martin, J.E. (1982). Use of psychotropic drugs by mentally retarded adults in community programs. *Journal of the Association for Persons with Severe Handicaps, 7*, 54–59.

Aman, M.G., & Singh, N.W. (1986). A critical appraisal of recent drug research in mental retardation: The Coldwater studies. *Journal of Mental Deficiency Research, 30*, 203–216.

Arnold, L. E. (1993). Clinical pharmacological issues in treating psychiatric disorders of patients with mental retardation. *Annals of Clinical Psychiatry, 5*, 189–197.

Avorn, J., Soumerai, S.B., Everitt, D.E., Ross-Degnan, D., Beers, M.H., Sherman, D., Shalom-Schatz, S.R., & Fields, D. (1992). A randomized trial of a program to reduce the use of psychoactive drugs in nursing homes. *The New England Journal of Medicine, 327*, 168-173.

Bishop, A.C. (1992). Empirical approach to psychopharmacology for institutionalized individuals with severe or profound mental retardation. *Mental Retardation, 30*, 283–288.

Bouras, N., Brooks, D., & Drummond, K. (1993). Community psychiatric services for people with mental retardation. In

N. Bouras (Ed.), *Mental health in mental retardation*. New York: Cambridge University Press.

Briggs, R. (1989). Monitoring and evaluating psychotropic drug use for persons with mental retardation: A follow-up report. *American Journal on Mental Retardation, 93,* 633–639.

Brown, G.W. (1990). Rule-making and justice: A cautionary tale. *Mental Retardation, 28,* 83–87.

Burd, L., Fisher, W., Vesely, B.N., Williams, M., Derbeshian, J., & Leech, C. (1991). Prevalence of psychoactive drug use among North Dakota group home residents. *American Journal on Mental Retardation, 96,* 119–126.

Chadsey-Rusch, J., & Sprague, R.L. (1989). Maladaptive behaviors associated with neuroleptic drug maintenance. *American Journal on Mental Retardation, 93,* 607–617.

Fawcett, J. (1995). Happy DSM-IV to all— Do we have a new baby or a Frankenstein? *Psychiatric Annals, 25,* 9–10.

Ficker-Terrill, C., & Rowitz, L. (1991). Choices. *Mental Retardation, 29,* 63–64.

Findholt, N.E. & Emmett, C.G. (1990). Impact of interdisciplinary team review on psychotropic drug use with persons who have mental retardation. *Mental Retardation, 28,* 41–46.

Gardner, J.F., & Chapman, M.S. (1993). *Developing staff competencies for supporting people with developmental disabilities: An orientation handbook* (2nd ed.). Baltimore, MD: Paul H. Brookes.

Glaser, B.A., & Morreau, L.E. (1986). Effects of interdisciplinary team review on the use of antipsychotic agents with severely and profoundly mentally retarded persons. *American Journal on Mental Retardation, 90,* 371–379.

Gowdey, C.W., Zarfas, D.E., & Phipps, S. (1987). Audit of psychoactive drug prescriptions in group homes. *Mental Retardation, 25,* 331–334.

Havercamp, S. (1996). *Psychiatric symptoms and mental retardation: Reliability of rating scales as a function of IQ.* Unpublished master's thesis, Department of Psychology, Ohio State University.

Kastner, T.A., & Walsh, K. (1994). Interdisciplinary team review of psychotropic drug use in community settings. *Mental Retardation, 32,* 243–245.

King, B.H., DeAntonio, C.A., McCracken, J.T., Forness, S.R., & Ackerland, V. (1994). Psychiatric consultation in severe and profound mental retardation. *American Journal of Psychiatry, 151,* 1802–1809.

LaMendola, W., Zaharia, E.S., & Carver, M. (1980). Reducing psychotropic drug use in an institution for the retarded. *Hospital and Community Psychiatry, 31,* 271–272.

Lepler, S., Hodas, A., & Cotter-Mack, A. (1993). Implementation of an interdisciplinary psychotropic drug review process for community-based facilities. *Mental Retardation, 31,* 307–315.

Lepler, S., Hodas, A., & Cotter-Mack, A. (1994). What input do community-based psychiatrists need from staff and families of our consumers? *Mental Retardation, 32,* 245–247.

Levitas, A.S., & Gilson, S.F. (1990). Toward the developmental understanding of the impact of mental retardation on assessment of psychopathology. In E. Dibble & D.G. Gray (Eds.), *Assessment of behavior problems in persons with mental retardation living in the community* (pp. 71–106). Rockville, MD: National Institute of Mental Health.

Lindsey, P. (1994). Assessing the ability of adults with mental retardation to give direct consent for residential placements: A follow-up study for the Consent Screening Interview. *Education and Training in Mental Retardation and Developmental Disability, 29,* 155–164.

Lindsey, P., & Luckasson, R. (1991). Consent Screening Interview for community residential placement: Report on the initial pilot study data. *Mental Retardation, 29,* 119–124.

Luckasson, R., Coulter, D.L., Polloway, E.A., Reiss, S., Schalock, R.L., Snell, M.E., Spitalnik, D.M., & Stark, J.A. (1992). *Mental retardation: Definition, classification, and systems of supports.* Washington, DC: American Association on Mental Retardation.

Morris, C.D., Niederbuhl, J.M., & Mahr, J.M. (1993). Determining the capability of individuals with mental retardation to give informed consent. *American Journal on Mental Retardation, 98,* 263–272.

New York State Association for Retarded Citizens v. Rockefeller, Nos. 72 Civ. 356, 72 Civ. 357 (E.D. N.Y., filed April 30, 1975).

Nirje, B. (1972). The right to self-determination. In W. Wolfensberger (Ed.), *Normalization* (pp. 176–200). Ontario, Canada: National Institute on Mental Retardation.

Perske, R. (1989). *Proceedings of the national conference on self-determination.* Minneapolis, MN: Institute on Community Integration.

Poindexter, A.R. (1989). Psychotropic drug patterns in a large ICF/MR facility: A ten-year experience. *American Journal on Mental Retardation, 93,* 624–626.

Reiss, S. (1992). Assessment of a man with a dual diagnosis. *Mental Retardation, 30,* 1–6.

Reiss, S. (1994). *Handbook of challenging behavior: Mental health aspects of mental retardation.* Worthington, Ohio: IDS Publishing Corporation.

Reiss, S., & Rojahn, J. (1993). Joint occurrence of depression and aggression in children and adults with mental retardation. *Journal of Intellectual Disability Research, 37,* 287–294.

Rinck, C., Guidry, J., & Calkins, C.F. (1989). Review of states' practices on the use of psychotropic medication. *American Journal on Mental Retardation, 93,* 627–632.

Schalock, R.L., Foley, J.W., Toulouse, A., & Stark, J.A. (1985). Medication and programming in controlling the behavior of mentally retarded individuals in community settings. *American Journal of Mental Deficiency, 89,* 503–509.

Sovner, R. (1986). Limiting factors in the use of DSM-III criteria with mentally ill/mentally retarded persons. *Psychopharmacology Bulletin, 22,* 1055-1059.

Sprague, R.L. (1977). Overview of psychopharmacology for the retarded in the United States. In P. Mittler (Ed.), *Research to practice in mental retardation: Biomedical aspects* (Vol. 3). Baltimore, MD: University Park Press.

Sprague, R.L., & Baxley, G.B. (1978). Drugs for behavior management. In J. Wortis (Ed.), *Mental retardation and developmental disabilities* (Vol. 10, pp. 92–129). New York: Brunner/Mazel.

Sprague, R.L., & Werry, J.S. (1971). Methodology of psychopharmacological studies with the retarded. In N.R. Ellis (Ed.), *International review of research in mental retardation* (Vol. 5, pp. 147–219). New York: Academic Press.

Szymanski, L.S., & Tanguy, P.E. (1980). *Emotional disorders of mentally retarded persons: Assessment, treatment and consultation.* Baltimore, MD: University Park Press.

Taylor, S.J., Bogdan, R., & Racino, J.A. (1991). *Life in the community: Case studies of organizations supporting people with disabilities.* Baltimore, MD: Paul H. Brookes.

Wolfensberger, W. (1972). *Normalization: The principle of normalization.* Toronto, Canada: National Institute on Mental Retardation.

Wyatt v. Stickney, 344 F. Supp. 387 (filed 1972).

Instruments for Assessing Effects of Psychotropic Medication

Anne DesNoyers Hurley[1], Steven Reiss[2], Michael G. Aman[3], Luis Salvador-Carulla[4], Howard Demb[5], Earl Loschen[6], and Stuart Einfeld[7]

INTRODUCTION

Since the mid-1980s, mental retardation researchers have been developing instruments for the assessment of psychopathology in people with an IQ below the range of 70 to 75. Among the earliest and best known of these instruments are the Aberrant Behavior Checklist (ABC; Aman & Singh (1986), the Psychopathology Inventory for Mentally Retarded Adults ([PIMRA]; Matson; 1997), and the Reiss Screen for Maladaptive Behavior (Reiss, 1988). Originally, the ABC was intended as an aid in the assessment of drug treatment effects, the PIMRA was intended as a research instrument, and the Reiss Screen as a cost-effective means to screen large numbers of people for possible eligibility for dual diagnosis (mental health/mental retardation) programs. Over time, however, these instruments, plus a number of newer instruments such as the Emotional Problems Scales: Self-Report Inventory and Behavior Rating Scales (Strohmer & Prout, 1991), have been used for a wider range of purposes than was originally envisioned.

SIGNIFICANCE OF INSTRUMENTS

Assessment instruments provide a systematic method for describing clinical phenomena. The basic elements of assessment instruments are test stimuli and responses. The test stimuli may be unstructured (e.g., pictures, inkblots) or structured (e.g., objective questions), and the responses may be unstructured (i.e., a person may report anything) or structured (e.g., multiple-choice format). An example of an instrument with unstructured stimuli and responses is the Thematic Apperception Test (Murray, 1943), in which the person makes up stories about a series of drawings of ambiguous scenes. An example of an instrument with unstructured stimuli and structured responses is the Apperceptive Personality Test/Mental Retardation (Reiss, Benson, & Szyszko, 1992), in which the person first makes up stories about four drawings of ambiguous stimuli and then completes

a multiple-choice questionnaire about the story characters and story themes. An instrument with both structured stimuli and unstructured responses is any diagnostic interview in which a specific schedule of questions is asked and the person can say anything in response. Examples of instruments with both structured stimuli and structured responses are the ABC, PIMRA, and Reiss Screen, in which specific questions are asked within a multiple-choice format.

All instruments can be interpreted either subjectively or objectively. Subjective interpretation is based on the opinions of a clinician who has had extensive experience examining test results from many people. Objective interpretation is based on objective rules applied to numerical scores. Users of standardized instruments compare the person's scores with those obtained from various reference or normative groups. If the instrument has been validated, objective scores indicate an observed clinical characteristic or treatment outcome.

DIAGNOSES AND TREATMENT

Ideally, the treating psychiatrist will prescribe drug therapy based on either a diagnosis or an objective description of the person's aberrant behavior. The physician uses the diagnosis as a guide in determining whether or not drug therapy will be used, in selecting medications and dosage levels, and in evaluating treatment effectiveness.

Clinicians must weigh at least five considerations when determining a psychiatric diagnosis. First, the same

1 Director of Clinical Services, Bay Cove Human Services, MR/DD Division and Assistant Professor of Psychiatry, Tufts University School of Medicine, Boston, MA

2 Professor of Psychology and Psychiatry and Director, Nisonger Center, The Ohio State University, Columbus, OH

3 Professor of Psychology and Psychiatry, Nisonger Center, The Ohio State University, Columbus, OH

4 Associate Professor of Medical Psychology, Universidad de Cadiz, Spain

5 Assistant Professor of Psychiatry, Albert Einstein College of Medicine, Bronx, NY

6 Chief, Department of Psychiatry, Southern Illinois University, Springfield, IL

7 Lecturer in Child Psychiatry, University of Sydney, Sydney, Australia

behavior considered to be a symptom of mental illness in a person with average intelligence is sometimes misattributed to mental retardation in a person with substantially below-average intelligence. This phenomenon, which has been called *diagnostic overshadowing* (Reiss, Levitan & Szysko, 1982), suggests a tendency to underdiagnose mental disorders in people with mental retardation. Second, people with cognitive impairment have difficulty complying with standard diagnostic interviews —questions during clinical interviews may be misunderstood (Sovner, 1986). Stress or mental illness may cause the person to function below the minimal degree of cognitive performance needed to respond effectively to diagnostic questions. Third, people with mental retardation may have aberrant behaviors that existed prior to a mental illness but that were intensified by mental illness. Diagnosticians often mistakenly assume that the aberrant behaviors began with the mental illness. For example, self-injurious behavior may increase dramatically in frequency or severity when a person is under stress or suffering from a mental illness. Fourth, many clinicians do not recognize symptoms of psychopathology when they are manifested within the context of limited developmental skills. For example, in some people with mental retardation, a feeling that one can drive a car may indicate grandiosity, which is symptomatic of mania. Fifth, in diagnostic interviews, people may hide mental health problems or feel embarrassed to ask for clarification of questions that are misunderstood (Reiss, 1994). Individuals with mental retardation are especially prone to hide their disability (Edgerton, 1967).

People with mental retardation may present with mental illness in unique ways that makes utilization of standard assessment techniques difficult or inappropriate. It is most important, then, that sound instrumentation be developed and used to aid in the diagnostic process and in evaluating treatment response specifically for this population. Potentially, instruments can provide objective information that may help clinicians determine a diagnostic formulation. When used in this manner, however, instruments *should not be the sole or exclusive basis for a diagnosis.* At best, instruments can provide sources of information to be considered in the context of all available information.

Additionally, the development of a diagnostic formulation is often complex because a person can have more than one psychiatric disorder at the same time (Bernstein, 1991; Biederman, Newcorn, & Sprich, 1991; Bird, Gould, & Staghezza, 1993; Keller et al., 1992; Pliszka, 1992). This occurrence has been most often referred to as comorbidity. For example, a high prevalence of comorbidity exists across three disruptive behavior disorders in childhood called attention deficit hyperactivity disorder (ADHD), oppositional defiant disorder, and conduct disorder (Biederman et al., 1991).

Comorbidity can occur as combinations of psychiatric disorders, neurodevelopmental disorders, and other neurobiological conditions. For instance, a person with mental retardation who has temporal lobe epilepsy caused by a lesion in the dominant hemisphere may show abnormal behavior intermittently depending on the timing of the epileptic discharges in the brain or how successful the antiepileptic drug treatment regiment has been in achieving remission of seizures. Such a brain lesion may cause dysphasia in some instances and lead to autistic behavior as well (Hauser, DeLong, & Rosman, 1975). Also, the level of intelligence may vary transitorily or show progressive decline because of a progressive underlying disorder such as neoplastic disease or antiepileptic drug intoxication (Iivanainen, Viukari, & Helle, 1977). Thus comorbidity, including neurobiological conditions, may further complicate treatment plans. Comorbidity also is common among various affective and anxiety disorders (Bernstein & Garfinkel, 1986; Kashani et al., 1987; Woolston et al., 1989). A good psychometric instrument should help clinicians avoid overlooking comorbid conditions. Because a number of scales should be elevated, the total score on the instrument should be high when comorbid conditions are present.

Instruments can play an important role in evaluating the treatment response of psychoactive agents. When an instrument is used to evaluate treatment effects, it should be administered prior to drug therapy to obtain baseline data and again at selected points during drug therapy. Weekly or monthly intervals are often used; if the ratings are taken too frequently, some staff may defer to checking automatically the same rating every time the scale is completed. Instruments also can be used to help evaluate side effects. For example, if a person with mental retardation suffering from depression is treated with a neuroleptic medicine, the presence of sedation may be indicated by a rise in the Lethargy/Social Withdrawal index on the ABC, a decrease on the Hyperactivity index, and no change on other measures.

Instruments can be used to help evaluate treatment responses. A custom-designed rating scale that includes items on observed affect, hours of sleep, percentage of food taken at each meal, and change in weight could be constructed by a clinician. The scale should use numeric anchor points to maximize possible reliability. In a case of depression, for example, a 5-point scale for observed affect based on crying/sad faces could be constructed using anchor points as follows: (1) *nearly all the time*, (2) *75% of the waking day*, (3) *50% of the waking day*, (4) *25% of the waking day*, and (5) *rarely*. The scale should be based on the specific presenting complaints of the person being treated. The monitoring of treatment response is difficult in cases in which behavioral symptoms occur intermittently (such as behavioral abnormalities associated with epilepsy, or are otherwise unstable, such as progressive symptoms). In such cases, it may be difficult to obtain reliable data.

EVALUATING AND SELECTING INSTRUMENTS

Types and Purposes of Instruments

A number of instruments have been developed to assess psychiatric and behavior disorders in people with mental retardation. These scales are standardized questionnaires completed by either the person (a self-report instrument) or by a caregiver or informant (a rating scale). When completed by the person, the instrument may assess feelings, thoughts, or behavior. When completed by caregivers, the instrument is focused on observable behavior.

Psychiatric and behavior instruments serve two purposes: They assist the clinician in quantifying observable symptoms and signs, and they assist the clinician in determining a psychiatric diagnosis using a conventional system such as the DSM-IV or ICD-10. Child rating scales, for example, may focus on behavioral manifestations such as hyperactivity, and these results can be used to diagnose psychiatric disorders such as ADHD. Rating scales may also enhance the study of treatment responses by providing multiple ratings over time, such as for changes in mood.

Psychometrically sound rating scales comprise multiple items that assess one or more domains (i.e., categories or scales) of behavior. A single-item scale is psychometrically unsound; usually, 5 to 20 items are used per scale so that there is adequate sampling of the behavioral class or diagnosis of interest. Many instruments use Likert scales, which provide numerical points. For example, a nurse may rate the frequency of behavior into five categories, such as 0 (*never*) to 4 (*frequently*). In this case, the Likert scale uses 5 points, with the number 0 representing *not present*. Rating scales vary by the number of different numerical categories they contain (Bech, 1993).

Characteristics of Informant Rating Scales

Rating scales completed by informants such as caregivers are often the instruments of choice when treating patients with mental retardation. The limitations and biases of such instruments are often less pronounced than are those associated with alternatives. A certain amount of subjectivity exists when using informants, because the rater is required to judge another person's level of internal feeling through external observations and the person's statements. Therefore, it is desirable to use average rating scores from multiple informants who have contact with the individual under a variety of conditions (Reiss, 1988). With children, information can be obtained from a parent, a teacher, a mental health worker, or a child care worker. With adults, information can be obtained from a supervisor at work, a teacher, a parent, a mental health worker, a spouse, or a worker in a group home or residential center.

Different raters often provide somewhat different information about the same person (Achenbach, 1991). In assessing childhood psychiatric disorders, for example, parents appear to be the best informants for observable behavior (e.g., poor peer relations or acting out), whereas children appear to be better informants of their own feelings and sleep patterns (Bird, Gould, & Staghezza, 1992; Fendrich, Weissman, & Warner 1991; Kashani, Orvaschel, Burk, & Reid, 1985; Weissman, Orvaschel, & Padian, 1980). When comparing child-parent to child-teacher ratings on the psychiatric instruments, researchers found that overall agreement between self-reported behavior on the one hand, and parents' and teachers' ratings on the other hand, were low (r = 0.13-0.35), although somewhat higher for child-parent than for child-teacher (Achenbach, McConaughy, & Howell, 1987; Williams, McGee, Anderson, & Silva, 1989). The Developmentally Delayed Children's Behavior Checklist (Einfeld & Tonge, 1991), a broad spectrum instrument designed to describe disturbed emotions and behaviors in children and young adults with moderate to severe mental retardation, was found to have high interrater reliability for raters within groups (e.g., within parents, teachers, or nurses only), but lower interrater reliability between groups (e.g., between teachers and aides and vice versa).

The relationship between reports of different raters (e.g., teacher and child) may vary with the type of behavior (e.g., aggression), the population of children (community, outpatient, inpatient), or the type of instruments used. There is, therefore, a need for rating instruments that can give reliable information across observers and classes of behaviors. Informants are essential aids to the clinician working with people with mental retardation. Individuals who observe the patient in many different settings, who are familiar with people with mental retardation generally, and who ideally have known the patient for a significant time, can supply information that the clinician must have in order to consider a psychiatric diagnosis and to judge the effectiveness of pharmacotherapy.

Raters differ on how well they know the consumer. Parents generally have an extensive knowledge of their child's behavior, although not necessarily of their child's mental state or feelings. When program staff are used as informants, problems regarding their knowledge of the consumer may arise. A staff member's knowledge of a consumer often differs from a parent's intimate, developmental knowledge. Additionally, each staff member has different types of contact, for example through vocational programs, day residential programs, or night programs. Reading level and educational level of staff also account for great variation in their ability to answer questions accurately on rating scales.

Rating scales also vary widely according to the qualifications of the intended rater. Some instruments were developed with a particular role or profession in mind, such as the Nurse's Observation Scale for Inpatient Observation (Honigfield & Klett, 1965). Even within that profession, however, qualifications can vary. Nurses may have little psychiatric experience or extensive experience in psychiatry. The answers given by nurses of different experiences will vary, because what an experienced nurse considers aberrant may be different from what an inexperienced nurse considers it to be.

Many rating scales used with people with mental retardation were designed for use with professional raters. However, some scales (such as the Reiss Screen for Maladaptive Behavior) were designed for use with caregivers who know the individual well. Because nonprofessional raters may be unfamiliar with technical language, the Reiss Screen supplies a word (such as *delusion*) followed by a simple definition, and the rater is required to rate it in accordance with definitions provided for *no problem, problem,* or *major problem.* The PIMRA, in contrast, is administered verbally, which allows the interviewer to explain the item and give examples.

Psychometric Issues

Reliability and Validity. Instruments have been evaluated in terms of their reliability and validity. Reliability refers to the degree to which an instrument consistently measures any symptoms or diagnostic category, whereas validity refers to the degree to which an instrument measures the specific symptoms or diagnostic category it purports to measure. When an instrument is unreliable, it tends to yield significantly different results when administered to the same individuals. When an instrument is reliable, but not valid, it tends to yield the same results over time, but the results inaccurately reflect the characteristic of interest.

Reiss (1994) has argued that, historically, certain psychometric criteria have been overemphasized, and others underemphasized, in the evaluation of psychiatric instruments. For example, Reiss has suggested that the criterion of internal reliability should be given substantial weight, because it determines the maximum possible validity coefficient. (Internal reliability is the extent to which various items within a scale measure the same characteristic.) It is recommended that only instruments with Cronbach alpha values of at least .7 be considered for use. Reiss (1994, 1997) also has suggested that factor analysis is widely misinterpreted and misused.

Researchers are still assessing the validity of the instruments currently available. A number of available instruments, however, provide extensive information on reliability and related psychometric properties. Acceptable levels of reliability vary considerably depending on the length of the scale (longer scales should have higher reliability then more brief scales) and the nature of the phenomena being measured (because mood varies considerably over time, acceptable test-retest reliabilities for mood scales are as low as .6).

Sensitivity and Specificity. Instruments must be used carefully to avoid the pitfalls of overdiagnosis and underdiagnosis of mental illness. Two concepts address this issue. *Sensitivity* indicates the percentage of people with a given disorder who are correctly detected by the instrument as having the disorder. *Specificity* is the percentage of people incorrectly classified as having a disorder they do not have. A test can be sensitive without being specific and vice versa. Sensitivity and specificity are calculated by estimating the actual occurrence of a disorder for each individual in a population and then comparing this with the results of a testing procedure in that population (Riegelman, 1981). When new instruments are developed and tested, investigators should provide sensitivity and specificity estimates in addition to data on reliability and validity. This information will be helpful to clinicians when they use the instrument.

Task Specificity. One factor to consider when selecting a dual diagnosis instrument is whether the instrument has subscales of particular interest in a given case. For example, the ABC has scales that measure irritability and hyperactivity, which are relevant to the treatment of ADHD; the Reiss Screen has scales that measure depression. Which instrument one selects may depend on whether the individual has an attention deficit disorder or is depressed. One disadvantage of developing one's own rating instrument that is tailored to the needs of a particular person is the absence of normative data. It is often helpful to be able to compare a person's behavior and symptoms to an appropriate reference group. This is one of the major advantages of standardized instruments.

Other relevant factors in selecting an instrument are length, cost, and demonstrated sensitivity to changes in behavior resulting from treatment. Another important consideration is the instrument's coverage of target behaviors. Some instruments are generic in structure, whereas others address specific diagnostic disorders. Some instruments are narrow and assess one or two specific problem areas, whereas others are multifaceted. For example, both the Beck Depression Inventory (Beck, Ward, Mendelson, Nock, & Erbaugh, 1961) and the Zung Depression Rating Scale (Zung, 1965) have been widely used in research studies on depression. The Zung scale has been modified for people with mild to moderate levels of mental retardation (Burt, Loveland, & Lewis, 1992).

Population Parameters. Each instrument must be selected for use based on the population for which it was developed. The standardization population should be representative of the people for whom the instrument will be used. For example, a test of schizophrenia should include a normative sample of patients with schizophrenia. The sample should exclude people with organic brain disorders, such as neoplasm or degenerative conditions manifesting predominantly as behavioral symptoms. A normative sample of mentally healthy control subjects is also needed. Additionally, the normative samples should be similar to the intended clinical populations in terms of cognitive level, gender, and ethnic composition, except where these factors have been found to be irrelevant.

Tests for people with mental retardation should include a normative sample of such people specified by their particular developmental level. For example, the Emotional Problems Scales (Strohmer & Prout, 1991) are intended to evaluate people with mild mental retardation or borderline normal intelligence. The DASH was designed for individuals with more significant levels of mental retardation (Matson, Coe, Gardner & Sovner, 1991).

Many rating scales developed for use with people who do not have mental retardation may be used with people with mild mental retardation. As the person's level of impairment increases, the use of such instruments becomes progressively less valid. People with mental retardation have many different neuropsychological profiles, which suggests a need for further stratification of the population. Problems in visual, auditory, communication, or visual-motor abilities may cause certain features of a disorder to develop with advancing age. In some cases, there is good empirical evidence that various behavioral disorders are associated with specific developmental disabilities, such as fragile X, Prader-Willi or Angelman syndromes. As was mentioned earlier, for some instruments, such as the Zung Depression Rating Scale, there are available modifications that extend the range of disability that may be assessed by the instrument (Burt et al., 1992). Clinicians must carefully consider the cognitive level required by these general instruments when using them with individuals with mental retardation.

RECOMMENDATIONS FOR USING MENTAL RETARDATION INSTRUMENTS

Whenever possible, rating instruments should be used to help evaluate the effects of psychoactive medications, including any changes in medication, such as changes in dosage levels. Specific recommendations are as follows:

1. Clinicians should familiarize themselves with the type of instruments available and become well acquainted with at least a few. Several authors have prepared summaries that describe many of the available instruments that can be used as a general introduction to what is available (Aman, 1991a, 1991b, 1993; Hogg & Raynes, 1987; Reiss, 1994). A number of instruments also are described in the next section of this chapter.

2. When first using an instrument, it is important to read carefully the instructions in the user guide or test manual and any other scientific literature that is readily available.

3. Instruments with good psychometric characteristics (reliability, validity, adequate sensitivity and specificity, sensitivity to changes in behavior resulting from treatment, etc.) will produce better results than those with less favorable properties.

4. The rating scale should be completed by competent and knowledgeable staff or family; these individuals

must be thoroughly introduced to the proper instructions to complete the scale.

5. Raters should be carefully chosen and well motivated to complete the scale, consistent with the requirements listed in the user guide or test manual.

6. Instructions to raters or self-raters should be read or presented carefully in accordance with requirements listed in the user guide or test manual.

7. Be on guard for halo and other bias effects. Halo effects are tendencies for informants to rate people based on their own feelings or on a stereotype rather than on observation. For example, a halo effect may be indicated when an informant consistently provides very high or very low ratings across all subscales. Ratings are also suspect when all items are rated exactly the same. Other sources of bias are fake-good responses, in which people rate themselves too positively, and fake-bad responses, in which people present themselves too negatively. Social desirability is a particularly important source of bias—it occurs when self-ratings are made based on what the person thinks is expected (what the examiner wants to find) rather than on personal opinion. Self-report forms always are suspect for social desirability, fake-good, and fake-bad biases. **The best way to minimize informant bias is to select two or more raters and use average scores.** This procedure also helps when ratings are taken over a long period of time and one of the raters becomes unavailable.

8. Regular follow-up assessments should be undertaken. These should occur before treatment, during pharmacotherapy, and at the conclusion of treatment.

9. Results of measures should be noted in the person's records and the physician's progress notes.

10. Diagnosis and treatment decisions should not be based solely on psychometric instruments. Instruments should be used as only one source of information in the decision-making process.

MENTAL RETARDATION RATING SCALES

The following is a brief review of the most commonly used rating scales developed specifically for individuals with mental retardation and developmental disabilities and used to assess behavior and psychiatric status.

Aberrant Behavior Checklist ([ABC]; Aman & Singh, 1986, 1994) The ABC is a 58-item informant rating scale specifically designed to assess treatment effects.

The original pool of items was factor analyzed after testing on 927 adolescents and adults. The five factorially derived subscales are (1) Irritability, Agitation and Crying (15 items); (2) Lethargy, Social Withdrawal (16 items); (3) Stereotypic Behavior (7 items); (4) Hyperactivity, Noncompliance (16 items); and (5) Inappropriate Speech (4 items). Each item is rated on a 4-point scale from 0 (*not present*) to 3 (*the problem is severe*). The factor structure has been replicated in a number of studies (Marshburn & Aman 1992; Rojahn & Helsel, 1991), and a newer version (the ABC-Community) has been normed with a community sample (Aman, Burrow, & Wolford, 1995; Aman & Singh, 1994).

The ABC was largely institutional in origin and derived with a sample of people with severe to moderate mental retardation. More recent data on the ABC are available; however, they pertain to a large community-based sample of children in special education placements, most with mild mental retardation (Marshburn & Aman, 1992). The newer ABC-Community was also studied with adults living in group homes (Aman et al., 1995). Validity data are available for the relationships of subscale scores to behavior problems (Rojahn & Helsel, 1991). The ABC has been used in at least 15 treatment and medication studies, and it has proved to be sensitive to behavior changes in the large majority of these (Aman, 1994).

AAMR Adaptive Behavior Scale — Residential and Community, Second Edition ([ABS-RC:Z]; Nihira, Leland, & Lambert, 1993). Part II of the revised version of the original AAMR Adaptive Behavior Scales consists of maladaptive behavior ratings for a large number of behaviors. The 14 domains include the following: (1) violent & destructive behavior, (2) anti-social behavior, (3) rebellious behavior, (4), untrustworthy behavior, (5) withdrawal, (6) stereotypic behavior & odd mannerism, (7) inappropriate interpersonal manners, (8) unacceptable vocal habits, (9) unacceptable or eccentric habits, (10) self-abusive behavior, (11) hyperactive tendencies, (12) sexually aberrant behavior, (13) psychological disturbances, and (14) use of medications. The items are rated as *do not apply, occasionally occurring,* or *occurring frequently.*

Assessment Information Rating Profile (Bouras, 1995). This instrument is a comprehensive psychiatric assessment form that provides a structure for organizing all information available about the individual from a variety of sources. Answers are coded numerically. Problem behaviors are rated in terms of frequency and severity, and the Clinical Psychopathology Learning Disabilities Rating Scale is included in which behavior is rated as *observed* or *not observed*. Data are available on more than 500 cases. At the present time, there is no manual available containing data regarding development of the instrument or reliability and validity.

The Diagnostic Assessment of the Severely Handicapped ([DASH]; Matson, Coe, Gardner & Sovner, 1991). The DASH is a 96-item informant rating scale, closely tied to the DSM-III-R, for assessing adults with severe to profound mental retardation. The standardization sample included 506 persons living in institutions. The internal reliability (alpha) coefficients for the 13 psychometric scales range from .20 to .84, with a median value of .52. More research and development is needed on this instrument. We are not aware of any research with the DASH for assessing medication effects.

Developmental Behaviour Checklist ([DBC; Einfeld & Tonge, 1994). The format for this instrument was based on the Child Behavior Checklist (Achenbach & Edelbrock, 1986 a, 1986b), which is a widely-researched and extensively used scale for children without disabilities. The Developmental Behaviour Checklist has two forms, one for caregivers and one for teachers. The original items were derived by studying case files, and factor analysis resulted in six subscales: (1) Disruptive Behavior (20 items), (2) Self-Absorbed Behavior (20 items), (3) Language Disturbance (9 items), (4) Anxiety (12 items), (5) Autistic Relating (9 items), and (6) Antisocial Behavior (4 items). A 3-point rating scale is used: *not true*, *sometimes true*, and *often/very true*. This scale has been used in a growing number of peer-reviewed studies (Einfeld, personal communication, November 1994; Einfeld & Tonge, 1995).

Emotional Problems Scales: Behavior Rating Scales (BRS) & **Self-Report Inventory** (SRI) (Strohmer & Prout, 1991). This instrument offers an informant rating scale and a self-rating scale companion set. The Behavior Rating Scales (BRS) were developed for individuals with mild mental retardation or borderline intelligence. The original pool of items was collected from 841 adolescents and adults and the normative samples contained individuals with psychiatric disorders as well as mentally healthy people. The BRS has 12 subscales, for which scores are plotted over a cumulative frequency distribution of percentiles: (1) Thought/Behavior Disorder (15 items), (2) Verbal Aggression (8 items), (3) Physical Aggression (19 items), (4) Sexual Maladjustment (8 items), (5) Noncompliance (15 items), (6) Hyperactivity (19 items), (7) Distractibility (19 items), (8) Anxiety (11 items), (9) Somatic Concerns (12 items), (10) Withdrawal (19 items), (11) Depression (11 items), and (12) Low Self-esteem (15 items). Also, selected subscales

can be totaled to calculate Externalizing Behavior Problems and Internalizing Behavior Problems. Items for this scale were selected by experienced clinicians and have a high degree of face validity. This scale takes some time to complete because of the large number of items. As with some of the other measures, the number of items in each subscale varies considerably, from 8 on Sexual Maladjustment and Verbal Aggression to 19 on Physical Aggression and Distractibility. It is recommended that raters be professionals in the field of mental retardation. The SRI has 162 items derived from the same sample as the BRS. Six scales were developed: (1) Thought and Behavior Disorder (20 items), (2) Impulse Control (33 items), (3) Anxiety (25 items), (4) Depression (36 items), (5) Low Self-Esteem (20 items), and (6) Lie Scale (12 items) to assess the validity of the patient's responses. Items are read to the consumer and the clinician marks "yes" or "no."

In his review of instruments, Aman (1991a) rated the data on standardization, interrater reliability, criterion group validity, and congruent validity as all good for the BRS. For the SRI, Aman commented favorably on the scale's internal consistency and test-retest reliability, but he characterized the available data on criterion group validity as being weak. These instruments are among very few in the field for which the content validity of items has been established in a formal way. Empirical data are generally weak thus far on the grouping of items within subscales (Aman, 1991a). Reiss (1994) has questioned the absence of peer-reviewed reports on the scale. We know of no empirical work in which these instruments have been used to select patients for pharmacotherapy or to assess the effect of pharmacotherapy.

The Psychopathology Inventory for Mentally Retarded Adults ([PIMRA]; Matson, 1997). This instrument is available both as a 56-item informant rating scale and as a 56-item inventory self-report scale. Each is designed to be individually administered to either the informant or to the consumer. The standardization sample had 398 people. Moreover, the user guide reports psychometric data on 508 adults with abilities ranging from severe mental retardation to borderline intelligence. The PIMRA, which was designed to correspond to DSM-III, has the following scales with seven items each: (1) Schizophrenia, (2) Affective Disorder, (3) Psychosexual Disorder, (4) Adjustment Disorder, (5) Anxiety Disorder, (6) Somatoform Disorder, (7) Personality Disorder, and (8) Inappropriate Adjustment. There is also a total score based on all 56 items. Items are judged as either being true or false. The self-report inventory is typically read aloud to the individual who rates himself or herself. This inventory is intended for adolescents or adults with mild mental retardation, although some adults with moderate mental retardation are able to complete the inventory. Respondents are required to answer yes or no.

Reviews of the PIMRA have been mixed. Aman (1991a) concluded that although it is promising as a screening instrument, the reliability, internal consistency, and validity data did not support the PIMRA as a principal tool to establish a diagnosis. Aman (1991) criticized the PIMRA for yielding low alpha coefficients (between .45 to .73 in one study) and noted that the self-report instrument correlated poorly with the informant version. Reiss (1994) noted both favorable and unfavorable reviews of the PIMRA. Reiss also said that the PIMRA is one of the more established instruments in terms of widespread use over a period of years, which suggests that it is of practical value.

The Reiss Screen for Maladaptive Behavior ([Reiss Screen]; Reiss, 1988). The Reiss Screen was developed as a screening tool to identify mental health problems in people with mild, moderate, and severe mental retardation. The items were selected based on judgments of experts. The scale contains 38 items, and the manual reports research data on about 2,000 persons. The scale is to be completed by two caregivers and the scores are averaged. Ratings are on a 3-point scale of *no problem*, *problem*, and *major problem*. A 26-item total score provides an index of the severity of a person's problem. This rating scale is well-designed and easy to use.

The scale scores were validated against psychiatric diagnoses. The Reiss Screen total score was able to discriminate between people with and without a psychiatric disorder. The validity of certain scales have also been established. The instrument has been used successfully in a number of drug studies (e.g., Branford, 1996a, 1996b). Svec, Bedard and Siegling (1991) found a good concordance of the Aggression scale with present and lifetime aggression. This is one of the oldest and most established instruments.

The Reiss Scale for Children's Dual Diagnosis (Reiss & Valenti-Hein, 1994). This scale is similar to the Reiss Screen in that two caregivers are asked to rate items on a 3-point scale. The standardization sample had 583 children and adolescents with mild to severe mental retardation. Ten scales were derived from factor

analysis, all with 5 items each: (1) Anger/Self-Control, (2) Anxiety Disorder, (3) Attention-Deficit, (4) Autism/Pervasive, (5) Conduct Disorder, (6) Depression, (7) Poor Self-Esteem, (8) Psychosis, (9) Somatoform Behavior, and (10) Withdrawn/Isolated. The instrument also assesses significant maladaptive behaviors such as crying spells, enuresis/encopresis, hallucinations, involuntary movements, lies, obesity, pica, sets fires, sexual problem, and verbal abuse. Cronbach's alpha coefficients were estimated at .91 for the total score and between .63 and .86 for the scales. As with the original Reiss Screen, the items were selected based on expert clinical judgments. The total score discriminated between children with and without a mental health diagnosis. We are not aware of any research with the Reiss Scale that assessed its use for diagnosing subjects of medication studies or for monitoring medication effects.

CONCLUSIONS

There is a need to develop more instruments and to study more extensively the ones that have been developed. Such research should address the central diagnostic issues in patients with mental retardation to develop meaningful criteria by which to judge the presence or absence of different mental illnesses.

The available instruments that were specifically designed for people with mental retardation have not demonstrated sufficient validity with respect to identifying any agreed upon diagnostic entity, but many show good promise. At the present time, then, it is wise to use these instruments carefully. It has been recommended that clinicians use qualitative interpretation and inspection of individual items to guide them rather than relying solely on suggested cut-off scores or scale measurements (Hurley & Sovner, 1992). Furthermore, it is recommended that several inventories be used simultaneously, and that, ideally, two caregivers complete each inventory. Although a number of instruments are widely used (the ABC, ABS, PIMRA, and Reiss Screen), there is no consensus in the field as to which instrument is best. There is a consensus that rating scales are one of the most economical, clinically relevant, and useful tools available to help clinicians in assessing treatment effects.

REFERENCES

Achenbach, T.M. (1991). Clinical data systems: Rating scales and interviews. In R. Michels, A.M. Cooper, S.B. Guze, L.L. Judd, G.L. Klerman, A.J. Solnit, & A.J. Stunkard (Eds.), *Psychiatry* (Vol. 2). Philadelphia: Lippincott.

Achenbach, T. M., & Edelbrock, C.S. (1986a). *Child Behavior Checklist and Youth Self-Report*. Burlington, CT: Author.

Achenbach, T.M. & Edelbrock, C.S. (1986b). *Teacher's Report Form*. Burlington, VT: Author.

Achenbach, T.M., McConaughy, S.H., & Howell, C.T. (1987). Child/adolescent behavioral and emotional problems: Implications of cross-informant correlations for situational specificity. *Psychological Bulletin, 101*, 213-232.

Aman, M.G. (1991a). *Assessing psychopathology and behavior problems in persons with mental retardation: A review of available instruments* (DHHS publication No ADM 91-1712). Rockville, MD: U.S. Department of Health and Human Services.

Aman, M.G. (1991b). Review and evaluation of instruments for assessing emotional and behavioral disorders. *Australia and New Zealand Journal of Developmental Disabilities, 17*, 127-145.

Aman, M.G. (1993). Monitoring and measuring drug effect: II. Behavioral, emotional and cognitive effects. In J.S. Werry & M.G. Aman (Eds.), Practitioner's guide to psychoactive drugs for children and adolescents (pp. 99-159). New York: Plenum Medical Books.

Aman, M.G. (1994). Instruments for assessing treatment effects in developmental disabled populations. *Assessment in Rehabilitation and Exceptionality, 1*, 1-20.

Aman M.G., Burrow, W.H., & Wolford, P.L. (1995). The Aberrant Behavior Checklist-Community: Factor validity and effect of subject variables for adults in group homes. *American Journal on Mental Retardation, 100*, 293–294.

Aman, M.G., & Singh, N.N. (l986) *Aberrant Behavior Checklist manual*. East Aurora, NY: Slosson Educational Publications.

Aman, M.G. & Singh, N.N. (1994). *Aberrant Behavior Checklist Community supplementary manual*. East Aurora, NY: Slosson Educational Publications.

Bech, P. (1993). *Rating scales for psychopathology, health status and quality of life: A compendium on documentation in accordance with the DSM-III-R and WHO Systems*. New York: Springer-Verlag.

Beck, A. T., Ward, C. H, Mendelson, M., Nock. J., & Erbaugh, J. (1961). An inventory for measuring depression. *Archives of General Psychiatry, 4*, 561-571.

Bernstein, G.A. (1991). Comorbidity and severity of anxiety and depressive disorders in a clinic sample. *Journal of the American Academy of Child and Adolescent Psychiatry, 30*, 43-50.

Bernstein, G.A. & Garfinkel, B.B. (1986). School phobia: The overlap of affective and anxiety disorders. *Journal of the American Academy of Child and Adolescent Psychiatry, 25*, 235-241.

Biederman, J., Newcorn, J., & Sprich, S. (1991). Comorbidity of attention deficit hyperactivity disorder with conduct, depressive, anxiety and other disorders. *American Journal of Psychiatry, 148*, 564-577.

Bird, H.R., Gould, M.S., & Staghezza, B. (1992). Aggregating data from multiple informants in child psychiatry epidemiological research. *Journal of the American Academy of Child and Adolescent Psychiatry, 31*, 78-85.

Bird, H.R., Gould, M.S., & Staghezza, B.M. (1993). Patterns of diagnostic comorbidity in a community sample of children aged 9 through 16 years. *Journal of the American Academy of Child and Adolescent Psychiatry, 32*, 361-368.

Bouras, N. (1995). *Psychiatric Assessment Rating Profile*. Unpublished manuscript, Guy's Hospital, Division of Psychiatry and Psychology, London.

Branford, D. (1996a). Factors associated with the successful or unsuccessful withdrawal of antipsychotic drug therapy prescribed for people with learning disabilities. *Journal of Intellectual Disability Research, 40*, 322-329.

Branford, D. (1996b). A review of antipsychotic drugs prescribed for people with learning disabilities who live in Leicestershire. *Journal of Intellectual Disability Research, 40*, 358-368.

Burt, D. B., Loveland, K. A., & Lewis, K. R. (1992). Depression and the onset of depression in adults with mental retardation. *American Journal on Mental Retardation, 96*, 502-511.

Edgerton, R. B. (1967). *The cloak of incompetence: Stigma in the lives of the mentally retarded*. Berkeley: University of California.

Einfeld, S.L., & Tonge, B.J., (1991). Psychometric and clinical assessment of psychopathology in developmentally disabled children. *Australia and New Zealand Journal of Developmental Disabilities, 17*, 147-154.

Einfeld, S.J., & Tonge, B.J. (1994): *Manual for The Developmental Behaviour Checklist (Primary Care Version)*. University of New South Wales and Monash University, Victoria, Australia.

Einfeld, S.L., & Tonge B.J. (1995). The Developmental Behaviour Checklist: The development and validation of an instrument for the assessment of behavioral and emotional disturbance in children and adolescents with mental retardation. *Journal of Autism and Developmental Disorders, 25*, 81–104.

Fendrich, M., Weissman, M.M., & Warner, V. (1991). Longitudinal assessment of major depression and anxiety disorders in children. *Journal of the American Academy of Child and Adolescent Psychiatry, 30*, 38-42.

Hauser, S.L, DeLong,G.R., & Rosman, N. (1975). Pneumographic findings in the infantile autism syndrome: A correlation with temporal lobe disease. *Brain, 98*, 667-688.

Hogg, J., & Raynes, N.B. (Eds.) (1987). *Assessment in mental handicap: A guide to assessment, practices, tests, and checklists*. London: Croom Helm Associates.

Honigfield, G., & Klett, C.J. (1965). The Nurses' Observation Scale for Inpatient Evaluation. *Journal of Clinical Psychology, 21*, 65-67.

Hurley, A.D., & Sovner, R. (1992). Inventories for evaluating developmentally disabled individuals. *Habilitative Mental Healthcare Newsletter, 11*, 42-50.

Iivanainen, M., Viukari, M., & Helle, E.P. (1977). Cerebellar atrophy in phenytoin-treated mentally retarded epileptics. *Epilepsia, 18*, 375-386.

Kashani, J.H., Beck, N.C., Hoeper, E.W., Fallahi, C., Corcoran, C.M., McAllister, J.A., Rosenberg, T.K., & Reid, J.C. (1987). Psychiatric disorders in a community sample of adolescents. *American Journal of Psychiatry, 144*, 584-589.

Kashani, J.H., Orvaschel, H., Burk, J.P., & Reid, J.C. (1985). Informant variance: The issue of parent-child disagreement. *Journal of the American Academy of Child Psychiatry, 24*, 437-441.

Keller, M.B., Lavori, P.W., Beardslee, W.R., Wunder, J., Schwartz, C.E., Roth, J., & Biederman, J. (1992). The disruptive behavioral disorder in children and adolescents: Comorbidity and clinical course. *Journal of the American Academy of Child and Adolescent Psychiatry, 31*, 204-209.

Marshburn, E. C. & Aman, M. G. (1992). Factor validity and norms for the Aberrant Behavior Checklist in a community sample of children with mental retardation. *Journal of Autism and Developmental Disorders, 22*, 357-373.

Matson, J.L. (1997). *The PIMRA manual* (2nd ed.). Worthington, OH: IDS Publishing Corporation.

Matson, J.L., Coe, A., Gardner, W.I., & Sovner, R. (1991). A factor analytic study of the diagnostic assessment for the severely handicapped scale. *The Journal of Nervous and Mental Disease, 179*, 553–557.

Murray, HA (1943). Thematic Apperception Test manual. Cambridge, MA: Harvard University Press.

Nihira, K., Leland, H., & Lambert, N. (1993). *Adaptive Behavior Scale—Residential and Community*. Washington, D.C.: AAMR.

Pliszka, S.R. (1992). Comorbidity of attention-deficit hyperactivity disorder and overanxious disorder. *Journal of the American Academy of Child and Adolescent Psychiatry 31*, 197–203.

Reiss, S. (1997). Comments on the Reiss Screen and its factor structure. *Journal of Intellectual Disability Research*.

Reiss, S. (1994). *Handbook of challenging behavior: Mental health aspects of mental retardation*. Worthington, OH: IDS Publishing Corporation.

Reiss, S. (1988). *Test manual for the Reiss Screen for Maladaptive Behavior*. Worthington, OH: IDS Publishing Corporation.

Reiss, S., Benson, B.A., & Szyszko, S. (1992). *The apperceptive personality test: mental retardation*. Worthington, OH: IDS Publishing Corporation.

Reiss, S., Levitan, D.W., & Szyszko, J. (1982). Emotional disturbance and mental retardation: Diagnostic overshadowing. *American Journal of Mental Deficiency, 86*, 567-574.

Reiss, S., & Valenti-Hein, D. (1994). Development of a psychopathology rating scale for children with mental retardation. *Journal of Consulting and Clinical psychology, 62*, 28-33.

Riegelman, R. K. (1981). Diagnostic discrimination of test. In R. K. Riegelman (Ed.), *Studying a study and testing a test* (pgs. 119-130). Boston: Little, Brown.

Rojahn, B., & Helsel, W.J. (1991). The Aberrant Behavior Checklist with children and adolescents with dual diagnosis. *Journal of Autism and Developmental Disorders, 21*, 17-28.

Sovner, R. (1986). Limiting factors in the use of DSM-III criteria with mentally ill/mentally retarded persons. *Psychopharmacology Bulletin, 22*, 1055-1059.

Strohmer, D.C., & Prout, H.T. (1991). *The Emotional Problems Scales*. Odessa, FL: Psychological Assessment Resources.

Svec, H.J., Bedard, C., & Siegling, S. (1991). Charting life histories of aggression with psychotropic medication for du-

ally diagnosed persons. *Clinical Bulletin of the Developmental Disabilities Program (Ontario) 2*, 1-2.

Weissman, M.W., Orvaschel, H., & Padian, N. (1980). Children's symptom and social functioning self-report scales: Comparison of mothers and children's reports. *Journal of Nervous and Mental Disease, 68*, 736-740.

Williams, S. McGee, R., Anderson, J., & Silva, P. (1989). The structure and correlates of self-reported symptoms in 11-year old children. *Journal of Abnormal Child Psychology, 17*, 55-71.

Woolston, J.L., Rosenthal, S.L., Riddle, M.A., Sparrow, S.S., Cicchetti, D., & Zimmerman, L.D. (1989). Childhood comorbidity of anxiety/affective disorders and behavior disorders. *Journal of the American Academy of Child and Adolescent Psychiatry, 28*, 707-713.

Zung, W.W.K. (1965). A self-rating depression scale. *Archives of General Psychiatry, 12*, 63-70.

Side Effects:
Recognition and Management

Jacquelyn Gardner Wilson[1], Rex S. Lott[2], and Luke Tsai[3]

What are *side effects* or *adverse drug reactions?* The two terms are used interchangeably in the literature but they do not mean the same thing. Adverse drug reactions are noxious, unintended, and occur at doses normally used for therapy (WHO, 1975). They represent the more serious or noxious events associated with the use of medication. In contrast, the term *side effects* does not necessarily imply noxious results. For example, the mood stabilizing effects of carbamazepine and valproic acid are side effects that are sometimes beneficial to the person.

Rosenheim and Moulton (cited in Davies, 1977, p. 10) and Linkewich (1981) proposed dividing adverse drug reactions into several subcategories including overdosage, intolerance, side effects, secondary effects, idiosyncrasy, and hypersensitivity. However, many would disagree with this classification system, and we do not use it in this chapter. Instead, we focus on the side effects that are usually significant (either because of their frequency or their potential severity) in the normal course of treatment. Such effects vary from mild to severe, from acute to chronic, and from reversible to irreversible.

In this chapter we delineate some general principles to consider when prescribing psychotropic medications for this population, and we discuss the various adverse drug reactions. However, we do not discuss the mechanisms of adverse drug reactions.

RECOGNIZING AND MANAGING SIDE EFFECTS

People with mental retardation and developmental disabilities are likely to experience the same spectrum of adverse effects from psychotropic drugs as does the general population. There are few, if any, situations in which these drugs seem to cause adverse effects that are unique to this population. Nevertheless, this population may be at an increased risk of experiencing side effects, which may be unrecognized or ignored for various reasons. One problem is that the person's functional handicap may distort or mask some signs of drug toxicity (Aman, Paxton, Field, & Foote, 1986). For example, if a person with moderate mental retardation, primary dysarthria, and difficulty ambulating develops signs of benzodiazepine, lithium, or phenytoin toxicity (e.g., slurred speech, confusion, and clumsiness), these signs may go unrecognized for some time because of the preexisting functional handicaps. Another problem is the person's inability to alert caregivers regarding adverse effects. People with mild to moderate mental retardation potentially may be able to report problems, but they may not be able to comprehend or recognize adverse effects as being drug-induced (e.g., akathisia or dizziness). Unless educated to do so, they may not alert their caregivers about the development of the adverse drug reactions (Aman & Singh, 1988; Zametkin & Yamada, 1993). Additionally, people with severe to profound mental retardation may be unable to report adverse effects because of impairments or deficits in speech. In these people, adverse reactions may be manifested as changes in behavior (e.g., increased aggression or self-injury).

Another problem in recognizing adverse effects concerns stereotypic behaviors, which are common in

1 Clinical Assistant of Pharmacy Practice and Psychiatry, Wayne State University, Detroit, MI
2 Associate Professor, Idaho State University, College of Pharmacy, Pocatello, ID
3 Professor and Director, Developmental Disorders Clinic, University of Michigan, Ann Arbor, MI

people with mental retardation and in children with autism (Baumeister & Forehand, 1973). Differentiating between these behaviors and drug-induced dyskinesia, even for experienced raters, may be difficult (Meiselas et al., 1989; Shay et al., 1993). Some other drug-induced movement disorders discussed later in this chapter also may be difficult to differentiate from stereotypies (Perry, Nobler, & Campbell, 1989). Furthermore, it is difficult to distinguish between the side effects of certain psychotropic medications and various psychiatric symptoms and coexisting medical problems (Arnold, 1993). For example, the SSRIs have side effects of insomnia, akathisia, hyperactivity, and agitation. Antipsychotic medication can also produce akathisia or Parkinsonian-like features. Drugs with high anticholinergic properties (e.g., benztropine, thioridazine, and doxepin) can produce agitation, confusion, hyperactivity, hallucinations, irritability, lethargy, and memory impairment, known as an anticholinergic psychosis. Severe intoxication with phenytoin or carbamazepine and possibly valproic acid may, on occasion, lead to increased seizure activity. Often these signs are misdiagnosed as a worsening of the preexisting disorder.

Individual variation in medication response is probably greater in people with mental retardation and developmental disabilities, such that side effects may be less predictable. Individual differences may be related in part to the impact of the developing brain on the pharmacodynamics of a given medication. Another factor is what Arnold (1993) called the "end-of-curve" phenomenon, in which unusual reactions are seen when patients fall at either extreme of the bell-shaped curve. Genetic features may also account for some individual differences in medication response. Recent findings suggest that mutations in chromosome 21 are important in the genesis of familial Alzheimer's disease (Golde, Estus, & Usiak, 1990; Hardy, 1994). Chromosome 21 trisomy is responsible for many cases of Down syndrome. It has been estimated that 25% of individuals with Down syndrome develop Alzheimer's almost two decades earlier than does the general population. Defects in cleaving beta amyloid proteins are involved in the pathophysiology of Alzheimer's; these proteins accumulate in neuritic plaques found in the brains of these patients (Golde et al., 1990; Hardy, 1994). Genetically determined degenerative changes such as these may impact an individual's response to medications. Most Alzheimer's patients are more sensitive to the CNS effects of psychotropic medications. Additionally, Alzheimer's is associated with a deficit in cholinergic neurotransmission in the CNS. Drugs with

potent CNS anticholinergic activity (many psychotropic medications) may aggravate the symptoms of Alzheimer's.

BEHAVIORAL SIDE EFFECTS

Behavioral side effects may develop insidiously over a long period of time or may occur in an idiosyncratic and unpredictable fashion.

Agitation and Restlessness

These effects may develop early in the course of treatment with tricyclic antidepressants (TCAs) or fluoxetine in people with autistic disorder or mental retardation (Cook, Rowlett, Jaselskis, & Leventhal, 1992). Other SSRIs (e.g., paroxetine, sertraline, and fluvoxamine) may also cause this effect, although many clinicians believe it to be more common with fluoxetine. SSRIs (occasionally) and antipsychotic medications (frequently) may cause akathisia as a prominent side effect. Similar reactions may be seen in patients with panic disorder or depression who are treated with antidepressants (Cole & Bodkin, 1990; Gorman et al., 1987). Shortly after ingesting the medication, the patient experiences a sudden onset of inner restlessness or a wired feeling, irritability, increased energy, and insomnia (Zitrin, Klein, & Woerner, 1980). The duration of the jitteriness reaction varies from a few hours to a day (Pohl, Yeragani, Balon, & Lycaki, 1988; Zubenko, Cohen, & Lipinski, 1987). Temporarily lowering the initial dose may be necessary, although tolerance occurs in most people. Low doses of benzodiazepines may help to alleviate the initial jitteriness (Klein, Gittelman, & Quitkin, 1980). When agitation associated with SSRI treatment causes sleep disturbance, many clinicians coadminister trazodone (Desyrel), a sedating antidepressant, in low doses to help counteract sleep disturbance.

Sedation

Sedation, which may be indicated by tiredness or sleep, is a side effect of many psychotropic and anti-epileptic medications. It is undesirable when it interferes with learning and functional abilities. The degree of sedation is often dose-related. Fortunately, tolerance to this effect usually occurs during long-term treatment. Low-potency antipsychotic medications (e.g., thioridazine, mesoridazine, and chlorpromazine) produce prominent sedation. All benzodiazepines produce sedation. Beta-blockers (e.g., propranolol and atenolol) have been noted to cause significant sedation in some people with mental retardation and developmental disabilities (Sovner, 1990). Carbamazepine, gabapentin, phenobarbital, and primidone are the more sedating antiepileptic medications. Sedation may be especially problematic at initiation of therapy or with dose escalation.

Tertiary-amine TCAs (e.g., amitriptyline and doxepin) are very sedating, whereas secondary ones (i.e., desipramine, amoxapine, and protriptyline) are less sedating. SSRIs, as a group, are much less sedating than are TCAs. Single bedtime doses of TCAs are often recommended both to capitalize on the sleep-promoting effects of these drugs and to lessen carry-over daytime sedation. However, large bedtime doses may cause nighttime dizziness, confusion, and ataxia, particularly in elderly or debilitated patients. This effect may necessitate use of these drugs in divided doses during the day or a switch to a less sedating TCA.

Impaired Memory

The use of benzodiazepines may lead to some impairment in memory. Acute, brief amnesia is possible depending on the dose, milligram potency, and route of administration of the drug. Chronic use of benzodiazepines can cause insidious memory impairment that may be more common and more severe among elderly people. Carbamazepine has been shown to impair memory in some people with mental retardation and developmental disabilities (Evans & Gualtieri, 1985). Many psychotropic medications possess potent anticholinergic properties (e.g., TCAs, low-potency antipsychotic medications, and anticholinergic anti-Parkinson medications), which may impair memory (Gelenberg et al., 1989). For people with mental retardation and developmental disabilities (for whom there is emphasis on learning and skill acquisition), these powerful anticholinergic drugs should be avoided whenever possible.

Hostility, Disinhibition, Aggression

These behaviors are occasionally encountered as paradoxical reactions to benzodiazepines and have been reported with all benzodiazepines, including alprazolam (Gardner & Cowdry, 1985). Most clinicians who treat people with mental retardation and developmental disabilities have observed possible examples of these reactions, although there is little research or clinical experience definitively characterizing them. Those who are treated with benzodiazepines should be observed for possible evidence of disinhibition, which may be noted as an increase in aggressive or self-injurious behavior. Should these paradoxical effects seem to occur, gradual, closely evaluated withdrawal of the benzodiazepine may be indicated. Carbamazepine has been reported to produce an amphetamine-like reaction, consisting of hyperactivity, self-injury, or aggression (Evans & Gualtieri, 1985; Friedman, Kastner, Plummer, Ruiz & Henning, 1992).

Switch Mania

Long-term studies suggest that TCAs and monoamine oxidase inhibitors (MAOIs) increase the risk of manic relapse among some patients with bipolar I disorders (Angst, 1985; Rabkin, Quitkin, McGrath, Harrison, & Tricamo, 1985). SSRIs may be somewhat less likely to precipitate manic episodes. Bupropion may be the safest antidepressant for patients in whom there is a risk of mania. Patients with rapid cycling are at risk for manic switches when given antidepressants (Wehr, Sack, Rosenthal, & Cowdry, 1988). When patients with bipolar depression are treated with a TCA or an MAOI, mood stabilizing medication (e.g., lithium, valproate, or carbamazepine) should be given simultaneously to reduce the risk of precipitating mania. Although valproic acid and carbamazepine have been reported to induce mania in people with mental retardation and developmental disabilities (Evans & Gualteri, 1985), such adverse effects are uncommon.

Sleep Disturbances

Sleep disturbances have been reported in patients receiving large single doses of TCAs at night (Flemenbaum, 1976; Pollack & Rosenbaum, 1987). Nightmares or disturbing dreams may occur, accompanied by temporary confusion, disorganization, and quasi-hallucinatory hypnagogic and hypnopompic episodes. These reactions are uncommon and may disappear spontaneously. If the disturbances persist, administration of medication as a single daytime dose may be helpful. Somnambulism (appearing confused and walking about in a quick, detached, and clumsy manner) has been reported to occur in patients treated with neuroleptic drugs, within two to three hours after sleep onset (Flemenbaum, 1976). Initial and middle insomnia and afternoon tiredness and sleepiness have been associated with MAOIs. Insomnia may respond to a short-acting hypnotic or antihistamine, or to a sedating antidepressant such as trazodone. MAOI-induced day-time somnolence may require discontinuation of the treatment.

Withdrawal Reactions

Rapid discontinuation of most psychotropic medications may precipitate withdrawal reactions. As a rule, unless toxic or allergic symptoms necessitate immediate withdrawal, these medications should be tapered and discontinued slowly. People with mental retardation and developmental disabilities, in the experience of many clinicians, may be especially susceptible to the effects of rapid discontinuation of psychotropic medication. Careful monitoring during tapering will allow adjustment of the speed of withdrawal to avoid unnecessary symptoms.

Some withdrawal symptoms are predictable. For example, rapid discontinuation of highly anticholinergic drugs after long-term therapy should be expected to produce signs and symptoms of cholinergic overactivity (i.e., diarrhea and intestinal cramping). Rapid withdrawal from sedating medication is likely to cause hyperactivity, sleep disturbance, and over-alertness. Discomfort associated with withdrawal symptoms may be manifested as a behavioral change for people with mental retardation and developmental disabilities who have limited verbal ability. TCA, anticholinergic, or MAOI withdrawal may cause nausea, vomiting, diarrhea, abdominal cramps, malaise, cold sweats, chills, dizziness, headache, and insomnia within two weeks of abrupt discontinuation (Dilsaver, 1989; Garner, Kelly, & Thompson, 1993; Klein et al., 1980; Naylor, Grunhaus, & Cameron, 1987). Pronounced anxiety, panic attacks, and autonomic hyperactivity (tachycardia, hypertension, sweating, and restlessness) have also been described (Dilsaver & Greden, 1983; Gawin & Markoff, 1981). If the withdrawal symptoms are mild, they usually subside within a few days. In more severe cases, a small dose of the discontinued antidepressant may be given and repeated after one hour if only partial improvement is obtained after the first dose.

SSRI withdrawal symptoms have been described in the general population. These symptoms should be expected in people with mental retardation and developmental disabilities if these medications are withdrawn abruptly. Influenza-like symptoms, dizziness, nausea, and insomnia are frequently reported by patients; these symptoms may occur even with gradual tapering of dosage (Lazowick & Levin, 1995).

Neuroleptic withdrawal symptoms of nausea, vomiting, anorexia, diaphoresis, behavioral worsening, insomnia, hyperkinesis, and seizures have been reported (Davis & Rosenberg, 1979; Gualtieri & Guimond, 1981; Gualtieri, Quade, Hicks, Mayo, & Schroeder, 1984; Lawrence, 1985; Mikkelsen, Albert, & Upadhyaya, 1987; Zimmerman & Heistad, 1982). These symptoms generally occur after long-term treatment and an abrupt discontinuation of therapy. They may be mild or severe and may last for a few days to as long as 16 weeks (Gualtieri et al., 1984). A gradual reduction of 10% to 25% of the original dose every 2 to 4 weeks may be helpful in avoiding or minimizing this withdrawal phenomenon. Low-dose lorazepam or propranolol may also be helpful in managing these side effects if the gradual reduction alone is not effective (Sovner, 1991).

In some circumstances, it may be difficult to differentiate between temporary withdrawal symptoms and a relapse of the behavioral symptoms that were treated with medication. One useful strategy for differentiation is to administer an acute dose of the medication that is being withdrawn. Especially in the case of antidepressants (which typically have a delayed onset of therapeutic effect), rapid relief of symptoms or resolution of the abnormal behavior suggests temporary withdrawal symptoms rather than a more lasting relapse in behavioral condition. In this case, reinstitution of the last dose of medication and a slower tapering of dosage will often allow for successful discontinuation of the medication.

CARDIOVASCULAR EFFECTS

Hypertensive Reaction

This reaction may develop during treatment with MAOIs (tranylcypromine and phenelzine). The reaction is usually associated with dietary indiscretion involving tyramine-containing foods (e.g., aged cheeses, aged meats, and broad beans) or with drug interaction (e.g., with amphetamines, methylphenidate, TCAs, L-dopa, cold pills, sinus medications, and diet aids). Clinicians should be aware that occasionally this reaction can occur spontaneously. The mild form of reaction may be manifested by mild headache or palpitation. The severe form, hypertensive crisis, is manifested by a sharp rise in blood pressure (often with systolic levels over 200 mm Hg and diastolic pressure levels over 120 mm Hg), accompanied by a severe throbbing headache. Patients may also experience flushing, sweating, palpitations, chest discomfort, a choking sensation, photophobia, nausea, and vomiting. If untreated and sustained, intracranial hemorrhage may occur, which may be fatal. In order to prevent the hypertensive reaction, patients who receive these drugs or their caregivers should be given clear verbal and written instructions about food, beverage, and drug restrictions. When the MAOI is discontinued, the dietary and medication restrictions should be maintained for at least two weeks. In mild cases of hypertensive reaction, the treatment includes rest, reassurance, observation with blood pressure monitoring, and discontinuation of the medications. In severe cases (e.g., severe pounding headache, systolic pressure above 200 mm Hg, and diastolic pressure above 115 mm Hg), pharmacological treatment (e.g., with phentolamine, diazoxide, or nifedipine) should be considered (Clary & Schweizer, 1987; Cockhill & Remick, 1987).

Orthostatic Hypotension

This reaction is common in patients treated with TCAs, maprotiline, trazodone, and MAOIs (phenelzine, tranylcypromine, isocarboxazid). Also, it commonly occurs during treatment with low-potency antipsychotic medications (e.g., chlorpromazine, clozapine, thioridazine, and others). Hypotension occurs in the early phase of treatment with TCAs, but it may not appear until the third to sixth week of treatment with MAOIs (Kronig, Rose, Walsh, Woodring, & Glassman, 1983). Elderly patients are more prone to develop this side effect, and they are at greater risk of injury. Orthostatic hypotension may be dangerous because it results in falls and serious physical injuries. Nortriptyline clearly causes less orthostatic hypotension than other TCAs. The newer, non-TCAs such as bupropion, the SSRIs (fluoxetine, sertraline, fluvoxamine, and paroxetine), venlafaxine, and nefazodone cause less orthostatic hypotension. However, limited data are available about the efficacy and safety of these newer agents for use with people with mental retardation and developmental disabilities.

Cardiac Conduction Delays

Manifested by increased PR, QRS, or QT intervals, cardiac conduction delays are often noted in patients treated with therapeutic doses of TCAs. Generally, these delays are not clinically significant. They may be dangerous, however, when they occur in patients with preexisting conduction disease, particularly bundle branch block (Glassman & Bigger, 1981). The newer antidepressants such as bupropion, and the SSRIs, may be the preferred drugs for treatment of depression in the presence of underlying significant cardiac conduction disease. Before initiation of treatment with TCAs, patients should be assessed for possible underlying cardiac disease.

ENDOCRINE AND METABOLIC EFFECTS

Psychotropic medications may interfere with a number of hormonal and metabolic functions and may also have profound effects on sodium, calcium, and water metabolism. Resulting complications are reversible with discontinuation of the psychotropic drugs; however, often the drugs cannot be discontinued, and the endocrine or metabolic dysfunction must be treated.

Hyperprolactinemia

This effect commonly occurs during treatment with classical (typical) neuroleptic drugs (Reichlin, 1992) and is much less likely to occur during treatment with clozapine. Elevated prolactin concentrations may return to normal in approximately one-third of patients despite continued antipsychotic treatment. Prolonged elevation of prolactin concentrations may cause gynecomastia (enlargement of the breast) and galactorrhea (an irregular flow of milk from the breast) in either sex. Ovarian or testicular function may be diminished because of a decline in FSH and LH released by the pituitary gland. Reduced gonadal function may lead to menstrual disturbances (e.g., amenorrhea) or infertility in women (Reichlin, 1992) and impotence with loss of libido, even in the presence of normal testosterone levels, in men (Ghadirian, Chouinard, & Annable, 1982). Prolactin levels usually increase within two weeks of the initiation of the neuroleptics and may tend to return toward normal after several months of continued treatment (Brown, 1983; Meltzer, 1985). When neuroleptic-induced hyperprolactinemia is suspected, other potential causes such as hypothyroidism (either idiopathic or lithium-induced) should be considered and investigated when appropriate (Thorner, Vance, Horvath, & Kovacs,

1992). Treatment for antipsychotic drug-induced hyperprolactinemia is not considered necessary unless clinically significant complications develop. When treatment is necessary, dosage reduction or drug discontinuation, when possible, are the approaches of first choice. If neuroleptic medication must be continued in patients with complications caused by hyperprolactinemia, bromocriptine or amantadine treatment may be helpful (Marken, Haykal, & Fisher, 1992; Thorner, McNeilly, Hagan, & Besser, 1974).

Hypothyroidism

Hypothyroidism has been noted in patients being treated with lithium. The reported incidence varies from 1% to 26% (Joffe, Kutcher, & MacDonald, 1988; Leroy, Villeneuve, & Lajeunesse, 1988; Myers et al., 1985; Yassa, Saunders, Nastase, & Camille, 1988). It has been suggested that the risk of lithium-induced hypothyroidism increases with increasing duration of treatment (Emerson, Dyson, & Utiger, 1973). People with mental retardation and developmental disabilities may not be able to report the relevant symptoms of this adverse reaction, suggesting the need to monitor thyroid functioning closely. Patients who develop hypothyroidism while responding positively to lithium can be treated with exogenous thyroid hormone (levothyroxine). This includes patients with asymptomatic, sustained elevation of TSH in the presence of normal thyroid hormone plasma concentrations. For such patients, levothyroxine dosage is adjusted to maintain normal TSH levels.

Nephrogenic Diabetes Insipidus

Nephrogenic diabetes insipidus (NDI) is frequently caused by lithium treatment. The diagnosis of NDI is confirmed by a water deprivation test (Reeves & Andreoli, 1992). Clinically, NDI is manifested by polyuria and polydipsia. Most patients with lithium-induced NDI tolerate the polyuria and require no intervention from a physician. Lithium should be discontinued in patients with severe NDI in which continued water intake cannot match with urine losses. People with mental retardation and developmental disabilities who are treated with lithium should be observed carefully for polyuria. Those who have severe disabilities may be unable to communicate increased thirst or to increase their fluid intake to compensate for polyuria. Additionally, increased urine volume may be difficult to identify in people who are incontinent and wear diapers or absorbent undergarments. These people may be at increased risk for dehydration and serious lithium intoxication. If the lithium cannot be discontinued, amiloride, a potassium-sparing diuretic (Kosten & Forrest, 1986), or indomethacin (Weinstock & Moses, 1990) can be used to treat NDI.

Hypercalcemia

Some patients taking chronic lithium therapy may develop hypercalcemia (Salata & Klein, 1987), which appears to be related to mild hyperparathyroidism. The increase in serum calcium level usually is mild. When the increase is more than 1.5 mg/dl or when patients become symptomatic (e.g., show polyuria, myopathy, anorexia, and possibly delirium or altered mental status), the drug should be discontinued. Although this adverse reaction to lithium is not common, the potential consequences are serious. Renal calcium stones and osteopenia have been reported. Laboratory monitoring is of primary importance.

Weight Gain

Weight gain may occur during treatment with MAOIs (more common with phenelzine), TCAs (especially amitriptyline), lithium, valproate, clozapine, and most neuroleptics (with the possible exception of molindone). Most commonly, weight gain is partly a result of increased food intake, often accompanied by a craving for sweets and other carbohydrates (Stein, Stein, & Linn, 1985). Drug-induced weight-gain can distress patients and leads to noncompliance with medication. Substantial weight gain may occur and place patients at increased cardiovascular risk; acute weight gain may occasionally precipitate cardiovascular symptoms. There is, in many cases, no satisfactory treatment for drug-induced weight gain, aside from substituting a different medication or discontinuing the causative drug.

REPRODUCTIVE AND ADVERSE SEXUAL EFFECTS

Psychotropic drugs are among the most common groups of drugs to adversely affect sexual and reproductive function. However, sexual side effects caused by psychotropic drugs tend to be underestimated because patients are reluctant to report such intimate issues. Communication difficulties for people with mental retardation and developmental disabilities may also interfere with identification of these adverse responses. Vulnerability to sexual dysfunction caused by psychotropic agents generally increases with age.

Psychotropic drug-induced sexual dysfunction may be manifested in a variety of ways. Changes in libido (most commonly, decreased) have been associated with TCAs, SSRIs, and benzodiazepines; nefazodone and bupropion may have less adverse effect. Priapism (prolonged, painful erection) has been associated with amitriptyline, desipramine, trazodone, clozapine, risperidone, and lithium. Impotence has been associated with MAOIs, TCAs, SSRIs, and antipsychotic medications. Ejaculatory and orgasmic disturbances (delayed, inhibited, or spontaneous orgasm) have been associated with antipsychotic medications (especially thioridazine), trazodone, and SSRIs. Additionally, as was mentioned earlier, antipsychotic medication-induced hyperprolactinemia may cause changes in sexual function. Occurrence of these side effects may negatively impact the general well-being and, occasionally, the physical health of any person. Physicians need to keep the risk of these side effects in mind and routinely monitor for their possible occurrence.

HEMATOLOGIC REACTIONS

Certain psychotropic drugs may produce hematopoietic toxicity when given to susceptible patients (i.e., with a specific pharmacologic or immunologic abnormality that underlies the sensitivity). Generally, hematologic disorders are expressed as a reduction in the number of any or of all blood cells.

Aplastic Anemia

In aplastic anemia, the bone marrow is completely empty, resulting in anemia, leukopenia, and thrombocytopenia. Aplastic anemia may cause symptoms of anemia (e.g., weakness, shortness of breath, palpitation, angina, and loss of energy), leukopenia-related bacterial and fungal infection, and thrombocytopenia with bleeding into the skin (ecchymoses or purpura) or from the mucous membranes and body apertures. Aplastic anemia is the most serious of the drug-induced disorders because of its high rate of mortality. Fortunately, aplastic anemia is rare and has seldom been linked to psychotropic drugs. It is

more frequently associated with anticonvulsants such as phenytoin, mephenytoin, carbamazepine, valproic acid, and felbamate. If a patient is proved to have aplastic anemia, the suspected drug should be discontinued immediately, and the patient should be promptly referred for a bone-marrow transplant.

Agranulocytosis

Agranulocytosis is characterized by a decrease in white blood cells. Patients may be asymptomatic initially but later develop symptoms such as sore throat, fever, chills, and drenching sweats. If the offending drug is continued, death from sepsis may occur. Agranulocytosis has been reported with the use of phenothiazines (e.g., chlorpromazine), clozapine, carbamazepine, phenytoin, mephenytoin, primidone, and meprobamate. Because of the risk of agranulocytosis during clozapine therapy (approximately 0.8%), weekly monitoring of white blood cell counts is required; early detection of clozapine-induced agranulocytosis with immediate discontinuation of the drug and institution of supportive treatment is associated with a decreased risk of fatal outcome. Frequent, routine monitoring of blood counts in people treated with other drugs (e.g., carbamazepine) is not helpful in reducing the risk of agranulocytosis nor in improving its detection. It is important that treated patients, when feasible, and caregivers be educated regarding the symptoms of agranulocytosis so that they seek medical attention immediately if the symptoms occur.

Leukocytosis

An increase in the number of polymorphonuclear neutrophils beyond normal limits, or leukocytosis, is relatively common during treatment with lithium. No symptoms or morbidity are known to result from this effect, except for possible confusion with infection. When lithium is discontinued, the white count quickly reverts to normal.

Eosinophilia

An increased percentage (>6%) of eosinophils in the peripheral blood, called eosinophilia, may be an important sign of a variety of drug-induced systemic disorders. It frequently occurs with skin rashes progressing to exfoliative dermatitis, but may occur in other hypersensitivity states, such as vasculitis, pulmonary infiltration, asthma, respiratory failure, pulmonary fibrosis, disseminated intravascular coagulation, and purpura fulminans. Eosinophilia may also occur as an isolated finding. Eosinophilia has been associated with clomipramine, phenothiazines, barbiturates, phenytoin, and carbamazepine.

Benign Leukopenia

Benign leukopenia, signalled by a total leukocyte count between 2.5 and 4.0 x 10⁹/l, usually has an asymptomatic course. It does not increase risk of infection. When the causative drug is discontinued, leukopenia will disappear over a period of days to a few weeks. Leukopenia has been associated with most antipsychotic drugs, clozapine, most TCAs, phenytoin, and carbamazepine. The significance of benign leukopenia lies in its possible confusion with agranulocytosis.

Thrombocytopenia

This condition, which is manifested by a diminished number of platelets, is occasionally caused by some psychotropic drugs such as barbiturates, carbamazepine, chlorpromazine, diazepam, phenytoin, fluphenazine, imipramine, and valproate. Valproate (Depakene or Depakote), when used in large doses that achieve plasma concentrations at or above approximately 100 mcg/ml, is frequently associated with reduced platelet counts. On occasion the reduction may be dramatic; bleeding complications, however, are uncommon. Under most circumstances, when the platelet count is significantly less than 20.0 x 10⁹/l, there is risk of severe hemorrhage from mucous membranes or possibly into the CNS. With milder thrombocytopenia, trauma may cause bleeding (petechiae, purpura, or ecchymoses) at sites of relatively minor injury. Treated patients and caregivers should be instructed to be alert for signs such as increased or new onset of bleeding associated with toothbrushing. If significant thrombocytopenia occurs in patients taking one of these drugs, the drug may need to be discontinued.

IMMUNOLOGIC AND GASTROINTESTINAL EFFECTS

Antipsychotic medications and some antiepileptic agents may affect cellular immune functions. For example,

antinuclear antibodies have been detected in the patients treated with phenothiazines (e.g., chlorpromazine, trifluoperazine; Conoso, DeOliveira, & Nixon, 1990). This immunologic abnormality has been associated with the development of systemic lupus erythematosus, polyarthritis, and polyserositis (Goldman, Hudson, & Weddington, 1980).

Xerostomia

Known as dry mouth, xerostomia commonly occurs during therapy with medications that have anticholinergic side effects. Therefore, it predictably occurs with TCAs, lower-potency antipsychotic drugs, clozapine, and anticholinergic/anti-Parkinson medications (e.g., benztropine or trihexyphenidyl). Of the antidepressants, trazodone, SSRIs, bupropion, and nefazodone are less likely to cause xerostomia. High-potency antipsychotics such as haloperidol, fluphenazine, or risperidone are less likely to cause xerostomia, but this advantage may be lost if anticholinergic medication must be coadministered to treat extrapyramidal side effects. Most patients develop some tolerance to this side effect over time. Persistent xerostomia may result in difficulties with chewing, swallowing, speaking, denture fit, increased risk of dental caries, candidiasis, or acute sialoadenitis. Treatment should begin with the elimination of medications known to induce xerostomia or with the substitution of drugs with less anticholinergic effect. Chewing sugarless gum or sucking on hard sugarless candy stimulates saliva production. Artificial saliva (e.g., Salivart and Moi-Stir) may be helpful in some patients. Use of sugarless preparations is important to reduce the likelihood of dental caries.

Dysphagia

Antipsychotic drugs may produce or aggravate dysphagia, a problem either with initiating swallowing or with transferring food from the mouth to the upper esophagus (Bucholz, 1995). Dysphagia may result in nasal or oral regurgitation, coughing while eating, significant weight loss, aspiration, and asphyxiation. Because dysphagia is relatively common in people with severe mental retardation, a possible causative or contributory role for medication should be considered when this problem is discovered.

Gastroesophageal Reflux

Psychotropic drugs with anticholinergic effects may impair esophageal motility, decrease lower esophageal sphincter pressure, or increase gastric volume, which results in gastroesophageal reflux. The reflux of gastric contents into the esophagus can produce regurgitation, a sour or bitter taste in the mouth, heartburn, chest pain, aspiration with choking, wheezing, and coughing. Prolonged gastroesophageal reflux can cause esophageal ulceration; it can also lead to bleeding or stricture formation (Spechler, 1989). For those individuals with significant gastroesophageal reflux, elimination of anticholinergic medications, when possible, may significantly improve clinical status. Additionally, the need for promotility medications such as metoclopramide and cisapride may be reduced or eliminated.

Nausea, Vomiting, and Gastrointestinal Discomfort

These are common side effects of lithium, valproic acid, clomipramine, and SSRIs. These side effects may be dose limiting or necessitate therapy changes during treatment with SSRIs. Gastrointestinal discomfort may also develop after abrupt withdrawal of TCAs, neuroleptics, and benztropine. It is often possible to minimize these side effects by administering the medication with or after meals or by using sustained-release (e.g., LithoBID) or enteric-coated (e.g., Depakote) medications.

Constipation or Abnormal Distension

This effect most commonly occurs as a complication of treatment with psychotropic drugs with anticholinergic effects (e.g., TCAs, lower-potency antipsychotics, and anticholinergic anti-Parkinson agents). Potentially serious sequelae may include paralytic ileus, megacolon, pseudo-obstruction, or actual mechanical obstruction. Constipation is a common problem in people with mental retardation and developmental disabilities and may be easily overlooked. Patients taking drugs with anticholinergic properties should be monitored carefully. If significant constipation occurs, dietary fiber, bulk laxatives, stool softeners, or osmotic agents (e.g., milk of magnesia) are often helpful. Fluid intake is very important in preventing constipation or impaction. Careful assessment may reveal that actual fluid intake is marginal; increase in fluid intake is often a relatively easy treatment for constipation. Eight to ten glasses of water per day is recommended, especially for individuals who are sedentary or nonambulatory.

Diarrhea

Diarrhea may occur in patients treated with lithium, particularly during the first six months of treatment and when serum lithium values exceed 0.8. This side effect is of significance, because gradual fluid and electrolyte loss may predispose treated people to gradual accumulation of lithium with potential intoxication. SSRIs also may produce diarrhea in the beginning of treatment. Gradual dose increases and administration with food may help reduce this side effect.

HEPATIC EFFECTS

Psychotropic drugs can produce liver disease that is clinically, biochemically, and sometimes pathologically difficult to distinguish from acute viral hepatitis, chronic hepatitis, obstructive jaundice, cirrhosis, or primary biliary cirrhosis (Ludwig & Axelsen, 1983). Drug-induced hepatic injury may be classified as predominantly hepatocellular or predominantly cholestatic. The symptoms of hepatocellular hepatotoxicity (nausea, fatigue, and anorexia) are similar to those of acute viral hepatitis (Lee, 1995; Zimmerman & Ishak, 1987). Hepatocellular degeneration, necrosis, or steatosis may result and may progress to death. Valproic acid has been reported to produce a fatal hepatotoxicity. It primarily occurs within the first six months of treatment. Important risk factors include age less than two years; the presence of developmental delay, congenital abnormalities, or other neurological disorders; and the use of other antiepileptic drugs in combination with valproic acid (Bryant & Dreifuss, 1996). Although frequent monitoring of laboratory tests of liver function is advocated, it is not likely to allow early detection of valproic acid-induced hepatotoxicity. Treated people and their caregivers should be educated regarding the need to seek medical attention if symptoms of abdominal pain, vomiting, and jaundice are noted. Hepatocellular hepatotoxicity is also associated with MAOIs. Clinically and biochemically, drug-induced cholestasis may mimic obstructive jaundice. It has most commonly been reported in patients who take phenothiazine antipsychotic drugs (e.g., chlorpromazine, fluphenazine, perphenazine, prochlorperazine, thioridazine, and trifluoperazine), although it is a relatively rare event. Other psychotropic drugs may very rarely cause cholestasis.

RENAL AND GENITOURINARY SYSTEM EFFECTS

Polyuria

Polyuria is often associated with the use of lithium (see earlier discussion of NDI). Education of patients and caregivers is an important aspect of managing lithium-induced polyuria. It is important to correct the possible misperception that polyuria results from excessive fluid intake and can therefore be managed by restricting fluids; this approach may predispose affected patients to serious lithium accumulation and potential intoxication. People with lithium-related polyuria should be allowed free access to liquids. Thiazide diuretics may help decrease urine volume to a tolerable level; however, because thiazides may increase serum lithium levels, lithium dosage may need to be reduced. Should diuretics not work or not be tolerated, indomethacin may be helpful. Indomethacin may also cause lithium accumulation. Patients receiving lithium in combination with either diuretics or indomethacin must be monitored carefully for symptoms of lithium intoxication and for unnecessarily elevated lithium plasma concentrations.

Incontinence and Enuresis

Although incontinence has been reported with most classes of neuroleptics, it does not appear to be a common side effect. The problem usually develops shortly after the start of neuroleptic treatment, sometimes remits spontaneously, but also may require drug discontinuation (Ambrosini & Nurnberg, 1980). Although incontinence is usually not associated with antidepressant medication, overflow incontinence can occur if anticholinergic activity causes urinary retention. Trazodone, carbamazepine, clonazepam, and phenytoin have occasionally been associated with incontinence. If the offending agent can be discontinued, no other treatment should be necessary and urodynamic evaluation would not be indicated. Even with drug continuation, some patients will spontaneously become continent.

If the problem persists, consultation with a urologist should be considered.

Urinary Retention

Urinary retention may be accompanied by other symptomatic complaints including decreased frequency of urination, difficulty voiding, suprapubic discomfort, and reduced bladder sensation. Psychotropic drugs with anticholinergic activity have been most commonly implicated in causing urinary retention. These drugs include phenothiazines, TCAs (amitriptyline and protriptyline are the most anticholinergic; desipramine, nortriptyline, and amoxapine are among the least). However, drugs with very low or negligible anticholinergic activity (e.g., MAOIs, benzodiazepines, trazodone, fluoxetine, bupropion, and sertraline) have also been linked to urinary retention. Dosage reduction or drug discontinuation usually should reverse the problem. Should difficulties arise for patients taking low-potency antipsychotics (e.g., clozapine, chlorpromazine, or thioridazine), either dosage reduction or changing to a less anticholinergic, higher-potency drug (e.g., haloperidol or thiothixene) may be all that is necessary. However, switching to a high-potency neuroleptic drug may increase the risk of extrapyramidal side effects leading to the use of anti-Parkinson drugs (potent anticholinergics). The use of an alternate such as amantadine could be considered. Acute episodes of retention may require catheter decompression of the bladder. If continuation of the causative drug is necessary, the use of a cholinergic agonist such as bethanechol will often relieve symptoms (Everett, 1975).

Renal Failure

As a complication of lithium therapy, renal failure is fortunately uncommon. Acute renal failure may occur following episodes of acute lithium toxicity, and hemodialysis may be necessary on a short-term basis. People with preexisting renal disease or episodes of lithium intoxication may be predisposed to the development of renal failure after long-term lithium treatment. Laboratory monitoring of renal function (serum creatinine) during ongoing lithium treatment is important. Additionally, close monitoring of people treated with lithium to avoid episodes of lithium intoxication may prevent eventual renal damage (Gitlin, 1993; Hetmar, Povlsen, Ladefoged, & Bolwig, 1991).

NEUROMUSCULAR EFFECTS

Myoclonus

Myoclonus has been associated with TCA or MAOI treatment. In most cases it has been mild and consisted of two to three very brief jerks of the lower extremities, usually in the evening during relaxation. Some more severe forms of myoclonus are repetitive jaw jerking, causing stuttering; sudden arm jerking, resulting in dropping objects; and nocturnal myoclonus (Garvey & Tollefson, 1987). Myoclonus usually develops after two to four weeks of treatment. People with mental retardation and developmental disabilities may have difficulty describing myoclonus, yet this effect may cause discomfort and interference with functional ability. In severe cases, clonazepam, valproic acid, or carbamazepine may be helpful and allow continued use of the causative drug.

Nocturnal Myoclonus

Repetitive, violent, jerky contraction of the legs may develop in patients taking antidepressants such as clomipramine, standard TCAs, and MAOIs. Although the patient may not be aware of this effect, it may be most disturbing to the bed partner (Casas et al., 1987). Nocturnal myoclonus sometimes responds to dose reduction, or to drugs for myoclonus such as carbamazepine, clonazepam, and valproate. A switch to another antidepressant is advised in cases that fail to respond.

Action (Intention) Tremor of Upper Extremities

This effect is relatively common during treatment with TCAs and lithium. Education of patients and caregivers regarding tremor is important. Fine tremor is not usually a sign of serious lithium intoxication. Patients and caregivers should be informed that coarsening and increasing amplitude of tremor may be a symptom of lithium intoxication requiring medical intervention. Because this tremor is most pronounced during voluntary use of the affected limbs, considerable interference with motor activities may occur. This is of special significance to people with mental retardation and developmental disabilities who already have an impairment in motor coordination. This tremor may be aggravated by

caffeine intake. For many affected people, tolerance with reduction of tremor occurs over time. If a dose reduction is not feasible or does not relieve the tremor, propranolol may be tried. Doses of propranolol required for relief of tremor are usually 40-160 mg/day (Gelenberg & Jefferson, 1995).

Acute Extrapyramidal Symptoms

The acute, dose-related neuroleptic-induced movement abnormalities are referred to as extrapyramidal symptoms because they result from disturbances in the brain structures affecting bodily movement, excluding motor neurons, the motor cortex, and the pyramidal tract. Distinction between these neuromuscular effects and the tardive syndromes is important. Acute extrapyramidal symptoms generally occur relatively early in the course of treatment with antipsychotic drugs, are more frequent or severe with larger daily doses, are reversible with discontinuation of medication, and are treatable with anticholinergic anti-Parkinson medications. The primary symptoms are acute dystonia, neuroleptic-induced Parkinsonism, and acute akathisia.

Acute dystonia involves intermittent or sustained muscular contraction or spasm that may produce an abnormal posture, involuntary movements, rigidity, or cramping in the muscles of the head, neck, or trunk. Bizarre postures or gait may be the results of the involvement of extremities. Sustained contraction of the masticatory muscles can produce facial grimacing, opening of jaw, and protrusion of the tongue. In oculogyric crisis, patients exhibit upward and lateral rotation of the eyes. Blepharospasm with sustained eye closure may occur. During these events, the head may be tilted backward (retrocollis) or sideways (torticollis).

Acute dystonia tends to occur during the first few days of treatment with antipsychotic medication or with a rapid increase in dose (Neppe & Ward, 1989). However, reactions may also develop after a switch to depot medication. Dystonia is more common with the use of high-potency typical antipsychotic drugs such as haloperidol or fluphenazine. Dystonic reactions may last for a few seconds to several hours. Treatment of the reactions with an anticholinergic anti-Parkinson agent (e.g., benztropine) or an anticholinergic antihistamine (diphenhydramine given either intravenously or intramuscularly) usually provides relief in minutes. Benzodiazepine may also be helpful. If the antipsychotic drug cannot be discontinued and the patient is not already on routine doses of an anti-Parkinson agent, one should be started.

A seven-day course of anti-Parkinson agents at the start of neuroleptic therapy has been recommended to prevent acute dystonic reaction (Winslow, Stiller, Coons, & Robison, 1986).

Neuroleptic-induced Parkinsonism is characterized by bradykinesia (slow movement) or akinesia (lack of movement), tremor, and rigidity. Akinesia is the earliest, most common, and frequently the only marked manifestation of drug-induced Parkinsonism (DeMario, 1988; Goetz & Klawans, 1981; Rifkin, Quitkin, & Klein, 1975). A blank, unblinking, mask-like facial appearance may commonly be observed, and the treated person may be incorrectly attributed as being over-drugged. The tremor is often described as a coarse "pill-rolling" or "to and fro" rhythmical movement that is greater at rest. Rigidity is most apparent in the limbs, where a cogwheeling resistance is noted during passive movement. All of these signs may present in varying degrees and combinations. Onset of this syndrome may occur after the first week of treatment, but usually within the first month (Kane, 1989). The anticholinergic-type anti-Parkinson drugs (benztropine, biperidin, trihexyphenidyl, and procyclidine) are the most extensively used drugs. Antihistamines with anticholinergic properties (e.g., diphenhydramine) and dopamine-releasing agents (e.g., amantadine) can be considered when the anticholinergic anti-Parkinson drugs are not effective or cause unacceptable side effects. Parkinsonian side effects are more common with higher-potency, typical antipsychotic medications. Changing medication to one with lower potency or to one of the newer atypical antipsychotics may be an effective strategy for relief of Parkinsonian symptoms.

Acute akathisia (an inability to sit still or an intense subjective sense of restlessness) usually occurs during the early phase of neuroleptic drug treatment, especially with rapid-dosage increases of high-potency neuroleptic drugs. Akathisia is the most common of the acute extrapyramidal symptoms, yet it is often the most difficult to assess and identify. In its most severe form, an individual is unable to maintain any position for more than a few moments. Aggression, assault, and suicide have been attributed to the pervasive discomfort of akathisia. SSRIs such as fluoxetine can cause akathisia (Lipinski, Zimmerman, & Pope, 1989). Diagnosis of drug-induced akathisia in people with mental retardation and developmental disabilities is even more difficult than in the general psychiatric population because it is often a subjective problem (Ganesh, Murti Rao, & Cowie, 1989). Akathisia is easily confused with the underlying agitation for which antipsychotic medication is

prescribed. At the present time, there is no universally acceptable objective definition of akathisia. Thus, treatment of this condition is challenging. Anticholinergic anti-Parkinson drugs are often only partly effective. Dosage reduction, discontinuation, or changing the causative antipsychotic to a medication with a lower likelihood of causing akathisia are preferred therapeutic approaches, but they are not always feasible or effective. Propranolol or other lipophilic beta-adrenergic blocking agents may be helpful (Fleischhacker, Roth, & Kane, 1990). Benzodiazepines such as clonazepam or lorazepam may be effective when other treatments are not. If other forms of extrapyramidal symptoms are present, anticholinergic anti-Parkinson drugs should be used first.

Recently, Gross, Hull, Lytton, Hill and Piersel (1993) reviewed drug-induced akathisia in individuals with mental retardation. They commented that the 13% prevalence of akathisia in individuals reported earlier (Stone, May, Alvarez, & Ellmann, 1989) probably was an underestimate. According to Gross et al., many individuals did not have expressive verbal skills and could not report the subjective feelings of neuroleptic-induced akathisia.

Tardive Symptoms

These late-onset neuromuscular symptoms may persist indefinitely in some people despite discontinuation of the causative drug. Clinically, they are differentiated from acute extrapyramidal symptoms by their late onset, clinical manifestations, lack of response to anticholinergic anti-Parkinson medications, and tendency to appear or worsen when the causative medication is withdrawn or the dose is reduced. The primary symptoms are tardive akathisia, tardive dystonia, and tardive dyskinesia.

Tardive akathisia refers to late-occurring akathisia that persists despite the withdrawal of an antipsychotic drug. When the drug is restarted, akathisia may improve temporarily. Reserpine and tetrabenazine seem to be effective drugs for suppressing chronic akathisia (Burke, Kang, Jankovic, Miller, & Fahn, 1989). Tardive dystonia develops after a median of five years of exposure to antipsychotic drugs (Kang, Burke, & Fahn, 1986). The abnormal movements in tardive dystonia are similar to those present in primary torsion dystonia, with the face and neck being the most frequently involved bodily regions.

Tardive dyskinesia is a movement disorder consisting of frequent, repetitive, involuntary movements of the lips, tongue, jaw, face, trunk, or limbs. The abnormal involuntary movements may increase with emotional arousal or during activities requiring repetition of motor activities or attention to fine motor tasks. Attempts at conscious control of the symptoms may be successful or may increase the movements. The movements may decrease with relaxation and are entirely absent during sleep. Tardive dyskinesia occurs after prolonged treatment with typical antipsychotic medications, amoxapine, and metoclopramide. There is little evidence to suggest that, of the typical antipsychotics, one agent is more or less likely to cause tardive dyskinesia. Some atypical antipsychotic agents (e.g., clozapine) may cause tardive dyskinesia, whereas others (e.g., risperidone) may be less likely to do so. The onset of symptoms is typically subtle but may be abrupt when the antipsychotics are suddenly withdrawn. The symptoms may persist for months or years following antipsychotic treatment.

Estimates of the incidence and prevalence of tardive dyskinesia vary greatly. Epidemiologic research consistently shows an annual incidence rate of approximately 4% and a prevalence of up to 30% to 35% of the antipsychotic-treated population. Patients with late-onset psychoses, people with affective disorders, women, and individuals over the age of 50 are more prone to developing the symptoms (Casey, 1993; Yassa, Nair, & Schwartz, 1986). Large doses of antipsychotic medication, amoxapine, or metoclopramide and long duration of treatment increase the risk of developing tardive dyskinesia. Long-term follow-up studies suggest that tardive dyskinesia is not usually progressive. It may follow a fluctuating course with spontaneous remissions and exacerbations (Gardos et al., 1988). Age may influence the likelihood of recovery from symptoms. In young patients, discontinuation of antipsychotic medication generally causes a temporary increase in symptoms, but there may be steady improvement over a period of months or years, provided that the antipsychotics are withheld. Most research shows that mild cases in the young are usually transient and reversible, with current remission rates of 50%-90% being reported. Severe cases of persistent tardive dyskinesia (approximately 3% of cases) may cause interference with breathing, speaking, and eating or may be disfiguring. Persistent tardive dyskinesia occurs less frequently than does withdrawal or transient tardive dykinesia, but its intensity is quite alarming and debilitating (Gualtieri, Schroeder, Hicks, & Quade, 1986; Kalachnik, 1991). Buccal-lingual-masticatory facial movements appear to be common in people with mental retardation and developmental disabilities (Cohen, Khan, Zheng, & Chiles, 1991; Gualtieri et al., 1986).

In the past, treatment consisted of either trying to reduce dopamine (DA) activity (e.g., by increasing the dose of the neuroleptic drug) or enhancing cholinergic activity (e.g., by administering physostigmine, which reduces acetylcholine metabolism, or lecithin, deanol, or choline, which are purported to increase brain acetylcholine synthesis). The former tactic leads to temporary relief and later to potential worsening of the condition. The latter tactic has produced only temporary or negligible benefits. Attempts to modify or amplify DA activity (such as with L-dopa) in order to desensitize DA receptors have, at times, led to encouraging findings. Several other drugs (clozapine, clonidine, propranolol, benzodiazepines, calcium channel blockers, and vitamin E) have shown some promise of efficacy, but further studies are needed to establish their usefulness in the treatment of tardive dyskinesia (Marken & Stanislav, 1995). In situations where tardive dyskinesia is present and antipsychotic medication must be continued, clozapine is considered a potentially useful treatment agent; clozapine does not worsen tardive dyskinesia.

At the present time, no proven safe and consistently effective treatments are available for tardive dyskinesia. Therefore, prevention and early diagnosis of this syndrome must be emphasized. Physicians should examine patients prior to initiation of potentially causative drugs and regularly during therapy (every three to six months). Effective prevention also lies in cautious use of neuroleptic drugs given at the lowest effective dose.

Neuroleptic Malignant Syndrome

Neuroleptic malignant syndrome (NMS) is a rare, but potentially fatal, side effect of antipsychotic medication (Boyd, 1993; Guze & Baxter, 1985; Shalev, Hermesh, & Munitz, 1989). Core features of this syndrome are severe muscle rigidity (lead pipe rigidity) or catatonia, instability of the autonomic nervous system (including hypertension or labile blood pressure, tachycardia or bradycardia, cardiac arrhythmias, dilated pupils, prominent diaphoresis, and incontinence of feces or urine), rapid onset of severe hyperthermia (body temperatures of 101°-104° F), and altered mental status (ranging from agitation and alert mutism to stupor or even coma). There may be associated choreiform movements, dyskinetic movements, a festinating gait, and flexor extensor posturing (Pope, Keek, & McElroy, 1986). All antipsychotic drugs (including the atypical agents) have been reported to induce NMS. Manifestations may develop within 45 minutes of initiating neuroleptic therapy, after months to years of treatment, or after a dosage increase (Moyes, 1973; Yeragani & Chaitin, 1987). The highest risk of developing NMS appears to occur when neuroleptics are either being initiated or increased. It typically occurs at doses within the currently accepted range (Shalev & Munitz, 1986). Severe, acute extrapyramidal symptoms may be accompanied by unrelated medical disorders that cause fever and other symptoms and signs mimicking NMS. In this setting, differential diagnosis of NMS may be quite difficult.

Early reports indicated that NMS was lethal in approximately 20%-30% of patients who developed this side effect, but recent reports suggest that lethality has decreased significantly. This improved prognosis may be related to increased awareness, earlier diagnosis, rapid drug discontinuation, earlier institution of intensive supportive care, and use of DA-augmenting drugs (e.g., amantadine, L-dopa, and bromocriptine) or muscle relaxants such as dantrolene (Caroff & Mann, 1988).

Boyd (1993) reviewed 29 published cases of NMS occurring in patients with mental retardation and developmental disabilities. He found that the fatality rate in this population (21%) was approximately double the rate reported for the general population. In the majority of cases (90%), the offending antipsychotic drug had been introduced for the first time or reintroduced after a drug-free period. Haloperidol and fluphenazine were the most frequently implicated drugs, with chlorpromazine a distant third. However, antipsychotic polypharmacy was found in approximately 55% of these cases. The mean number of days to onset of NMS was about 8 days. Using commonly accepted population estimates, Boyd (1993) projected that approximately 7,500 individuals with mental retardation and developmental disabilities would develop NMS annually in the United States; of these cases, 750 would result in fatality. The potential for morbidity and mortality is clearly significant. Patients receiving antipsychotic drugs should be monitored for the onset of symptoms suggesting NMS. Caregivers should be educated regarding the significance of symptoms such as sudden onset of high fever, muscle rigidity, and change in mental status, and they should be instructed to seek medical attention immediately if these symptoms occur. Antipsychotic medication should be used as judiciously as possible.

CONVULSIVE EFFECTS

Seizures are uncommon but significant side effects of many psychotropic drugs (Messing, Clossom, & Simon,

1984). Drug-induced seizures may be of special concern for people with mental retardation and developmental disabilities because of the high prevalence of epilepsy in this population. Estimation of the relative tendency of specific drugs to induce seizures can be difficult. Seizures are more likely to be reported with newly marketed drugs than with older agents for which the risk of seizures is known and accepted (Dessain, Schatzberg, Woods, & Cole, 1986). Generally, lower-potency antipsychotic medications are more likely to induce epileptic seizure activity (Baldessarini, 1985). Clozapine, loxapine, and chlorpromazine are commonly implicated in seizure induction; thioridazine, although a low-potency agent, appears less likely to induce seizures (Cold, Wells, & Foemming, 1990). Amoxapine, maprotiline, clomipramine, and bupropion are the antidepressants most frequently associated with induction of seizures (Rosenstein, Nelson, & Jacobs, 1993). Factors that may predispose patients to drug-induced seizures include present or past history of seizures, family history of epilepsy, use of multiple psychotropic drugs, postnatal brain damage, and administration of high doses of a potentially causative drug. Prevention or avoidance of drug-induced seizures can be enhanced by (a) ensuring that antiepileptic treatment is optimized prior to initiating therapy with potentially epileptogenic drugs for patients with preexisting seizure disorders; (b) avoiding high doses or rapid upward titration; (c) avoiding psychotropic polypharmacy; and (d) using drugs with a high epileptogenic potential cautiously, if at all.

Not every paroxysmal event in a patient receiving a psychotropic agent is a seizure, and misidentifying other conditions as epilepsy can lead to unnecessary and potentially harmful treatment. If a patient on a psychotropic drug has a seizure, one must screen for medical or neurological illness before assuming that the seizure is due to the drug. One must approach an event that appears to be a seizure in a methodical and rational manner and not abruptly change therapy. In many situations, seizure control can be acceptably maintained despite the use of potentially epileptogenic drugs.

MONITORING GUIDELINES

General principles that will aid in the early recognition or detection of medication side effects are shown in Table 7-1 (adapted from Zametkin and Yamada, 1993).

Table 7-1. Guidelines for Monitoring Side Effects

1. A baseline physical assessment and laboratory screening should occur before the medication is implemented, to reduce or prevent false attributions of effects to the medication.

2 Perform follow-up assessments and laboratory monitoring at regular intervals during the titration phase and maintenance therapy, to monitor organ systems that are known to be adversely affected by the medication.

3. Observe the person closely prior to initiating medication therapy. A baseline behavioral assessment is essential for recognizing changes from usual (past) levels for a particular individual.

4. Expect and look for side effects. Remember that people with mental retardation and developmental disabilities may not be able to complain; therefore, practitioners should be aware that an increase in problem behavior may be secondary to the side effects of a medication.

5. Be familiar with the potential side effects and routinely see patients to assess such problems. Some people may be much more sensitive to the effects of medications than others.

6. Parents and caregivers can play a vital part in the monitoring process. Educate and alert them to the potential positive and negative effects of the medication. However, parents' or caregivers' assessments should not be routinely substituted for a formal assessment by the practitioner.

7. Educate the individual whenever possible. People with mild to moderate mental retardation should be informed of the treatment plan at a level they can understand. Ensuring their understanding of the potential positive and negative effects of the medication will enhance compliance.

8. Ask open-ended questions whenever possible when screening for side effects, to prevent getting an echolalic response from a person whose verbal skills are limited.

9. Use rating scales, which are especially helpful because this population is less likely to provide information.

RATING SCALES OF ADVERSE EFFECTS

Objective instruments should be routinely employed to monitor for side effects. Researchers have repeatedly demonstrated that systematic questionnaires or checklists are more reliable for detecting adverse drug reactions than is spontaneous reporting (Bennett & Lipman, 1977; Herranz, Artega, & Armijo, 1982). Without systematic questioning, important reactions may go unreported or unrecognized (Corso, Pucino, DeLeo, Calis, & Gallelli, 1992). It is not feasible to review all available standardized rating scales in this chapter. The purpose of this review is to highlight certain rating scales that are commonly used or were developed primarily for this population.

There are three different types of rating scales used to detect adverse drug reactions (Kalachnik, 1995): medication-specific, general purpose, and side effect-specific. Medication-specific scales are designed to pick up the significant side effects of one medication or a medication class. Many of these are based on the most-frequently occuring symptoms described in the *Physicans' Desk Reference* and other standard sources (Medical Economics Data, 1996). They lose their utility when multiple medications are employed or added.

General Purpose Rating Scales

General purpose rating scales can be used with people who take several medications. They provide an organized, detailed review of body parts and may require a high level of cooperation from the rater or patient. Before using these scales, it is very important to obtain a pretreatment assessment to decrease the likelihood of a false positive. The following is a list of some general purpose rating scales:

1. Adverse Drug Reaction Detection Scale ([ADRDS]; Corso et al., 1992). *Advantages:* The ADRDS is an in-depth and organized review of all body parts that is suitable for use in a research or clinical-practice setting. *Disadvantages:* The ADRDS questionnaire is long and may take some time to complete; therefore, it may be more suitable for verbal individuals with mild to moderate mental retardation.

2. The Dosage Record and Treatment Emergent Symptom Scale ([DOTES]; Guy, 1976b). DOTES was developed by the Early Clinical Drug Evaluation Unit of the National Institute of Mental Health (NIMH). *Advantages:* It is widely used with children and adults, provides a systemic review of all body parts, and includes a physical examination and inquiry. Additionally, it assesses some behavioral side effects, allows for the recording of daily medication dosages, and evaluates the relationship and the intensity of the symptom to medication. *Disadvantages:* It was developed for research purposes. Its coding system is somewhat cumbersome and it may be more suitable for verbal individuals.

3. Monitoring of Side Effects Scales ([MOSES]; Kalachnik, 1988). *Advantages:* MOSES was developed by a Minnesota task force of health care professionals primarily for people with mental retardation and developmental disabilities. It is an in-depth scale that uses lay terminology and targets antiepileptic and psychotropic medications. It also has an extrapyramidal symptom subscale. *Disadvantages:* It is long and only assesses the presence or absence of symptoms.

4. Subjective Treatment Emergent Symptoms Scale ([STESS]; Guy, 1976c). *Advantages:* The STESS was designed for children up to 15 years of age. It features lay terminology such that it can be completed by the child, parent, or supervising adult. It can be used as a screening tool in clinical settings to evaluate the presence and severity of physical complaints. *Disadvantages:* It does not permit assessment of the relationship of physical complaints to medication and does not assess the duration of symptoms.

5. Treatment Emergent Symptoms Scale ([TESS]; Guy, 1976d). *Advantages:* TESS is a short, 6-item scale used in conjunction with the DOTES. The presence and severity of symptoms not on the DOTES are rated. TESS is used to assess the relationship of symptoms to prescribed medication. *Disadvantages:* It was developed

for research purposes, must be used in conjunction with the DOTES, and may be more suitable for verbal individuals. A special coding system has been designed; the coded entries on the DOTES and TESS must match.

Side Effect-Specific Scales

Side effect-specific scales provide for detailed ratings for a single type of a commonly known side effect. The scales described here were developed to assess the acute and chronic extrapyramidal symptoms produced by most neuroleptic medications (described in detail earlier in this chapter). Although most of them were developed as research instruments and may be more appropriate for verbal individuals, they can be used in clinical practice and offer helpful collateral information. It is very important to obtain a pretreatment assessment, because, unfortunately, extrapyramidal symptoms (especially tardive dyskinesia) are often unrecognized or misdiagnosed (Meiselas et al., 1989).

1. Abnormal Involuntary Movement Scale ([AIMS]; Guy, 1976a). *Advantages:* The AIMS is the most widely recognized and utilized rating scale for routine screening and early detection of tardive dyskinesia. It is a 12-item scale that provides for ratings of the presence, severity, impairment, and patient's awareness of movements. Dental status is also assessed to reduce false positives on oral-facial movements. *Disadvantages:* The AIMS may require the rater to be a little creative at times to activate movements in individuals who are more severely impaired. This may reduce the reliability of the assessment if different raters are employed. Additionally, it is unable to capture tardive dystonias or tardive akathisia.

2. Barnes Akathisia Rating Scale ([BARS]; Barnes, 1989). *Advantages:* The BARS has both objective and subjective components. The objective component is performed with the subjects in several different positions and settings. *Disadvantages:* It is a relatively new research instrument, and it is still used primarily by researchers. It does not evaluate all important types of extrapyramidal symptoms, necessitating the use of at least one additional scale.

3. Curtis, Love, Mahood, Platman, and Sherr Abnormal Movement Scale ([CLAMPS]; Curtis, Love, Mahood, Platman, & Sherr, 1992). This instrument was developed by an interdisciplinary task force of professionals at Rosewood Center in Owings Mills, MD, a residential treatment facility for persons with mental retardation and developmental disabilities. *Advantages:* The CLAMPS was designed to rate dystonic, Parkinsonian, and dyskinetic movements.

Tremors are rated separately from choreoathetoid movements. *Disadvantages:* The scale is still new. Psychometric data on its validity and reliability has not been published.

4. Dyskinesia Identification System: Condensed User Scale ([DISCUS]; Sprague and Kalachnik, 1991). *Advantages:* The DISCUS is used to detect the presence and overall intensity of symptoms. Reliability and validity data are available for use with people with mental illness and people with mental retardation. A high total score is correlated with a diagnosis of tardive dyskinesia (Sprague & Kalachnik, 1991). *Disadvantages:* It cannot be used to assess the severity of a specific symptom or the subjective concerns of the individual. It does not capture tardive akathisia.

5. Extrapyramidal Symptom Rating Scale ([ESRS]; Chouinard, Ross-Chouinard, Annable, & Jones, 1980). *Advantages:* This instrument, which consists of both objective and subjective components, assesses the presence or absence of acute and chronic extrapyramidal symptoms. *Disadvantages:* A major portion of the ESRS must be completed by a physician. The ESRS does not assess the severity of symptoms.

6. Simpson-Angus Neurological Rating Scale ([NRS]; Simpson & Angus, 1970). *Advantages:* The NRS is an objective scale, designed to measure Parkinsonian side effects and akathisia. It has been used in many research studies. *Disadvantages:* It does not capture the true severity of akathisia and does not assess dystonias or dyskinesias.

Several other scales are worth mentioning here. The Systematic Assessment for Treatment Emergent Effects (SAFTEE) was developed by the NIMH (1986) as a research instrument. It uses a very comprehensive, organ-system approach that also elicits detection of some unanticipated side effects. The UKU Side Effect Scale (Lingjaerde, Anfors, Bech, Dencker, & Elgin, 1987), developed by the Scandinavian Society of Psychopharmacology, is a cross between a general scale and a side effect-specific scale. It was developed for the assessment of side effects produced by psychotropic medication and is recommended for use in both clinical trials and practice settings. The Withdrawal Emergent Symptom Checklist ([WESC]; Engelhardt, 1974) is useful for assessing behavioral effects when withdrawing medications. (For a more comprehensive review of the techniques and analysis of rating instruments presented in this chapter, see Kalachnik, 1988; Munetz & Benjamin, 1988; NIMH, 1985).

There is a need for more research regarding the efficacy and safety of psychotropic medications in people with mental retardation and developmental disabilities. There also is a need for better assessment tools in the research setting as well as in general practice.

CONCLUSION

A number of significant adverse effects of psychotropic drugs occur in people with mental retardation and developmental disabilities. A wide range of prevalence estimates of these effects has been reported (Casey, 1991). A full appreciation of these potential adverse effects is important when weighing the benefit-to-risk ratio of using any particular medication.

There is a paucity of systematic and well controlled studies of psychotropic drug-induced side effects, particularly with regard to the immune system, hematology, and reproductive and sexual functions. The conclusions published in most relevant reports, especially those pertaining to people with mental retardation and developmental disabilites, are based on small uncontrolled studies or case reports. For most psychotropic drugs, therefore, it is currently not possible to predict, based on scientific research, which patients are at risk of developing clinically relevant complications.

Standardized, user-friendly rating scales for monitoring various drug-induced side effects are needed. Such scales are essential for future prospective and systematic research in terms of collecting reliable and usable data and for enhancing the quality of psychiatric care for this population. The purpose of reviewing some existing scales in this chapter was not to recommend or endorse any particular scale but to encourage practitioners to incorporate a formal monitoring program. Most of the rating scales can be used by trained practitioners or health care workers, with the results subject to review by a psychiatrist, trained psychiatric pharmacist, or nurse specialist. Techniques and norms for measuring the blood concentrations of psychotropic drugs also need to be further characterized. Such information is critical for the development of objective measures and to assist with the diagnoses of these side effects.

REFERENCES

Aman, M.G., Marks, M.B., Turbott, S.H., Wilsher, C.P., & Merry, S.N. (1991). Methylphenidate and thioridazine in the treatment of intellectually subaverage children: Effects on cognitive motor performance. *Journal of American Academy of Child and Adolescent Psychiatry, 30*, 816–824.

Aman, M.G., Paxton, J.W., Field, C.J., & Foote, S.E. (1986). Prevalence of toxic anticonvulsant drug concentrations in mentally retarded persons with epilepsy. *American Journal of Mental Deficiency, 90*, 643–650.

Aman, M.G., & Singh, N.N. (1988). *Psychopharmacology of the developmental disabilities.* New York: Springer-Verlag.

Ambrosini, P.J., & Nurnberg, H.G. (1980). Enuresis and incontinence occurring with neuroleptics [Letter to the Editor]. *American Journal of Psychiatry, 137*, 1278–1279.

Angst, J. (1985). Switch from depression to mania: A record study over decades between 1920 and 1982. *Psychopathology, 18*, 140–154.

Arnold, L.E. (1993). Clinical pharmacological issues in treating psychiatric disorders of patients with mental retardation. *Annals of Clinical Psychiatry, 5*, 189–198.

Baldessarini, R.J. (1985). *Chemotherapy and psychiatry.* Cambridge, MA: Harvard University Press.

Barnes, T.R.E. (1989). A rating scale for drug-induced akathisia. *British Journal of Psychiatry, 154*, 672–676.

Baumeister, A.A., & Forehand, R. (1973). Stereotyped acts. In N.R. Ellis (Ed.), *International review of research in mental retardation,* (Vol. 6, pp. 55–96). New York: Academic Press.

Bennett, B.S., & Lipman, A.G. (1977). Comparative study of prospective and voluntary reporting in determining the incidence of adverse drug reactions. *American Journal of Hospital Pharmacy, 34*, 931–936.

Boyd, R.D. (1993). Neuroleptic malignant syndrome and mental retardation: Review and analysis of 29 cases. *American Journal on Mental Retardation, 98*, 143–155.

Brown, W.A. (1983). Prolactin levels and effects of neuroleptics. *Psychosomatics, 5*, 317–322.

Bryant, A.E., & Dreifuss, F.E. (1996). Valproic acid hepatic fatalities: III. U.S. experience since 1986. *Neurology, 46*, 465–469.

Bucholz, D.W. (1995). Oropharyngeal dysphagia due to iatrogenic neurological dysfunction. *Dysphagia, 10*, 248–254.

Burke, R.E., Kang, U.J., Jankovic, J., Miller, L.G., & Fahn, S. (1989). Tardive akathisia: An analysis of clinic features and response to open therapeutic trials. *Movement Disorders, 4*, 157–175.

Caroff, S.N., & Mann, S.C. (1988). Neuroleptic malignant syndrome. *Psychopharmacology Bulletin, 23*, 514–518.

Casas, M., Garcia-Ribera, C., Alvarez, E., Udina, C., Queralto, J.M., & Grau, J.M. (1987). Myoclonic movements as a side effect of treatment with therapeutic doses of clomipramine. *International Clinical Psychopharmacology, 2*, 333–336.

Casey, D.E. (1991). Neuroleptic drug-induced extrapyramidal syndromes and tardive dyskinesia. *Schizophrenia Research, 4*, 109–120.

Casey, D.E. (1993). Neuroleptic-induced acute extrapyramidal symptoms and tardive dyskinesia. *Psychiatric Clinics of North America, 16*, 589.

Chouinard, G., Ross-Chouinard, A., Annable, L., & Jones, B.D. (1980). Extrapyramidal symptom rating scale. *Canadian Journal of Neuroscience, 5*, 164–166.

Clary, C., & Schweizer, E. (1987). Treatment of MAOI hypertensive crisis with sublingual nifedipine. *Journal of Clinical Psychiatry, 48*, 249–250.

Cockhill, L.A., & Remick, R.A. (1987). Blood pressure effects of monoamine oxidase inhibitors — the highs and lows. *Canadian Journal of Psychiatry, 32*, 803–808.

Cohen, S.A., Khan, A., Zheng, Y., & Chiles, J. (1991). Tardive dyskinesia in the mentally retarded: Comparison of prevalence, risk factors and topography with a schizophrenic population. *Acta Psychiatrica Scandinavica, 83*, 234–237.

Cold, J.A., Wells, B.G., & Foemming, J.H. (1990). Seizure activity associated with antipsychotic therapy. *DICP: Annals of Pharmacotherapy, 24*, 601–606.

Cole, J.O., & Bodkin, J.A. (1990). Antidepressant drug side effects. *Journal of Clinical Psychiatry, 51*, 21–26.

Cook, E.H., Jr., Rowlett, R., Jaselskis, C., & Levanthal, B.L. (1992). Fluoxetine treatment of children and adults with autistic disorders and mental retardation. *Journal of the American Academy of Child and Adolescent Psychiatry, 31*, 734–745.

Conoso, R.T., De Oliveira, R.M., & Nixon, R.A. (1990). Neuroleptic associated auto-antibodies: A prevalence study. *Biological Psychiatry, 27*, 863–870.

Corso, D.M., Pucino, F., DeLeo, J.M., Calis, K.A., & Gallelli, J.F. (1992). Development of a questionnaire for detecting potential adverse drug reactions. *Annals of Pharmacotherapy, 26*, 890–896.

Curtis, J.L., Love, R.C., Mahood, P., Platman, S.R., & Sherr, J.D. (1992). *Curtis, Love, Mahood, Platman, and Sherr Abnormal Movement Scale (CLAMPS).* Unpublished manuscript.

Davies, D.M. (Ed.). (1977). *Textbook of adverse drug reactions.* London: Oxford University Press.

Davis, K.L., & Rosenberg, G.S. (1979). Is there a limbic system equivalent of tardive dyskinesia? *Biological Psychiatry, 14*, 699–703.

DeMaio, D. (1988). Notes on human behavioral pharmacotoxicology. In C. Radovco-Thomas & F. Garcin (Eds.), *Progress in neuropsychopharmacology and biological psychiatry* (pp. 33–40). Elmsford, NY: Pergamon Press.

Dessain, E.C., Schatzberg, A.F., Woods, B.T., & Cole, J.O. (1986). Maprotiline treatment in depression: A perspective on seizures. *Archives of General Psychiatry, 43*, 86–90.

Dilsaver, S.C. (1989). Antidepressant withdrawal syndromes: Phenomenology and pathophysiology. *Acta Psychiatrica Scandinavica, 79*, 113–117.

Dilsaver, S.C., & Greden, J.F. (1983). Antidepressant withdrawal phenomena. *Biological Psychiatry, 19*, 237–256.

Emerson, C.H., Dyson, W.L., & Utiger, R.D. (1973). *Journal of Clinical Endocrinology and Metabolism, 36*, 338–346.

Engelhardt, D.M. (1974). *Withdrawal Emergent Symptoms (WES) Checklist.* State University of New York, Downstate Medical Center, Department of Psychiatry.

Evans, R.W., & Gualtieri, C.T. (1985). Carbamazepine: A neuropsychological and psychiatric profile. *Clinical Neuropharmacology, 83*, 221–286.

Everett, H.C. (1975). The use of bethanechol chloride with tricyclic antidepressants. *American Journal of Psychiatry, 132*, 1202–1204.

Fleischhacker, W.W., Roth, S.D., & Kane, J.M. (1990). The pharmacologic treatment of neuroleptic-induced akathisia. *Journal of Clinical Psychopharmacology, 10*, 12–21.

Flemenbaum, A. (1976). Pavor nocturnus: A complication of single daily tricyclic or neuroleptic dosage. *American Journal of Psychiatry, 133*, 570–572.

Friedman, D.L., Kastner, T., Plummer, A.T., Ruiz, M.Q., & Henning, D. (1992). Adverse behavioral effects in individuals with mental retardation and mood disorders treated with carbamazepine. *American Journal on Mental Retardation, 96*, 541–546.

Ganesh, S., Murti Rao, J.M., & Cowie, V.A. (1989). Akathisia in neuroleptic medicated mentally handicapped subjects. *Journal of Mental Deficiency Research, 33*, 323–329.

Gardner, D.L., & Cowdry, R.W. (1985). Alprazolam induced dyscontrol in borderline personality disorder. *American Journal of Psychiatry, 142*, 98–100.

Gardos, G., Cole, J.O., Haskell, D., Marby, D., Schneibolk-Paine, S., & Moore, P. (1988). The natural history of tardive dyskinesia. *Journal of Clinical Psychopharmacology, 8*(Suppl. 4), 31–33.

Garner, E.M., Kelly, M.W., & Thompson, D.F. (1993) Tricyclic antidepressant withdrawal syndrome. *Annals of Pharmacotherapy, 27*, 1068–1072.

Garvey, M.J., & Tollefson, G.D. (1987). Occurrence of myoclonus in patients treated with cyclic antidepressants. *Archives of General Psychiatry, 44*, 269–272.

Gawin, F.H., & Markoff, R.A. (1981). Panic anxiety after abrupt discontinuation of amitriptyline. *American Journal of Psychiatry, 138*, 117–118.

Gelenberg, A.J., & Jefferson, J.W. (1995). Lithium tremor. *Journal of Clinical Psychiatry, 56*(Suppl. 7), 283–287.

Gelenberg, A.J., Van Putten, T., Lavori, P.W., Wojcik, J.D., et al. (1989). Anticholinergic effects on memory: Benztropine versus amantadine. *Journal of Clinical Psychopharmacology, 9*, 180–185.

Ghadirian, A.M., Chouinard, G., & Annable, L. (1982). Sexual dysfunction and plasma prolactin levels in neuroleptic-treated schizophrenic outpatients. *Journal of Nervous and Mental Disease, 170*, 463–367.

Gitlin, M.J. (1993). Lithium-induced renal insufficiency. *Journal of Clinical Psychopharmacology, 13*, 276–280.

Glassman, A.H., & Bigger, J.T., Jr. (1981). Cardiovascular effects of therapeutic doses of tricyclic antidepressants: A review. *Archives of General Psychiatry, 38*, 815–820.

Goetz, C.G., & Klawans H.L. (1981). Drug-induced extrapyramidal disorders: A neuropsychiatric interface. *Journal of Clinical Psychopharmacology, 1*, 297–303.

Golde, T.E., Estus, S., & Usiak, M. (1990). Expression of beta amyloid protein precursor mRNAs: Recognition of a novel alternatively spliced form and quantitation in Alzheimer's disease using PCR. *Neuron, 4*, 253–267.

Goldman, L.S., Hudson, J.L., & Weddington, W.W. (1980). Lupus-like illness associated with chlorpromazine. *American Journal of Psychiatry, 12*, 1613–1614.

Gorman, J.M., Liebowitz, M.R., Fyer, A.J., Goetz, D.H., Campeas, R.B., Fyer, M.R., Davies, S.O., & Klein, D.F. (1987). An open trial of fluoxetine in the treatment of panic attacks. *Journal of Clinical Psychopharmacology, 7*, 329–332.

Gross, E.J., Hull, H.G., Lytton, G.J., Hill, J.A., & Piersel, W.C. (1993). Case study of neuroleptic-induced akathisia: Important implications for individuals with mental retardation. *American Journal on Mental Retardation, 98*, 156–164.

Gualtieri, C.T., & Guimond, M. (1981). Tardive dyskinesia and the behavioral consequences of chronic neuroleptic treatment. *Developmental and Behavioral Pediatrics, 4*, 202–209.

Gualtieri, C.T., Quade, D., Hicks, R.E., Mayo, J.P., & Schroeder, S.R. (1984). Tardive dyskinesia and other clinical consequences of neuroleptic treatment in children and adolescents. *American Journal of Psychiatry, 141*, 20–23.

Gualtieri, C.T., Schroeder, S.R., Hicks, R.E., & Quade, D. (1986). Tardive dyskinesia in young mentally retarded individuals. *Archives of General Psychiatry, 43*, 335–340.

Guy, W. (1976a). Abnormal Involuntary Movement Scale. In *ECDEU assessment manual for psychopharmacology (revised)* (DHEW Publication No. ADM 76–338, pp. 534–537). Washington, DC: U.S. Government Printing Office.

Guy, W. (1976b). Dosage Record and Treatment Emergent Symptom Scale. In *ECDEU assessment manual for psychopharmacology (revised)* (DHEW Publication No. ADM 76–338, pp. 223–244). Washington, DC: U.S. Government Printing Office.

Guy, W. (1976c). Subjective Treatment Emergent Symptom Scale. In *ECDEU assessment manual for psychopharmacology (revised)* (DHEW Publication No. ADM 76–338, pp. 347–350). Washington, DC: U.S. Government Printing Office.

Guy, W. (1976d). Treatment Emergent Symptom Scale. In *ECDEU assessment manual for psychopharmacology (revised)* (DHEW Publication No. ADM 76–338, pp. 341–345). Washington, DC: U.S. Government Printing Office.

Guze, B.H., & Baxter, L.R. (1985). Current concepts: Neuroleptic malignant syndrome. *The New England Journal of Medicine, 313*, 163–166.

Handen, B.L., Feldman, H., Gosling, A., Breaux, A.M., McAuliffe, S. (1991). Adverse side effects among mentally retarded children with ADHD. *Journal of the American Academy of Child and Adolescent Psychiatry, 30*, 241–245.

Hardy, J. (1994). Alzheimer's disease: Clinical molecular genetics. *Clinics in Geriatric Medicine, 10*, 239–247.

Herranz, J.L., Artega, R., & Armijo, J.A. (1982). Side effects of sodium valproate in monotherapy controlled by plasma levels: A study in 88 pediatric patients. *Epilepsia, 23*, 203–214.

Hetmar, O., Povlsen, U.J., Ladefoged, J., & Bolwig, T.G. (1991). Lithium: Long-term effects on the kidney. A prospective follow-up study ten years after kidney biopsy. *Bristish Journal of Psychiatry, 158*, 53–58.

Joffe, R.T., Kutcher, S., & MacDonald, C. (1988). Thyroid function and bipolar affective disorder. *Psychiatry Research, 25*, 117–121.

Kalachnik, J.E. (1988). Medication monitoring procedures: Thou shall, here's how. In K.D. Gadow & A.G. Poling (Eds.), *Pharmacotherapy and mental retardation* (pp. 231–268). Boston: Little, Brown.

Kalachnik, J.E. (1991). *Tardive dyskinesia monitoring and the Dyskinesia Identification System: Condensed User Scale (DISCUS)*. Sandoz.

Kalachnik, J.E. (1995). *Standardized monitoring for psychotropic medication side effects*. Paper presented at the Indiana Association of Rehabilitation Facilities Conference & Exposition, Indianapolis.

Kane, J.M. (1989). Schizophrenia: Somatic treatment. In H.I. Kaplan & B.J. Sadock (Eds.), *Comprehensive textbook of psychiatry* (Vol. 2, 5th ed., pp. 781–783). Baltimore: William & Wilkins.

Kang, U.J., Burke, R.E., & Fahn, S. (1986). Natural history and treatment of tardive dystonia. *Movement Disorders, 1*, 193–208.

Klein, D., Gittelman, R., & Quitkin, F. (1980). *Diagnosis and drug treatment of psychiatric disorder: Adults and children* (2nd ed.). Baltimore: Williams & Wilkins.

Kosten, T.R., & Forrest, J.N. (1986). Treatment of severe lithium induced polyuria with ameloride. *American Journal of Psychiatry, 143*, 1563–1568.

Kronig, M.H., Rose, S.P., Walsh, B.T., Woodring, S., & Glassman, A.H. (1983). Blood pressure effects of phenelzine. *Journal of Clinical Psychopharmacology, 3*, 307–310.

Lawrence, J.M. (1985). Reactions to withdrawal of antidepressants, antiparkinsonian drugs, and lithium. *Psychosomatics, 26*, 869–877.

Lazowick, A.L., & Levin, G.M. (1995). Potential withdrawal syndrome associated with SSRI discontinuation. *Annals of Pharmacotherapy, 29*, 1284–1285.

Lee, W.M. (1995). Drug-induced hepatoxicity. *New England Journal of Medicine, 333*, 1118–1127.

Leroy, M.C., Villeneuve, A., & Lajeunesse, C. (1988). Lithium, thyroid function and antithyroid antibodies. *Progress in Neuro-Psychopharmacology and Biological Psychiatry, 12*, 483–490.

Lingjaerde, O., Ahfors, U.G., Bech, P., Dencker, S.J., & Elgen, K. (1987). The UKU Side Effect Rating Scale: A new comprehensive rating scale for psychotropic drugs and a cross-sectional study of side effects in neuroleptic treated patients. *Acta Psychiatrica Scandinavica, 334*, (Suppl.), 1–100.

Linkewich, J.A. (1981). Adverse Reaction Review (ARR). *Hospital Pharmacy, 16*, 549–553.

Lipinski, J.F., Jr., Zimmerman, M.G., & Pope, P. (1989). Fluoxetine-induced akathisia: Clinical and theoretical implications. *Journal of Clinical Psychiatry, 50*, 339–342.

Ludwig,, J., & Axelsen, R. (1983). Drug effects on liver: An updated tabular compilation of drugs and drug related hepatic disease. *Digestive Disease and Science, 28*, 651–666.

Marken, P.A., Haykal, R.F., & Fisher, J.N. (1992). Management of psychotropic-induced hyperprolactinemia. *Clinical Pharmacy, 11*, 851–856.

Marken, P.A., & Stanislav, S.W. (1995). Schizophrenia. In L.Y. Young & M.A. Koda-Kimble (Eds.), *Applied therapeutics: The clinical use of drugs* (6th ed., chap, 75 pp. 1–26). Vancouver, WA: Applied Therapeutics, Inc.

Medical Economics Data. (1996). *Physicians' desk reference* (50th ed.). Monvale, NJ: Author.

Meiselas, K.D., Spencer, E.K., Oberfield, R., Peselow, E.D., Angrist B., & Campbell, M. (1989). Differentiation of stereotypies from neuroleptic-related dyskinesias in autistic children. *Journal of Clinical Psychopharmacology, 9,* 207–209.

Meltzer, H.Y. (1985). Long-term effects of neuroleptic drugs on the neuroendocrine system. *Advances in Biochemical Psychopharmacology, 40,* 50–68.

Messing, R.O., Closson, R.C., & Simon, R.P. (1984). Drug induced seizures: A 10 years experience. *Neurology, 34,* 1582–1586.

Mikkelsen, E.J., Albert, L.G., & Upadhyaya, A. (1987). Neuroleptic withdrawal cachexia. *New England Journal of Medicine, 319,* 929.

Moyes, D.G. (1973). Malignant hyperpyrexia caused by trimeprazine. *British Journal of Anesthesiology, 45,* 1163–1164.

Munetz, M.R., & Benjamin, S. (1988). How to examine patients using the Abnormal Involuntary Movement Scale. *Hospital and Community Psychiatry, 39,* 1172–1177.

Myers, D.M., Carter, R.A., Burns, B.H.,Armond, A., Hussain, S.B., & Chengapa, V.K. (1985). A prospective study of the effects of lithium on thyroid function and on the prevalence of antithyroid antibodies. *Psychological Medicine, 15,* 55–61.

National Institute of Mental Health. (1985). Rating scales and assessment instruments for use in pediatric psychopharmacology research. *Psychopharmacology Bulletin, 21*(4).

National Institute of Mental Health. (1986). Systematic Assessment for Treatment Emergent Effects (SAFTEE). *Psychopharmacology Bulletin, 22,* 347–381.

Naylor, M., Grunhaus, L., & Cameron, O. (1987). Myoclonic seizures after abrupt withdrawal from phenelzine and alprazolam. *Journal of Nervous and Mental Disease, 75,* 111–114.

Neppe, V.M., & Ward, N.G. (1989). The evaluation and management of neuroleptic-induced acute extrapyramidal syndromes. In V.M. Neppe (Ed.), *Innovative psychopharmacotherapy* (pp. 152–176). New York: Raven Press.

Perry, R., Nobler, M.S., & Campbell, M. (1989). Tourette-like symptoms associated with neuroleptic therapy in an autistic child. *Journal of the American Academy of Child and Adolescent Psychiatry, 28,* 93–96.

Pohl, R., Yeragani, V.K., Balon, R., & Lycaki, H. (1988). The jitteriness syndrome in panic disorder patients treated with antidepressants. *Journal of Clinical Psychiatry, 49,* 100–104.

Pollack, M.H., & Rosenbaum, J.F. (1987). Management of antidepressant-induced side effects: A practical guide for the clinician. *Journal of Clinical Psychiatry, 48,* 3–8.

Pope, H.G., Keek, P.E., & McElroy, S.L. (1986). Frequency and presentation of neuroleptic malignant syndrome in a large psychiatric hospital. *American Journal of Psychiatry, 143,* 1227–1233.

Rabkin, J., Quitkin, F.M., McGrath, P., Harrison, W., & Tricamo, E. (1985). Adverse reactions to monoamine oxidase inhibitors: Part II. Treatment correlates and clinical management. *Journal of Clinical Psychopharmacology, 5,* 2–9.

Reeves, W.B., & Andreoli, T.E. (1992). The posterior pituitary and water metabolism. In *Williams' textbook of endocrinology* (8th ed., pp. 311–356). Philadelphia: W.B. Saunders.

Reichlin, S. (1992). Neuroendocrinology. In *Williams' textbook of endocrinology* (8th ed., pp. 135–219). Philadelphia: W.B. Saunders.

Rifkin, A., Quitkin, F., & Klein, D.F. (1975). Akinesia. *Archives of General Psychiatry, 32,* 672–674.

Rosenstein, D.L., Nelson, J.C., & Jacobs, S.C. (1993). Seizures associated with antidepressants: A review. *Journal of Clinical Psychiatry, 54,* 289–299.

Salata, R., & Klein, I. (1987). Effect of lithium on the endocrine system: A review. *Journal of Laboratory and Clinical Medicine, 110,* 130–136.

Shalev, A., Hermesh, H., & Munitz, H. (1989). Mortality from neuroleptic malignant syndrome. *Journal of Clinical Psychiatry, 50,* 18–25.

Shalev, A., & Munitz, H. (1986). The neuroleptic malignant syndrome: Agent and host interaction. *Acta Psychiatrica Scandinavica, 73,* 337–347.

Shay, J., Sanchez, L.E., Cueva, J.E., Armenteros, J.L., Overall, J.E., & Campbell, M. (1993). Neuroleptic-related dyskinesia and stereotypies in autistic children: Videotaped ratings. *Psychopharmacology Bulletin, 29,* 359–363.

Simpson, G.M., & Angus, J.W.S. (1970). A rating scale for extrapyramidal side effects. *Acta Psychiatrica Scandinavica, 212,* 11–19.

Sovner, R. (1990). Drug profile V: Beta blockers. *The Habilitative Mental Healthcare Newsletter, 9,* 73–78.

Sovner, R. (1991). *An overview of psychotropic drug therapy for the treatment of emotional and behavioral disturbances in persons with developmental disabilities.* Paper presented at the meeting of the American Society of Hospital Pharmacists, New Orleans.

Spechler, S.J. (1989). Gastroesophageal reflux disease and other disorders of the esophagus. In S. Chopra & R.J. May (Eds.), *Pathophysiology of gastrointestinal disease* (pp. 37–70). Boston: Little, Brown.

Sprague, R.L., & Kalachnik, J.E. (1991). Reliability and a total score cutoff for the Dyskinesia Identification System: Condensed User Scale (DISCUS) with mentally ill and mentally retarded populations. *Psychopharmacology Bulletin, 27,* 51–58.

Stein, E.M., Stein, S., & Linn, M.W. (1985). Geriatric sweet tooth: A problem with tricyclics. *Journal of the American Geriatrics Society, 33,* 687–692.

Stone, R.K., May, J.E., Alvarez, W.F., & Ellman, G. (1989). Prevalence of dyskinesia and related movement disorders in a developmentally disabled population. *Journal of Mental Deficiency Research, 33,* 41–53.

Thorner, M.O., McNeilly, A.S., Hagan, C., & Besser, G.W., (1974). Long-term treatment of galactorrhea and hypogonadism with bromocriptine. *British Medical Journal, 2,* 419–422.

Thorner, M.O., Vance, M.L., Horvath, E., & Kovacs, K. (1992). Anterior pituitary. In *Williams' textbook of endocrinology,* (8th ed., pp. 221–310). Philadelphia: W.B. Saunders.

Wehr, T.A., Sack, D.A., Rosenthal, N.E., & Cowdry, R.W. (1988). Rapid cycling affective disorder: Contributing factors and treatment responses in 51 patients. *American Journal of Psychiatry, 145,* 179–184.

Weinstock, R.S., & Moses, A.M. (1990). Desmopressin and indomethacin therapy for nephrogenic diabetes insipidus in patients receiving lithium carbonate. *Southern Medical Journal, 83,* 1475–1477.

Winslow, R.S., Stiller, V., Coons, D.J., & Robison, M.W. (1986). Prevention of acute dystonic reactions in patients beginning high potency neuroleptics. *American Journal of Psychiatry, 143,* 706–710.

Yassa, R., Nair, V., & Schwartz, G. (1986). Early versus late onset psychosis and tardive dyskinesia. *Society of Biological Psychiatry, 21,* 1291–1297.

Yassa, R., Saunders, A., Nastase, C., & Camille, Y. (1988). Lithium-induced thyroid disorders: A prevalence study. *Journal of Clinical Psychiatry, 49,* 14–16.

Yeragani, V.K., & Chaitin, P. (1987). A prostaglandin theory of neuroleptic malignant syndrome. *Medical Hypotheses, 24,* 143–149.

Zametkin, A.J., & Yamada, E.M. (1993). Monitoring and measuring drug effects. In J.S. Werry & M.G. Aman (Eds.), *Practitioner's guide to psychoactive drugs for children and adolescents* (pp. 86–91). New York: Plenum Press.

Zimmerman, H.K.,& Ishak, K.G. (1987). The hepatic injury of monoamine oxidase inhibitors. *Journal of Clinical Psychopharmacology, 7,* 211–213.

Zimmerman, R.L., & Heistad, G.T. (1982). Studies of the long-term efficacy of antipsychotic drugs in controlling the behavior of institutionalized retardates. *Journal of the American Academy of Child Psychiatry, 21,* 136–43.

Zitrin, C.M., Klein, D.F., & Woerner, M.G. (1980). Treatment of agoraphobia with group exposure in vivo and imipramine. *Archives of General Psychiatry, 37,* 63–72.

Zubenko, G.S., Cohen, B.M., & Lipinski, J.F. (1987). Antidepressant-related akathisia. *Journal of Clinical Psychopharmacology, 7,* 254–257.

Drug Interactions with Psychotropic Medications

Roger W. Sommi[1], William H. Benefield, Jr.[2], Judy L. Curtis[3],
Rex S. Lott[4], Judith J. Saklad[5], and James Wilson[6]

The probability of using more than one drug in the population of patients with developmental disabilities is high. The coexistence of medical problems such as seizure disorders and cardiovascular disorders is relatively high, as is the use of medications to control symptoms associated with these disorders. Furthermore, many of the behavioral issues that are addressed in this population are complicated, and multiple drug therapy is often attempted. These considerations suggest a high likelihood of drug interactions, with potentially serious outcome effects on patients. Whenever a person is taking more than one drug, the clinician should be vigilant for the possibility of a drug interaction. Attention also should be paid to changes in a person's response to stable drug therapy, because of the possibility of interactions with food or surreptitious use of an interacting drug.

The authors of this chapter hope that a higher degree of vigilance and understanding of drug interactions will prevent many potential interactions and improve outcomes. To that end, we present an overview of drug interactions with psychopharmacological agents. Only clinically important interactions are addressed.

DEFINITIONS, CLASSIFICATION, AND IDENTIFICATION

Drug interactions are defined as those changes that occur in drug action or in the way the drug passes through the body when two or more drugs (or a drug and a food) are coadministered. The numbers of people affected by various interactions are unknown at this time. However, the more drugs an individual takes, the greater the risk of important interactions. The clinical importance of any specific interaction may depend on the current status of the individual's medical condition, the timing and duration of coadministration, the age of the person, the person's consumption of alcohol and tobacco, the

person's diet, the person's genetic makeup, and the therapeutic index (toxic concentration/therapeutic concentration) of the agents involved. All of these data are not routinely available, however, when assessing a potential drug interaction.

Drug interactions are classified in many ways that help the clinician to determine what action to take when a drug interaction arises. They are differentiated by mechanism (pharmacokinetic versus pharmacodynamic), onset (delayed or immediate), effect (additive/synergistic, antagonist, or neither), and outcome (beneficial, detrimental, or inconsequential). Further classification into drug-drug, drug-lab, and drug-food interactions is also useful. It is beyond the scope of this chapter to discuss in detail issues of pharmacodynamics and pharmacokinetics as they relate to drug interactions; therefore, the discussion is focused on applications to psychotropic medications. For additional information, the reader is directed to resources on drug interactions listed in the references that are updated quarterly (see Hansten & Horn 1994; Tatro & Olin 1994).

Anytime a person is taking more than one drug, the clinician should be vigilant for the possibility of a drug interaction. Similarly, changes in a person's response to stable drug therapy may indicate surreptitious use of an interacting drug or food product. Most drug interactions can be prevented or the adverse consequences minimized. Depending on the drug interaction and the person's medical problems, one or more of the following interventions can be used to minimize or avoid the interaction:

1 Associate Professor of Pharmacy Practice and Psychiatry, University of Missouri at Kansas City, Kansas City, MO
2 Clinical Pharmacologist, San Antonio State School, San Antonio, TX
3 Assistant Professor of Pharmacy Practice and Science, University of Maryland at Baltimore, Baltimore, MA
4 Associate Professor, Idaho State University, College of Pharmacy, Pocatello, ID
5 Clinical Assistant Professor of Pharmacy, The University of Texas Health Sciences Center at Houston, Houston, TX
6 Clinical Pharmacologist, San Antonio State School, San Antonio, TX

- Change the administration times so that the interacting drugs are not given together.
- Change one of the drugs to another with similar therapeutic effects that do not interact.
- Change the dose of the drug to account for differences in drug disposition.
- Discontinue one of the drugs.
- Make no changes in the dose or regimen of the drugs, but increase monitoring of the person for adverse consequences of the interaction.
- Use a different route of administration or dosage form.

The action that should be taken in any specific case depends on many factors, which are discussed in the following sections.

PHARMACOKINETIC INTERACTIONS

Pharmacokinetic drug interactions result from changes in the absorption, distribution, metabolism, and excretion of one or more drugs. Because changes in any of these processes affect the blood concentration or elimination of the drug, they also affect the intensity or duration of the drug's action. One important concept in assessing risk for a pharmacokinetic interaction is a preexisting reduction in capacity in any of the four kinetic processes. With a preexisting reduction in capacity, small changes in any pharmacokinetic process results in a larger percentage change in the drug's effect. Patients with gastrointestinal, hepatic disorders, or renal disorders are at higher risk for pharmacokinetic interactions, because these diseases compromise one or more pharmacokinetic processes. Elderly patients are also at risk due to decrements in renal and hepatic function associated with increased age.

Absorption

The classic example of absorption interactions is tetracycline (an antibiotic) and cations (antacids or calcium from dairy products). The cations bind to the tetracycline molecule in the gut to form a much larger, less lipophyllic (fat soluble) compound that is not absorbed into the general circulation. The effect is a drastic reduction in anti-infective efficacy, because the tetracycline does not reach the site of the infection.

Although there are few clinically important interactions involving the absorption of psychotropic medication, such interactions can occur in two ways. First, the interaction may reduce the total amount of a drug absorbed, as in the tetracycline example. Second, the interaction may reduce the rate at which a drug is absorbed. A reduced rate of absorption increases the length of time required to reach maximal plasma concentration (T max) and reduces the maximal plasma concentration (Cp max) after oral dosing. These changes are important for agents given on a PRN (as needed) basis because the therapeutic effect is dependent on achieving a target concentration of drug in the blood. Delaying T max and reducing Cp max can change the subjective response to medication. These changes are not usually significant for chronic therapy because there is little therapeutic effect derived from the peak plasma concentration. Steady-state plasma concentration (Cpss) is proportionally related to the amount of drug absorbed and, thus, will not be affected significantly by interactions that affect only the rate of absorption.

Antacids and food can increase pH level in the stomach, which can reduce the dissolution rate of products given in tablet form. Basic chemical compounds (e.g., antidepressants, benzodiazepines, and stimulants) are most affected. Generally, reduction of the dissolution rate results in a reduction in the rate of absorption, not the extent of absorption. An example is the coadministration of chlordiazepoxide (librium) and antacids. People taking chlordiazepoxide with water experience a more rapid and intense effect compared to those who take the drug with an antacid. The total amount of drug that is absorbed, however, is similar. The presence of food can delay gastric emptying time which also affects primarily the rate but not the extent of absorption. Most drugs when given with food will show an extension of T max and reduction in Cp max.

An absorption interaction between phenytoin (Dilantin) and certain foods, antacids, and enteral feedings has also been identified, although the mechanism is unknown. Puddings and enteral feedings such as Osmolyte and Ensure have been reported to decrease the oral absorption of phenytoin and thus the plasma concentration. People receiving oral supplements should receive phenytoin doses one hour prior to or two hours after supplementation. People receiving tube feedings should have the tube flushed and clamped for two hours before and two hours after the phenytoin dose. Administration times of antacids should also be adjusted so that the phenytoin dose is administered three to four hours apart from the antacid (Cacek,

1986; Jann, Bean, & Fidone, 1986; Saklad, Graves, & Sharp, 1986).

Many psychotropic drugs have significant anticholinergic effects. The anticholinergic effect can reduce gastric motility and hence the rate of absorption. Some drugs, especially ones that do not dissolve well, are absorbed in a limited area of the bowel (e.g., digoxin) or are degraded in gastrointestinal fluids (e.g., levodopa), and the rate and extent of their absorption may be changed when they are coadministered with an anticholinergic agent. Simply changing administration times such that the drug is given one hour prior to or two hours after consumption of food or antacids should prevent interactions that involve the binding of drugs. Giving the psychotropic drug by injection or using a therapeutically equivalent noninteracting drug will also avert absorption problems.

Distribution

Once in the systemic circulation, drugs are distributed to tissue compartments, primarily organs with high blood flow such as the brain, kidney, and liver. A portion of the drug is bound to plasma proteins such as albumin, alpha-1-acid glycoprotein, and lipoproteins. The fraction that is unbound (free fraction) is the active portion of the drug that can interact with receptor sites where the drug exerts its effects. Most distributional type interactions involve competition between two highly protein-bound drugs for protein binding sites, resulting in displacement of the drug from plasma proteins. This increases the free fraction and the effect of the drug. Most drugs are bound to albumin; therefore, changes in the amount of albumin can lead to changes in protein binding. People with cirrhosis or chronic renal disease and elderly individuals tend to have lower protein binding capacity and higher free fractions; these people are at higher risk for protein displacement type interactions.

Most psychotropic drugs are highly protein bound (>85%), with the exception of lithium, which is not bound to plasma proteins. As a class, the antiepileptic drugs are most associated with clinically-important protein binding interactions. This is probably due to the low therapeutic index of antiepileptics, whereby small changes can have significant effects on a patient's response to medication. Tricyclic antidepressants (TCAs) are bound primarily to alpha-1-acid glycoprotein and are less likely to interact with other drugs.

One confusing aspect of protein binding displacement interactions is that the total blood concentration of the drugs decreases slightly, whereas the concentrations of unbound, pharmacologically active drugs are increased or unchanged at equilibrium (MacKichan, 1992). For example, a person receiving phenytoin in combination with warfarin may appear to have many signs of phenytoin (Dilantin) toxicity, even though the blood concentration of phenytoin is in the reported therapeutic range. The toxicity is due to the higher free fraction of phenytoin due to displacement, not to higher total blood concentrations. Most blood concentrations used for therapeutic drug monitoring measure both bound and unbound drug levels, and thus do not indicate the change that occurs in free fraction. It is possible to measure the free fraction, which is probably a better indicator of a drug's effect.

Distributional interactions are difficult to assess. Changes in a person's response to a drug when another highly protein-bound drug is added to his or her regimen should lead one to suspect a protein binding interaction. Simply measuring a total blood concentration will not indicate the extent of change in free fraction. Obtaining a free concentration of drug may be useful, but few drugs have a free concentration readily available at commercial laboratories, and the assays are expensive. The physician should reduce the dose of the affected drug based on the patient's response or use a drug combination without an interaction.

Metabolism

Metabolism is an important step in the movement of drugs through the body. Metabolism inactivates drugs and increases water solubility, which allows for excretion into the urine. There are two phases of drug metabolism. Phase I metabolism (biotransformation) changes the chemical structure of the drug. The most common types of changes include oxidation (into hydroxymetabolites), acetylation (into N-acetyl metabolites), and demethylation (into desmethyl- or nor-metabolites) of the drug. Biotransformation often leads to the formation of an active metabolite. Active metabolites are common to psychotropic drugs and often account for a significant portion of the drug's overall effect. Phase II metabolism (conjugation) results in the addition of a hydrophilic moiety onto the drug or drug metabolite, which enhances the ability of the kidney to filter the drug into the urine.

Generally, drug interactions involve changes in the biotransformation of psychotropic drugs. Biotransformation of the compound often is associated with a set of metabolic enzymes. An important group of enzymes is the mixed oxidase system, or cytochrome P-450 (CYP). So-called enzyme inducers increase the metabolic conversion of the drug. Enzyme induction will cause a drug to clear faster from the body (reflected in a decrease in the drug's half-life) and cause steady-state concentrations to become lower, possibly to subtherapeutic levels. Conversely, drugs that inhibit enzyme activity (enzyme inhibitors) can extend the target drug's half-life and lead to an accumulation of the drug in the body, potentially to toxic concentrations. In addition, there may be either an increased or decreased formation of active metabolites, thereby changing the ratio of parent drug to active metabolites. The clinical significance of this change is dependent on the toxicity and therapeutic effect profile of the parent drug and the metabolite. Phase II metabolism is not usually induced or inhibited. Conjugation reactions are not generally involved in psychotropic drug interactions except in the case of severe dietary restrictions and overdose. The distinction in the metabolic pathway is important primarily with benzodiazepines, because some undergo Phase I and II metabolism and others only Phase II. Avoiding a metabolic interaction with benzodiazepines may simply mean choosing one that undergoes only Phase II metabolism.

The relationship between the initiation of an enzyme inducer or inhibitor and the resultant change in clinical effect of the target drug is dependent on the half-life of the inducer or inhibitor, the extent of the inhibition or induction, the doses of the agents given, the half-life of the target drug, and the therapeutic index of the target agent. (The target drug is the drug for which the metabolic parameters have been changed.) The onset of metabolic inhibition or induction is generally apparent within 24 hours of initiating drug therapy. Maximal enzyme activity change will occur sometime after steady-state has been reached for the inhibitor or inducer (four to five times the drug's half-life). After the metabolic activity change has been stabilized, the effect on the target drug will maximize when the new steady-state concentration is achieved. The degree of inhibition or induction will determine the extent of the change that occurs. Generally, the amount of enzymatic activity change increases as the dose of the inhibitor or inducer increases. In addition, most psychotropic drugs that cause enzyme inhibition or induction are themselves metabolized by CYP enzymes. In some cases, the drug can inhibit (auto-inhibition) or induce (auto-induction) its own metabolism. This process can change the time frames for maximal change in inhibition and induction (Hansten & Horn, 1994).

Age is an important factor in assessing risk for an interaction. Although the amount of enzyme inhibition caused by a drug is relatively the same for older and younger people, older people will have a greater percentage change in metabolic capacity because they have a lower overall capacity for Phase I metabolism. Thus, the older person has a higher risk of experiencing a significant change in metabolism (Cohen, Johnson, Berardi, Hyneck, & Achem, 1985; Feely, Pereira, Gut, & Hockings, 1984).

The influence of genetic differences in metabolism on the risk for drug interactions is becoming increasingly apparent. Genetic polymorphism (the presence of multiple forms of enzymes that are responsible for drug metabolism) generally results in two phenotypes: people who do not metabolize a certain drug efficiently (poor metabolizers) and people who metabolize the drug normally (extensive metabolizers). Poor metabolizers may have an abnormal form of a specific hepatic enzyme, a decreased rate of formation of the enzyme, or an increased rate of enzyme clearance. Poor metabolizers are persons at risk for toxicity at drug doses within the normal range. The prevalence of either phenotype is known to vary by racial and ethnic group. The importance of polymorphism in explaining interracial and interethnic differences in response to drugs is obvious. In terms of drug interactions, it is likely that people who are extensive metabolizers of a particular agent are likely to be more at risk for enzyme inhibition interactions and subsequent acute toxicity, because the proportional change in plasma concentration is likely to produce larger pharmacodynamic effects (Levy, 1993; Preskorn & Fast, 1991, 1992; Preskorn & Jerkovich, 1990; Preskorn & Magnus, 1994).

Biotransformation and changes in biotransformation have a complex relationship to the effect of a drug on an individual person. Biotransformation relies heavily on the hepatic CYP enzyme system. CYP is responsible for the metabolism of endogenous substances, such as hormones, and in metabolizing drugs and other foreign substances. The cytochrome system comprises many isoenzymes that are genetically determined. Three families of CYP isoenzymes (1, 2, and 3) are associated with drug metabolism in humans. These isoenzymes are distinct, yet they have a structural similarities. Structural similarity is important in that a drug that is known to affect one isoenzyme may also affect the activity of another with structural similarities (Nelson et al., 1993; Nerbert et al., 1991). Knowledge of CYP-mediated interactions is growing rapidly. Common substrates (drugs metabolized primarily by an isoenzyme), inducers, and inhibitors are summarized in Table 8-1.

Table 8-1. Common Substrates, Inducers and Inhibitors of CYP Isoenzymes

CYP 2D6	CYP 3A3/4		CYP 1A2	CYP 2C9/10	CYP 2C19
SUBSTRATES					

Antidepressants
paroxetine sertraline
venlafaxine
m-CPP metabolite
  of nefazodone
  and trazodone
desipramine
clomipramine
imipramine
nortriptyline
 	
Antiarrhythmics
encainide flecainide
propafenone
 	
Antipsychotics
clozapine
risperidone
thioridazine
perphenazine
haloperidol
 	
Beta-blockers
propranolol
metoprolol
timolol
 	
Opiates
Codeine
Dextromethorphan
	Antidepressants
	amitriptyline
	clomipramine
	imipramine
	desipramine
	nortriptyline
	sertraline
	trimipramine
	
	Benzodiazepines
	alprazolam
	triazolam
	midazolam
	clonazepam
	
	Antihistamines
	terfenadine
	aztemizole
	
	**Ca Channel
	Antagonists**
	diltiazem
	felodipine
	nifedipine
	nimodipine
	verapamil
	
	Antiarrhythmics
	lidocaine
	propafenone
	quinidine
	amiodarone
	disopyramide
		Other
		cisapride
		acetaminophen
		erythromycin
		estrogen
		cyclosporine
		carbamazepine
			Antidepressants
			imipramine
			amitriptyline
			clomipramine
			
			Antipsychotics
			clozapine
			
			Other
			propranolol
			caffeine
			theophylline
			tacrine
			R-warfarin
				**Nonsteroidal anti-
				inflammatory Agents**
				diclofenac
				mefenamic acid
				piroxicam
				naproxen
				ibuprofen
				
				Other
				phenytoin
				S-warfarin
				tolbutamide
					Antidepressants
					imipramine
					clomipramine
					
					Barbiturates
					hexobarbital
					
					Other
					propranolol
					diazepam
					mephenytoin
					omeprazole

INDUCERS					
	carbamazepine phenobarbital dexamethasone phenytoin rifampin		smoking (arryl compounds) omeprazole		rifampin
INHIBITORS					
fluoxetine paroxetine norfluoxetine quinidine sertraline (moderate) thioridazine perfenazine	ketoconazole itraconazole erythromycin azithromycin grapefruit juice (naringenin) nefazodone fluvoxamine fluoxetine (weak) sertraline (weak) paroxetine (weak)		fluvoxamine fluoroquinolones	fluoxetine sulfaphenazole	ketoconazole omeprazole fluoxetine fluvoxamine

Note. Adapted from Ketter et al., 1995; Preskorn, 1996; Riesenman, 1995.

Enzyme Inhibition

The classic drugs that cause enzyme inhibition are the H2 antagonists. Cimetidine (Tagamet) is the most widely reported metabolic inhibitor. Cimetidine and other H2 antagonists are relatively nonselective in their effect on CYP isoenzymes; therefore, their ability to antagonize the metabolism of drugs is widespread. Other common inhibitors include ciprofloxacin (Cipro), diltiazem (Cardizem), disulfiram (Antabuse), erythromycin, fluconazole (Diflucan), isoniazid (INH), ketoconazole (Nizoral), metronidazole (Flagyl), miconazole (Monistat), omeprazole (Prilosec), and verapamil (Calan, Isoptin). Each of these agents has differing potential to interact with psychotropic drugs (Hansten & Horn 1994). The potential to interact depends greatly on the selectivity of the drug to inhibit specific isoenzymes.

The metabolism of psychotropic drugs is affected by isoenzymes in two primary ways: preferential metabolism by one isoenzyme and selective isoenzyme inhibition. Furthermore, most drugs are metabolized through the CYP 3A3/4 or CYP 2D6 systems. Simply looking at the number of drugs in each category in Table 8-1 gives the reader some degree of appreciation for the importance of these two isoenzymes. Comparing CYP 3A3/4 to CYP 2D6, one finds that CYP 2D6 accounts for 2% of the enzymatic activity, whereas CYP 3A3/4 accounts for 30% of the activity. Therefore, on a relative basis, CYP 3A3/4 is probably more important overall in metabolic drug interactions.

Many TCAs, some phenothiazines, and other selected drugs are metabolized by one isoenzyme system predominantly. TCAs and the phenothiazines are metabolized predominately by CYP 2D6; theophylline, clozapine, and tacrine by CYP 1A2; benzodiazepines by CYP 2C; and terfenadine (Seldane), astemizole (Hismanal), cisapride (Propulsid), and triazolobenzodiazepines (alprazolam) by CYP 3A3/4. The newer antidepressants and, potentially, risperidone have the ability selectively to inhibit one or more of these enzymes. Fluoxetine has been implicated in inhibiting CYP 2C, CYP 2D6, and CYP 3A3/4. Fluvoxamine has been reported to inhibit CYP 1A2 (Brosen, Skejelbo, Rasmusse, Poulsen, & Loft, 1993; Crewe, Lennard, Tucker, Woods, & Haddock, 1992; Greenblatt, Preskorn, Cotreau, Horst, & Harmatz, 1992; Lasher, Fleishaker, Steenwyk, & Antal, 1991; Lemberger, Rowe, Bosomworth, Tenbarge, & Bergstrom, 1988; von Moltke et al., 1994).

The degree to which these enzymes are inhibited varies with the agent. In terms of higher to lower potency in inhibiting CY P2D6, paroxetine is a more potent inhibitor than fluoxetine, which is a more potent inhibitor than sertraline (Shank et al., 1988). Potency, however, does not correlate well with incidence of clinically relevant interactions. Differences in plasma concentration (highest with fluoxetine at clinically effective doses), and duration (longest with fluoxetine and its metabolite norfluoxetine) account for the differences in the incidence of drug interactions observed clinically (Preskorn, 1994). Indeed, a brief review of the literature suggests that the incidence of drug interactions is highest with fluoxetine. It is also apparent that the other agents can cause clinically significant interactions, and clinicians should be cognizant of this potential when treating patients receiving any of these agents.

Enzyme Induction

Enzyme induction is the process by which a drug can increase the metabolic activity of the CYP system. Reactions include a faster clearance of drugs, a reduction in the target drug's half-life, a decrease in blood concentration, and potentially a loss of therapeutic effect. In addition, formation of metabolites will be increased, and potentially the overall character of response to the medication can be changed.

Most enzyme induction reactions have been reported with antiepileptic drugs. Carbamazepine (Tegretol) and the barbiturates are classic examples of inducer drugs. Other common inducers include phenytoin (Dilantin), primidone (Mysoline), and rifampin (Rifadin, Rimactane). Little is known about the selectivity of these drugs for specific isoenzymes. It is likely that induction occurs for specific isoenzymes, but further study is required to delineate the importance of this effect (Hansten & Horn, 1994).

Another common enzyme inducer is cigarette smoking. Cigarette smoke contains a number of polycyclic hydrocarbons that are capable of inducing CYP1A enzyme activity, which may last several weeks after the person has stopped smoking (Jusko, 1978, 1979). Smoking is known to increase the clearance of TCAs (Linnoila, George, Guthrie, & Leventhal, 1981; Perel, Hurwicz, & Kanzler, 1975), antipsychotics (Swett, 1974, 1977; Vinarova, Vinar, & Kalvach, 1984), and benzodiazepines (Boston Collaborative Drug Surveillance Program, 1973; Greenblatt, Allen, Harmatz, & Shader, 1979). People who smoke may require higher doses of a given drug to achieve a desired effect. Smoking interactions seem to be most important for people who smoke more than 20 cigarettes daily (Hansten and Horn, 1994; Swett, 1974).

Generally, the adverse effects of interactions that involve enzyme induction can be prevented by increasing the dose of the target drug. However, physicians should be conservative when making dose adjustments for drugs with active metabolites.

Excretion

Drugs are removed from the body in the urine. The parent drug and metabolites are filtered at the glomerulus, and they can then be secreted into the urine through an active process at the renal tubules or passively reabsorbed back into the bloodstream. In order for the kidney to filter a drug, the drug must not be protein-bound, because albumin and other proteins are not filtered through the kidney. Thus, any drug that changes the degree of protein binding or the amount of blood that is filtered through the glomerulus (glomerular filtration rate [GFR]) can change the clearance of a drug. Changes in blood pressure or in the constriction of the afferent or efferent renal arterioles can change GFR. Interactions resulting in a reduction in GFR decrease the clearance of renally eliminated drugs, extending their half-life, increasing plasma concentrations, and potentially leading to toxicity. Of the psychotropic drugs, lithium is almost 100% dependent on renal elimination, and changes in GFR can drastically change the clearance of lithium (Hansten & Horn, 1994).

Active tubular secretion is a process that takes place in the proximal portion of the renal tubule. Some drugs (primarily organic acids and organic bases) are actively transported from the blood, through the cells of the lining of the renal tubule into the fluid that has been filtered through the glomerulus. Inhibition of this process can lead to reduced drug clearance, prolonged half-life, accumulation of drug, and potentially, drug toxicity. Sometimes, this interaction mechanism is used as a benefit. Probenecid (Benemid) competes with penicillins and cephalosporins for tubular secretion. This results in a prolonged effect of the antibiotic, which is desirable in certain circumstances.

In the case of psychotropic agents, thiazide diuretics interact with lithium. Chronic use of thiazide diuretics results in decreased distal tubular reabsorption of sodium, causing sodium depletion. This increases the passive reabsorption of sodium back into the bloodstream at the proximal tubule. Because lithium is reabsorbed like sodium at the proximal tubule, the net result is a passive increase in the reabsorption of lithium back into the bloodstream, decreased lithium clearance, increased lithium concentration, and possibly lithium toxicity (Ciraulo, Shader, Greenblatt, & Creelman, 1989; Hansten & Horn, 1994)

The degree of passive tubular reabsorption of any drug is determined by a combination of factors: urinary pH, whether the drug is a weak acid or weak base, and the lipophylicity of the drug. A drug will undergo passive diffusion back into the blood if it is lipophyllic and in the non-ionized form. The degree of ionization is primarily a factor of urinary pH. An acidic drug will be more ionized in a basic (higher) pH and less ionized in an acidic (lower) pH. Increasing urinary pH (with sodium bicarbonate or acetazolamide, for example) will increase the reabsorption of weak bases (e.g., TCAs, phenothiazines, antihistamines, pseudoephedrine, or amphetamine) and lead to accumulation in the blood, increase in half-life, and, potentially, toxicity. Increasing urinary pH will also increase the urinary excretion of weak acids (e.g., lithium or tranylcypromine) and reduce the blood concentration and drug half-life and potentially lead to loss of therapeutic effect. Decreasing the urinary pH (with ammonium chloride, vitamin C, or methenamine for example) will have the opposite effect (Ciraulo et al., 1989; Hansten & Horn, 1994).

Decreasing or increasing renal blood flow can significantly change the real elimination of drugs. As was discussed previously, lithium is most susceptible to this type of interaction. Nonsteroidal anti-inflammatory drugs (NSAIDS) such as indomethacin (Indocin), ibuprofen (Motrin, Rufen, Advil, and others), naproxen (Naprosyn, Anaprox, and Aleve), piroxicam (Feldene), and diclofenac (Voltaren) interfere with the production of prostaglandin E2 (PGE_2). PGE_2 is in part responsible for the dilatation of the renal artery; inhibiting it can result in a vasoconstriction, decreased renal blood flow, and a subsequent decrease in GFR. Over a period of five to ten days, lithium can accumulate, possibly to a level of toxicity, because of the decrease in excretion. Similarly, some ACE inhibitors such as captopril (Capoten) and lisinopril (Prinivil or Zestril) can decrease GFR and result in lithium accumulation and possibly toxicity (Ciraulo et al., 1989; Hansten & Horn, 1994; Tatro & Olin, 1994).

In summary, the excretion interactions are most important for lithium, because it is almost totally dependent on renal excretion for elimination from the body. Changes in GFR, active tubular secretion, or passive tubular reabsorption can dramatically influence the pharmacokinetics of lithium and potentially lead to toxicity or loss of effect. Alterations in urinary pH, with subsequent changes in the passive reabsorption of drugs, is commonly used in situations such as overdose to enhance elimination of drugs, but altering urinary pH is not likely to be a common issue in most other situations.

Pharmacodynamics

In contrast to pharmacokinetic interactions, pharmacodynamic interactions are less well defined. They include interactions of drugs with similar pharmacological activity (e.g., competing for the same receptors) or similar effects mediated by different pathways (e.g., dopaminergic effects of benzodiazepines mediated via GABA mechanisms interacting with levodopa). In either case, the result could be an increased (additive or synergistic) or decreased (antagonistic) effect.

Whereas pharmacokinetic interactions can easily be broken down into the components of absorption, distribution, metabolism, and excretion, pharmacodynamic interactions are more difficult to model. Three pharmacodynamic models have been proposed for the study of changes in pharmacologic activity: E max, hysteresis, and mixed effect models (Fuseau & Sheiner, 1984; Holford & Sheiner, 1981; Sheiner, Stanski, Vozeh, Miller, & Ham, 1979; Unadkat, Bartha, & Sheiner, 1986). Essentially, these models were designed to quantify the change that results in the concentration response relationships of an agent. Researchers define a specific drug action and then compare the concentration response relationships with and without the interaction. Changes in the concentration needed to achieve a certain degree of effect suggest a pharmacodynamic interaction. In many cases, pharmacodynamic and pharmacokinetic interactions occur simultaneously. For example, the interaction between haloperidol and carbamazepine results in increased metabolic clearance of haloperidol (pharmacokinetic) and an increase in sedation (pharmacodynamic).

SPECIAL CONSIDERATIONS FOR PEOPLE WITH DEVELOPMENTAL DISABILITIES

Very few data are available addressing issues specific to drug interactions in people with mental retarda-tion and developmental disabilities. Most clinicians are left to extrapolate from data from studies of people who have psychiatric conditions but no developmental disability. Given that 20% to 40% of people with mental retardation and developmental disabilities in various service programs are receiving one or more psychotropic medications (Aman, Field & Bridgeman, 1985; Aman, Sarphare, & Burrow, 1995; Hill, Balow, & Bruininks, 1985; Intagliata & Rinck, 1985; Pary, 1993; Rinck & Calkins, 1989), the potential for interactions is great. When one considers the medical complications prevalent in this population and the complications that arise with the aging process, the potential for drug interactions is further increased.

Nutritional problems arise often in this population. With ongoing malnutrition or undernutrition, reductions in plasma proteins can arise, which can increase a person's risk for protein displacement interactions. Supplements (liquids, puddings, or tube feedings) can facilitate the maintenance of nutritional needs, but they can interact with phenytoin when given together. Also common in this population are coexisting seizure disorders, which are often difficult to control and at times require multiple drug therapy. Antiepileptic drugs, well known for having potential drug interactions, pose yet another risk for this population.

There appears to be a high incidence of peptic ulcer and gastroesophageal reflux disease among people with mental retardation and developmental disabilities. Treatment with antacids and H2 antagonists, agents known to have significant interactions, can put clients at risk for interactions. Frequent use of antibiotics, especially macrolide agents, such as erythromycin and clarithromycin, is commonplace and can lead to inhibition of drug metabolism and toxicity. Tuberculosis may become more common— especially among institutionalized individuals. Likelihood of administration of rifampin to people receiving psychotropic drugs may increase the chances of enzyme induction interactions.

Currently, researchers are studying the polymorphic metabolism of drugs and the delineation of the role of specific isoenzymes in drug metabolism. This process is genetically controlled. The high incidence of genetic changes in people with mental retardation and developmental disabilities suggests that there are specific deficiencies of certain types of metabolic enzymes that increase risk for altered metabolism. Further research is needed to clarify this issue.

SIGNIFICANT INTERACTIONS BY DRUG CLASS[7]

Neuroleptics

The conventional antipsychotics undergo hepatic metabolism and have a number of interactions (see Table 9-3). The length of time it takes for significant interactions varies with the specific agents and dosages. Most significant interactions occur within several days after drug treatment is initiated, although some are seen within hours.

Some noteworthy interactions are as follows. The side effects of neuroleptics can be enhanced by the concurrent use of other drugs with similar effects; for example, benzodiazepines and anti-Parkinson agents enhance sedative and anticholinergic side effects. Because of their action at adrenergic receptors, neuroleptics (especially atypical antipsychotics such as clozapine, risparidone and olanzapine) can interact with antihypertensive agents, which may cause hypotension. Stimulants, such as amphetamine, can interfere with the antipsychotic action of neuroleptics. Antidepressants, such as amitriptyline, imipramine, and fluoxetine, interact with neuroleptics to inhibit each other's metabolism, resulting in greater blood concentrations. On the other hand, anticonvulsants such as carbamazepine and the barbiturates induce the liver enzymes that metabolize neuroleptics, thereby reducing the antipsychotic effects of these drugs. Lithium, a mood stabilizer, has been reported to result in neurotoxicity in some patients on neuroleptics. The newer atypical antipsychotics (clozapine and risperidone) have significantly different pharmacological profiles and thus have different risks in terms of drug interactions.

Anticholinergics

Anticholinergic drugs (benztropine/Cogentin and trihexyphenidyl/Artane) are used primarily to reverse the extrapyramidal side effects of the conventional antipsychotics. As such, the drug interaction is beneficial. However, the anticholinergic effects are widespread and can be additive to the existing anticholinergic effects of other psychotropic agents such as antipsychotics and antidepressants. Enhanced anticholinergic effects may include constipation, urinary retention, intolerable dry mouth, and blurred vision. Of particular importance for people with mental retardation and developmental disabilities is the negative effect anti-cholinergics can have on cognition. If the anticholinergic effects are excessive, delirium can result.

Anticonvulsants

As was noted earlier in this chapter, the anticonvulsants have the most potential by far for interactions, protein displacement, primarily enzyme inhibition, enzyme induction, and additive CNS depression interactions. Tables 10-4 and 10-5 show some relevant interactions with anticonvulsants; Table 10-4 shows the interactions of anitconvulsant drugs with each other. **Because of the high potential for interaction, the physician should consult standard reference sources to determine if a drug-drug interaction might be anticipated before prescribing an anticonvulsant drug to a patient who already is taking another drug for any reason.**

Monoamine Oxidase Inhibitors (MAOIs)

The monoamine oxidase inhibitors (MAOIs) include phenelzine (Nardil), isocarboxazid (Marplan), and tranylcypromine (Parnate). A resurgence in the use of the MAOIs has increased concern about potential drug interactions with food, over-the-counter drugs, and other medications. Monoamine oxidase (MAO) is an enzyme responsible for the metabolism of a large number of amine compounds. Dopamine, norepinephrine, and serotonin are common substrates for MAO in the brain and throughout the body. MAO is in part responsible for the regulation of these catecholamines. Fermented foods (beers, cheeses, smoked meats, etc.) contain large amounts of tyramine which can cause significant increases in blood pressure if absorbed in sufficient quantity. Normally MAO in the gut wall and liver metabolize tyramine and prevent this effect.

MAO exists in at least two forms: MAO-A and MAO-B. MAO-A is found primarily in the intestines, brain, and liver. Whereas there is more MAO-B in the brain, most platelet MAO is MAO-B. MAO-B is also found in the lung and liver. MAO-B seems to be more selective for dopamine and tyramine, whereas MAO-A has an effect on norepinephrine, serotonin, tyramine, and dopamine.

---

7 The tables in this section are used to identify the major interactions with various psychotropic drugs. They do not provide exhaustive lists of all potential or reported drug interactions. The interactions listed are those considered to be most common and those of clinical significance (i.e., interactions with a likelihood of increased toxicity, loss of therapeutic effect, or with life-threatening potential).

MAOIs are generally nonselective in their action on MAO-A or B, although selegiline (Eldepryl) is more selective for MAO-B. This difference is important in that intestinal MAO is not inhibited with MAO-B selective inhibitors. Thus these agents are less likely to inhibit the degradation of tyramine and are less likely to produce the hypertensive reactions. Many of the new psychotropic MAOIs are selective for either A or B.

Another important difference in agents is whether the MAO inhibition is reversible or irreversible. Some agents (i.e., isocarboxazid, phenelzine, selegiline, and tranylcypromine) irreversibly inhibit MAO. In order for the MAO activity to return to pretreatment levels, the body has to regenerate the enzyme, which takes approximately two weeks. The newer agents (e.g., moclobemide) tend to be reversible inhibitors, and MAO activity will return to baseline as the drug is eliminated from the body. The type of inhibition (reversible versus irreversible) is important in that despite discontinuation of the MAOI, a drug that interacts with the MAOI can still do so for up to two weeks after discontinuing the MAOI (Hansten & Horn, 1994).

Interactions with MAOIs fall into three categories: (a) exacerbation or prolongation of the normally occurring side effects of the drug; (b) hypertensive crisis caused by the release and potentiation of catecholamines; and (c) serotonin syndrome, with the concomitant use of serotonin active agents (Blackwell & Schmidt, 1984; Kapur & Kambhampat, 1992). Hypertensive crisis, a rapid and intense increase in blood pressure, is the most well known and feared consequence of drug interactions with MAOIs. The drugs that may cause a hypertensive crisis when used in combination with an MAOI are direct- or indirect-acting sympathomimetics (ephedrine, pseudoephedrine, phenylpropanolamine, and phenylephrine); MAOI will intensify the noradrenergic effect of these drugs. However, if an accidental exposure should occur, phentolamine is antidotal. Other drugs suspected to interact with MAOIs to cause hypertensive crisis include Levodopa and dopamine; tricyclic antidepressants (TCAs) such as amitriptyline, desipramine, amoxapine, clomipramine, doxepin, imipramine, nortriptyline, and protriptyline; and stimulants and anorexiants such as amphetamine, dextroamphetamine, and fenfluramine (Blackwell et al., 1992; Tatro & Olin, 1994).

Certain foods contain large amounts of tyramine, which may also cause a hypertensive crisis. Inhibition of MAO in the gut wall and liver can cause tyramine to accumulate. Tyramine is an indirect-acting sympathomimetic and can cause a rapid and intense hypertensive episode. Foods that contain large amounts of tyramine should not be consumed during MAOI treatment. These include smoked, aged or pickled meat or fish; sauerkraut; aged cheeses such as Swiss and Cheddar; yeast extracts; and fava beans (see Shulman et al., 1989). Foods with moderate amounts of tyramine are beer, avocados, meat extracts, and red wines such as Chianti; these may be consumed in moderate quantities during MAOI treatment. Foods with low amounts of tyramine include beverages that contain caffeine (coffee, cola), distilled spirits, chocolate, soy sauce, cottage and cream cheese, and yogurt and sour cream; these may be consumed during MAOI treatment.

The combination of serotonin-active agents such as selective serotonin reuptake inhibitors (SSRIs) with the MAOIs may also cause a condition of serotonin excess referred to as the serotonin syndrome. Symptoms that may be present during this reaction include the following: confusion, agitation, chills, shivering, difficulty in coordination, memory changes, myoclonus, hyperreflexia, restlessness, sweating, fever, nausea, vomiting, aggressiveness, tremor, and coma. Although rare, this reaction can be fatal. Treatment involves discontinuing the drugs involved and supporting the patient.

When sulfonylureas or insulin is given with an MAOI, the physician should monitor for symptoms of hypo- or hyperglycemia. Generally, combination therapy with the SSRIs should be avoided; clinicians should wait at least 5 weeks after stopping fluoxetine or 2 weeks after stopping other agents before initiating an MAOI. They also should wait at least 2 weeks after stopping MAOI before initiating other agents.

Other Antidepressants

The tricyclic antidepressants (TCAs) include: amitriptyline, desipramine, amoxapine, clomipramine, doxepin, imipramine, nortriptyline, protriptyline, and trimipramine. The heterocyclic antidepressants include trazodone (Desyrel). The SSRIs include fluoxetine (Prozac), fluvoxamine (Luvox), sertraline (Zoloft), and paroxetine (Paxil). Presently, the only selective serotonin and norepinephrine reuptake inhibitors that is available commercially is venlafaxine (Effexor). The serotonin S2 antagonists include nefazodone (Serzone).

Most antidepressant interactions involving TCAs and heterocyclic agents are pharmacodynamic in nature. Additive sedative, cardiovascular, and anticholinergic effects are the most common and predictable interactive side effects involving these agents. More recently, the importance of enzyme inhibition interactions has surfaced as newer, more selective agents have come to the market. Cimetidine (Tagamet) and other H2 blockers, quinidine (a heart beat regulator), and SSRIs inhibit or interfere with the metabolism of TCAs, possibly producing several fold increases in plasma concentrations. This increases risk of cardiac symptoms and also of toxicity. Physicians may need to switch from cimetidine to ranitidine, famotidine, or nizatidine when TCA toxicity is seen with the combination.

SSRIs are known to impair oxidative metabolism in the liver (Barros, 1993; Ciraulo et al., 1990a; Gilbaldi, 1992; Preskorn et al., 1994). Most of the drug interactions have been reported with fluoxetine. However, it appears that any SSRI will inhibit the metabolism of drugs that undergo metabolism through CYP 2D6 (Preskorn et al., 1994). Drugs that are known to be metabolized by CYP 2D6 (e.g., dextromethorphan, desipramine, encainide haloperidol, imipramine, metoprolol, propranolol, perphenazine, and thioridazine) are predicted to have a lower clearance when administered with these antidepressant drugs. The importance of the CYP 3A3/4 and CYP 1A2 enzymes has come to light more recently with the marketing of fluvoxamine and nefazodone. Both of these agents inhibit CYP 3A3/4. CYP 3A3/4 inhibition reduces the metabolism of terfenadine (Seldane) and astemizole (Hismanal) and the benzodiazepines, alprazolam and triazolam. Interactions with the nonsedating antihistamines have resulted in cardiovascular complications (QT prolongation and torsades de pointes). Additionally, most of the SSRI antidepressants inhibit CYP 3A3/4 to some extent and thus have the potential to impair significantly the metabolism of these agents as well. Metabolism interactions are discussed more fully in an earlier section of this chapter.

The interaction of cyproheptadine with antidepressant medication may reduce the effectiveness of the antidepressant drug. When this happens, cyproheptadine should be discontinued if possible. The mechanism of the interaction is unknown but may be caused by antagonism of serotonergic action of antidepressant drugs.

Table 11-5 (see Chapter 11) shows additional interactions of antidepressant medications. Antidepressants (especially fluoxetine) can interact with beta blockers (e.g., metoprolol, propranolol) to cause severe bradycardia. When antidepressants are given to patients taking beta blockers, blood pressure and heart rate should be monitored. Antidepressants also can have adverse effects in persons being treated with neuroleptic drugs, especially for elderly persons.

Anxiolytics

The benzodiazepines can be classified in many ways with regard to drug interactions. The metabolic pathways (Phase I versus Phase II) are important in determining whether an agent poses a risk for metabolic interactions. Some of the benzodiazepines (diazepam, chlordiazepoxide, desmethyldiazepam, alprazolam, triazolam, clonazepam, flurazepam, nitrazepam, and others) undergo oxidative metabolism, often to desmethyldiazepam or desmethylflurazepam. Both of these active metabolites have a very long half-life relative to the parent drug, and they are common metabolites for many benzodiazepines. Inhibition of the metabolism can result in accumulation of high concentrations of long-acting metabolite and of excess CNS depression, respiratory depression, and cognitive dysfunction. Other agents either do not undergo oxidative metabolism (oxazepam, femazepam) or the active metabolites do not have extended half-lives relative to the parent agent (alprazolam, triazolam, and lorazepam). In the case of agents that do not undergo oxidative metabolism, enzyme inducers or inhibitors have no effect on the elimination rate. In the case of agents with half-lives similar to the parent compound, elimination may be affected, but the degree of change in clinical effects would not be as prominent as with the longer-acting agents.

Anxiolytic drugs (alprazolam, chlordiazepoxide, clonazepam, diazepam, desmethyldiazepam, flurazepam, midazolam, and triazolam) interact with cimetidine, macrolide antibiotics (erythromycin, clarithromycin), and nefazodone (Divoll, Greenblatt, Abernethy, & Shader, 1982; Greenblatt, Abernethy, Morse, Harmatz, & Shader, 184; Klotz & Rimann, 1980; Ruffalo, Thompson, & Segal, 1981). The interaction increases the plasma concentration of benzodiazepines that undergo oxidative hepatic metabolism. Excessive or increased sedation is possible within a few hours to a few days of taking the medications on a regular basis. The actual clinical significance of the interaction is usually minor and not well documented for most benzodiazepines. Clinicians may need to use an alternate H2 blocking drug such as ranitidine or reduce the dose of benzodiazepine.

The interaction of benzodiazepines and rifampin may reduce the anti-anxiety, antiepileptic, or sedative effects of these medications. Although the interaction is likely, the actual clinical significance is usually minor. Physicians may need to adjust upward the dose of benzodiazepine.

Fluoxetine and buspirone may interact, reducing the

clinical effectiveness in the treatment of anxiety disorders. Thus far, only isolated cases have been reported. No special precautions are indicated other than monitoring for possible occurrence.

Two cases have been reported of an adverse reaction to the interaction of clozapine and diazepam (see Sassim & Grohman, 1988). One person experienced a loss of consciousness, apnea, and mental confusion; the other became delirious. Both patients recovered spontaneously within a few minutes. Benzodiazepines should be avoided if possible during the initiation of clozapine. If used in combination, the person should be monitored for respiratory difficulties.

Finally, consumption of large quantities of ethyl alcohol while on benzodiazepine therapy may produce a combined CNS depressant effect (Dorian et al., 1985; Erwin, Linnoila, Hartwell, Erwin, & Guthrie, 1986; Seller & Busto, 1982). The onset of an adverse reaction may be minutes to hours after drinking.

Lithium

Lithium is particularly sensitive to changes in renal excretion. Any drug capable of changing renal blood flow (GFR), active tubular secretion, or passive tubular reabsorption is likely to change the renal elimination of lithium. Additionally, changes in sodium intake or excretion (e.g., via use of diuretics or excessive water intake) will also effect lithium elimination. Generally, increases in dietary sodium enhance lithium excretion, whereas decreases reduce elimination. Because lithium is not metabolized by the liver, it is not associated with metabolic interactions.

Lithium has a half-life of 16 to 24 hours in the average person. Any changes in the clearance of lithium will change the half-life and, subsequently, the steady-state concentration. The new steady-state concentration will be established, and hence the maximal effect occurs approximately four to five days after the interaction (i.e., it takes 4 to 5 half-lives to reach steady state).

Some important drug interactions with lithium are shown in Table 8-2. The interactions that result in excess concentrations of lithium (>1.4 mEq/L) can present as gastrointestinal distress (nausea, vomiting, and diarrhea), hand tremors, confusion, dysphoria, muscle weakness, ataxia, slurred speech, seizures, coma, and death. Clinicians should watch for these signs and, when indicated, adjust dose to achieve pre-interaction concentration. Monitoring is needed after 3 and 5 days and then on a regular basis. Encephalopathy has been report-

ed for people given lithium and antipsychotic medication (see Baastrop, Hollnagel, Sorenson, & Schou, 1976; Goldney & Spence, 1986; Juhl, Tsuang, & Perry, 1977; Krishna et al., 1978).

Stimulants

The stimulants include pemoline (Cylert), methylphenidate (Ritalin), and dextroamphetamine (Dexedrine). Because they are metabolized to inactive metabolites, metabolic inhibition or induction interactions are unlikely to be clinically significant. Most stimulants are excreted into the urine as a metabolite or unchanged drug. The amount excreted can change depending on the pH of the urine. Generally the more acidic the urine (lower pH), the more drug that is excreted. Urinary alkalinizers such as sodium bicarbonate may increase the effects of stimulants by decreasing urinary clearance and prolonging half-lives.

Pharmacodynamically, stimulants can interact with MAOI-type antidepressants. The sympathomimetic effect of the stimulants can cause a hypertensive crisis interaction if they are combined with an MAOI; for this reason, the combination is contraindicated. In fact, stimulants should not be used until 2 weeks after MAOI therapy has been discontinued. Stimulants also may interact with clonidine in patients with pre-existing cardiovascular disease. Death has been reported in cases of combined stimulant and clonidine use in the treatment of hyperactivity.

Opioid Antagonists

Naltrexone has relatively specific pharmacologic activity and thus is not likely to have many pharmacodynamic interactions. Generally, the only interactions of clinical significance are with the opioid analgesics. Naltrexone will reduce the analgesic response for some people receiving analgesics such as codeine, propoxyphene, morphine, and meperidine for pain. The narcotic antagonist properties of naltrexone occur within hours to 1-2 days of administration of the first dose. The use of non-opioid analgesics such as ibuprofen, ketorolac, or naproxen may provide adequate pain relief as an alternative to the narcotic analgesics. Assessment of pain response for clients with mental retardation and developmental disabilities is often difficult. Caregivers who are familiar with the client's communication may be helpful in assessment of response to analgesic medication.

Table 8-2. Agents that Interact with Lithium[8]

Interacting Agents	Onset	Severity	Mechanism	Presentation	Management
DRUGS AFFECTING LITHIUM					
thiazide diuretics	delayed	moderate	decreased lithium clearance caused by reduction in tubular secretion and increased passive tubular reabsorption	possible excessive lithium concentration and toxicity	monitor lithium concentration after 3 and 5 days; adjust dose to achieve preinteraction concentration; monitor for signs and symptoms of toxicity
Nonsteroidal anti-inflammatory drugs ibuprofen (Motrin) naproxen (Naprosyn) indomethacin (Indocen) ketoprofen (Orudis) piroxicam (Feldene)	delayed	moderate-severe	decreased lithium clearance concentrations increase 50%-60%	possible excessive lithium concentration and toxicity	monitor lithium levels after 5 days and weekly until stable; adjust dose to achieve preinteraction concentration; monitor for signs of toxicity; use of aspirin or sulindac is less likely to cause interaction
ACE Inhibitors enalapril captopril lisinopril	delayed	moderate	decreased glomerular filtration rate and reduced lithium excretion	possible increased toxicity from dehydration	monitor lithium concentration after 3 and 5 days; adjust dose to achieve preinteraction concentration; monitor for signs and symptoms of toxicity
Sodium (restricted from diet)	delayed	moderate	decreased sodium intake results in increase in reabsorption of lithium in distal tubule and subsequent increase in lithium concentrations	may be severe often occurs when person is put on a salt-restricted diet for medical problems	minimize changes in dietary sodium, any weight loss diet should be closely monitored for sodium-restricted items; monitor lithium concentration; adjust dose to achieve preinteraction concentration; monitor for signs and symptoms of toxicity
loop diuretics furosemide (Lasix) bumetanide (Bumex)	delayed	minor	increased lithium levels (mechanism unknown)	possible interaction (not as well documented as with thiazide diuretics)	monitor lithium concentration after 3 and 5 days; adjust dose to achieve preinteraction concentration; monitor for symptoms of toxicity

8 See Baldwin and Safferman (1990), Ciraulo et al. (1989), Cook (1985), Correa and Eiser (1992), Gelenberg (1998), Goldney and Spence (1986), Huang (1990), Juhl, Tsuang, and Perry (1977), Kapur and Kambhampat (1992), Krishna et al. (1978), Kristoff et al. (1992), Ragheb (1990), Tatio and Olin (1994).

Table 8-2. Continued

Interacting Agents	Onset	Severity	Mechanism	Presentation	Management
Fluoxetine (Prozac)	delayed	moderate	increased lithium levels (mechanism unknown)	possible interaction possible toxicity	monitor lithium concentration after 3 and 5 days adjust dose to achieve preinteraction concentration monitor for symptoms of toxicity
Theophylline caffeine	delayed	minor	increased renal clearance of lithium reduced half-life reduced steady-state concentrations	concentrations may decrease up to 20% possible reemergence of symptoms	monitor clinically for emergence of psychiatric symptomatology monitor lithium concentration after 3 and 5 days adjust dose to achieve preinteraction concentration
Acetazolamide (Diamox)	delayed	minor	possible impaired proximal tubular reabsorption increased renal clearance of lithium reduced lithium concentration	relatively small change in serum concentration of lithium possible loss of therapeutic effect	monitor clinically for emergence of psychiatric symptomatology monitor lithium concentration after 3 and 5 days adjust dose to achieve preinteraction concentration
Sodium (high dietary intake)	delayed	moderate	increased renal clearance reduced lithium concentrations	modest changes in concentration of lithium and subsequent loss of effect	minimize changes in dietary sodium monitor clinically for emergence of psychiatric symptomatology monitor lithium concentration after 3 and 5 days adjust dose to achieve preinteraction concentration
Methyldopa (Aldomet)	delayed	moderate	? (unknown)	possible sedation, confusion, ataxia, and dysphoria no changes in lithium concentration	monitor clinically for signs of toxicity may consider alternative therapy for hypertension may require stopping one or both drugs

Table 8-2. Continued

Interacting Agents	Onset	Severity	Mechanism	Presentation	Management
Ca channel antagonists Verapamil (Calan, Isoptin) diltiazem (Cardizem)	delayed	moderate	? (unknown)	neurotoxicity (EPS, choreoathetosis), bradycardia, and return of psychiatric symptoms reported decreases in lithium concentrations reported	monitor clinically for signs of toxicity consider alternative therapy for Ca channel antagonists
Antipsychotics	delayed	moderate	? (unknown)	encephalopathy (fever, lethargy, confusion, leukocyctosis, seizures, severe EPS, elevated liver enzymes) similar to NMS in some cases risk is variable; may be more readily reversible with phenothiazines retrospective reviews suggest that encephalopathy is uncommon but possible	use combinations of lithium and neuroleptics judiciously clinically monitor for emergence of encephalopathy discontinue agents if suspected
Carbamazepine (Tegretol)	delayed	moderate	? (unknown)	neurotoxicity (sedation, lethargy, ataxia, tremor, hyperreflexia, and muscle weakness) despite therapeutic levels of each drug risk factors associated with toxicity not known some individuals tolerate the combination	monitor for signs of neurotoxicity

Fenfluramine

The primary interaction with fenfluramine is with MAOI-type antidepressants. The sympathomimetic effects of fenfluramine in combination with an MAOI can cause a hypertensive crisis reaction. The effect may be delayed up to 2 weeks after discontinuation of MAOI. Fenfluramine should not be used in combination with MAOIs. Fenfluramine also has mild to moderate interactions with oral sulfonylureal hypoglycemic agents. Physicians should monitor blood glucose regularly for hypoglycemia when initiating fenfluramine for people with diabetes.

CONCLUSION

Knowledge of drug interactions is crucial to the selection of a psychoactive medication. Although our current knowledge of these interactions is limited, researchers are reporting new information at a rapid rate, especially in regard to the metabolic isoenzymes. Since new psychotropic drugs and other medications will continue to be introduced at a significant rate, clinicians need to remain vigilant to the possibility of serious, unknown interactions. **The key to managing drug interactions is being able to predict and prevent an interaction, and to identify when an interaction is occurring and to take action.**

REFERENCES

Aman, M.G., Field, C.J., & Bridgeman, G.D. (1985). City-wide survey of drug patterns among non-institutionalized retarded persons. *Applied Research in Mental Retardation*, 5, 159–171.

Aman, M.G., Sarphare, G., & Burrow, W.H. (1995). Psychotropic drug use in group homes: Prevalence and relationship to demographic/psychiatric variables. *American Journal on Mental Retardation*, 99, 500–509.

Baastrup, P.C., Hollnagel, P., Sorenson, R., & Schou, M. (1976). Adverse reactions in treatment with lithium carbonate and haloperidol. *Journal of the American Medical Association*, 236, 2645–2646.

Baldwin, C.M., & Safferman, A.Z. (1990). A case of lisinopril-induced lithium toxicity. *DICP, The Annals of Pharmacotherapy* 5, 946–947.

Barros J. (1993). An interaction of sertraline and desipramine. *American Journal of Psychiatry*, 150, 1751.

Blackwell, B., & Schmidt, G.L. (1984). Drug interactions in psychopharmacology. *Psychiatric Clinics of North America*, 7, 625–637.

Bodkin, J.A., & Teicher, M.H. (1989). Fluoxetine may antagonize the anxiolytic action of buspirone. *Journal of Clinical Psychopharmacology*, 9, 150–151.

Boston Collaborative Drug Surveillance Program. (1973). Clinical depression of the central nervous system due to diazepam and chlordiazepoxide in relation to cigarette smoking and age. *New England Journal of Medicine*, 288, 871–878.

Brockmeyer, N.H. et al. [PLEASE PROVIDE ALL AUTHOR NAMES] (1990). Comparative effects of rifampin and/or probenecid on the pharmacokinetics of temazepam and nitrazepam. *International Journal of Clinical Pharmacology, Therapeutics and Toxicology*, 28, 387–393.

Brosen, K., Skejelbo, E., Rasmusse, B.B.,

Poulsen, H.E., & Loft, S. (1993). Fluvoxamine is a potent inhibitor of cytochrome P-450 1A2. *Biochemical Pharmacology*, 44, 349–355.

Cacek, A.T. (1986). Review of alterations in oral phenytoin bioavailability associated with formulation, antacids and food. *Therapeutic Drug Monitoring*, 8, 166–171.

Ciraulo, D.A., & Shader, R.I. (1990a). Fluoxetine drug-drug interactions: I. Antidepressants and antipsychotics. *Journal of Clinical Psychopharmacology*, 10, 48–50.

Ciraulo, D.A., & Shader, R.I. (1990b). Fluoxetine drug-drug interactions II. *Journal of Clinical Psychopharmacology*, 10, 213–217.

Ciraulo, D.A., Shader, R.I., Greenblatt, D.J., & Creelman, W. (Eds). (1989). *Drug interactions in psychiatry*. Baltimore: Williams & Wilkins.

Cohen, I.A., Johnson, C.E., Berardi, R.R., Hyneck, M.L., & Achem, S.R. (1985). Cimetidine-theophylline interaction: Effects of age and cimetidine dose. *Therapeutic Drug Monitoring*, 33, 426–434.

Cook, B.L., Smith, R.E., Perry, P.J., & Calloway, R.A. (1985). Theophylline-lithium interaction. *Journal of Clinical Psychiatry*, 46, 278–279.

Correa, F.J., & Eiser, A.R. (1992). Angiotensin-converting enzyme inhibitors and lithium toxicity. *American Journal of Medicine*, 93, 108–109.

Crewe, H.K., Lennard, M.S., Tucker, G.T., Woods, F.R., & Haddock, R.E. (1992). The effect of selective serotonin reuptake inhibitors on cytochrome P-450 2D6 (CYP 2D6) activity in human liver microsomes. *British Journal of Clinical Pharmacology*, 34, 262–265.

Divoll, M., Greenblatt, D.J., Abernethy, D.R., & Shader, R.I. (1982). Cimetidine impairs clearance of antipyrine and desmethyldiazepam in the elderly. *Journal of the American Geriatric Society*, 30, 684–689.

Dorian, P., Sellers, E.M., Kaplan, H.L.,

Hamilton, C., Greenblatt, D.J., & Abernethy, D. (1985). Triazolam and ethanol interaction: Kinetic and dynamic consequences. *Clinical Pharmacology and Therapeutics*, 37, 558–562.

Erwin, C.W., Linnoila, M., Hartwell, J., Erwin, A., & Guthrie, S. (1986). Effects of buspirone and diazepam, alone and in combination with alcohol, on skilled performance and evoked potentials. *Journal of Clinical Psychopharmacology*, 6, 199–209.

Feely, J., Pereira, L., Gut, E., & Hockings, N. (1984). Factors affecting the response to inhibition of drug metabolism by cimetidine-dose response and sensitivity of elderly induced subjects. *British Journal of Clinical Pharmacology*, 17, 77–81.

Fuseau, E., & Sheiner, L.B.(1984). Simultaneous modeling of pharmacokinetics and pharmacodynamics with a non-parametric pharmacodynamic model. *Clinical Pharmacology and Therapeutics*, 35, 733–741.

Gelenberg, A.J. (1988). ACE inhibitors and lithium toxicity. *Biological Therapeutic Psychiatry*, 11, 43.

Gibaldi, M. (1992). Drug interactions: Part 1. *Annals of Pharmacotherapy*, 26, 709–713.

Goldney, R.D., & Spence, N.D. (1986). Safety of the combination of lithium and neuroletic drugs. *American Journal of Psychiatry*, 143, 882–884.

Grady, T.A., Pigott T.A., L'Heureux, F., & Murphy, D.L. (1992). Seizure associated with fluoxetine and adjuvant buspirone therapy. *Journal of Clinical Psychopharmacology*, 12, 70–71.

Greenblatt, D.J., Abernethy, D.R., Morse, D.S., Harmatz, J.S., & Shader, R.I. (1984). Clinical importance of the interaction of diazepam and cimetidine. *New England Journal of Medicine*, 310, 1639–1643.

Greenblatt, D.J., Allen, M.D., Locniskar, A., Harmatz, J.S., & Shader, R.I. (1979). Lorazepam kinetics in the elderly. *Clinical Pharmacolgy and Therapeutics*, 26, 103–113.

Greenblatt, D.J., Allen, M.D., Harmatz, J.S., & Shader, R.I. (1980). Diazepam disposition determinants. *Clinical Pharmacology and Therapeutics, 27*, 301–312.

Greenblatt, D.J., Preskorn, S.H., Cotreau, M.M., Horst, W.D., & Harmatz, J.S. (1992). Fluoxetine impairs clearance of alprazolam but not of clonazepam. *Clinical Pharmacology and Therapeutics, 52*, 479–486.

Hansten, P.D., & Horn, J.R. (Eds). (1994). *Drug interactions and quarterly updates.* Vancouver, WA: Applied Therapeutics, Inc.

Hill, B.K., Balow, E.A., & Bruininks, R.H. (1985). A national study of prescribed drugs in institutions and community residential facilities for mentally retarded people. *Psychopharmacological Bulletin, 21*, 279–284.

Hiller, A., Olkkola, K.T., Isohanni P., & Saarnivaara, L. (1990). Unconsciousness associated with midazolam and erythromycin. *British Journal of Anaesthesiology, 65*, 826–828.

Holford, N.H.G., & Sheiner, L.B. (1981). Understanding the dose-effect relationship: Clinical application of pharmacokinetic-pharmacodynamic models. *Clinical Pharmacokinetics, 6*, 429–453.

Huang, L.G. (1990). Lithium intoxication with coadministration of a loop-diuretic. *Journal of Clinical Psychopharmacology, 3*, 228.

Intagliata, J., & Rinck, C. (1985). Psychoactive drug use in public and community residential facilities for mentally retarded persons. *Psychopharmacology Bulletin, 21*, 268–278.

Jann, M.W., Bean, J., & Fidone, G.S. (1986). Interaction of dietary pudding with phenytoin. *Pediatrics, 78*, 952–953.

Juhl, R.P., Tsuang, M.T., & Perry, P.J. (1977). Concomitant administration of haloperidol and lithium carbonate in acute mania. *Diseases of the Nervous System, 38*, 675–676.

Jusko, W.J. (1978). Role of tobacco smoking in pharmacokinetics. *Journal of Pharmacokinetics and Biopharmaceutics. 6*, 7–39.

Jusko, W.J. (1979). Influence of cigarette smoking on drug metabolism in man. *Drug Metabolism Review, 9*, 221–236.

Kapur, S., & Kambhampati, R.K. (1992). Drug interactions in psychopharmacology. In M.S. Keshavan & J.S. Kennedy (Eds.), *Drug-induced dysfunction in psychiatry* (pp. 21–37).

Ketter, T.A., Flockhart, D.A., Post, R.M., Denicoff, K., Pazzaglia, P.J.,

Marangell, L.B., George, M.S., & Callahan, A.M. (1995). The emerging role of cytochrome P450 3A in psychopharmacology. *Journal of Clinical Psychopharmacology, 15*, 387–398.

Klotz, U., & Reimann, I. (1980). Delayed clearance of diazepam due to cimetidine. *New England Journal of Medicine, 302*, 1012–1014.

Kristoff, C.A., Hayes, P.E., Barr, W.H., Small,

R.E., Townsend, R.J., & Ettig, P.G. (1986). Effects of ibuprofen on lithium plasma and red blood cell concentrations. *Clinical Pharmacy, 7*, 51–55.

Lasher, T.A., Fleishaker, J.C., Steenwyk, R.C., & Antal, E.J. (1991). Pharmacokinetic pharmacodynamic evaluation of the combined administration of alprazolam and fluoxetine. *Psychopharmacology, 104*, 323–327.

Lemberger, L., Rowe, H., Bosomworth, J.C., Tenbarge, J.B., & Bergstrom, R.F. (1988). The effect of fluoxetine on the pharmacokinetics and psychomotor responses of diazepam. *Clinical Pharmacology and Therapeutics, 43*, 412–419.

Levy, R.A. (1993). Ethnic and racial differences in response to medicines: Preserving individualized therapy in manged pharmaceutical programs. Reston, VA: National Pharmaceutical Council.

Linnoila, M., George, L. Guthrie, S., & Leventhal, B. (1981). Effect of alcohol consumption and cigarette smoking on antidepressant levels of depressed patients. *American Journal of Psychiatry, 138*, 841.

Ludden, T.M. (1985). Pharmacokinetic interactions of the macrolide antibiotics. *Clinical Pharmacokinetics, 10*, 63–79.

MacKichan, J.J. (1992). Influence of protein binding and the use of unbound (free) drug concentrations. In W.E. Evans, J.J. Schentag, & W.J. Jusko (Eds.), *Applied pharmacokinetics: Principles of therapeutic drug monitoring* (3rd ed., Chap. 5). Vancouver WA: Applied Therapeutics.

McEvoy, G.K (ed.). (1994). *AHFS drug information 94.* Bethesda, MD: American Society of Hospital Pharmacists.

Nelson, D.R., Kamataki, T., Waxman, D.J., Guenerich, F.P., Estabrook, R.W., Feyersisen, R., Gonzalez, F.J., Coon, M.J., Gunsalus, I.C., & Gotoh, O. (1993). The P450 superfamily: Update on new sequences, gene mapping, accession numbers, early triorial names of enzymes and nomenclature. *DNA and Cell Biology, 12*, 1–51.

Nerbert, D.W., Nelson, D.R., Coon, M.J., Estabrook, R.W., Feyereisen, R., Fuji-Kuriyama, Y., Gonzalez, F.J., Guengerich, F.P., Gunsalus, I.C., & Johnson, E.F. (1991). The P450 superfamily: Update on new sequences, gene mapping, and recommended nomenclature. *DNA and Cell Biology, 10*, 1–14.

Ochs, H.R., Greenblatt, D.J., Roberts, G.M., & Dengler, H.J. (1981). Diazepam interaction with antituberculosis drugs. *Clinical Pharmacology and Therapeutics, 29*, 671–678.

Ohnhaus, E.E., Brockmeyer, N., Dylewicz, P., & Habicht, H. (1987). The effect of antipyrine and rifampin on the metabolism of diazepam, *Clinical Pharmacology and Therapeutics 42*, 148–156.

Olkkola, K.T., Aranko, K., Luurila, H., Hiller, A., Saarnivaara, L., Himberg, J.J., & Neuvonen, P.J. (1993). A potentially hazardous interaction between erythromycin and midazolam. *Clinical Pharmacology and Therapeutics, 53*, 298–305.

Pary, R. (1993). Psychoactive drugs used with adults and elderly adults who have mental retardation. *American Journal of Mental Retardation, 98*, 121–127.

Perel, J.M., Hurwicz, M.J., & Kanzler, M.B. (1975). Pharmacodynamics of imipramine in depressed patients. *Psychopharmacology Bulletin, 11*, 16–18.

Phillips, J.P., Antal, E.J., & Smith, R.B. (1986). A pharmacokinetic drug interaction between erythromycin and triazolam. *Journal of Clinical Psychopharmacology, 6*, 297–299.

Preskorn, S.H., Alderman, J., Chung, M., Harrison, W., Messia, M., & Harris, S. (1994). Pharmacokinetics of desipramine coadminstered with sertraline or fluoxetine. *Journal of Clinical Psychopharmacology, 14*, 90–98.

Preskorn, S.H., & Fast, G.A. (1991). Therapeutic drug monitoring for antidepressants: Efficacy, safety, and cost effectiveness. *Journal of Clinical Psychiatry, 52*, 23–33.

Preskorn, S.H., & Fast, G.A. (1992). Tricyclic antidepressant-induced seizures and plasma concentrations. *Journal of Clinical Psychiatry, 53*, 160–162.

Preskorn, S.H., & Jerkovich, G.S. (1990). Central nervous system toxicitiy of tricyclic antidepressants: Phenomenology, course, risk factors, and role of therapeutic drug monitoring. *Journal of Clinical Psychopharmacology, 10*, 88–95.

Preskorn, S.H., & Magnus, R.D. (1994). Inhibition of hepatic P-450 isoenzymes by serotonin selective reuptake inhibitors: Invitro and invivo findings and their implications for patient care. *Psychopharmacology Bulletin, 30*, 251–259.

Preskorn, S.H. (1996). Reducing the risk of drug-drug interations: a goal of rational drug development. *Journal of Clinical Psychiatry, 57(suppl 1)*, 3–6.

Raghab, M. (1990). The clinical significance of lithium-nonsteroidal anti-inflammator drug interactions. *Journal of Clinical Psychopharmacology, 10*, 350–4.

Riesenman, C. (1995). Antidepressant drug interactions and the cytochrome P450 system: A critical appraisal. *Pharmacotherapy, 15 (6 pt. 2)*, 84S–99S.

Rinck, C., & Calkins, C. (1989). Patterns of psychotropic medication use among older persons with developmental disabilities. *Journal of Applied Gerontology, 8*, 216–228.

Ruffalo, R.L., Thompson, J.F., & Segal, J. (1981). Cimetidine-benzodiazepine drug interaction. *American Journal of Hospital Pharmacy, 38*, 1365–1366.

Saklad, J.J., Graves, R.H., & Sharp, W.P. (1986). Interaction of oral phenytoin and enteral feedings. *Journal of Parenteral and Enteral Nutrition, 10*, 322–323.

Sassim, N., & Grohmann, R. (1988). Adverse

drug reactions with clozapine and simultaneous application of benzodiazepines. *Pharmacopsychiatry, 21,* 306–307.

Shulman, K.I., Walker, S.E., Mackenzie, S., & Knowles, S. (1989). Dietary restriction, tyramine, and the use of monoamine oxidase inhibitors. *Journal of Clinical Psychopharmacology, 9,* 397.

Sellers, E.M., & Busto, U. (1982). Benzodiazepines and ethanol: Assessment of the effects and consequences of psychotropic drug interactions. *Journal of Clinical Psychopharmacology, 2,* 249–262.

Shader, R.I. (1994). Question the experts. *Journal of Clinical Psychopharmacology, 14,* 293.

Shank, R.P., Vaught, J.L., Pelley, K.A., Sether, P.E., McComsey, D.F., & Maryanott, B.E. (1988). McN-5652: A highly potent inhibitor of serotonin uptake. *Journal of Pharmacology and Experimental Therapeutics, 247,* 1032–1038.

Sheiner, L.B., Stanski, D.R., Vozeh, S., Miller R.D., & Ham, J. (1979). Simultaneous modeling of pharmacokinetic and pharmacokinetics: Application to d-tubocurarine. *Clinical Pharmacology and Therapeutics, 25,* 358–371.

Sovner, R., & Davis, J.M. (1991). A potential drug interaction between fluoxetine and valproic acid. *Journal of Clinical Psychopharmacology, 11,* 389.

Swett, C. (1974). Drowsiness due to chlorpromazine in relation to cigarette smoking. *Archives of General Psychiatry, 31,* 211–214.

Swett, C. (1977). Side effects of chlorpromazine in relation to cigarette smoking. *Psychopharmacology Bulletin, 13,* 57–58.

Tatro, D.S., & Olin, B.R. (Eds.). (1994). *Drug interaction facts.* St. Louis: Facts and Comparisons (A Wolters Kluwer Co.).

Unadkat, J. O., Bartha, F., & Sheiner, L.B. (1986). Simultaneous modeling of pharmacokinetics and pharmacodynamics with nonparamentric kinetic and dynamic models. *Clinical Pharmacology and Therapeutics, 40,* 86–83.

Vinarova, E., Vinar, O., & Kalvach, Z. (1984). Smokers need higher doses of neuroleptic drugs. *Biological Psychiatry, 19,* 1265–1268.

von Moltke, L.L., Greenblatt, D.J., Coutreau-Bibbo, M.M., Duan, S.X., Harmatz, J.S., & Shader, R.I. (1994). Inhibition of desipramine hydroxylastion in vitrop by serotonin-reuptake inhibitor antidepressants and by quinidine and ketoconazole: A model system to predict drug interactions in vivo. *Journal of Pharmacology and Experimental Therapeutics, 268,* 1278–1283.

Neuroleptics

Alan A. Baumeister[1], Jay A. Sevin[2], Bryan H. King[3]

Neuroleptics were first received with enthusiasm. This new class of drugs was credited with revolutionizing psychiatric care for children with mental retardation—it opened doors to community placements and replaced alternative treatments such as electroconvulsive and insulin-shock therapies (Abbott, Blake, & Vincze, 1965). Initially the drugs appeared to be effective for treating many symptoms, including hyperactivity, aggression, tantrums, agitation, insomnia, and self-injury. One early investigator went so far as to suggest that thioridazine (Mellaril) is "virtually free of side effects" (LeVann, 1969). Unfortunately, the initial optimism was somewhat misplaced. These drugs have significant side effects, and some authorities have questioned their use with people with mental retardation, except for those with mild cognitive impairment for whom a diagnosis of schizophrenia is unequivocal.

Despite the controversy that has surrounded the use of these drugs in recent years, neuroleptics remain the most widely prescribed class of psychotropic medication for people with mental retardation. Some clinicians are quite comfortable prescribing these drugs for treating severe maladaptive behaviors that may vary widely in terms of severity and topography. In clinical practice it is not uncommon to come across people with mental retardation who may have been receiving a neuroleptic drug for a number of years for the treatment of behaviors like running away or noncompliance, for which very little clinical evidence can be marshaled in terms of efficacy. One can also find people who were placed on a neuroleptic so many years ago that no one distinctly remembers what had prompted the initial drug trial.

The first modern neuroleptic, chlorpromazine (Thorazine), was introduced in 1952 (Swazey, 1974). More than a dozen other neuroleptics have been marketed since then. Historically, chlorpromazine and related drugs have been referred to by numerous labels. The term *neuroleptic*, which means "to seize the neuron," was proposed in 1955 by Delay and Deniker to distinguish these drugs from traditional sedative-hypnotic compounds (Swazey, 1974). Today, the term is often used to refer to both the antipsychotic and the neurologic effects of these medications. Another early term applied to these drugs was *ataractic*, which means "equanimity or freedom from perturbation." Drugs in this group have also been called tranquilizers. With the advent of anxiolytic medications, chlorpromazine and related drugs became known as major tranquilizers, and the anti-anxiety drugs were designated minor tranquilizers. It is now recognized that drugs like chlorpromazine differ from tranquilizers in that they have specific antipsychotic actions that are unrelated to sedation; moreover, their hypnotic effect is relatively weak and reversible. Another commonly used label for these medications is *antipsychotic*. The problem with this term is that it implies a range of applications that is too narrow, because the medications are used for severe behavior disorders that may not represent a true psychosis.

Although neuroleptic drugs can be organized into eight chemical classes (see Table 9-1), chemical classification has little clinical utility because it is unrelated to antipsychotic efficacy, except in regard to clozapine. The selection of a neuroleptic drug in treatment is based on considerations other than chemical classification, particularly the patient's medication history, the physician's prior experience with particular neuroleptics, and the drug's side effects.

Clozapine was the first fundamentally different antipsychotic drug to be introduced after chlorpromazine. Because of its unique pharmacological profile, clozapine is often referred to as an atypical neuroleptic. Clozapine may be effective in reducing symptoms of schizophrenia in patients who do not respond well to other antipsychotics. It is unclear whether clozapine is more effective than traditional neuroleptics; however, it has fewer neurologic side effects.

Another atypical antipsychotic is risperidone, which

1 Assistant Professor of Psychology, Louisiana State University, Baton Rouge, LA
2 Psychologist, Developmental Neuropsychiatric Unit, Southeast Louisiana Hospital, Mandeville, LA
3 Assistant Professor of Psychiatry, UCLA, Los Angeles, California
Other committee members: A. Langa, Consultant Psychiatrist, Lynebank Hospital; and Michael J. Levine, Medical Director, Developmental Disabilities Services, Louisiana Healthcare Authority

Table 9-1. Doses and Side Effects of Neuroleptic Chemical Classes

Chemical Class (Proprietary Name)	Doses (mg)		Side Effects		
	Adults	Children	Sedation	Autonomic	Motor
Phenothiazines chlorpromazine (Thorazine) thioridazine (Mellaril)	200 - 800	10 - 200	+++	+++	+
Thioxanthines thiothixene (Navane)	5 - 30	1 - 6	+ to ++	++	++
Butyrophenones haloperidol (Haldol)	2 - 20	0.25 - 6	+	+	+++
Diphenylbutylpiperidine pimozide (Orap)	2 - 6	1 - 6	+	?	+++
Dibenzoxazapine loxapine (Loxitane)	60 - 100	Not Known	++	+ to ++	++
Dihydroindolone molindone (Moban)	50 - 225	1 - 155	++	++	++
Dibenzodiazepine clozapine (Clozaril)	100 - 700	Not Known	+++	+++	0
Benzisocazole risperidone (Risperdal)	2 - 16	Not Known	+	++	+

Note. +=low, ++=medium, +++=high. Data are from Baldessarini (1990), Campbell et al. (1993), and Marder and Van Putten (1995).

was only recently marketed and, like clozapine, appears to have comparatively fewer neurologic side effects. Because atypical antipsychotics differ in this respect from conventional neuroleptics, they have been labeled nonneuroleptic antipsychotics (Davis, Janicak, Preskorn, & Ayd, 1994). Risperidone may also have superior antipsychotic efficacy, although the data are too limited to draw any firm conclusions at this time. Open clinical trials indicate that clozapine may be effective in controlling aberrant behavior in people with mental retardation (Rubin & Langa, 1995); however, systematic data on the use of clozapine and risperidone with this population are not available.

Sertindole is another atypical neuroleptic. As this book was being prepared for publication, the drug was about to be marketed. Extrapyramidal side effects appear to be no greater than those attributable to placebo at any dose studied thus far. However, the possibility of prolongation of the QT interval as measured on an EKG, with the associated risk of arrhythmia, may limit the use of this drug.

PHARMACOLOGY

Pharmacodynamics

The potency of a neuroleptic is determined by the amount of drug required to produce a criterion antipsychotic effect. Potencies of neuroleptics vary widely. The typical adult daily doses of low-potency drugs such as chlorpromazine range from 200 to 600 mg; for high-potency drugs such as haloperidol, the daily doses range from 5 to 20 mg. The side effect profiles of neuroleptics are correlated with their antipsychotic potency. Low-potency neuroleptics tend to have relatively strong sedative, anticholinergic, and hypotensive side effects but cause fewer extrapyramidal symptoms; the reverse is true for high-potency drugs. Neuroleptics interact with receptors for a variety of brain neurotransmitters, including dopamine, serotonin, acetylcholine, histamine, and norepinephrine (Peroutka & Snyder, 1980). Their ability to antagonize, or block, dopamine receptors appears to correlate well with the efficacy of these drugs.

Most neuroleptic drugs in clinical use today show two pharmacological actions: (a) amelioration of schizophrenic symptoms and (b) evocation of extrapyramidal symptoms. Both effects appear to be related to the blockade of dopamine receptors in the brain, producing the desired therapeutic effects as well as unwanted effects. A particular type of dopamine receptor, called the D2 receptor, appears to be important in mediating the antipsychotic effect of most neuroleptics. The extent to which a neuroleptic blocks D2 receptors correlates strongly with the drug's antipsychotic potency (Peroutka & Snyder, 1980). An important exception to this general principle is clozapine, which has weak affinity for D2 receptors but strongly antagonizes D4 receptors and 5-HT2 serotonin receptors. Neuroleptic drugs also interfere with cholinergic receptors in the brain (Kito, Sejawa, Kuriyama, Yamamura, & Altman, 1984; Snyder,

Benerjee, Jamamura, & Greenberg, 1974). The anticholinergic activity of neuroleptics varies widely. Affinity for cholinergic receptors is inversely correlated with the neuroleptic drug's propensity to induce extrapyramidal side effects.

Pharmacokinetics

Although neuroleptics are generally well absorbed when taken orally, they may be extensively metabolized when they first pass through the liver before reaching general circulation (first-pass metabolism). For example, chlorpromazine and fluphenazine are metabolized to a significant extent when they pass through the gut and liver. When injected intramuscularly, drugs avoid this breakdown. This is one reason for using depot antipsychotic medications (e.g., flupenthixol and fluphenazine), which are injected intramuscularly in preparations that are absorbed slowly. Other neuroleptics, such as haloperidol, undergo relatively little first-pass metabolism.

The half-lives of these drugs vary, but generally are about 20 to 40 hours (see Table 9-2 for pharmacokinetic parameters of selected drugs). Because of their high lipid solubility, however, they may take at least four times longer to reach a pharmacodynamic equilibrium, and at least several days of cessation to lose pharmacological

Table 9-2. Pharmacokinetic Parameters of Orally Administered Neuroleptics

Drug	tmax* (h)	F** (%)	t1/2*** (h)	Vd**** (L/kg)	fu*****
chlorpromazine	2-4	25-65	12-36	10-35	0.05-0.01
clozapine	1-6	40-60	12-36	4-8	0.05
flupenthixol	3-8	30-70	24-36	10-20	0.01
fluphenazine	2-5	1?-50	8-32	5?-60?	<0.10
haloperidol	3-6	40-80	15-30	15-20	0.08
pimozide	4-8	15-25	30-150	20-40	0.03
risperidone	1-3	6-8	3-22	0.7-0.8	.10
sulpiride	2-6	15-65	6-15	3	—
thioridazine	2-4	10-60	10-30	10	0.03

*   time to reach peak plasma concentration
**   bioavailability
***   elimination half-life
****   volume of distribution
***** unbound fraction of the drug

Note. Data are from Balant-Gorgia et al. (1993), De Coster (1988), and Jann et al. (1993).

effects. They are long-acting drugs, in terms of both pharmacodynamic equilibrium and elimination (Campbell, Gonzalez, Ernst, Silva, & Werry, 1993). More than 160 metabolites have been postulated for chlorpromazine, of which about 100 have been detected in blood or urine. With the possible exception of haloperidol, several studies have failed to show significant correlation between plasma drug concentration and any measure of pharmacological effect, including clinical improvement, increase in CSF homovanillic acid concentration, or increase in plasma prolactin concentration. Thus, in clinical practice there is seldom a good reason to obtain blood neuroleptic levels.

After neuroleptics enter the bloodstream, they are transported throughout the body to an apparent volume of distribution that depends on the specific drug. Most neuroleptics are lipid soluble and pass readily into the CNS. At a given time, however, only a fraction of the total amount of the drug in the body is at the site of action. The rest might be excreted without ever reaching the site of action (Baldessarini, Coyne, & Teicher, 1988; Bowers, 1974).

Like most drugs, neuroleptics bind, to a greater or lesser degree, to plasma and tissue proteins. The extent of this binding is important, because only the unbound drug is active. An increase in the unbound fraction of the drug may produce an increase in therapeutic or toxic effect. This may result either from a change in the concentration of plasma proteins or from displacement by other drugs from binding sites on proteins.

Biotransformation of most neuroleptics occurs in the liver, involving a variety of chemical reactions such as oxidation, reduction, hydrolysis, and conjugation. The cytochrome P450-mediated system consists of many isoenzymes, which selectively use drugs as their substrates. Some of these reactions follow a polymorphic pattern. These processes can change neuroleptics such as chlorpromazine and thioridazine into biologically active metabolites, producing substances that essentially act as new drugs. Biotransformation of haloperidol results in a series of metabolites that have no pharmacological activity (Forsman & Ohman, 1977).

Steady-state blood levels of neuroleptics may vary by as much as 20- to 25-fold between individuals on a fixed daily dose. Most of this variability is due to differences in rates of metabolism (Baldessarini et al., 1988). Metabolism can be affected by genetic, environmental, and physiological factors; individual differences in distribution and protein binding are relatively unimportant. The kidneys are the primary site of neuroleptic drug excretion. This activity may be impaired in the very young and very old, especially those with liver or kidney problems.

SYSTEM/PHYSICAL EFFECTS

The most important pharmacological actions of the neuroleptics are those on the CNS, cardiovascular system, autonomic nervous system, and endocrine functions. Minor dermatologic and respiratory effects have also been noted. Side effects are usually extensions of these many pharmacological actions.

Neuroleptics affect various levels of the nervous system. Most neuroleptics lower the seizure threshold. The aliphatic phenothiazines (e.g., chlorpromazine) and clozapine are the most troublesome in this regard. Proconvulsive effects appear to be relatively low for piperazine phenothiazines and for the thioxanthenes such as fluphenazine and thiothixene. Haloperidol has variable and unpredictable effects on seizure thresholds. Neuroleptic agents should be used with caution for patients with untreated epilepsy. This point is important because a substantial proportion of people with mental retardation suffer from epilepsy (James, 1986). The majority of neuroleptics have a protective action against nausea. The anti-emetic effect of most neuroleptics occurs with very low doses. The exception to this is thioridazine, which has no clinical efficacy as an anti-emetic in humans. Other CNS effects, like drug-induced Parkinsonism and extrapyramidal symptoms, are discussed later as possible side effects.

Cardiovascular effects include mild hypotension, orthostatic hypotension (caused by adrenolytic actions), and reflex tachycardia (caused by anticholinergic effects). Chlorpromazine may also increase coronary blood flow. Possible EKG changes include the following: (a) prolongation of the Q-T and P-R intervals, (b) blunting of the T wave, and (c) depression of the S-T segment (Baldessarini et al., 1988). Thioridazine in particular might cause high incidence of Q-T and T wave changes. It can also produce ventricular arrhythmias and sudden death.

Neuroleptics can have complex and unpredictable effects in the autonomic nervous system. They also may have complicated antihistaminic effects. Chlorpromazine can block the pressor effects of noradrenalin. It can also produce miosis (constriction of the pupil) in humans, whereas other neuroleptics (especially thioridazine) can cause cycloplegia (impairment of visual accommodation) and mydriasis (dilation of the pupil) via blockade of muscarinic receptors. Some neuroleptics can also cause constipation, dry mouth, blurred vision, difficulty urinating, and decreased sweating that are due to anticholinergic effects. Urinary retention is especially common in men with prostatism (Carlsson, 1978; Kito et al., 1984). Neuroleptics can decrease sex drive and impair aspects of sexual functioning in men and women. Impotence in men may appear rapidly but usually disappears with discontinuation of the drug. Thioridazine in particular is associated with delayed or retrograde ejaculation in men.

Neuroleptic use can result in increased prolactin secretion, which can cause secretion of milk and breast enlargement in both men and women. Chlorpromazine can reduce the level of gonadotropins (sex hormones) as well as estrogens and progestins. This particular action might contribute to amenorrhea (absence of menstruation) that is sometimes seen in women. Sexual disturbance with loss of libido may occur in men (Baldessarini et al., 1988; Creefe, Burt, & Snyder, 1978).

Breast milk from mothers taking chlorpromazine contains both the parent compound and some of its metabolites. The concentration of chlorpromazine in breast milk is in the same order of magnitude as that in plasma. Similar reports are available for other neuroleptics. This is not surprising in view of the high lipophilicity of these substances. In some cases pharmacological effects have been observed in neonates. Chlorpromazine and its metabolites can cross the placenta to the fetus (O'Donoghue, 1974).

Nonreproductive endocrinological functions can also be affected. Neuroleptics are known to inhibit the release of growth hormone, and chlorpromazine may reduce the secretion of other hormones in response to stress. Other endocrine effects include weight gain and increase in appetite, which can occur with all neuroleptics but are less common with molindone and haloperidol. Chlorpromazine may also impair glucose tolerance.

Although skin reactions may be observed shortly after administration of neuroleptics, they generally are resolved with time. Such reactions are reported in about 5% of patients receiving phenothiazines. If these side effects occur, it is usually within the first five weeks of drug use. Increased sensitivity of skin to the sun is also reported in some cases. Opacities of the cornea and lens of the eye can occur with prolonged use. Long-term neuroleptic use can result in abnormal concentrations of melanin (pigment) in the skin, although this phenomenon is rare. Jaundice is observed in less than 1% of cases. Neuroleptics usually have little effect on respiration, although vasomotor reflexes mediated by the brain stem might be depressed by low doses of chlorpromazine, which can cause a centrally mediated fall in blood pressure in some cases.

SIDE EFFECTS

In many respects neuroleptics are safe medications. Many have a high therapeutic index (the ratio of lethal to therapeutic doses), which enhances their safety. The medications have minimal abuse potential; generally, they do not result in psychological dependence. However, they can produce a number of side effects sufficiently serious to warrant limiting their use.

Effects on Behavior and Learning. Drowsiness is a commonly reported side effect. In some cases, sedative effects may be associated with impairments in learning, school performance, verbal expression, social interaction, and the acquisition of new adaptive behaviors. Tolerance to the sedating effects of neuroleptics is often observed.

Research studies on the effects of neuroleptics on learning have provided mixed results. Some researchers have found that neuroleptics can impair learning, especially when given in doses high enough to produce sedative effects. The drugs have been found to impair performance on IQ tests (Aman, 1984), suppress conditioned avoidance responses (Thompson, Hackenberg, & Schaal, 1991), and interfere with reinforcement procedures (see Aman & Singh, 1986). Other researchers have found that neuroleptics can facilitate discrimination learning (Anderson et al., 1984), language-based therapy programs (Campbell et al., 1978; Fisher, Kerbeshian, & Burd, 1986), and reinforcement-based learning programs (Ferster & DeMyer, 1961). Other researchers have found no effects on learning (Sandford & Nettlebeck, 1982). In their review of the literature, Aman and Singh (1986) concluded that the effects of neuroleptics on learning may depend on dosage, the characteristics of patients (e.g., some of the studies showing positive effects included participants with autism), and the specific neuroleptic agent (e.g., low-potency neuroleptics may impair learning more than high-potency compounds).

The effects of neuroleptics on adaptive behavior are undetermined. There are many anecdotal reports of people who showed improved adaptive behavior when problem behavior was reduced with neuroleptics. The improvements in adaptive behavior included social interactions, work and school performances, and self-help skills. However, the relatively few researchers who systematically evaluated adaptive behavior found that neuroleptics either have no effect on adaptive behavior or cause adaptive behavior to deteriorate (Baumeister, Todd, & Sevin, 1993).

Extrapyramidal Effects. Some of the most common and disturbing side effects of neuroleptics are movement disorders. As was previously noted, a major advantage of the new atypical neuroleptics—clozapine, sertindole, and risperidone—is that motor side effects may be reduced. Motor side effects occur because conventional neuroleptics affect the extrapyramidal motor system of the brain. Extrapyramidal side effects occur in approximately 15%-30% of all patients treated with neuroleptics (Appleton, 1981). High-potency neuroleptics are most likely to produce these effects. Extrapyramidal side effects include pseudo-Parkinsonism, akathisia, acute dystonias, and tardive dyskinesia.

Pseudo-Parkinsonism. Neuroleptics can produce motor side effects that are indistinguishable from the symptoms of idiopathic Parkinson's disease. These include tremors, rigidity (increased resistance to passive motion), bradykinesia (extreme slowness of movement), shuffling gait, and akinesia (muscle weakness or absence of voluntary movement). Tremor is greater at rest than during active movement and can involve a variety of muscle groups in the upper and lower extremities and head and mouth. Rhythmic motions of the thumb against the index finger (pill rolling) are characteristic. Tremor in conjunction with rigidity produces cogwheeling, a jerky or ratchety motion that occurs when the muscle is passively extended or flexed. In some cases, drooling may occur and facial expressions may be mask-like. The symptoms of pseudo-Parkinsonism may wax and wane over time and may increase with emotional stress and decrease with sleep or sedation. Extrapyramidal symptoms can generally be reduced by lowering dosage or adding anti-Parkinson drugs (e.g., diphenhydramine or benztropine). Sometimes a change in medication is necessary, for example, from a high-potency to a low-potency agent.

Akathisia. Akathisia is a syndrome characterized by motor restlessness and an inability to sit still. Patients often have difficulty concentrating, may engage in frequent pacing, and may appear generally agitated. Because the symptoms resemble anxiety or psychotic relapse, diagnosis is often missed, and neuroleptic dosage is sometimes increased inappropriately in an attempt to reduce agitation. Akathisia usually worsens with increasing dose. Symptoms may disappear with lower doses, and short-term treatment with benzodiazepines or beta-blockers may provide patients with

relief. Akathisia usually occurs within the first six to eight weeks of neuroleptic treatment.

Acute Dystonias. Dystonias are characterized by extreme muscle rigidity or muscle spasms, often affecting the tongue, eyes, neck, jaw, and back, and usually occur within the first 5 days of neuroleptic treatment (Ayd, 1961). Dystonia may be both frightening and painful for an affected individual, particularly in the case of nonverbal persons who may not understand why or how their muscles are contracting outside of their control. Younger patients and males are more likely to experience dystonias, which are rare in persons over 50. Immediate injections of diphenhydramine are usually prescribed once a diagnosis is made.

Tardive Dyskinesia. Tardive dyskinesia is a neurologic side effect caused by chronic exposure to neuroleptic drugs (usually at least a year). It consists of frequent, repetitive, involuntary movements of the lips, jaw, face, and, sometimes, trunk and limbs. The tongue may protrude involuntarily. Breathing may be affected in some cases. Slow, writhing athetoid movements are not uncommon. Symptoms usually decrease with sleep and sedation and may increase during stress (see American Psychiatric Association, 1992, for an overview).

It is generally reported that the risk of developing tardive dyskinesia increases with chronic neuroleptic use, with symptoms usually appearing within the first five years of neuroleptic use (Appleton, 1981). Tardive dyskinesia is more common with late onset psychosis and in women (Yassa, Camille, & Belzile, 1986). Many researchers have found that advancing age is the single greatest risk factor for developing this condition. Symptoms are also less likely to remit spontaneously in older patients.

In some patients, extrapyramidal symptoms are not evident until neuroleptics are withdrawn. In these cases, tardive dyskinesia is referred to as "withdrawal dyskinesia." In some cases, symptoms may remit with the reintroduction of the medication. However, there is generally no effective treatment. Drug-free periods (drug holidays) in the course of treatment may actually be accompanied by an increased risk of subsequent tardive dyskinesia for reasons as yet unclear (Yassa et al., 1986).

Tardive dyskinesia occurs in approximately 20%-30% of people with mental retardation who have been treated chronically with neuroleptics. Some data suggest a relationship between cumulative drug exposure and risk for developing tardive dyskinesia. However, such a relationship has been inconsistently found (Aman & Singh, 1985; Kane & Smith, 1982).

Withdrawal Symptoms

In addition to movement disorder, neuroleptic withdrawal can be followed by a number of other symptoms. Weight loss, insomnia, anticholinergic rebound (characterized by vomiting, diarrhea, and diaphoresis), and a broad spectrum of behavioral problems such as aggression, self-injury, hyperactivity, and noncompliance have been reported by various researchers (Gualtieri, 1993; Gualtieri, Quade, Hicks, Mayo, & Schroeder, 1984; Poindexter, 1994; Sovner, 1995). As was noted earlier, there is little evidence that neuroleptics cause physical or psychological dependence, and it is not at all uncommon for individuals without mental retardation to discontinue neuroleptic drugs abruptly without concern for adverse physical effects. Conversely, Gualtieri et al. (1984) reported that discontinuing a neuroleptic dose abruptly or in 25% decrements over four to eight weeks produced clinically significant symptoms in 44% of a sample of children and adolescents with and without mental retardation. In all cases, withdrawal dyskinesia, nondyskinetic symptoms, and behavioral deterioration remitted spontaneously within eight weeks. Abrupt withdrawal was not associated with any greater likelihood of withdrawal symptoms than was gradual taper. Only 29% of these subjects required resumption of neuroleptic medication, presumably because of the reemergence of disorders that existed before neuroleptic medication was begun rather than because of withdrawal symptoms. Neuroleptic withdrawal symptoms may be reduced by treatment with clonidine (Sovner, 1995).

Recognizing withdrawal symptoms in the context of mental retardation is an enormous challenge. If aggression or self-injury increases in the context of a neuroleptic taper, is this evidence of withdrawal or confirmation that the drug had been effective in attenuating these symptoms at a higher dose? If these symptoms spontaneously remit, does this indicate withdrawal or acquisition of better coping strategies by an individual having to deal with an urge that had been suppressed by medication? If an individual adds a new behavior to his or her repertoire in the context of a medication reduction, is this a withdrawal phenomenon or the expression of a new creativity emerging without the potential cognitive fetters of a neuroleptic drug? These questions cannot adequately be answered given our present state of knowledge. Drawing comparisons from the larger population of individuals treated with neuroleptics for mental disorder, significant nondyskinetic withdrawal symptoms are probably rare, as are tardive dyskinesia variants like tardive akathisia, tardive myoclonus, and tardive tics.

Neuroleptic Malignant Syndrome and Agranulocytosis

Neuroleptic malignant syndrome (NMS) is characterized by muscle rigidity, severe extrapyramidal symptoms, fever, autonomic instability (such as tachycardia or hypertension), altered consciousness, grand mal seizures, and, in some cases, coma. It is a rare phenomenon, probably occurring only in about 1% of patients receiving neuroleptics. However, it can be fatal if not identified and treated. Moreover, for reasons which are not clear, mortality rates for people with NMS have been reported to be twice as high in people with mental retardation than in the general population (i.e., 20% vs. 10%; see Boyd, 1993).

Agranulocytosis refers to a reduction in the formation of white blood cells. This is a serious condition in which the patient becomes susceptible to life-threatening infections. Agranulocytosis is associated most strongly with clozapine, occurring in 1% to 2% of patients on this medication. Weekly white blood cell counts must be performed for patients taking clozapine so that agranulocytosis can be detected early if it occurs.

DRUG INTERACTIONS

Additional medications may be prescribed to patients who are receiving neuroleptics to treat psychiatric disorders or to treat neuroleptic-induced side effects. Such concurrent use of medications may result in untoward drug interactions. For example, anticonvulsants such as carbamazepine and the barbiturates, which may be used to stabilize mood or control seizures in patients receiving neuroleptics, induce the liver enzymes that metabolize antipsychotics and can lower the level of neuroleptics in blood and tissue. The mood stabilizer lithium has been reported to be associated with a severe syndrome of neurotoxicity in some patients on neuroleptics. This reaction is rare and its basis unknown.

Antidepressants such as amitriptyline, imipramine, and fluoxetine are often used with neuroleptics for patients who have both depressive and psychotic symptoms. These two types of medications can inhibit each other's metabolism, resulting in greater blood concentrations, which have to be considered for possible toxicity. The side effects of neuroleptics can be enhanced by concurrent use of other drugs with similar effects; for example, sedation and anticholinergic side effects are enhanced with concurrent use of benzodiazepines and anti-

Parkinson agents that are used to treat the extrapyramidal side effects of neuroleptics. Because of their action at adrenergic receptors, neuroleptics can interact with antihypertensive agents, which may cause increased hypotension. Conversely, neuroleptics reduce the antihypertensive action of guanethidine. Neuroleptics may reduce the effects of anti-Parkinsonian drugs, such as L-dopa, and stimulants, such as amphetamine, can interfere with the antipsychotic action of neuroleptics. These and other drug interactions are shown in Table 9-3.

Table 9-3. Some Drug Interactions with Neuroleptics

Drug	Interaction
amphetamines	may reduce antipsychotic effect of neuroleptics
antacids	may decrease absorption of neuroleptics
anticholinergics	may inhibit response to neuroleptics; excess anticholinergic effects may occur
barbiturates	serum neuroleptic levels may be reduced
benzodiazepines	respiratory depression, stupor, hypotension may be increased
beta-adrenergic blockers	may increase hypotension; neuroleptics antagonize effects of bromocriptine
buspirone	may increase plasma neuroleptic levels
carbamazepine (Tegretol)	neuroleptics may increase carbamazepine levels
chlorphentermine	anorectic effect of chlorphentermine may be reduced
clonidine (Catapres)	hypotension and delirium have been reported
contraceptives	may increase likelihood of extrapyramidal symptoms
diazoxide	may interact to produce hyperglycemia
epinephrine	pressor effect of epinephrine may be reversed by neuroleptics
ethanol	sedative effects of alcohol are potentiated by neuroleptics
fluoxetine (Prozac)	may increase plasma neuroleptic levels
fluvoxamine (Luvox)	may increase likelihood of hyperprolactinemia from neuroleptics
guanethidine (Ismelin)	may inhibit antihypertensive response to guanethidine
H2-receptor antagonists	antihistaminic effect may be increased by neuroleptics
hydroxyzine (Atarax, Vistaril)	may reduce antipsychotic effect of neuroleptics
Kaopectate	may reduce serum neuroleptic levels
levodopa (Larodopa)	may inhibit anti-Parkinsonian effect of levodopa
lithium (Eskalith, Lithane, Lithobid)	may lower serum concentrations of both drugs
meperidine	may increase lethargy, orthostatic hypotension, respiratory depression
methyldopa (Aldomet)	may produce hypertension
monoamine oxidase inhibitors (MAOIs)	effect of MAIO may be reduced by neuroleptics
nonsteroidal anti-inflammatory drugs	may increase side effects of drowsiness, fatigue, confusion
oral anticoagulants	effects of oral anticoagulant may be reduced by neuroleptics
orphenadrine (Norflex, Norgesic)	may reduce plasma neuroleptic and increase anticholinergic side effects
phenylpropanolamine	sudden death
phenytoin (Dilantin)	metabolism of phenytoin may be inhibited by neuroleptics; may elicit or exacerbate extrapyramidal effects
smoking	may reduce plasma level of neuroleptic; may increase likelihood of akathisia
succinylcholine (Anectine)	may potentiate effect of succinylcholine
trazodone (Desyrel)	combined use may increase risk of liver toxicity
tricyclic antidepressants	sedative effect of antidepressants may be potentiated

CLINICAL INDICATIONS EXCLUSIVE OF MENTAL RETARDATION

Neuroleptics are among the most frequently prescribed psychotropic medications. The empirical literature is most supportive of their efficacy for treating people with schizophrenia or other psychotic disorders. Clinical reports have also indicated that neuroleptics suppress many of the symptoms associated with Tourette syndrome, attention-deficit disorder with hyperactivity, autism, and mood disorders.

Schizophrenia

Early researchers studying the effects of phenothiazine treatment with people with schizophrenia reported significant improvements in many symptoms including decreases in hallucinations, delusions, physical aggression, property destruction, agitation, irritability, and social withdrawal. Also reported were a decrease in the need to use seclusion and restraint as well as an increase in the number of people who left inpatient facilities subsequent to treatment. Since the 1960s, numerous researchers have examined the clinical efficacy of neuroleptics in the treatment of schizophrenia. Controlled group outcome studies have generally supported the use of neuroleptics over placebos; about three out of four persons with schizophrenia show a beneficial clinical response to treatment with neuroleptics, with considerable variability in symptom remission occurring across patients (National Institute of Mental Health, 1964; Poling, Gadow, & Cleary, 1991).

Although most patients show substantial gains, about 20% may show only minimal improvements. Patients often show greater changes in the positive symptoms of schizophrenia (e.g., motor agitation, hallucinations, and delusions) than in the negative symptoms (e.g., lack of reaction to the environment and blunted affect). Delusions, hallucinations, hostility, agitation, impulsive behavior, and disorganized thinking are often markedly reduced. Clinical gains have been reported in all subtypes of clinical schizophrenia, such as the paranoid subtype. In some cases, poor self-care, appetite, and insomnia also improve. Some withdrawn patients may become more alert and communicative. However, improvements in judgment and memory are less commonly reported.

Neuroleptic therapy, with or without psychotherapy, has been found to be more effective than electrocon-vulsive therapy or psychotherapy alone. Some patients show a better response to one neuroleptic than another. Separate trials of different antipsychotics for individual patients is a common psychiatric practice.

Some patients show dramatic decreases in agitation and hyperactivity after only a few days. Cooperation and socialization often improve prior to the remission of delusions and other symptoms related to thought disorder. Most improvements usually occur within the first six weeks of treatment (Appleton, 1981). In some cases, however, psychotic symptoms may actually be exacerbated.

Long-term pharmacotherapy for schizophrenia is usually required; many researchers conducting well-controlled studies found a significant difference in relapse rates for patients on maintenance doses of antipsychotics versus those on placebos (Davis, 1986). Prognosis is more favorable for patients with an abrupt onset of symptoms, onset precipitated by an external stressor, onset in midlife, and good premorbid social and occupational functioning. The efficacy of neuroleptics in treating childhood schizophrenia is less well-documented, although some researchers have reported positive results. However, many children experience untoward sedation and continue to show clinically significant impairments despite a statistically significant remission of symptoms.

Other Indications

A few studies of chlorpromazine and haloperidol indicated decreases in aggression in children with hyperactivity or conduct disorders (Campbell et al., 1984; Werry, Sprague, & Cohen, 1975). Neuroleptics have been used with mixed results to treat hyperactivity in children who do not have mental retardation. Several clinical trials with low-dose neuroleptic treatment indicated beneficial effects including decreased fidgetiness and increased attention and memory (Gittelman-Klein, Klein, Katz, Saraf, & Pollack, 1976). However, stimulant medication (e.g., methylphenidate) is generally considered to be superior to low-dose neuroleptics for decreasing hyperactivity and distractibility and increasing attention; detrimental effects on attention and learning are often reported with higher doses of neuroleptics.

Because of their rapid calming effects, neuroleptics are occasionally used in combination with lithium as an initial treatment for mania in people with bipolar disorder. People with mood disorders that have psychotic features may also receive neuroleptics. Neuroleptics are also used in some cases as a pre-anesthetic to decrease patients' apprehension over impending surgery. Low doses of high-potency neuroleptics, such as haloperidol, are often used to treat elderly people with organic mental syndromes and disorders. High-potency neuroleptics are also the treatment of choice for amphetamine psychoses. Stuttering and intractable hiccups have also been treated with neuroleptics.

INDICATIONS IN MENTAL RETARDATION

Labeled Indications

Neuroleptic medications may be therapeutically useful for a variety of psychiatric disorders irrespective of the concurrent presence of mental retardation. These labeled indications have been approved by the U. S. Food and Drug Administration (FDA) based on controlled studies that demonstrated significant benefit for a given medication in the treatment of specific symptoms or illnesses. However, virtually all of the studies on which FDA approval of neuroleptic drugs is based specifically excluded people with mental retardation. The package inserts for several neuroleptic drugs contain specific disclaimers denoting the absence of research with people with mental retardation.

The labeled indications for neuroleptics are shown in Table 9-4. These indications include the treatment of psychotic disorders, particularly schizophrenia, as well as the attenuation of symptoms of anxiety, hyperactivity, and conduct disorders, and some severe behavior problems in children, manifested by combative and explosive behavior. As regards use in the treatment of anxiety, hyperactivity, and combative behavior, many newer drugs with fewer associated side effects have been introduced since these particular indications were approved, so that the neuroleptics are second- and third-line interventions at best. The package insert for haloperidol, for example, specifically cautions against the use of this agent prior to exploring alternatives (psychotherapy or other medications) for hyperactivity or combative behavior. Additionally, the diagnostic classification of particular psychiatric disorders has changed significantly since the original studies that supported the use of neuroleptics for personality disorders were conducted, calling into question the rationale for prescribing neuroleptics for the treatment of these disorders as defined in current psychiatric nosology.

An additional complication regarding the use of neuroleptics with people with dual diagnoses of psychiatric illnesses and mental retardation derives from the problem of diagnostic precision. The diagnosis of schizophrenia denotes the presence of a specific constellation of symptoms and signs highlighted by impairment in reality testing, or by psychosis, as exemplified by hallucinations and delusions. Although a diagnosis of schizophrenia presupposes the presence of psychosis, the diagnosis of psychosis does not equate with schizophrenia. Individuals with bipolar disorders, or individuals with particular drug intoxications, for example, may have psychoses without manifesting schizophrenia.

There is no question that schizophrenia can be diagnosed in some individuals with mental retardation (Reid, 1989; Turner, 1989). When a diagnosis of schizophrenia can be made with confidence, there is a general consensus that neuroleptics are indicated. However, some authorities have argued that true psychosis can be diagnosed only in people who can express delusional thought and who can acknowledge hallucinations, thus excluding virtually all individuals with severe and profound mental retardation (Reid, 1983). Other authorities argue that schizophrenia can be diagnosed in this group (e.g., Werry & Taylor, 1994). The DSM-IV (American Psychiatric Association, 1994) requires the presence of two or more of the following symptoms for a diagnosis of schizophrenia: delusions, hallucinations, disorganized speech, disorganized or catatonic behavior, and negative symptoms. Three of these symptoms—hallucinations, disorganized or catatonic behavior, and negative symptoms—are manifested in overt behavior and can, in theory, be diagnosed in nonverbal people. For example, some individuals display presumptive evidence of response to hallucinations (e.g., striking out at or talking to empty space) or adopt catatonic postures that appear to be psychotic in origin. In these cases, the presence of psychosis may be considered.

Haloperidol is the treatment of choice for Tourette syndrome. The results of most studies indicate that approximately 80% of people with Tourette show some initial response (Poling et al., 1991; Shapiro, Shapiro, & Wayne, 1973). Some researchers examining the effects of pimozide on tic disorders have found it to be less sedating than haloperidol and only slightly less effective (Shapiro et al., 1989).

Unlabeled Indications

Unlabeled indications are those not listed on the FDA-approved label, but they are "based on rational scientif-

Table 9-4. FDA Labeled Indications for Neuroleptics

Indication	Drug
Psychosis	
manifestations of psychotic disorders	chlorpromazine (Thorazine) trifluoperazine HCl (Stelazine) thiothixene (Navane) chlorprothixene (Taractan) haloperidol (Haldol) loxapine (Loxitame) molindone (Moban) fluphenazine (Prolixin) risperidone (Risperdal) thioridazine (Mellaril) mesoridazine (Serentil)
treatment of schizophrenia	
severely ill schizophrenic patients who fail to respond adequately to standard antipsychotic drug treatment	clozapine (Clozaril)
manic type of manic illness	chlorpromazine (Thorazine)
Motor and Vocal Tics	
tics and vocal utterances of Tourette disorder in children and adults	haloperidol (Haldol) pimozide (Orap)
Combative, Explosive Behavior	
severe behavioral problems in children marked by combativeness or explosive hyperexcitable behavior out of proportion to immediate provocation	chlorpromazine (Thorazine) haloperidol (Haldol) thioridazine (Mellaril)
Hyperactivity	
short-term treatment of hyperactive children who show excessive motor activity with accompanying conduct disorders consisting of some or all of the following symptoms: difficulty sustaining attention, aggressivity, mood lability, and poor frustration tolerance	chlorpromazine (Thorazine) haloperidol (Haldol) thioridazine (Mellaril)
Anxiety	
pre-operative relief of restlessness and apprehension	chlorpromazine (Thorazine)
short-term treatment of generalized non-psychotic anxiety	trifluoperazine HCl (Stelazine) prochlorperazine (Compazine) thioridazine (Mellaril)
short-term treatment of moderate to marked depression with varying degrees of anxiety in adults	
agitation, anxiety, depressed mood, tension, sleep disturbances, and fears in geriatric patients	thioridazine (Mellaril)
anxiety, tension, depression, nausea, and vomiting in acute and chronic alcoholics; anxiety and tension associated with personality disorders	mesoridazine (Serentil)
Mental Retardation	
hyperactivity and uncooperativeness associated with mental deficiency and chronic brain syndrome	mesoridazine (Serentil)
specific disclaimer regarding use in mental retardation	mesoridazine (Serentil) trifluoperazine HCl (Stelazine) perphenazine (Trilafon) prochlorperazine (Compazine) thiothixene (Navane) chlorprothixene (Taractan) fluphenazine (Prolixin)
Medical Indications	
acute, intermittent porphyria	chlorpromazine (Thorazine)
adjunct in the treatment of tetanus	chlorpromazine (Thorazine)
intractable hiccups	chlorpromazine (Thorazine)
control of nausea and vomiting	chlorpromazine (Thorazine) perphenazine (Trilafon)

ic theory, reliable medical opinion, or controlled clinical studies" (American Medical Association, 1986, p. 9). Neuroleptics are most frequently prescribed to people with mental retardation for unlabeled indications— particularly for reduction of problem behaviors that do not fall neatly into any diagnostic category. Behavior problems most frequently treated with neuroleptics are aggression, self-injury, and hyperactivity. Thioridazine is the drug most frequently used for this purpose, followed by haloperidol, chlorpromazine, and a variety of other medications. Mesoridazine, the only neuroleptic for which management of problem behavior in people with mental retardation is a labeled indication, is used infrequently. In the empirical literature there is no relationship between the medication used and the type of behavior problem targeted for reduction, nor is there any compelling evidence that one neuroleptic is more effective than another.

The use of neuroleptics to control problem behavior is consistent with their well-established efficacy in reducing psychomotor agitation and aggression in other clinical populations. The effects of neuroleptics on problem behavior in people with mental retardation have been examined in numerous studies. These studies are summarized in Tables 9-5 through 9-8. It is difficult to draw firm conclusions from this literature because much of the research is flawed methodologically (see Baumeister et al., 1993). The evidence for efficacy is strongest with respect to stereotyped behavior. The majority of studies summarized in Table 9-6 showed that neuroleptics suppressed stereotyped behavior, and some of these studies are methodologically sound. The evidence pertaining to other problem behaviors such as aggression, destructiveness, agitation, and self-injury is less compelling. Nevertheless, the majority of studies have indicated that neuroleptics can reduce these behaviors as well. Thus, the drugs appear to be nonselective in that they often suppress a broad range of behaviors (Baumeister et al.,

Table 9-5. Neuroleptics and Self-Injurious Behavior[a]

Reference	IQ	N	Drug	Method Sound[b]	Effect
Abbott et al. (1965)	0-90	141	thioridazine	no	↓
Aman & White (1988)	0-50	11	thioridazine	yes	↓
Burns (1980)	?	1	droperidol	no	↓
Connolly (1968)	≤50	132	thioridazine	no	59%↓, 10%↑,
Durand (1982)	< 20	1	haloperidol	no	NE
Goldstein et al. (1985)	< 50	1	fluphenazine	yes	↓
Grabowski (1973b)	< 35	2	haloperidol	no	↓
Gualtieri & Schroeder (1989)	< 35	15	fluphenazine	no	73%↓, 27%NE
Haegeman & Duyck (1978)	<36	19?	pipamperone	no	↓
Kaplan (1969)	< 50	8	thioridazine	no	25%↓, 75%NE
Le Vann (1969)	?	54?	haloperidol	no	↓
Le Vann (1959)	< 70	33?	trifluoperazine	no	↓
Llorente (1969)	50% < 50	65?	thioridazine	no	↓
Lowther (1960)	0 - 70	57?	trifluoperazine	no	↓
McDougle et al. (1995)	< 35	1	risperidone	no	↓
Mikkelsen (1986)	< 35	6	haloperidol	no	100%↓
Pregelj & Barkauskas (1967)	?	98	thioridazine	no	91%↓
Rubin & Langa(1995)	35 - 70	4	clozapine	no	100%
Singh & Aman (1981)	<30	19	thioridazine	yes	NE
Sprogis et al. (1957)	?	77?	chlorpromazine	no	↓
Wolfson (1957)	<20	1	chlorpromazine	no	↓

a Adapted from A.A. Baumeister, M.E. Todd, & J.A. Sevin (1993), "Efficacy and specificity of pharmacological therapies for behavioral disorders in persons with mental retardation," *Clinical Neuropharmacology, 16*, 217-294. Copyright 1993 by Raven Press. Reprinted with permission.

b Methodologically sound means that the study employed either (1) an experimental design in which the subjects were randomly assigned to concurrently run drug or placebo groups or (b) quasiexperimental within-subject designs in which at least one reversal of the drug effect was demonstrated.

Table 9-6. Neuroleptics and Stereotyped Behavior[a]

Reference	Dx	N	Drug	Method Sound[b]	Effect
Aman et al. (1984)	MR (IQ < 20)	4	chlorpromazine	yes	↓
Aman et al. (1989)	MR (IQ 0-50)	20?	haloperidol	yes	↓
Anderson et al. (1984)	MR (IQ < 70)	40?	haloperidol	yes	↓
Campbell et al. (1982)	Autism	33	haloperidol	yes	↓
Campbell et al. (1978)	Autism	40	haloperidol	yes	↓
	<4.5 yrs.				NE
	≥4.5 yrs.				↓
Cohen et al. (1980)	Autism	10	haloperidol	yes	↓
Davis et al. (1969)	MR (IQ <35)	9	thioridazine	no	↓
Heistad et al. (1982)	MR	100	thioridazine	yes	↓
Heistad et al. (1979)	?	60	thioridazine	yes	↓
Hollis (1968)	MR (IQ < 35)	1	chlorpromazine	no	↓
Hollis & St. Omer (1972)	?	2	chlorpromazine	no	↓
Lewis et al. (1986)	?	6	thioridazine	yes	33%↑, 17%↓, 50%NE
Singh & Aman (1981)	IQ≤30	19	thioridazine	yes	↓
Singh et al. (1993)	MR (IQ < 20)	3	thioridazine	yes	↓

a Adapted from A.A. Baumeister, M.E. Todd, & J.A. Sevin (1993), "Efficacy and specificity of pharmacological therapies for behavioral disorders in persons with mental retardation," *Clinical Neuropharmacology*, 16, 217-294. Copyright 1993 by Raven Press. Reprinted with permission.
b Methodologically sound means that the study employed either (1) an experimental design in which the subjects were randomly assigned to concurrently run drug or placebo groups or (b) quasiexperimental within-subject designs in which at least one reversal of the drug effect was demonstrated.

Table 9-7. Neuroleptics and Aggression[a]

Reference	MR Level	N	Drug	Method Sound[b]	Effect
Connolly (1968)	≤50	316	thioridazine	no	52%↓, 12%↑, 36%NE
Elie et al. (1980)	x =33	51	thioridazine	yes	↑
Haegeman & Duyck (1978)	IQ<36	19?	pipamperone	no	↓
LeVann (1959)	0 - 70	20	trifluoperazine	no	↓
LeVann (1971)	50- 70	7	haloperidol	no	86%↓, 0%↑, 14%NE
		10	chlorpromazine		20%↓, 20%↑, 60%NE
Llorente (1969)	0 - 70	65?	thioridazine	no	↓
Lowther (1960)	0 - 70	57?	trifluoperazine	no	↓
Lynch et al. (1985)	?	28?	pipothiazine	yes	↓
McConahey et al. (1976)	13-59	22	chlorpromazine	yes	NE
McDougle et al. (1995)	20-70	3	risperidone	no	100%↓
Pregelj & Barkauskas (1967)	?	92	thioridazine	no	↓
Rubin & Langa (1995)	50-70	6	clozapine	no	100%↓
Rudy et al. (1958)	0-70	25	chlorpromazine	no	88%↓
		23	promazine	no	
Sprogis et al. (1957)	?	77?	chlorpromazine	no	↓
Ucer & Kreger (1969)	40-70	25	haloperidol	no	52%↓, 16%↑, 32%NE
		21	thioridazine		14%↓, 5%↑, 81% NE

a Adapted from A.A. Baumeister, M.E. Todd, & J.A. Sevin (1993), "Efficacy and specificity of pharmacological therapies for behavioral disorders in persons with mental retardation," *Clinical Neuropharmacology*, 16, 217-294. Copyright 1993 by Raven Press. Reprinted with permission.
b Methodologically sound means that the study employed either (1) an experimental design in which the subjects were randomly assigned to concurrently run drug or placebo groups or (b) quasiexperimental within-subject designs in which at least one reversal of the drug effect was demonstrated.

Table 9-8. Neuroleptics and Hyperactivity[a]

Reference	Dx	N	Drug	Method Sound[b]	Effect
Abbott et al. (1965)	MR (IQ 0-90)	141	thioridazine	no	↓
Alexandris & Lundell (1968)	MR (IQ 55-86)	21	thioridazine	yes	↓
Aman et al. (1991)	ADHD (IQ < 46)	13	thioridazine	yes	23%↓
	ADHD (IQ 46-90)	17			29%↓
Aman & White (1988)	MR (IQ < 50)	11	thioridazine	yes	↓
Anderson et al. (1984)	Autism	40?	haloperidol	yes	↓
Campbell et al. (1982)	Autism	33	haloperidol	yes	↓
Campbell et al. (1978)	Autism	40?	haloperidol	yes	NE
Connolly (1968)	MR (IQ≤50)	396	thioridazine	no	61%↓,11%↑, 28%NE
Grabowski (1973a)	MR (IQ < 36)	25	haloperidol	no	96%↓, 4%↑
Haegeman & Duyck (1978)	MR (IQ < 36)	19?	pipamperone	no	↓
Kaplan (1969)	MR (IQ 20-50)	31	thioridazine	no	58%↓, 0%↑,42%NE
LeVann (1959)	MR (IQ < 70)	14	trifluoperazine	no	79%↓,21%NE
LeVann (1969)	?	54?	haloperidol	no	↓
LeVann (1970)	?	59?	thioridazine	yes	↓
			chlorprothixene		↓
LeVann (1971)	MR (IQ 35 -70)	13	haloperidol	no	100%↓
		12	chlorpromazine		33%↓, 8%↑, 58%NE
Llorente (1969)	MR (IQ < 70)	65?	thioridazine	no	↓
Lowther (1960)	MR (IQ < 70)	57?	trifluoperazine	no	?↓
Pregelj & Barkauskas (1967)	?	104	thioridazine	no	79%↓
Schulman & Clarinada (1964)	MR	6	promazine	yes	NE
Singh & Aman (1981)	MR (IQ≤30)	19?	thioridazine	yes	↓
Ucer & Kreger (1969)	MR (IQ 36-70)	25	haloperidol	no	52%↓, 20%↑, 28%NE
		20	thioridazine		10%↓, 10%↑, 80%NE
Young (1970)	?	60	fluphenazine	no	↓

a Adapted from A.A. Baumeister, M.E. Todd, & J.A. Sevin (1993), "Efficacy and specificity of pharmacological therapies for behavioral disorders in persons with mental retardation," Clinical Neuropharmacology, 16, 217-294. Copyright 1993 by Raven Press. Reprinted with permission.
b Methodologically sound means that the study employed either (1) an experimental design in which the subjects were randomly assigned to concurrently run drug or placebo groups or (b) quasiexperimental within-subject designs in which at least one reversal of the drug effect was demonstrated.

1993). However, there is great individual variation in response to these medications. Many people show little or no improvement, and occasionally problem behavior is actually exacerbated. At this time there is no way to predict who will respond and who will not.

Typically, in those studies indicating beneficial effects on problem behavior, average daily doses ranging from 50 to 250 mg chlorpromazine equivalents were used (see Baumeister et al., 1993). In studies indicating effects on stereotyped behavior, average doses (approximately 100 mg/day) tended to be lower than those used in studies indicating effects on other behaviors (approximately 200 mg/day). This may indicate greater potency with respect to reducing stereotypy. However, in rare studies in which doses were directly compared, low doses (50–115 mg/day) have been found to be as effective as higher doses (175–230 mg/day) in reducing hyperactivity and aggression (e.g., Singh & Aman, 1981). Singh and Aman (1981) presented data suggesting that dose titration based on global impressions of behavior change provided to physicians by direct-care staff resulted in the use of doses that were higher than necessary. This finding points to the importance of basing medication decisions on direct objective behavioral measures.

Several researchers have examined the efficacy of neuroleptics in treating people with autism. Trials of low-potency neuroleptics, such as chlorpromazine, have generally yielded poor results: Few favorable effects and frequent negative side effects such as sedation are typically reported (Campbell, Perry, Small, & Green, 1987). However, the results of studies of high-potency neuroleptics have been more positive. Decreases in social withdrawal, hyperactivity, aggressiveness, stereotypic behavior, and inappropriate affect have been reported for children with autism following treatment with haloperidol (Anderson et al., 1984; Campbell et al., 1978, 1993). Moreover, the beneficial effects of haloperidol in this group occur at conservative doses that minimize side effects. Haloperidol is useful for reducing some problem behaviors in children with autism. It does not correct the core problem in this disorder.

CONCLUSIONS

Neuroleptics are prescribed to people with mental retardation for both labeled and unlabeled indications. Although the principal labeled indication is psychosis, particularly schizophrenia, this use of neuroleptics accounts for only a small percentage of the prescriptions written for people with mental retardation. Instead, the large majority of these people receive neuroleptics for unlabeled indications, for the purpose of controlling aberrant behavior, which in many instances is not part of any well-defined psychiatric syndrome.

Any use of neuroleptics is of concern because of their potential for producing untoward effects, which may include permanent and debilitating movement disorders, life-threatening toxic reactions, and interference with adaptive behavior and cognitive functioning. In healthy people without mental retardation, neuroleptics can produce very unpleasant subjective effects. These effects include inner restlessness combined with external inhibition of movement, anxiety, dejection, and slowed, confused thought (Spiegel, 1989; Swazey, 1974). It is reasonable to assume that such effects would also occur in people with mental retardation, although they may be difficult to detect in nonverbal individuals who have difficulty expressing their internal psychological states.

The efficacy of neuroleptics in treating schizophrenia is well established. There is consensus among professionals that treatment with neuroleptics is indicated for people with mental retardation who display unambiguous symptoms of schizophrenia. Moreover, because schizophrenia is typically a chronic disease, many patients require long-term, if not lifelong, treatment with neuroleptics. However, professionals disagree about the use of neuroleptics with nonverbal patients. Some believe that schizophrenia cannot be diagnosed in people who are unable to express themselves verbally or who are unable to acknowledge hallucinations and delusions.

Others feel that the diagnosis can be made in this group on the basis of nonverbal behavioral symptoms. Still others are willing to concede that trials of neuroleptics are warranted for the treatment of psychotic symptoms even when true schizophrenia cannot be diagnosed.

Professional disagreement exists regarding the use of neuroleptics to reduce aberrant behavior in people with mental retardation. The evidence regarding efficacy for such therapy is weak. Effects on the behavior of people with mental retardation are highly variable and unpredictable. There is no neuroleptic with effects specific to a particular behavior, and neuroleptics may exert nonspecific effects on behavior or cognition generally. We recommend that long-term maintenance therapy with neuroleptics be utilized only after due consideration of other pharmacological and behavioral treatments. When maintenance therapy is necessary, the lowest effective dose should be used to minimize the risk of adverse reactions. Additionally, treatment response and side effects should be monitored systematically using objective, reliable, and valid measures, and the need for continuing therapy should be evaluated on a regular basis.

When appraising ongoing need for neuroleptics, clinicians should review the person's psychiatric diagnosis, and they should answer the following questions. Is this medication effective? Is the patient's habilitative function optimized? Is this the best that can be expected from any drug trial? Are the risks of continued drug exposure still outweighed by the benefits of treatment and the risks of no treatment? If there is some ambiguity, medication effectiveness should be tested, either by significant increases or decreases in dosage. Clinicians should be prepared to use alternatives in the absence of convincing evidence of medication responsiveness.

There are minimal data regarding the optimal rate for discontinuation of neuroleptics. Some clinicians will abruptly stop a drug, and others will extend a taper over several months to years. Given that detoxification and withdrawal from well-known addictive drugs is usually accomplished over the course of one or two months, it is unlikely that neuroleptic withdrawal strategies need be stretched out over years, and such continued drug administration in the absence of necessity merely exposes an individual to risks without benefit. Generally, neuroleptics should not be terminated abruptly. Clinicians should be prepared to modify the rate of neuroleptic withdrawal flexibly so as to minimize unnecessary drug exposure and to limit the severity or extent of withdrawal-emergent symptoms should they appear.

REFERENCES

Abbott, P., Blake, A., & Vincze, L. (1965). Treatment of mentally retarded with thioridazine. *Diseases of the Nervous System, 26,* 583–585.

Alexandris, A., & Lundell, F.W. (1968). Effect of thioridazine, amphetamine and placebo on the hyperkinetic syndrome and cognitive area in mentally deficient children. *Canadian Medical Association Journal, 98,* 92–96.

Aman, M.G. (1984). Drugs and learning in mentally retarded persons. In G.D. Burrows & J.S. Werry (Eds.), *Advances in human psychopharmacology.* (Vol. III). Greenwich, Conn.: JAI Press.

Aman, M.G., Marks, R.E., Turbott, S.H., Wilsher, C.P., & Merry, S.N. (1991). Clinical effects of methylphenidate and thioridazine in intellectually subaverage children. *Journal of the American Academy of Child and Adolescent Psychiatry, 30,* 246–256.

Aman, M.G., & Singh, N.N. (1985). Dyskinetic symptoms in profoundly retarded residents following neuroleptic withdrawal and during methylphenidate treatment. *Journal of Mental Deficiency Research, 29,* 187–195.

Aman, M.G., & Singh, N.N. (1986). A critical appraisal of recent drug research in mental retardation: The Coldwater studies. *Journal of Mental Deficiency Research, 30,* 203–216.

Aman, M.G., Teehan, C.J., White, A.J., Turbott, S.H., & Vaithianathan, C. (1989). Haloperidol treatment with chronically medicated residents: Dose effects on clinical behavior and reinforcement contingencies. *American Journal on Mental Retardation, 93,* 452–60.

Aman, M.G., & White, A.J. (1988). Thioridazine dose effects with reference to stereotypic behavior in mentally retarded residents. *Journal of Autism and Developmental Disorders, 18,* 355–366.

Aman, M.G., White, A.J., & Field, C. (1984). Chlorpromazine effects on stereotypic and conditioned behaviour of severely retarded patients– a pilot study. *Journal of Mental Deficiency Research, 28,* 253–260.

American Medical Association. (1986). *Drug evaluations* (6th ed.). Philadelphia: W.B. Saunders Company.

American Psychiatric Association. (1992). *Tardive dyskinesia: A task force report of the American Psychiatric Association.* Washington, DC: Author.

American Psychiatric Association. (1994). *Diagnostic and statistical manual of mental disorders* (4th ed.). Washington, DC: Author.

Anderson, L.T., Campbell, M., Grega, D.M., Perry, R., Small, A.M., & Green, W. H. (1984). Haloperidol in the treatment of infantile autism: Effects on learning and behavioral symptoms. *American Journal of Psychiatry, 141,* 1195–1202.

Appleton, W.S. (1981). *Practical clinical psychopharmacology* (3rd ed.). Baltimore, MD: Williams & Wilkins.

Ayd, F.J. (1961). A survey of drug-induced extrapyramidal reactions. *Journal of the American Medical Association, 175,* 1054–1060.

Baldessarini, R.J. (1990). Drugs and the treatment of psychiatric disorders. In A.G. Gilman, T.W. Rall, A.S. Nies, & P. Taylor (Eds.), *Goodman and Gilman's the pharmacological basis of therapeutics* (8th ed., pp. 383–435). New York: Pergamon Press.

Baldessarini, R.J., Coyne, B.M., & Teicher, M.H. (1988). Significance of neuroleptic dose and plasma levels in the pharmacological treatment of psychosis. *Archives of General Psychiatry, 45,* 79–91.

Balant-Gorgia, A.E., Balant, L.P., & Andreoli, A. (1993). Pharmacokinetic optimization of the treatment of psychosis, *Clinical Pharmacokinetics, 25,* 217–236.

Baumeister, A.A., Todd, M.E., & Sevin, J.A. (1993). Efficacy and specificity of pharmacological therapies for behavioral disorders in persons with mental retardation. *Clinical Neuropharmacology, 16,* 271–294.

Bowers, B. (1974). Thioridazine: Central dopamine turnover and clinical effects of anti-psychotic drugs. *Clinical Pharmacology and Therapeutics, 17,* 73–78.

Boyd, R.D. (1993). Neuroleptic malignant syndrome and mental retardation: Review and analysis of 29 cases. *American Journal on Mental Retardation, 98,* 143–155.

Burns, M.E. (1980). Droperidol in the management of hyperactivity, self-mutilation and aggression in mentally handicapped patients. *Journal of Internal Medicine Research, 8,* 31–33.

Campbell, M., Anderson, L.T., Meier, M., Cohen, I.L., Small, A. M., Samit, C., & Sachar, E.J. (1978). A comparison of haloperidol and behavior therapy and their interaction in autistic children. *Journal of the American Academy of Child and Adolescent Psychiatry, 17,* 640–655.

Campbell, M., Anderson, L.T., Small, A.M., Perry, R., Green, W.H., & Caplan, R. (1982). The effects of haloperidol on learning and behavior in autistic children. *Journal of Autism and Developmental Disorders, 12,* 167–175.

Campbell, M., Gonzalez, N.M., Ernst, M., Silva, R., & Werry, J.S. (1993). Antipsychotics (neuroleptics). In J.S. Werry & M.G. Aman (Eds.), *Practitioner's guide to psychoactive drugs for children and adolescents* (pp. 269–296). New York: Plenum.

Campbell, M. Perry, R., Small, A.M., & Green, W.H. (1987). Overview of drug treatment in autism. In E. Schopler & E. Mesibov (Eds.), *Neurobiological issues in autism.* New York: Plenum Press.

Campbell, M., Small, A.M., Green, W. H.,

Jennings, S.J., Perry, R., Bennett, W.G., & Anderson, L. (1984). Behavioral efficacy of haloperidol and lithium carbonate: A comparison in hospitalized aggressive children with conduct disorder. *Archives of General Psychiatry, 41,* 650–656.

Carlsson, A. (1978). Mechanism of action of neuroleptic drugs. In M.A. Lipton, A. DiMascio, & K.L. Killam (Eds.), *Psychopharmacology: A generation of progress* (pp. 1057–1070). New York: Robin Press.

Cohen, I.L., Campbell, M., Posner, D., Small, A.M., Triebel, D., & Anderson, L.T. (1980). Behavioral effects of haloperidol in young autistic children. *Journal of the American Academy of Child Psychiatry, 19,* 665–677.

Connolly, J.R. (1968). Behavior disorders in mental retardates. *Pennsylvania Medicine, 71,* 67–69.

Creefe, I., Burt, B., & Snyder, S.H. (1978). Biochemical actions of neuroleptic drugs: Progress on dopamine receptors. In L.L. Iverson, F.D. Iverson, & S.H. Snyder (Eds.), *Handbook of psychopharmacology* (Vol. 10, pp. 37–89). New York: Plenum Press

Davis, J. (1986). Maintenance therapy and the natural course of schizophrenia. *Journal of Clinical Psychiatry, 46,* 18–21.

Davis, J.M., Janicak, P.G., Preskorn, S., & Ayd, F.J. (1994). Advances in the pharmacotherapy of psychotic disorders. In P.G. Janicak (Ed.), *Principles and practice of psychopharmacotherapy: Update* (Vol. 1, No. 1). Baltimore, MD: Williams & Wilkins.

Davis, K.V., Sprague, R.L., & Werry, J.S. (1969). Stereotyped behavior and activity level in severe retardates: The effect of drugs. *American Journal of Mental Deficiency, 76,* 397–407.

De Coster (1988). *Effects of a single oral dose administration of risperidone on plasma prolactin, growth hormone, and cortisol levels in healthy male volunteers* (Clin. Res. Rep. No. R64766/7). Beerse, Belgium: Janssen Research Foundation.

Durand, V.M. (1982). A behavioral/pharmacological intervention for the treatment of severe self-injurious behavior. *Journal of Autism and Developmental Disorders, 12,* 243–251.

Elie, R., Langlois, Y., Cooper, S.F., Gravel, G., & Albert, J. (1980). Comparison of SCH-12679 and thioridazine in aggressive mental retardates. *Canadian Journal of Psychiatry, 25,* 484–491.

Ferster, C.B., & DeMyer, M.K. (1961). Increased performances of an autistic child with prochlorperazine administration. *Journal of the Experimental Analysis of Behavior, 4,* 84.

Fisher, W., Kerbeshian, J., & Burd, L. (1986). A treatable language disorder: Pharmacological treatment of pervasive developmental disorder. *Developmental and Behavioral Pediatrics, 7,* 73–76.

Forsman, A., & Ohman, R. (1977). Applied pharmacokinetics of haloperidol in man. *Current Therapeutic Research, 21*, 396.

Gittelman-Klein, R., Klein, D.F., Katz, S., Saraf, K., & Pollack, E. (1976). Comparative effects of methylphenidate and thioridazine in hyperkinetic children. *Archives of General Psychiatry, 33*, 1217–1231.

Goldstein, M., Anderson, L.T., Reuben, R., & Dancis, J. (1985). Self-mutilation in Lesch-Nyhan disease is caused by dopaminergic denervation. *Lancet, 1*, 338–339.

Grabowski, S.W. (1973). Haloperidol for control of severe emotional reactions in mentally retarded patients. *Diseases of the Nervous System, 34*, 315–317.

Grabowski, S.W. (1973). Safety and effectiveness of haloperidol for mentally retarded behaviorally disordered and hyperkinetic patients. *Current Therapeutic Research, 15*, 856–861.

Gualtieri, C.T. (1993). The problem of tardive akathisia. *Brain and Cognition, 23*, 102–109.

Gualtieri, C.T., Quade, D., Hicks, R.E., Mayo, J.P., & Schroeder, S.R. (1984). Tardive dyskinesia and other clinical consequences of neuroleptic treatment in children and adolescents. *American Journal of Psychiatry, 141*, 20–23.

Gualtieri, C.T., & Schroeder, S.R. (1989). Pharmacotherapy for self-injurious behavior: Preliminary tests of the D-1 hypothesis. *Psychopharmacology Bulletin, 25*, 364–371.

Haegeman, J., & Duyck, F. (1978). A retrospective evaluation of pipamperone (Dipiperon) in the treatment of behavioural deviations in the severely mentally handicapped. *Acta Psychiatry Belg, 78*, 392–398.

Heistad, G.T., & Zimmermann, R.L. (1979). Double-blind assessment of mellaril in a mentally retarded population using detailed evaluations. *Psychopharmacological Bulletin, 15*, 86–88.

Heistad, G.T., Zimmermann, R.L., & Doebler, M.I. (1982). Long-term usefulness of thioridazine for institutionalized mentally retarded patients. *American Journal of Mental Deficiency, 87*, 243–251.

Hollis, J.H. (1968). Chlorpromazine: Direct measurement of differential behavioral effect. *Science, 159*, 1487–1489.

Hollis, J.H., & St. Omer, V.V. (1972). Direct measurement of psychopharmacologic response: Effects of chlorpromazine on motor behavior of retarded children. *American Journal of Mental Deficiency, 76*, 397–407.

James, D.H. (1986). Neuroleptics and epilepsy in mentally handicapped patients. *Journal of Mental Deficiency Research, 30*, 185–189.

Jann, M.W., Grinsley, S.R., Gray, E.C., & Chang, W. (1993). Pharmacokinetics and pharmacodynamics of clozapine. *Clinical Pharmacokinetics, 24*, 161–176.

Kane, J.M., & Smith, J.M. (1982). Tardive dyskinesia: Prevalence and risk factors, 1959–1979. *Archives of General Psychiatry, 39*, 473–481.

Kaplan, S. (1969). Double blind study at state institution using thiorodazine in program simulating outpatient clinic practice. *Pennsylvania Psychiatry Quarterly, 9*, 24–34.

Kito, F., Sejawa, T., Kuriyama, K., Yamamura, H.I., & Altman, R.W. (Eds.). (1984). *Neurotransmitter receptors.* New York: Plenum Press.

LeVann, L.J. (1959). Trifluoperazine dihydrochloride: An effective tranquilizing agent for behavioral abnormalities in defective children. *Canadian Medical Association Journal, 80*, 123–124.

LeVann, L.J. (1969). Haloperidol in the treatment of behavioural disorders in children and adolescents. *Canadian Psychiatric Association Journal, 14*, 217–220.

LeVann, L.J. (1970). Clinical experience with tarasan and thioridazine in mentally retarded children. *Applied Therapeutics, 12*, 30–33.

LeVann, L.J. (1971). Clinical comparison of haloperidol with chlorpromazine in mentally retarded children. *American Journal of Mental Deficiency, 75*, 719–723.

Lewis, M.H., Steer, R.A., Favell, J., McGomsey, J., Clontz, L., Trivett, C., Jordy, W., Schroeder, S.R., Kanoy, R.C., & Mailman, R.B. (1986). Thioridazine metabolism and effects on stereotyped behavior in mentally retarded patients. *Psychopharmacology Bulletin, 22*, 1040–1044.

Llorente, A.F. (1969). The management of behavior disorders with thioridazine in the mentally retarded. *Journal of the Maine Medical Association, 60*, 229–231.

Lowther, G.H. (1960). Clinical experience with trifluoperazine in low-grade mental defectives. *Canadian Medical Association Journal, 82*, 1158–1160.

Lynch, D.M., Eliatamby, C.L.S., & Anderson, A.A. (1985). Pipothiazine palmitate in the management of aggressive mentally handicapped patients. *British Journal of Psychiatry, 146*, 525–529.

Marder, S.R., & Van Putten, T. (1995). Antipsychotic medications. In A.F. Schatzberg & C.B. Nemeroff (Eds.), *Textbook of psychopharmacology* (pp. 247–280). Washington, DC: American Psychiatric Press.

McConahey, O.L., Thompson, T., & Zimmermann, R. (1976). A token system for retarded women: Behavior therapy, drug administration, and their combination. In T. Thompson & J. Grabowski (Eds.), *Behavior modification of the mentally retarded* (2nd Ed., pp.167–234). New York: Oxford University Press.

McDougle, C.J., Brodkin, E.S., Yeung, P.P.,

Naylor, S.T., Cohen, D.J., & Price, L.H. (1995). Risperidone in adults with autism or pervasive developmental disorder. *Journal of Child and Adolescent Psychopharmacology, 5*, 273–282.

Mikkelsen, E.J. (1986). Low-dose haloperidol for stereotypic self-injurious behavior in the mentally retarded. *New England Journal of Medicine, 315*, 398–399

Mlele, T.J.J., & Wiley, Y.V. (1986). Clopenthixol decanoate in the management of aggressive mentally handicapped patients. *British Journal of Psychiatry, 149*, 373–376.

National Institute of Mental Health, Psychopharmacology Service Center Collaborative Study Group. (1964). Phenothiazine treatment in acute schizophrenia: Effectiveness. *Archives of General Psychiatry, 10*, 246–261.

O'Donoghue, S.E.F. (1974). Metabolic activity in the human foetus and neonate as shown by administration of chlorpromazine. *Journal of Physiology, 242*, 105P–106P.

Peroutka, S.J., & Snyder, S.H. (1980). Relationship of neuroleptic drug effects at brain dopamine, serotonin, or-adrenergic, and histamine receptors to clinical potency. *American Journal of Psychiatry, 137*, 1518–1522.

Poindexter, A.R. (1994). Weight changes with neuroleptic withdrawal. *National Association for the Dually Diagnosed Newsletter, 11*, 7–8.

Poling, A., Gadow, K.D., & Cleary, J. (1991). *Drug therapy for behavior disorders: An introduction.* New York: Pergamon Press.

Pregelj, S., & Barkauskas, A. (1967). Thioridazine in the treatment of mentally retarded children: A four-year retroactive evaluation. *Canadian Psychiatric Association Journal, 12*, 213–215.

Reid, A.H. (1983). Psychiatry of mental handicap: A review. *Journal of the Royal Society of Medicine, 76*, 587–591.

Reid, A.H. (1989). Schizophrenia in mental retardation: Clinical features. *Research in Developmental Disabilities, 10*, 241–249.

Rubin, M., & Langa, A. (1995). Clozapine, mental retardation and severe psychiatric illness: Clinical response in the first year. *Harvard Review of Psychiatry, 2*, 293–294.

Rudy, L.H., Himwich, H.E., & Rinaldi, F. (1958). A clinical evaluation of psychopharmacological agents in the management of disturbed mentally defective patients. *American Journal of Mental Deficiency, 62*, 855–860.

Sandford, D., & Nettlebeck, T. (1982). Medication and reinforcement within a token programme for disturbed mentally retarded residents. *Applied Research in Mental Retardation, 3*, 21–36.

Schulman, J.L., & Clarinada, M. (1964). The effect of promazine on the activity level of retarded children. *Pediatrics, 33*, 272–275.

Shapiro, A.K., Shapiro, E., & Wayne, H. (1973). Treatment of Tourette syndrome with haloperidol: Review of 34 cases. *Archives of General Psychiatry, 28,* 92–97.

Shapiro, E., Shapiro, A.K., Fulop, G., Hubbard, M., Mandeli, J., Nordlie, J., & Philips, R.A. (1989). Controlled study of haloperidol, pimozide, and placebo for the treatment of Gilles de la Tourette syndrome. *Archives of General Psychiatry, 46,* 722–730.

Singh, N.N., & Aman, M.G. (1981). Effects of thioridazine dosage on the behavior of severely mentally retarded persons. *American Journal of Mental Deficiency, 85,* 580–587.

Singh, N.N., Landrum, T.J., Ellis, C.R., & Donatelli, L.S. (1993). Effects of thioridazine and visual screening on stereotypy and social behavior in individuals with mental retardation. *Research in Developmental Disabilities, 14,* 163–177.

Snyder, S.H., Benerjee, S.T., Jamamura, H., & Greenberg, D. (1974). Drugs, neurotransmitters and schizophrenia. *Science, 184,* 1243–1253.

Sovner, R. (1995). Thioridazine withdrawal-induced behavioral deterioration treated with clonidine: Two case reports. *Mental Retardation, 33,* 221–225.

Spiegel, R. (1989). *Psychopharmacology.* New York: Wiley.

Sprogis, G.R., Lezdins, V., White, S.D., Ming, C., Lanning, M., Drake, M.E., & Wyckoff, G. (1957). Comparative study on thorazine and serpasil in the mental defective. *American Journal of Mental Deficiency, 61,* 737–742.

Swazey, J.P. (1974). *Chlorpromazine in psychiatry: A study of therapeutic innovation.* Cambridge, MA: MIT Press.

Thompson, T., Hackenberg, T.D., & Schaal, D.W. (1991). Appendix D: Pharmacological treatments for behavior problems in developmental disabilities. In NIH Consensus Development Conference (Ed.), *Treatment of destructive behaviors in persons with developmental disabilities.* Bethesda, MD: National Institutes of Health.

Turner, T.H. (1989). Schizophrenia and mental handicap: An historical review, with implications for further research. *Psychological Medicine, 19,* 301–314.

Ucer, E., & Kreger, K.C. (1969). A double-blind study comparing haloperidol with thioridazine in emotionally disturbed, mentally retarded children. *Current Therapy Research, 11,* 278–283.

Werry, J.S., Sprague, R.L., & Cohen, N.M. (1975). Conners' Teacher Rating Scale for use in drug studies with children: An empirical study. *Journal of Abnormal Child Psychology, 3,* 217–229.

Werry, J.S., & Taylor, E. (1994). Schizophrenic and allied disorders. In M. Rutter, E. Taylor, & L. Hersov (Eds.), *Child and Adolescent Psychiatry* (pp. 594–615). London: Blackwell Scientific Publications.

Wolfson, I.N. (1957). Clinical experience with serpasil and thorazine in treatment of disturbed behavior of mentally retarded. *American Journal of Mental Deficiency, 62,* 276–283.

Yassa, R., Camille, Y., & Belzile, L. (1986). Tardive dyskinesia in the course of antidepressant therapy: A prevalence study and review of the literature. *Journal of Clinical Psychopharmacology, 7,* 243–246.

Young, E. (1970). Hospital experience with fluphenazine enanthate. *Diseases of the Nervous System, 31,* 705–709.

Antiepileptics

Norberto Alvarez[1], Richard A. Kern[2], Nancy N. Cain[3], David L. Coulter[4],
Matti Iivanainen[5], and Alice T. Plummer[6]

DEFINITION, CLASSES, AND NAMES

Antiepileptic drugs are used to treat seizures, which result from abnormal synchronous and rhythmic discharges of electrical energy by groups of neurons in the brain. These abnormal firings cause characteristic transient changes in motor and/or cognitive behavior. Seizures can be triggered by external events such as electroshock or chemical irritation, or by intrinsic factors such as damage or malformation of brain tissue on either a gross or a cellular level. *Epilepsy* is a disorder of brain function in which seizures recur intermittently and unpredictably.

The major antiepileptic drugs are listed in Table 10-1. These drugs are effective in preventing the occurrence of seizures in individuals prone to manifest them. However, none of these drugs has been shown to prevent the emergence of epilepsy in persons who may, by virtue of their histories or their genetic backgrounds, be at risk to do so (Temkin et al., 1990). Thus, it would be more precise to call these drugs "anti-seizure" rather than "antiepileptic," but the latter term will be used here because it is better known.

Antiepileptic drugs were first discovered in the early 1900s, when phenobarbital (Luminal, Gardenal), a barbiturate in use as a sedative at that time, was found to have seizure-preventing properties. As shown in Table 10-1, some of these drugs come from classes of chemicals that are structurally related to phenobarbital. Others belong to entirely different drug classes such as the benzodiazepines, iminostilbenes, branched-chain fatty acids, phenyltriazine, amino acid analogs, and a carbonic anhydrase inhibitor.

PHARMACOLOGY

Pharmacodynamics

Phenobarbital and clonazepam enhance GABA-mediated inhibition of neuronal high-frequency firing by acting at the GABA-A receptor on the cell membrane. The drugs appear to prolong the time the chloride channel remains open after it is opened by endogenous GABA. Phenobarbital may decrease voltage-dependent calcium conductance and block excitatory transmission, but these effects may not be clinically relevant. Primidone is oxidized to phenobarbital, and its mechanism of action is therefore likely to be similar.

Both phenytoin and carbamazepine are thought to block high-frequency firing of neurons. This is done by direct inhibition and blockage of the voltage-gated sodium channel in the neuronal cell membrane and by delaying the cell's reactivation. The drugs may further stimulate sodium/potassium-activated ATPase processes, which would stabilize the cell membrane. They may decrease voltage-dependent calcium conductance. Oxcarbazepine's mechanism of action is poorly understood and is probably related to interactions with sodium and potassium channels (Schmutz, Brugger, Gentsch, McLean, & Olpe, 1994).

Ethosuximide is unique because its clinically important mechanism of action is linked to a decrease in voltage-dependent calcium conductance and blockage of excitatory transmission. The mechanism of action of valproic acid is poorly understood, but data suggest that it may block voltage-gated sodium channels and also enhance GABA-mediated inhibition. The precise mechanism by which it does this is unclear; some of the putative mechanisms (such as inhibition of GABA degradation) do not appear to be clinically relevant.

The pharmacology of the benzodiazepines (e.g., clonazepam, diazepam) is discussed in Chapter 12 on anxiolytics. Only aspects of benzodiazepine use that are specific to seizure control are discussed in this chapter.

The mechanism of action of gabapentin, lamotrigine,

---

1 Assistant Professor of Neurology, Harvard University Medical School, Boston, MA
2 Medical Director, Ohio State University Nisonger Center, Columbus, OH
3 Clinical Associate Professor of Psychiatry, University of Rochester School of Medicine and Dentistry, Rochester, NY
4 Associate Professor of Pediatrics and Neurology, Boston University School of Medicine, Boston, MA
5 Professor of Child Neurology, University of Helsinki Medical School, Helsinki, Finland
6 Associate Clinical Director, Christian Health Care Center, Wyckoff, NJ

Table 10-1. Antiepileptic Medications

Class	Generic Name	Trade Name	Abbreviation	Laboratory
Barbiturates	phenobarbital	Luminal	PB	Various
	primidone	Mysoline	PRM	Wyeth-Ayerst
	mephobarbital	Mebaral	MPB	Winthrop
Hydantoins	phenytoin	Dilantin	PHT	Parke-Davis
	ethotoin	Peganone	ETH	Abbott
	mephenytoin	Mesantoin	MHT	Sandoz
	phenacemide	Phenurone	PAC	Abbott
Succinimides	methsuximide	Celontin	MSM	Parke-Davis
	phensuximide	Milontin	PSM	Parke-Davis
	ethosuximide	Zarontin	ESM	Parke-Davis
Benzodiazepines	clonazepam	Klonopin	CZP	Roche
	clorazepate	Tranxene		Abbott
	diazepam	Valium	DZP	Various
	lorazepam	Ativan	LZP	Wyeth-Ayerst
Iminostilbenes	carbamazepine	Tegretol	CBZ	Ciba-Geigy
	oxcarbazepine	Trileptal	OCBZ	Ciba-Geigy
Fatty acids	valproic acid	Depakene	VPA	Abbott
	divalproex sodium	Depakote	VPA	Abbott
Oxazolidindiones	trimethadione	Tridione	TMO	Abbott
	paramethadione	Paradione	PMO	Abbott
Amino acid	gabapentin	Neurontin	GBP	Parke-Davis
Phenyltriazine	lamotrigine	Lamictal	LTG	Glaxo-Wellcome
Carbonic anhydrase	acetazolimide	Diamox		Lederle
Dicarbamate	felbamate	Felbatol	FBM	Wallace

and felbamate are not well understood. Although gabapentin was developed to mimic the action of GABA, it does not actually interact with any GABA receptors in the brain, and its mechanism of action is unknown. Gabapentin's action might be related to the enhancement of this amino acid in the brain, but this has not been established. However, it has been established that the antiepileptic action of gabapentin is related to the concentration of the drug in neurons and that the clinical effect is directly related to dose.

Lamotrigine is thought to inhibit glutamate-mediated excitotoxicity and may also act at voltage-gated sodium channels to inhibit repetitive neuronal firing. Felbamate may act at the N-methyl-D-aspartate (NMDA) receptor to decrease glutamate-mediated excitotoxicity. It also may have a separate effect via GABA-mediated inhibition of repetitive neuronal firing. This dual mechanism may be related to felbamate's effec-

tiveness against both partial and generalized seizures.

Topiramate has multiple mechanisms of action. The effects on non-NMDA glutamate receptors and on voltage-sensitive sodium channels could explain the antiseizure efficacy (White, 1997). Generally, the pharmacodynamic and neurotoxic effects of two drugs used together are additive rather than potentiated (Leppik & Wolff, 1993; Wyllie, 1993).

Pharmacokinetics

Information on pharmacokinetics is summarized in Table 10-2. The anticonvulsant drugs bind to protein, specifically albumin, so that the free (unbound) fraction in the blood is in equilibrium with the amount in the brain. The drug bound to albumin does not cross the blood-brain barrier and thus is not therapeutically active or capable

Table 10-2. Pharmacokinetic Properties of Anticonvulsant Drugs

Drug/Parameter	Dose	%Prot	Vol Distr	T max	T½	Tss	Th. R
Phenobarbital	2-5	45	0.55	0.5-4	65-110	15-20	10-30
Primidone	6-12	<20	0.75	2-4	8-15	4-7	6-12
Phenytoin	5-10	7-90	0.7-1	0.5-4	10-60	15-20	10-20
Methsuximide	10-75	20	0.65	1-4	30-60	7-10	40-100
Ethosuximide	10-75	20	0.65	1-4	30-60	7-10	40-100
Clonazepam	0.10-0.15	85	3	1-4	20-40	6	20-75
Clorazepate	0.3-3	90-95		1	50-150	21	1-2
Lorazepam	0.05				8-25	7	20-30
Carbamazepine (CBZ)	10-30	75	0.8-2	4-12	20-50	20-30	4-12
Oxcarbazepine	15-30						15-30
10-OH (CBZ)		10-15			2	8-20	ND
Valproate	15-30	70-93	0.1-0.4	1-2	5-15	2	50-100
Gabapentin	1800-2400*	0	0.65-1	2-3	5-7	1-2	ND
Lamotrigine	100-200*	55	1	4-12	24	4	ND
Felbamate	3000*	25-35	1	6-20	19	4	ND

Note. Dose expressed in mg/kg per day. % Prot = Percentage of drug bound to protein. Vol D= Volume of distribution in l/kg. T Max = Time to maximal serum concentration in hours. T½ = Elimination half-life in hours. Tss = Steady state time in days. Th. R = Therapeutic range in μg/ml. ND = Not defined. * = Total daily dose.

of producing toxicity. As the free drug is metabolized, some of the bound drug will be released to maintain equilibrium. If two drugs with a high degree of protein binding are used together, such as phenytoin and valproic acid, the unbound fraction is increased. For example, if phenytoin is 90% protein bound, and the total blood level of phenytoin is 15 μg/ml, then 1.5 μg/ml is free. If valproic acid is added to the therapeutic plan, it will displace some phenytoin from albumin, resulting in an elevation of the free fraction. The increase might easily be as much as 20% to 30% to the total blood concentration, which would be an increase from about 3 μg/ml to about 4.5 μg/ml, well within the toxic range when the total is 15 μg/ml. This may result in clinical neurotoxicity when the total (bound plus unbound) drug concentration is at the therapeutic level. Additionally, more phenytoin will be metabolized in the liver, and a new equilibrium will occur with a lower blood level of total phenytoin. Such interactions must be considered in making therapeutic decisions.

Phenobarbital is available in tablets and as intramuscular and intravenous preparations. Phenobarbital is metabolized mostly in the liver, with approximately 25% eliminated through the kidneys. Phenobarbital is an inducer of the P450 enzymatic group. Because it can induce its own metabolism, the half-life of phenobarbital may shorten after chronic use. Phenobarbital has a long half-life, between 60 and 140 hours in adults and between 37 and 73 hours in children under 15 years. Because of the long half-life, blood levels tend to be stable, and dosage can be once or twice a day. Occasional failures in compliance will not produce marked changes in blood levels. Phenobarbital is a weak acid, and 40% to 60% is bound to plasma proteins. It has a linear kinetic metabolism, with plasma levels directly related to the total dose.

Phenytoin is available in oral and injectable forms and as a slow release formulation with a serum peak concentration of 4 to 12 hours. The acid absorbs much faster, and the peak serum is around 2 to 3 hours. The injectable form, due to the high pH, is used mainly as an intravenous preparation in the treatment of status epilepticus or when loading doses of phenytoin are needed. A prodrug, phosphenytoin, recently introduced in the United States, can be given through intravenous or intramuscular routes. After absorption, 70% to 90% of the phenytoin is bound to albumin; 95% is excreted as metabolites. The main metabolic pathway is through the P450 oxidase system in the liver. This is a rate-limited metabolism that is saturated at certain doses; when this happens, small increases in the total dose of phenytoin are associated with high blood levels and the potential for toxic effects. The half-life is more prolonged in neonates (30 to 70 hours) and might also be prolonged in elderly people.

Primidone is available as tablets and in suspension

form. Its metabolites include phenobarbital and phenylethylmalonide (PEMA); PEMA has mild antiepileptic and toxic activity. The peak level of primidone occurs approximately 3 hours after ingestion in adults and 4 to 6 hours after ingestion in children. The plasma protein binding is less than 10%, and the elimination half-life in monotherapy is between 10 to 15 hours and may be decreased to half that when used in combination with other antiepileptic medications. Most of the drug is excreted in the urine. Clinical toxicity can occur with blood levels of primidone in the therapeutic range.

Carbamazepine is available in normal tablets, controlled-release tablets, and in liquid forms. Absorption is similar for the various pharmaceutical forms but fastest with the suspension form; absorption may be improved with food (Levy, Pitlick, Troupin, Green, & Neal, 1975). The drug can be used rectally, but this is uncommon. The drug is metabolized through different pathways. The main compound is an epoxide which has the same antiepileptic, analgesic, and toxic effects as carbamazepine. This metabolite can contribute to clinical intoxication even when the dose of carbamazepine remains constant. Valproate inhibits the metabolism of the epoxide, increasing the metabolite's concentration (McKauge, Tyrer, & Eadie, 1981). Peak plasma concentrations occur 4 to 8 hours after ingestion. The free fraction in plasma is approximately 30%. Carbamazepine is present in tears and saliva. It is also present in breast milk, but this is not considered an impediment to breast feeding (Yerby, 1987). The relationship between the oral dose and the blood concentration has been difficult to establish (Strandjord & Johannessen, 1980; Tomson, Svensson, & Hilton-Brown, 1989). Additionally, several studies did not find a relationship between blood serum level and clinical efficacy. Thus, the clinical response is more important than the blood level in adjusting the dose of carbamazepine. Generally, blood levels between 5 µg/ml and 10 µg/ml offer the maximal antiepileptic protection with minimal side effects (Schmidt & Jacob, 1993).

Oxcarbazepine is rapidly metabolized to the active metabolite, 10-hydroxy carbamazepine (monohydroxy derivative, MHD), by reduction reactions not dependent on the hepatic P450 system (Schmutz et al., 1994). The half-life is 1 to 2 hours, but since the active metabolite MHD has a half-life of around 8 to 10 hours, twice-daily administration is enough. Both compounds are 40% to 60% bound to plasma proteins. Serum levels do not have a simple relationship with toxicity.

Valproate is available in syrup, tablet, and capsule form. It is rapidly absorbed through the whole intestinal tract and is found in the brain and in the spinal fluid (Rosenfeld, Leppik, Eates, & Mireles, 1987). Peak absorption varies between 1 hour for valproic acid syrup and 5 hours for the divalproex tablets. The divalproex sprinkle forms are associated with smaller fluctuations in serum concentrations (Cloyd et al., 1992). However, this preparation can produce complications in patients with feeding tubes, especially the "button" type (Jones-Saete, Kriel, & Cloyd, 1992). Administration with meals might delay absorption of valproate (Mattson, Cramer, Williamson, & Novelly, 1978). The drug is mostly bound to protein, although the free fractions (approximately 5% to 20%) are difficult to predict in individual cases because the relationship between total and free is not linear when the binding sites are saturated. The half-life is approximately 6 to 12 hours when used in monotherapy and 8 to 9 hours when used in polytherapy. Higher doses are needed in patients in polytherapy. Rectal administration, which can result in therapeutic blood levels (Cloyd & Kriel, 1981), might be indicated in the treatment of status epilepticus (Snead & Miles, 1985) or in other situations such as intractable vomiting, surgery, and feeding disorders.

After oral administration, gabapentin is easily absorbed from the gastrointestinal tract. Most of the gabapentin is not bound to protein and is excreted unchanged by the kidneys. The peak levels are directly related to the total dose (up to 600 mg given three times a day) but are less than expected after doses as high as 4,800 mg/day, suggesting a limit in the maximal effect. The half-life is relatively short (6 hours), and multiple daily doses are needed. Gabapentin does not induce hepatic microsomal enzymes and does not interact with the other major antiepileptic medications such as phenobarbital, phenytoin, carbamazepine, and valproic acid (McLean, 1994).

Lamotrigine is available as tablets. The absorption is rapid and not affected by food. The peak concentration is approximately 2 hours after ingestion. Blood levels are directly related to the total dose in a linear fashion. Protein binding is 55%. Most of the drug is metabolized in the liver, with no evidence of enzyme saturation even with high dose. Only 5% is eliminated unchanged. The half-life after a single dose in monotherapy is 32 hours (range 14-103) and decreases to 25 hours (range 11 to 61) when given in multiple doses. Medications that induce liver enzymes (such as phenobarbital, phenytoin, carbamazepine) reduce the half-life to 15 hours, but valproic acid can prolong the half-life to 60 hours.

Vigabatrin exists as a mixture of two isomers, R(–)

and S(+), but only the S(+) component is active. The drug, which is highly soluble in water, has dose-linear kinetics with rapid absorption after oral ingestion. Peak blood levels occur about two hours after ingestion, and food has no effect on absorption. The half-life is 7 to 9 hours in adults and 5 to 6 hours in children (Richens, 1991). The clinical effect depends on the irreversible inhibition of the GABA-T enzyme and not on the half-life of the drug. Browne et al. (1987) found that it took between 2 to 10 days for clinical effects to become apparent after changes in dosage. There is no correlation between plasma levels and clinical efficacy. Only 5% of vigabatrin is protein bound. Because vigabatrin does not interfere with the cytochrome P450-dependent liver enzymes, it should not affect the pharmacokinetics of the other major antiepileptic medications. The usual dose in adults is 2 to 3 g per day given in 1 or 2 doses. In children the recommended dose is 0.5 to 1 g per day.

Topiramate, which is available in tablets, has a rapid absorption with 80% bioavailability. The maximum peak is 1-4 hours after oral administration; the half-life is 21 hours. Only a small fraction is metabolized, and 80% is eliminated in the urine. Protein binding is less than 15%. The pharmacokinetics are linear.

SIDE EFFECTS

The side effects of anticonvulsant medications are summarized in Table 10-3. This list is not exhaustive and should be supplemented with other resources. Most of the central nervous system (CNS) side effects are dose related and can be ameliorated by decreasing dosages. Often, side effects have been reported with blood levels within the therapeutic range. For example, clinicians have reported cases of tremors induced by therapeutic levels of valproic acid and behavior changes associated with therapeutic levels of phenobarbital and benzodiazepines. As with all drugs, any patient can have unpredictable adverse effects.

Most, if not all, antiepileptic medications have sedative effects. This effect is largely dose related, but it is more evident with the barbiturates (phenobarbital, mephobarbital, primidone, benzodiazepines, clorazepate, dibenzodiazepine, and clonazepam). The sedative effects are one of the limiting factors in the use of these medications. However, the major antiepileptic medications are not considered good sedative-hypnotics, and presently they are not used as such.

Mothers with epilepsy are up to three times more likely than mothers without epilepsy to have children with major malformations (Monson et al., 1973; Shapiro et al., 1976). The most typical major malformations are oral clefts and cardiac defects. It is unclear if antiepileptic drugs play a role in the occurrence of these malformations because many other factors are present, including a possible genetic link, lower socioeconomic status, the occurrence of seizures during pregnancy, complications of pregnancy, and paternal epilepsy. The so-called "fetal hydantoin syndrome," which includes growth deficiency and structural malformations (Gaily, 1990), does not seem to be specific for phenytoin but may also be seen with other antiepileptic medications. Spinal dysraphism (i.e., defective fusion) has been reported in newborns exposed to valproic acid during the pregnancy.

Phenobarbital

The systemic side effects of phenobarbital are minimal even after many years of use. However, decreased libido and impotence occur in about 16% of patients (Mattson et al., 1985). Compared with other antiepileptic medications, phenobarbital has fewer hematological, hepatic, and gastrointestinal effects. Phenobarbital activates hepatic enzymes, which could result in major changes in the metabolism of other drugs administered simultaneously. As will be discussed later, cognitive and behavioral side effects are a major concern with phenobarbital; there is concern that normal clinical doses may cause some loss of IQ. However, there are methodological shortcomings in some of the studies reporting these side effects.

Heller et al. (1995) compared phenobarbital, phenytoin, carbamazepine, and valproic acid in adults recently diagnosed with epilepsy. Although the clinical efficacy of the four drugs was the same, more frequent and more serious side effects (mostly lethargy, drowsiness, and dizziness) occurred with phenobarbital (22% of the patients). In all, 3% of phenytoin patients, 5% of valproate patients, and 11% of carbamazepine patients had unacceptable side effects.

Forsythe and Sills (1984) found that 30% of children treated with phenobarbital developed hyperactivity, irritability, aggressiveness, or depression. Brent et al. (1987, 1990) found depressive disorder in 6 of 15 children treated with phenobarbital; the depression improved after phenobarbital was stopped. In this study, insomnia and irritability were considered as symptoms of a depressive disorder.

Table 10-3. Side Effects of Common Antiepileptic Medications

Medication	Systemic/Physical Effects	CNS Effects
Phenobarbital	Nonspecific	Sedation Overactivity Irritability
Phenytoin	Hirsutism Gingival hyperplasia (Stinnet et al., 1987) Low folate (Berg et al., 1988) Low vitamin D (Lifshitz & Maclare, 1978) Rash	Ataxia (Kutt et al., 1964; Reynolds, 1989) Nystagmus Vomiting Sedation Dyskinesia (Krishnamoorthy et al., 1983) Arrhythmia Seizures
Ethosuximide	Rash (Sherwin, 1993) Anemia Leukopenia	Lethargy Nausea Dizziness Vomiting Visual changes
Clonazepam	Drooling (Browne, 1978)	Sedation Aspiration Disinhibition Hallucinations Hypotonia Ataxia Nystagmus
Carbamazepine	Hepatitis Anemia SIADH (Kalff et al., 1984) Leukopenia Low thyroid Low vitamin D	Diplopia (Pellock, 1987) Ataxia (Pellock, 1987) Nausea Sedation Dyskinesia Arrhythmia (Boesen et al., 1983)
Valproic Acid	Hepatitis (Dreifuss et al., 1989) Pancreatitis (Camfield, 1979) Hyperammoniemia (Williams et al., 1984) Low carnitine (Bohen et al., 1992) Leukopenia (Jaeken et al., 1979) Low platelet (Loiseau, 1981) Obesity (Dinesen et al., 1984) Alopecia (hair loss) Tremor (Hyuman et al., 1979) Nausea	Sedation (Dreifuss & Langer, 1988) Vomiting Cerebral edema (Bigler, 1985)
Gabapentin	Weight gain Leukopenia Rash Low platelets (rare) ECG changes (rare)	Lethargy (McLean, 1995) Fatigue Dizziness Ataxia Headache Nausea Diplopia Tremor

Table 10-3. (Continued).
Side Effects of Common Antiepileptic Medications

Medication	Systemic/Physical Effects	CNS Effects
Lamotrigine	Rash (Messenheimer, 1995) Hepatitis	Lethargy Blurred vision Dizziness Ataxia Headache Nausea Diplopia
Felbamate	Aplastic anemia Hepatitis Rash Body odor	Anorexia Vomiting Insomnia Lethargy Headache Weight loss

Primidone

The side effects of primidone are similar to those of phenobarbital. Mattson et al. (1985) found that decreased libido and increased impotence occurred more frequently with primidone than with three other anticonvulsants. Other side effects included motor disturbances, gastrointestinal problems, and idiosyncratic reactions such as rashes. In the Mattson et al. study, there were no serious side effects except for two cases of transient psychosis that improved after primidone was discontinued.

In children, behavioral and cognitive side effects include depression (Rodin, Rim, Kitano, Lewis, & Rennick, 1976) and possibly decreased IQ (Trimble & Corbett, 1980). Herranz, Armijo, and Arteaga (1988) found behavioral effects similar to those produced by phenobarbital, primarily irritability and hyperactivity in 22% of children with epilepsy or febrile seizures. In 8% of the children, the side effects necessitated withdrawal of the treatment.

Phenytoin

The most common side effects of phenytoin are presented in Table 10-3. Idiosyncratic reactions such as agranulocytosis, Stevens-Johnson syndrome, aplastic anemia, liver failure, skin rash, serum sickness, and/or pancreatitis are sometimes seen at the beginning of therapy and might be an indication to discontinue the drug. Clinical toxicity, even with low phenytoin levels in serum, may develop unexpectedly due to a number of factors. These factors include (a) saturation kinetics of phenytoin, (b) individual metabolic differences, (c) inhibitory effects of certain simultaneously ingested drugs (e.g., cimetidine, warfarin, isoniazid) on the metabolism of phenytoin, and (d) the ability of certain drugs (e.g., aspirin, valproic acid) to displace phenytoin from protein binding, leading to increases in the serum free phenytoin level.

With multiple drug therapy, patients with severe brain damage are especially susceptible to phenytoin toxicity even at low serum concentration. Clinically, phenytoin toxicity may be accompanied by deterioration of intellectual and cognitive functioning, drowsiness, progressive difficulties in maintaining balance, deterioration in coordination, muscle hypotonia, abnormal weight loss, and loss of locomotion. EEG activity is slowed and reaction times are lengthened during intoxication.

The danger of chronic phenytoin intoxication in multiple drug therapy was demonstrated in a study of 131 phenytoin-treated persons with mental retardation and epilepsy (Iivanainen, Viukari, & Helle, 1977). In this study, phenytoin intoxication was diagnosed retrospectively in 73 people (56%), 18 of whom developed persistent loss of locomotion after about 22 months of clinical intoxication. The shortest duration of phenytoin intoxication until permanent loss of locomotion was only one month.

Another example of an insidious and dangerous effect of phenytoin was documented by the changed course of Baltic myoclonus epilepsy (Iivanainen & Eldridge, 1987). Its rather benign course worsened during phenytoin treatment, so that the patients became bedridden and pseudoretarded and their life span shortened from 50-to-60 years to under about 30 years. When these patients were treated with valproate instead of phenytoin, their life expectancy was not shortened. In some of these patients, the loss of locomotion was not reversible after valproate replaced phenytoin (Eldridge, Iivanainen, Stern, Koerber, & Wilder, 1983; Iivanainen & Himberg, 1982). In a third study, Aman, Paxton, Field, and Foote (1986) surveyed phenytoin and carbamazepine drug concentrations in saliva. Of 54 subjects taking phenytoin, at least one of two samples taken exceeded the therapeutic range for 15 patients (28% of sample).

Phenytoin can produce bone disorder by affecting calcium and vitamin D metabolism. The drug sometimes produces a reduction in the serum calcium level and, rarely, osteomalacia. Clinical manifestations of drug-induced bone disorder include rickets, increased risk of pathological fractures, increased seizure frequency due to hypocalcemia (Hahn, 1976), and prolonged hypocalcemia with tetany in infants born to mothers treated with phenytoin (Friis & Sardemann, 1977). Because hypocalcemia can increase seizure frequency, the need for additional antiepileptic drugs may be erroneously concluded, leading to a further reduction in serum calcium levels and producing a vicious cycle.

Phenytoin-induced liver disease is rare and occurs most frequently in adolescents or young adults. This side effect is equally likely for males and females. When hepatotoxicity develops, it occurs within 6 weeks of the first phenytoin exposure and may not be dose dependent. Liver biopsies of these patients show hepatitis with cell necrosis and eosinophilia with or without cholestasis.

Phenytoin affects endocrinological and other metabolic functions. Laboratory tests on thyroid functioning may become unreliable during phenytoin therapy because the drug decreases the serum thyroid hormone (T4) level. Phenytoin induces hyperglycemia. The drug should be monitored carefully in patients with risk factors for diabetes (Gharib & Munoz, 1974), as hyperglycemia may occur with a relatively low dose. Impotency and infertility have been attributed to phenytoin treatment.

Phenytoin produces immunoglobulin-A (IgA) deficiencies in serum, saliva (Aarli & Tinder, 1975), and nasal secretions (Gilhus & Aarli, 1981). This may predispose patients to recurrent infections. The average period from initiation of therapy until the deficiency state is reached is about 3 to 4 months. This IgA deficiency may increase susceptibility to gingival inflammation and lead to gingival hyperplasia during long-term phenytoin treatment.

Hematologic toxicity may be indicated by megaloblastic anemia or lymphadenopathy with a histologic picture suggestive of lymphomas or Hodgkin's disease. Folic acid deficiency or failure to utilize folic acid prob-

ably represents the basic mechanism in the development of megaloblastic anemia. Occasionally, phenytoin provokes a lupus-like or hypersensitivity syndrome (Iivanainen & Savolainen, 1983). A few cases of acute renal failure, vasculitis, fulminant purpura, disseminated intravascular coagulation, and myositis syndrome have been reported.

Intravenous administration of phenytoin may cause venous irritation, phlebitis (Jamerson et al., 1994), induration, and, in extreme cases, frank tissue necrosis (Hayes & Chesney, 1993). Fasciotomies and amputation of fingers may be needed (Sintenie, Tuinebreijer, Kreis, & Breederveld, 1992) but may be insufficient to prevent permanent disuse of the hand and forearm (Hanna, 1992). This complication is most often apparent in newborn babies. Fosphenytoin administration resulted in significantly less venous irritation and phlebitis compared with an equimolar dose of phenytoin (Jamerson et al., 1994).

Researchers have evaluated the possibility that phenytoin causes brain damage. In a study of individuals with mental retardation and epilepsy, phenytoin levels were associated with brain damage, although neither high plasma phenytoin levels nor frequent seizures proved to be the direct cause of the brain damage (Iivanainen et al., 1977).

Chronic phenytoin intoxication syndrome is associated with increased frequency of seizures, muscular hypotonia, choreoathetoid movements, orofacial dyskinesia, and psychiatric disorders. Rarely, asterixis, ophthalmoplegia, and spasticity occur. Although phenytoin intoxication syndrome is expressed as a functional disturbance of the cerebellum and cerebrum, it has been termed "phenytoin encephalopathy." If phenytoin is withdrawn in time, the neurological performance may improve within about 2 weeks, as the drug slowly clears from the central nervous system. Cerebellar atrophy is seen in phenytoin-treated patients with epilepsy in the absence of generalized tonic-clonic seizures or preexistent brain damage (Ney, Lantos, Barr, & Schaul, 1994). As degeneration of Purkinje cells was observed in the brains of epileptic patients before phenytoin was introduced as an antiepileptic drug, it is possible that a pre-existing cerebellar lesion may be a predisposing factor to further cerebellar damage during phenytoin overdosage. The higher the plasma phenytoin level, the more rapid is the development of persistent loss of locomotion (Iivanainen et al., 1977). There is experimental evidence that phenytoin distribution in Purkinje cell fraction is higher than in other cerebellar or cerebral neurons (Savolainen,   Iivanainen,   Elovaara,   &

Tammisto, 1980). The hypothesis that phenytoin toxicity may lead to cerebellar atrophy is supported by a recent case report. Iivanainen (personal communication, 1995) treated an 11-year-old boy with epilepsy. Magnetic resonance imagery revealed a normal cerebellum prior to therapy but cerebellar atrophy after phenytoin treatment was initiated.

In order to avoid aplastic anemia during phenytoin treatment, leukocyte analysis of sequential blood samples is needed. If the white cell count reaches 1,500/mm³, the drug should be discontinued. Some data suggest that riboflavin may be beneficial in preventing pure red blood cell aplasia. Although spontaneous recovery from phenytoin-induced liver disease may occur, immediate cessation of phenytoin exposure is necessary. Thorough brushing of the teeth and good oral hygiene are helpful in preventing gingival hyperplasia (growth of the gums) during long-term phenytoin therapy. The immunological or "lymphoproliferative" manifestations reverse when phenytoin is discontinued but readministration of the drug quickly reactivates these symptoms. To minimize fetal exposure to phenytoin, low-dosage monotherapy is favored for pregnant epileptic women. Recovery is maintained, even though phenytoin is continued, as long as folic acid is prescribed.

Carbamazepine

Carbamazepine is a relatively safe drug, with less toxicity than many other antiepileptic drugs (Mattson, Petroff, Rothman, & Behar, 1994; Smith et al., 1987). However, some investigators have found side effects in up to 50% of the patients exposed to carbamazepine (Heller et al., 1995; Herranz et al., 1988; Pellock, 1987), but discontinuance of the medication was needed in only a minority of cases (Heller et al., 1995; Herranz et al., 1988). Skin disorders, such as rash and pruritus, were the most common reason for termination of treatment (Ramsay, Wilder, Berger, & Bruni, 1983; Verity, Hosking, & Easter, 1995); exfoliative dermatitis was rarely a side effect.

Hematological complications such as aplastic anemia, agranulocytosis, and thrombocytopenia are unpredictable side effects of carbamazepine (Pellock, 1987). In the vast majority of cases, these side effects are transient and have no clinical significance (Verity et al., 1995); in a small number of cases, however, they may lead to death. The risk is mostly in the first two months of treatment and with elderly patients. The most commonly observed neurotoxic effects of carbamazepine are drowsiness,

sleepiness, ataxia, and visual disturbances. These are dose related and improve without sequelae with discontinuance of the medications (Ramsay et al., 1983).

Carbamazepine has antidiuretic properties, producing low blood levels of sodium. In a few cases, it may become necessary to discontinue the drug. The sodium effect is masked by lithium and phenytoin and enhanced by valproate and phenobarbital (Kalff et al., 1984; Sordillo, Sagransky, Mercado, & Michelis, 1978).

The cognitive side effects of carbamazepine have been studied on many occasions and found to be mostly dose related and not severe. Carbamazepine often has a positive effect on behavior and is used in the treatment of mood disorders (see Chapter 13); however, there are reports that carbamazepine sometimes leads to behavior problems. In persons with developmental disabilities, some investigators suggested that exacerbation of pre-existing behaviors such as self-injury and irritability may occur with cambamazepine (Evans & Gualtieri, 1985; Reid, Naylor, & Kay, 1981). Others documented the onset of aggression, hyperactivity, agitation, and insomnia (Dally, 1971; Evans & Gualtieri, 1985; Friedman, Kastner, Plummer, Ruiz, & Hanning, 1992; Myers & Carrera, 1989; Reid et al., 1981). Even though these problems have been described in persons with and without mental retardation, they may be more frequent in persons with developmental disabilities (Reid et al., 1981; Silverstein, Parrish, & Johnston, 1982). These adverse effects improve when carbamazepine is discontinued.

Valproate

Valproic acid usually is well tolerated and has few significant side effects when blood levels are within the 50 to 100 μg/ml range (Devinsky, 1995; Herranz et al., 1988; Verity et al., 1995). The most serious side effect is sudden hepatic failure, which cannot be anticipated by laboratory monitoring (Willmore, Triggs, & Pellock, 1991). The problem is usually reversible when valproate is stopped, but some deaths have occurred. Early reports suggested a high incidence of fatal hepatic failure in children younger than 2 years on polytherapy due to epileptic disorders (Dreifuss, Langer, Moline, & Maxwell, 1989; Dreifuss et al., 1987). The number of fatalities from polytherapy decreases with age, but some fatalities still occur in older children and in adults (Konig et al., 1994). The most frequent early signs of hepatic failure are vomiting, nausea, loss of appetite, apathy, seizure exacerbation, and fever. When these symptoms occur, valproate should be discontinued.

There is no explanation for the hepatic failure. Since valproate affects mitochondrial functions, unknown metabolic disorders (especially in children) may explain some of the cases (Dreifuss et al., 1987; Koskiniemi & Hakamies, 1979). Carnitine depletion has been considered as a potential explanation (Coulter, 1991), but it occurs with other antiepileptic medications that do not produce serious liver damage (Hug, McGraw, Bates, & Landrigan, 1991). There is no evidence that simultaneous treatment with carnitine will prevent fatalities (Coulter, 1991; Laub, Paetzke-Brunner, & Jaeger, 1986). Another potential severe side effect is pancreatitis (Coulter & Allen, 1980). However, it is not as frequent as hepatotoxicity.

Coagulation deficiencies are rare side effects due to thrombocytopenia and interference with platelet aggregation. This side effect needs to be considered in patients with self-injurious behaviors and also in patients about to undergo surgery. Other hematological complications are leukopenia and neutropenia, which improve when valproate is discontinued. Asymptomatic hyperammoniemia frequently occurs after the initiation of therapy with valproate (Murphy & Marquardt, 1982).

Several endocrine disorders have been described in women taking valproate alone or in combination with other drugs. Either polycystic ovaries or high serum levels of testosterone were reported in 80% of women treated with valproate before the age of 20 years (Isojarvi, Laatikainen, Pakarinen, Juntunen, & Myllyla, 1993). Tremors, weight gain, and hair loss are dose-related side effects that improve when valproate is discontinued. The combination of lithium, a tremorogenic drug, with valproate can induce serious tremors and requires discontinuing one of the drugs. Valproate may also be associated with encephalopathy (Pakalnis, Drake, & Denio, 1989; Sackellares, Soo, & Dreifuss, 1979) and with reversible dementia and brain atrophy (Papazian et al., 1995).

Herranz et al. (1988) found behavior problems in 17% of 110 children with febrile seizures during treatment with valproate. Drowsiness, which affected about 5% of the patients, was probably dose related. Hyperactivity, which affected about 3% of the patients, was not related to dose. Other investigators also found hyperactivity in a small percentage of patients on polytherapy (Barnes & Bower, 1975).

Gabapentin

Clinical studies indicate that gabapentin is well toler-
ated, with few significant side effects (Crawford, Ghadualis, Lane, Blumhardt, & Catwalk, 1987; U.K. Gabapentin Study Group, 1990; U.S. Gabapentin Study Group No. 5, 1993). The most commonly reported side effects are somnolence (19%), dizziness (17%), ataxia (12%), fatigue (11%), and tremor (6%). Generally, these side effects are mild—after 2 years, withdrawal of medication was required in only about 4% of patients in one study (U.S. Gabapentin Study Group, 1994).

There is no information regarding teratogenesis because very few pregnant women have been exposed to gabapentin. There is also little information regarding toxicity in overdose. In one extreme case of a 16-year-old girl who intentionally ingested 49 grams of gabapentin, the side effects were minimal (Fisher, Barr, Rogers, Fischer, & Trudeau, 1994).

Lamotrigine

When used as monotherapy, the incidence of side effects was less than for phenytoin or carbamazepine (Brodie, Richens, & U.K. Lamotrigine/Carbamazepine Monotherapy Trial Group, 1994; Steiner, Silviera, & Yuen, 1994). When used as an add-on medication, the rates at which medication withdrawal was required due to side effects varied across different studies from about 5% (Messenheimer et al., 1994) to about 9% (Matsuo et al., 1993). The most frequent reason for withdrawal was rash, which occurred in approximately 5% of patients, usually within the first month. Because these idiosyncratic reactions can be very severe, mostly in children younger than 16, the use of lamotrigine is not recommended for children.

Other side effects are dizziness, headaches, diplopia, ataxia, nausea, amblyopia, and somnolence. However, these are usually mild, and they are usually reversible when the medication is withdrawn. There are some reports of dizziness, ataxia, and diplopia when lamotrigine was given in combination with carbamazepine and oxcarbazepine. These side effects can be avoided if the drugs are given one hour apart. Two cases of overdose (1500 mg and 4000 to 5000 mg) were not associated with any serious consequences.

The frequency of systemic effects on liver, kidney, and blood cells is so low that there is no need to perform routine monitoring. Blood levels of lamotrigine are directly related to total dose. Lamotrigine has not shown any serious negative effect on behavior or cognition. Some preliminary studies in persons with epilepsy

Table 10-4. Interactions Between Antiepileptic Drugs

Original/ Added Drug	PB	PRM	PHT	CBZ	VPA	GBP	CZP	DZP	LTG	FBM
PB			NS	dual	+	NS			NS	
PRM		+a	dual							
PHT	dual	–		dual	– Total + Free	NS	–	–	NS	+
CBZ	–	NS	– 50%		b	NS	–	–	NS	–c
VPA	–	+	– 50%	–		NS			–	+
GBP	NS		NS	NS	NS					
LTG	–		–	–	+					
FBM			–	–	NS					

Original drugs appear in rows. New (or added drugs) are presented in columns together with changes that occur in the original drug.
   NS not significant.
   (–) decrease blood level.
   (+) increase blood level.
Dual refers to interactions that are variable; the blood level of the original drug might increase, decrease, or remain the same. Blank spaces appear when no information is available.
a Phenytoin induces PRM and there is a higher blood level of phenobarbital.
b Valproic acid increases the epoxide of carbamazepine, but does not change significantly the blood level of carbamazepine.
c Felbamate increases the epoxide of carbamazepine and decreases blood levels of carbamazepine.

suggested that lamotrigine might have some positive behavioral effects (Messenheimer, 1995).

Vigabatrin

This drug is tolerated very well. For only a few patients is it necessary to discontinue the medication due to side effects (Dulac et al., 1991). The most common side effects are drowsiness, fatigue, irritability, ataxia (Browne et al., 1987; Dam, 1991), and hyperkinesia (Dulac et al., 1991). Reversible depression and psychosis have been reported for a few patients (Browne et al., 1987; Grant & Heel, 1991). Neuropsychological testing has indicated no or minimal cognitive side effects (Kalviainen et al., 1991; Mumford & Cannon, 1994). In some animal studies, vigabatrin produced a dose-related microvascularization of the myelin. However, these lesions have not been observed in humans (Browne et al., 1991; Cannon, Butler, Mumford, & Lewis, 1991).

Topiramate

The most common side effects observed in double-blind trials were dizziness, somnolence, abnormal thinking, and fatigue. Other reported side effects were ataxia,

confusion, paresthesia, and impaired concentration. The side effects were dose related. In a few cases, chronic use was associated with weight loss and nephrolithiasis (Shorvon & Stefan, 1997).

DRUG INTERACTIONS

Antiepileptic drugs interact with each other by three principal mechanisms: enzyme induction, enzyme inhibition, and altered protein binding. Enzyme induction and inhibition refer to the property of certain drugs of stimulating or inhibiting the activity of liver enzymes, which affects the metabolism of other drugs. The degree of protein binding of various antiepileptic drugs is shown in Table 10-2. Generally, the free (unbound) fraction in the blood is in equilibrium with the brain concentration and is considered physiologically relevant. This free fraction can be measured in commercial laboratories. If two drugs with high degrees of protein binding are used together (such as phenytoin and valproic acid), one should expect some displacement of each drug from protein and a consequent increase in the unbound fraction. This may result in neurotoxicity, although the total (bound plus unbound) drug concentration may appear to be at "therapeutic" levels.

Phenobarbital and phenytoin induce a wide range of

Table 10-5. Drug Interaction Effects of Antiepileptic Drugs on Other Drugs

Drug	Increase Effect	Decrease Effect
Phenobarbital	Acetaminophen metabolities	Antidepressants, coumadin, warfarin, antipyrine, lidocaine, quinidine, steroids, griseofulvine, theophylline, cimetidine, vitamin D, haloperidol, methadone, thioridazine, cyclosporine
Phenytoin	Phenobarbital	Cyclosporine, digoxin, chloramphenicol, lidocaine, meperidine, theophylline, vitamin D, prednisone, steroids, haloperidol, folic acid, thioridazine, levodopa, tricyclics, oral contraceptives
Valproic Acid	Antypyrine	
Carbamazepine	Lithium, digitalis	Theophylline, warfarin, steroids, cyclosporine, haloperidol, doxycycline

enzymatic activity. Carbamazepine induces its own enzymatic metabolism and may induce metabolism of phenytoin and valproic acid, resulting in lower concentrations of each. Valproic acid inhibits the metabolism of both phenobarbital and the epoxide of carbamazepine, resulting in higher concentrations of each.

Phenytoin is a potent inductor of primidone, carbamazepine, and valproic acid biotransformation. The amount of phenobarbital derived from primidone may increase twofold, and the blood levels of carbamazepine and valproate can be reduced by 50%. (See Table 10-4 for a summary of interactions between anticonvulsants.)

When phenobarbital, primidone, or phenytoin are added to the therapy of a person already taking carbamazepine, the level of carbamazepine decreases and the level of the epoxide may increase. Valproic acid does not affect carbamazepine but decreases the clearance of the epoxide. Carbamazepine induces the metabolism of phenobarbital, primidone, valproic acid, benzodiazepines, ethosuximide, and sometimes phenytoin. Fluoxetine increases the plasma level of carbamazepine, while carbamazepine decreases the level of haloperidol.

Primidone and phenobarbital have similar drug interactions. Any drug that induces the hepatic enzymes involved in the biotransformation of primidone should affect the ratio between phenobarbital, primidone, and PEMA. Both phenytoin and carbamazepine cause a marked acceleration of the biotransformation of primidone.

Valproic acid added to a regimen with phenytoin results in decreases of the total phenytoin with simultaneous increases of the free fraction, such that toxicity may occur. There are no clinically significant interactions with the phenobarbital, benzodiazepines, gabapentin, and lamotrigine. Generally phenothiazines, methylphenidate, and imipramine do not significantly alter plasma levels of phenytoin. Antacids may reduce phenytoin absorption, resulting in low blood levels; cimetidine decreases phenytoin clearance, resulting in high levels.

Gabapentin is not metabolized at all and is excreted unchanged in the urine. It interacts with none of the known anticonvulsant drugs and has no effects on their blood levels. Lamotrigine is metabolized in the liver and interacts significantly with valproic acid but not with phenytoin. Valproic acid inhibits the metabolism of lamotrigine, resulting in a longer half-life and higher blood levels of lamotrigine as well as lower levels of valproic acid. Lamotrigine does not affect the blood level of carbamazepine, but it may increase the concentration of the epoxide metabolite of carbamazepine in some patients. Lamotrigine does not interfere with the metabolism of phenytoin or carbamazepine. Lamotrigine might have a pharmacodynamic potentiation of side effects with carbamazepine and oxcarbazepine. Enzyme-inducing drugs reduce the half-life, which is prolonged by drugs such as valproic acid. Felbamate is metabolized in the liver and interacts with virtually all of the known anticonvulsant drugs. It raises the blood levels of phenytoin and valproic acid and increases the concentration of the epoxide metabolite of carbamazepine.

Topiramate has no clinically significant interactions when given to patients on antiepileptic drugs. However, the clearance of topiramate is reduced when concomitant phenytoin or carbamazepine is discontinued (Shorvon & Stefan, 1997).

Anticonvulsant drugs also interact with many other drugs not used for the treatment of epilepsy, following

Table 10-6. Interaction Effects of Other Drugs on the Antiepileptic Drugs

Drug	Increase Effect	Decrease Effect
Phenobarbital	Propoxyphene, isoniazid, chloramphenicol, phenylbutazone	Dicumarol
Phenytoin	Cimetidine, anticoagulants, sulfa drugs, aspirin, ibuprofen, imipramine, propranolol,	Ethanol, nicotine, phenothiazine, antacids, phenylbutazone, salicylates, calcium supplements, rifampin, sucralfate
Valproic Acid	Acetylsalicylic acid	Ethanol
Carbamazepine	Propoxyphene, erythromycin, verapamil, diltiazem, isoniazid, cimetidine, imipramine, fluoxetine, haloperidol	Theophylline

similar mechanisms of interactions to those already noted. Some of these interactions are summarized in Table 10-5. Conversely, many non-antiepileptic drugs also influence the blood levels and the action of antiepileptic drugs, and some of these are listed in Table 10-6. The complex interactions make it necessary to consult standard reference sources to determine if a drug-drug interaction might be anticipated.

UNINTENDED COGNITIVE-MOTOR EFFECTS

Although there is evidence that unwanted psychoactive effects accompany several of the antiepileptic drugs, these effects were not discussed earlier with side effects. This is because they do not present as "side effects" in the usual way—that is, as a complaint of the patient. Rather, these are effects that may go undetected unless the clinical team is informed and vigilant.

Multi-Drug Monotherapy Comparisons

Over the years, there have been a number of attempts to compare effects of different drugs on both clinical and cognitive variables. Smith et al. (1987) compared the safety and efficacy of phenobarbital, primidone, phenytoin, and carbamazepine in 622 adults. The results indicated that, compared with a group of normal controls, all four drugs had negative effects on motor skills, cogni-

tion, and mood. More important are the results comparing the four drugs. After 1 and 3 months of treatment, significant differences emerged between the drugs. Patients receiving carbamazepine and primidone showed the least deterioration; those taking phenobarbital and phenytoin showed significantly more deterioration. No specific pattern characterized any of the drugs on the 9 neuropsychological tests.

Gallassi et al. (1992) discontinued phenobarbital, phenytoin, carbamazepine, and valproic acid monotherapy in patients whose seizures were well controlled to evaluate effects on cognitive functioning and behavior. Performance was compared to that of normal controls who received no medication. The phenobarbital group differed from the controls only on two tasks: the Trail Making task and the Corsi Block Recall task. The phenytoin group differed from controls on the Raven Progressive Matrices (a nonverbal IQ test) and on the Trail Making task. These differences occurred while patients were on their full dose and disappeared as phenytoin was phased out. Patients receiving carbamazepine did not show any deficits relative to controls; subjects taking valproate had significant deficits on 4 of the 9 neurological tasks, and these deficits disappeared as the drug was discontinued.

Pulliainen and Jokelainen (1994) compared phenytoin and carbamazepine over time in patients initiating therapy, as well as no drug in controls who were included to assess the impact of practice. They found that phenytoin slowed motor responses and impaired visual memory more than carbamazepine. The healthy volunteers showed greater gains with practice (time) than either drug group. Thus phenytoin impeded performance significantly on 2 of 24 variables, although the differences could have been caused by constitutional factors in the subjects with epilepsy.

Trimble and Corbett (1980) studied 312 children with epilepsy who were living in an institution and treated with a variety of anticonvulsants. The average IQ was 66. A decrease of 10 points or more was found for 31 children. Sodium valproate, sulthiame, primidone, and phenytoin, in that order, were the drugs most commonly associated with decreased IQ scores. Carbamazepine and (notably) phenobarbital were the drugs least associated with IQ decreases. The drugs most commonly associated with psychiatric depression were phenobarbital followed by sodium valproate and phenytoin; most commonly associated with conduct disorder were phenobarbital (50% of the children) followed by valproic acid (approximately 45% of the children). Valproic acid was often prescribed in the most difficult cases. Since this was a correlational study, however, causation cannot be inferred from the results.

Calandre, Domingues-Granados, Gomez-Rubio, and Molina-Font (1990) compared phenobarbital and valproic acid in children with epilepsy and with no treatment in a normal control group. They reported that the controls and the valproate group showed significant gains in performance IQ, whereas the phenobarbital group did not. This suggests that phenobarbital may have offset the practice effect often seen with repeated testing. Another study with children generally failed to show differential improvement in psychomotor performance after phenytoin, carbamazepine, and valproic acid monotherapy were withdrawn from patients with well-controlled seizures (Aldenkamp et al., 1993). Patients showed gains on only one of 12 measures (finger tapping with dominant hand) as compared with controls. There were no differences between phenytoin and carbamazepine, but this comparison was complicated by the fact that different drugs were used for different types of epilepsy (Aldenkamp et al., 1993).

Crossover Monotherapy Studies

Another popular strategy is to compare the effects of several different drugs within the same group of patients or in normal volunteers. Thompson, Huppert, and Trimble (1980) compared the effects of placebo, phenytoin, and carbamazepine on verbal recall and on self-ratings of mood. Phenytoin caused a significant reduction in immediate and delayed recall that was strongly related to blood levels; phenytoin also caused significant increases in self-ratings of fatigue. Carbamazepine was related to poorer performance than placebo, but none of the differences reached significance. Trimble and Thompson (1986) described two crossover investigations in which doses of phenytoin, carbamazepine, and valproate were manipulated to produce low and high drug concentrations in patients receiving monotherapy. High concentrations of phenytoin and valproate produced significant deterioration on several neuropsychological tests (primarily in memory, concentration, and decision-making speed). Higher concentrations of carbamazepine produced nonsignificant improvement on several tasks, although one measure of concentration and another of motor speed deteriorated at higher concentrations.

Meador, Loring, Huh, Gallagher, and King (1990) assessed the cognitive effects of phenobarbital, phenytoin, and carbamazepine in 15 patients who received each drug for 3 months. Although subjects taking phenobarbital performed more poorly than those on other drugs, the authors concluded that the differences on the test battery were small. Meador et al. (1995) also compared the cognitive effects of phenobarbital, phenytoin, and valproic acid in 59 normal volunteers. As compared with no medication, the three antiepileptic drugs impaired cognitive functioning on over half of the neuropsychological variables. Of the three antiepileptic drugs, subjects performed worst with phenobarbital and best with valproate. The authors commented that there was no "clinically significant" difference between phenytoin and valproate, meaning that the statistical differences were minor.

Vining et al. (1987) compared the effects of phenobarbital and valproic acid on cognitive functioning and behavior in 21 children with epilepsy but without mental retardation. All children eventually received both drugs given separately for six months each. The children showed significantly worse performance on about 20% of neuropsychological tests when taking phenobarbital. On the Wechsler Intelligence Scale for Children—Revised, the children performed better on the Performance scale and on the Full Scale IQ score. The children with phenobarbital also showed more conduct and overactivity problems as rated by their parents. As judged by routine clinical assessment, phenobarbital appeared to be no more sedating than valproic acid.

Phenobarbital

Hutt, Jackson, Belsham, and Higgins (1968) assessed the

effects of 180 mg of phenobarbital on perceptual-motor performance in four healthy volunteers. Phenobarbital depressed performance significantly on key pressing and verbal learning, and rate of speaking increased dramatically with medication. The study by Meador et al. (1995), in which the cognitive effects of phenobarbital, phenytoin, and valproate were compared in healthy adults, was described earlier. Although all three antiepileptic drugs had some adverse effects on cognitive performance relative to no drug, phenobarbital was the worst of the three drugs.

There is some evidence that phenobarbital may lower intellectual functioning and other types of cognitive performance. Camfield et al. (1979) conducted a double-blind placebo-controlled randomized study of the effects of phenobarbital in 79 children with febrile seizures. There was no difference in IQ due to drug condition, but there was a significant negative correlation between serum levels of phenobarbital and scores on a subtest of memory. Phenobarbital was also associated with daytime fussiness and sleep disturbance. However, Fishman (1979) challenged the memory results because he believed that the use of the memory subtest was invalid.

Farwell et al. (1990) compared the effects of phenobarbital and placebo in 217 children with febrile seizures, between 8 and 36 months of age. They found that active drug was associated with IQ scores that were lower by 8.4 points at the end of treatment and by 5.2 points 6 months after phenobarbital was discontinued. This study received much attention in both the medical and the lay press. Although many accepted the results as evidence that chronic phenobarbital may reduce IQ, others disagreed citing methodological shortcomings pertaining to the assignment of children to different drug conditions and poor medication compliance (Addy, 1990).

In contrast, some studies found that the effects of phenobarbital were no worse than with other anticonvulsant medications. Mitchell and Chavez (1987) compared the IQ performance and behavioral effects of phenobarbital and carbamazepine in newly medicated children. The drugs did not have any measurable effects on behavior or cognition. Young, Alger, Bauer, and Lauderbaugh (1986) compared mephobarbital and phenobarbital and found no significant differences between the two drugs. However, this may not be very remarkable—as a barbiturate, mephobarbital is likely to share any adverse effects that are caused by phenobarbital. A number of uncontrolled clinical studies found no negative effects on cognitive performance with phenobarbital monotherapy (Feely, O'Callagan, Duggan,

& Callaghan, 1980; Somerfeld-Ziskind & Ziskind, 1940; Wapner, Thurston, & Holowach, 1962) or with phenobarbital in combination with phenytoin (Dodrill & Wilensky, 1992).

Primidone

There have been few studies of the effects of primidone on cognitive-motor functioning. Since primidone is metabolized in part to phenobarbital, it may share some of phenobarbital's possible adverse effects. Although an association between primidone and IQ loss was found in the correlational study of Trimble and Corbett (1980), primidone was the second best drug in terms of neuropsychological effects in the extensive Veterans Administration study conducted by Smith et al. (1987).

Phenytoin

Phenytoin sometimes has been reported to have cognitive side effects, even when patients are carefully monitored and the drugs are given within the assumed therapeutic range. In the study by Thompson et al. (1980) phenytoin impaired memory and self-ratings of fatigue. Trimble and Thompson (1986) reported deterioration on several neuropsychological tests at higher concentration of phenytoin. In the Gallassi et al. (1992) study described earlier, phenytoin appeared to impede nonverbal IQ performance and performance on the Trail Making task. These deficits disappeared when the drug was withdrawn. Pulliainen and Jokelainen (1994) observed slow rates of responding and impaired memory with phenytoin relative to carbamazepine.

In a previously discussed study, Meador et al. (1990) compared phenobarbital, phenytoin, and carbamazepine in 15 adult patients. Whereas phenobarbital caused worse performance on one cognitive task, phenytoin and carbamazepine did not differ from one another on any task. Meador et al. (1991) compared the cognitive effects of carbamazepine and phenytoin in healthy adults. Only two significant differences were found between the two drugs: a motor task favored carbamazepine and an interference test (the Stroop Reaction Time Test) favored phenytoin.

Butlin, Danta, and Cook (1984) found no impairment on memory tasks in epileptic patients on monotherapy with either carbamazepine or valproic acid, but mild impairment was found on some tests for phenytoin. Similar findings were reported by Marchesi et al. (1980). The discrepancies among these studies may be explained by the pharmacokinetics of carbamazepine. Patients performed better on memory testing while taking controlled-release tablets, which produced much smaller daily fluctuations in the blood levels, than on the regular carbamazepine tablets (Aldenkamp, Alpherts, Moerland, Ottenvanger, & Van Parys, 1987).

As noted earlier, Aldenkamp et al. (1993) observed no differences between groups of children discontinuing phenytoin and carbamazepine. Aman, Werry, Paxton, and Turbott (1994) studied phenytoin's effects in 50 children taking monotherapy and whose seizures were well controlled. By giving medication before assessment or withholding medication until after testing, they assessed the effects of high and low drug concentrations, respectively. Fluctuations in phenytoin concentrations, of the order of 50%, had minimal effects on cognitive-motor performance. Division of subjects into those with low and high drug concentrations revealed no relationships with altered cognitive-motor performance.

A number of other studies found no significant differences between phenytoin and carbamazepine in patients with epilepsy as assessed by psychological tests (Brodie, McPhail, MacPhee, & Gray, 1987; Gillham et al., 1990; Meador et al., 1995; Verma, Yusko, & Greiffenstein, 1993). Although further studies are needed, it appears that a small majority of the available studies showed deterioration of cognitive-motor performance with phenytoin relative to the newer antiepileptic drugs. Although the drug may cause some interference, this is judged to be very minor.

Ethosuximide

For some reason, the succinimides have been infrequently studied for their neuropsychological side effects (see Aman, 1984; Smith, 1991). There are only about five relevant studies and most of these have indicated improvement (Aman, 1984; Smith, 1991). Since ethosuximide is usually employed for treating absence seizures, there is a chance that any positive effects may have been the indirect result of improved seizure control. On the other hand, Trimble and Reynolds (1976) referenced a French publication (Soulayrol & Roger, 1970) that reported that intellectual efficiency fell in the majority of children treated with ethosuximide.

Benzodiazepines

The cognitive-motor effects of benzodiazepines are discussed in Chapter 12. These drugs are thought to interfere with memory and other cognitive functions, especially in low-anxious persons.

Carbamazepine

Carbamazepine may have few potential cognitive-motor side effects. As we noted previously, this drug had few effects in direct comparisons of various forms of monotherapy (Aldenkamp et al., 1993; Gallassi et al., 1992; Meador et al., 1990; Trimble & Corbett, 1980). In crossover studies, carbamazepine had no more cognitive-motor effects (Andrewes, Bullen, Tomlinson, Elwes, & Reynolds, 1986; Butlin et al., 1984; Meador et al., 1990, 1991) than other antiepileptic drugs or had fewer cognitive-motor effects than other agents (Gallassi et al., 1992; Pulliainen & Jokelainen, 1994; Thompson et al., 1980; Trimble & Thompson, 1986).

Aman, Werry, Paxton, Turbott, and Stewart (1990) studied carbamazepine in 50 children with well-controlled seizures. Drug concentration was manipulated by giving carbamazepine before test sessions (producing peak concentrations) and delaying medication until after sessions (producing trough concentrations). The children performed significantly better after taking carbamazepine (at peak concentration) on measures of seat activity, attention span, and motor steadiness.

Thus, carbamazepine is one of the least worrisome drugs in terms of effects on CNS functioning. However, in a crossover trial with healthy volunteers, carbamazepine did have some adverse effects in relation to a no drug comparison (Meador et al., 1995).

Sodium Valproate

The relevant literature on neuropsychological effects has already been discussed in the preceding sections and will not be repeated here. In one study, valproate had more severe neuropsychological side effects than carbamazepine, phenobarbital and phenytoin. Gallassi et al. (1992) found that valproate had the most significant side effects compared with carbamazepine, phenobarbital, and phenytoin, whereas Meador et al. (1995) found that valproate had the least significant side effects compared with phenytoin and phenobarbital. In other investigations, valproate was found to have fewer side effects than phenytoin and phenobarbital, but more side effects than carbamazepine (Butlin et al., 1984; Calandre et al., 1990; Trimble & Thompson, 1986; Vining et al., 1987). Aman, Werry, Paxton, and Turbott (1987) found that high doses led to impairments in psychomotor speed and in some cognitive tests in children taking valproate. However, these studies did not find that any specific pattern of neuropsychological impairment or enhancement consistently characterized valproate as different from the other antiepileptic drugs.

New Antiepileptic Drugs

Because there are relatively few data on the new anticonvulsants (vigabatrin, gabapentin, lamotrigine), impressions must be treated as somewhat tentative. In general, these agents are regarded as relatively free of neuropsychological effects. Vining, Carpenter, and Aman (in press) concluded that vigabatrin may impair vigilance, motor dexterity, and memory, but they also noted reports of psychomotor enhancement. Behaviorally, the drug has been reported to cause reversible hyperactivity, excitement, agitation, and insomnia in children. Reversible depression and psychosis sometimes occur in small percentages of treated patients.

Vining et al. (in press) found a dearth of evidence on gabapentin. Drowsiness and dizziness sometimes occur, which could affect learning. Behavioral symptoms that have been reported in children include reversible hyperactivity, oppositional behavior, and what were characterized as bizarre behaviors. Vining et al. (in press) could find very little evidence regarding neuropsychological effects of lamotrigine. There are anecdotal reports of brightened mood and enhanced cognitive-motor performance, but these need to be investigated scientifically.

Conclusion

Although this literature is inconclusive, phenobarbital appears to be the most problematic antiepileptic drug in terms of neuropsychological effects. Some specific functions, such as memory, have been found to be impaired in isolated studies. Of greatest concern are the studies that suggest a small but significant loss of IQ in phenobarbital-treated children. Phenytoin and, perhaps to a lesser degree, valproate were also associated with cognitive-motor deterioration in some studies, and this was most evident at higher plasma concentrations. Carba-

mazepine appeared to have the fewest neuropsychological effects of the well-established antiepileptic drugs; in a few cases it even appeared to facilitate performance. Primidone and ethosuximide are relatively unstudied, although (by virtue of its relationship to phenobarbital) primidone may also be found to have adverse effects. The jury is still out on the new antiepileptics, although there is some early evidence that some of these will be found to have very mild adverse effects on cognitive-motor performance. In general, the studies on cognitive side effects had methodological shortcomings.

Many individuals react idiosyncratically to the antiepileptics, such that they may have adverse responses to drugs with the best reputations (e.g., carbamazepine) or beneficial reactions to agents with a bad name (e.g., phenobarbital). As noted by the American Academy of Pediatrics Committee on Drugs (1995), the "cognitive and behavioral side effects of anticonvulsant drugs are subtle and may be discrete, affecting isolated functions rather than overall performance."

CLINICAL INDICATIONS

The principal indication for these drugs is in the treatment of epileptic disorders. Outside this group of disorders, the indications are very limited for most antiepileptics. Over the years, antiepileptic medications were tried in the treatment of psychiatric disorders. In most instances, however, they did not prove useful. Recently three antiepileptic drugs, carbamazepine, valproic acid, and clonazepam, have found a role in the treatment of mood disorders and sometimes a less certain role in other behavior disorders. The remaining antiepileptic drugs have few established behavioral or psychiatric indications.

General Principles

The indications for antiepileptic medications depend primarily on an accurate diagnosis of the seizure type and do not depend on IQ level (Coulter, 1993). By definition, epilepsy is a chronic condition, the result of excessive abnormal activity of cerebral neurons. The abnormal activity has clinical and electroencephalographic effects. The identification of these effects is essential for valid diagnosis and appropriate treatment. However, individual differences occur in the clinical manifestations of an epileptic disorder.

Table 10-7. Classification of Epileptic Seizures

I. Partial (Focal, Local) Seizures
    A. Simple partial seizures (consciousness not impaired)
        1. With motor symptoms
        2. With somatosensory or special sensory symptoms
        3. With autonomic symptoms
        4. With psychic symptoms
    B. Complex partial seizures (with impairment of consciousness)
        1. Beginning as simple partial seizures and progressing to impairment of consciousness
        2. With impairment of consciousness at onset
    C. Partial seizures secondarily generalized

II. Generalized Seizures (Convulsive or Nonconvulsive)
    A. Absence and atypical seizures
        1. Absence seizures
        2. Atypical absence seizures
    B. Myoclonic seizures
    C. Clonic seizures
    D. Tonic seizures
    E. Tonic-clonic seizures
    F. Atonic seizures

III. Unclassified Epileptic Seizures

Most efforts to classify seizures are based on morphological descriptions of the epileptic event. New technology that allows simultaneous video recording of the electroencephalogram and the epileptic seizure has contributed to the understanding and definition of these events. A summary of the International Classification of Epileptic Seizures is presented in Table 10-7 (Commission on Classification and Terminology of the International League Against Epilepsy, 1981). This classification is based on the description of clinical events and associated EEG changes. The epileptic seizures are divided into two principal groups, partial and generalized, with a third option for those cases that cannot be classified. The partial seizures are those in which there is initial activation of a system of neurons limited to part of one cerebral hemisphere. These seizures are further divided into two groups depending on whether or not consciousness is impaired at the time of the seizure. A partial seizure might also evolve into a generalized seizure, indistinguishable clinically from a generalized seizure without a focal component. Generalized seizures are those in which the first clinical changes indicate initial involvement of both hemispheres of the brain.

Epileptic syndromes are divided into localized (partial or "focal") and generalized epilepsies (see Table 10-8). Within these two groups, the syndromes are further subdivided into idiopathic (unknown cause, probably genetic) and cryptogenic or symptomatic (organic cause is suspected or known) (Dreifuss, 1993). The clinical history and the electroencephalogram are the two most important elements in the diagnosis of epilepsy.

Electroencephalograms (EEGs) are very useful in the diagnosis of epilepsy and should be employed in all individuals with a suspected seizure disorder. Some epileptic seizures do not have a manifestation in the EEG, but this is the exception. It is very difficult to obtain an EEG in some persons with severe behavior disorders who are uncooperative, but it is often possible to obtain an EEG in such patients with simple techniques such as sleep deprivation, sedation, and special adapted hats (Alvarez & Sullivan, 1993). The best way to diagnose epileptic seizures is through long-term monitoring of the EEG with simultaneous video recording of the EEG and the patient. With this technique, a composite image can be obtained in a split video (Porter, Penry, & Wolfe, 1976; Sato, Penry, & Dreifuss, 1976; Sutula, Sackellares, Miller, & Dreifuss, 1981).

Once the diagnosis of epilepsy is confirmed, treatment is started with only one medication. If this medication does not control the epileptic disorder, a second medication is introduced. If this medication is effective, then the first medication is withdrawn. Very few patients will

Table 10-8. International Classification of Epilepsies and Epileptic Syndromes

1.0   Localization-related (focal, local, partial) epilepsies and syndromes
    1.1   Idiopathic (with age-related onset)
        a. Benign childhood epilepsy with centro-temporal spikes
        b. Childhood epilepsy with occipital paroxysms
    1.2   Symptomatic
    1.3   Unknown as to whether the behavior is symptomatic or idiopathic

2.0   Generalized epilepsies and syndromes
    2.1   Idiopathic (with age-related onset, listed in order of age)
        a. Benign neonatal familial convulsions
        b. Benign neonatal convulsions
        c. Benign myoclonic epilepsy of infancy
        d. Childhood absence epilepsy (pyknolepsy)
        e. Juvenile absence epilepsy
        f. Juvenile myoclonic epilepsy (impulsive petit mal)
        g. Epilepsy with grand mal (GTCS) seizures on awakening
    2.2   Cryptogenic or symptomatic (in order of age)
        a. West syndrome (infantile spasm)
        b. Lennox-Gastaut syndrome
        c. Epilepsy with myoclonic-astatic seizures
        d. Epilepsy with myoclonic absence
    2.3   Symptomatic
        2.3.1 Nonspecific etiology
            a. Early myoclonic encephalopathy
        2.3.2 Specific syndromes
            a. Epileptic seizures may complicate many disease states

3.0   Epilepsies and syndromes undetermined whether focal or generalized
    3.1   With both generalized and focal seizures
        a. Neonatal seizures
        b. Severe myoclonic epilepsy in infancy
        c. Epilepsy with continuous spike-wave during slow wave sleep
        d. Acquired epileptic aphasia (Landau-Kleffner syndrome)

4.0   Special syndromes
    4.1   a. Febrile convulsions

need a combination of two antiepileptic medications, and even fewer need three medications. Some cases of refractory epilepsy may require surgery.

Prior to 1975, it was common practice to resort to polytherapy in order to control difficult epileptic disorders. Since these drugs have different modes of action, polytherapy was thought to increase the chances of beneficial effects. Similar thinking is used to treat other disorders, such as polypharmacy in the treatment of cancer. However, the cumulative experience with patients with epilepsy is that the side effects outweigh the benefits when anticonvulsants are used in polytherapy, and several investigators have found that polypharmacy is not needed in persons with mental retardation (Beghi et al., 1987; Coulter, 1988). The same guidelines on polytherapy with regard to persons with epilepsy in general are also valid for persons with epilepsy and mental retardation.

Since the medications presently available do not cure epileptic disorders, most of the people found to have epilepsy can expect years of daily treatment. At least two years free of seizures are necessary before a decrease in medications should be considered. Attempts to discontinue antiepileptic medications without further seizures may be less successful in persons with mental retardation than in patients without retardation (Alvarez & Hazlett, 1983; Coulter, 1989; Mirza, Credeur, & Penry, 1993).

Fewer severe side effects and at least equal antiepileptic efficacy are reasons for choosing carbamazepine or valproate as a first choice over other drugs, although drugs such as phenobarbital and phenytoin have a good antiepileptic effect and are much cheaper. Additionally, phenobarbital has minimal systemic effects. Lerman and Lerman-Sagie (1995) have suggested the use of phenobarbital monotherapy when it controls seizures at low doses.

Choice of Antiepileptic Drug

Antiepileptic medications are not uniformly helpful for all types of epilepsy. The primary antiseizure indications for individual agents are listed below. The choice of antiepileptic drug depends on its therapeutic effects, side effects, and cost. Other applications are also summarized.

Phenobarbital. Phenobarbital is as effective as other major antiepileptic medications in generalized tonic, clonic, tonic-clonic seizures, or partial epilepsy with or without generalized seizures (Heller et al., 1995). It is one of the drugs of choice in the treatment of status epilepticus and in the treatment of neonatal seizures. For many years it was the drug of choice in the prevention of febrile seizures; however, today its use in febrile seizures is limited to very specific cases (Freeman, 1980).

Primidone. The indications for primidone are similar to those for phenobarbital; for practical purposes, primidone may be considered a barbiturate. Mattson et al. (1985) found that primidone was effective in generalized tonic-clonic as well as in complex partial seizures. However, the side effects were higher with primidone than with several other drugs examined. Patients who were able to tolerate primidone therapy had equivalent seizure control as with the other medications. Similar results were reported in studies conducted by Rodin et al. (1976) and by White, Plott, and Noton (1966). Primidone has also been used with some success in the treatment of essential tremors.

Phenytoin. Phenytoin is indicated in generalized tonic-clonic seizures, partial seizures with or without generalization, and status epilepticus developed from these seizure types. One advantage of phenytoin compared with other anticonvulsant drugs is its cost effectiveness. It is not indicated in the primary generalized epilepsies. It also may be used in cardiac arrhythmias and atrial fibrillation, although other drugs are more effective.

Benzodiazepines. Benzodiazepines are also discussed in Chapter 12. Diazepam (Valium) and lorazepam (Ativan) are used in the treatment of status epilepticus. Clonazepam (Klonopin), nitrazepam (Mogadan), and clorazepate (Tranxene) have a broad antiepileptic effect. They are effective in generalized tonic-clonic seizures, myoclonic seizures, typical and atypical absences, and simple and complex partial seizures with or without secondary generalization. They are mostly used in conjunction with other antiepileptic medications, and there is limited experience with the use of these drugs in monotherapy. Rapid eye movement (REM) onset sleep disorders have been successfully treated with clonazepam. Clonazepam might be particularly effective in the management of Lennox-Gastaut syndrome (Homan & Rosenberg, 1993). However, tolerance is a limiting factor with chronic use. Diazepam (Valium) and lorazepam (Ativan) are indicated in the treatment of status epilepticus. Diazepam and lorazepam are very effective in generalized tonic-clonic status and in partial motor and complex status (Browne & Penry, 1973). There is little indication for these drugs in the chronic treatment of epilepsy.

Carbamazepine. The two main indications for carbamazepine are in the treatment of epilepsy and mood disorders. Therapeutic effects are similar to those of the other major antiepileptic medications in the treatment of generalized tonic-clonic seizures and focal seizures with or without generalization (Heller et al., 1995; Mattson et al., 1985). Carbamazepine is not indicated in the treatment of absence seizures, myoclonic seizures, atonic, or akinetic seizures. Other indications are trigeminal and glossopharyngeal neuralgia (Rushton, Stevens, & Miller, 1981), a sleep disorder called nocturnal paroxysmal dystonia (Maccario & Lutsman, 1990), and some cases of multiple sclerosis (Schapiro, 1994). Oxcarbazepine is as effective as carbamazepine in partial and generalized tonic-clonic seizures. The drug appears to be effective in refractory partial and secondary generalized tonic-clonic seizures (Fisher & Blum, 1995).

Valproic Acid. Valproate is used in the treatment of both epileptic and mood disorders. Valproate is as effective as the other major antiepileptic medications in the treatment of simple and complex partial seizures with and without secondary generalization (Heller et al., 1995; Verity et al., 1995). Some researchers have suggested that carbamazepine is more effective than valproate in the treatment of complex partial seizures. Valproate is as effective as ethosuximide in the treatment of absence seizures and is the drug of choice when absence seizures are associated with generalized tonic-clonic seizures. Valproate is superior to other antiepileptic medications in the treatment of generalized epilepsies (Jeavons, Clark, & Maheswari, 1977). It is particularly effective in the treatment of photoconvulsive epilepsies (Jeavons, Bishop, & Harding, 1986), juvenile myoclonic epilepsy (Penry, Dean, & Riela, 1989), and certain epileptic syndromes in which myoclonic, tonic, or atonic-akinetic seizures are predominant. This includes the Lennox-Gastaut syndrome, a frequent cause of intractable seizures in persons with brain damage and mental retardation. Other potential indications are in the management of migraine disorders (Mathew et al., 1995) and possibly in the prevention of febrile seizures.

Gabapentin. Gabapentin has been used as add-on medication mostly in cases of refractory epilepsy. It is particularly effective in patients with partial seizures with or without generalization (Anhut et al., 1994; Chadwick, 1993; Crawford et al., 1987; Ramsay, 1994; Sivenius, Kalviainen, Mine, & Riekkinen, 1991; U.K. Gabapentin Study Group, 1990; U.S. Gabapentin Study Group No. 5, 1993). Presently there is limited information to support the efficacy of gabapentin in monotherapy (McLean, 1995). Periodic monitoring of blood counts and liver function tests are advisable when this medication is used. Anecdotal experience suggests that gabapentin can be used in children with partial seizures, but the lack of a liquid preparation or chewable tablet often makes this difficult.

Lamotrigine. This medication has been approved in the United States for the treatment of partial seizures. It is also useful in the treatment of primary generalized epilepsies including myoclonic, tonic-clonic, and absence seizures, and in cases with infantile spasms and Lennox-Gastaut syndrome (Matsuo et al., 1993; Messenheimer et al., 1994; Schapel et al., 1993; Schlumberger et al., 1994; Steiner, Silviera, & Yuen, 1994). Clinical improvement may be observed with doses of 300 mg/day but usually is better with doses of 500 mg per day (Dren, Moore, & U.S. Lamictal Protocol 05 Clinical Trial Group, 1991). It can be used as an add-on medication or in monotherapy. Some studies found that lamotrigine can reduce polypharmacy in cases with refractory seizures (Schlumberger et al., 1994). Lamotrigine has been used successfully in children with the Lennox-Gastaut syndrome. Other studies have shown that lamotrigine is effective in generalized and in focal seizures, suggesting an action very similar to valproate but with less severe side effects. Periodic monitoring of blood counts and liver function tests are advisable when this medication is used.

Vigabatrin. Vigabatrin is used to treat complex partial seizures, secondary generalized seizures, and generalized tonic-clonic seizures (Browne et al., 1987, 1991; Dam, 1991). It is also effective in the treatment of infantile spasms (Mattson et al., 1994), cryptogenic and sympto-

matic partial epilepsy in children, and Lennox-Gastaut syndrome in children (Dulac et al., 1991; Uldall, Alving, Gram, & Beck, 1991). However, seizure frequency may increase in some children with myoclonic epilepsy (Dulac et al., 1991). Vigabatrin has been used with mixed results to treat motor disorders, such as tardive dyskinesia and spasticity (Grant & Heel, 1991).

Felbamate. Felbamate is the only new drug that is approved for use in children, *but the risk of severe adverse effects is such that it is now used only as a last choice for patients with refractory seizures who have not responded to other drugs.* Felbamate can be very useful in children with Lennox-Gastaut syndrome who have incapacitating atonic seizures. Felbamate, gabapentin, and lamotrigine are all approved for the treatment of adolescents and adults with partial seizures. Felbamate was thought to be very safe when it was introduced, but it has been found to cause severe adverse effects that were discussed previously in this chapter. With felbamate therapy, periodic monitoring of blood counts and liver function tests are required.

Topiramate. This medication is effective as adjunctive therapy in adults with partial seizures with and without generalization. It is also effective in children with Lennox-Gastaut syndrome.

CONSIDERATIONS IN MENTAL RETARDATION

Antiepileptic medications are used in essentially the same ways in people with mental retardation as in the general population. However, the presence of other drugs or other physical conditions may complicate their use. Here we discuss clinical indications and research findings with special implications for the treatment of patients with developmental disabilities.

People with mental retardation are at high risk for epilepsy. The risk is strongly tied to the level of mental retardation, with far more of those with profound retardation having epilepsy (Pond, 1979) than those with mild retardation. Pond (1979) reviewed a number of prevalence studies and found that 3% to 6% of people having IQs between 50 to 70 have epilepsy, but the prevalence of seizures was as high as 42% in one report of people with more severe mental retardation.

Epilepsy can be difficult to diagnose in people with mental retardation. The clinician must depend on relatives or other professionals involved in the care of the patient. Some persons with mental retardation have abnormal behaviors that resemble epileptic disorders.

Many of the behavioral changes associated with epilepsy are not specific to the epileptic disorders. Without a good clinical history, behaviors that are not necessarily of epileptic origin may be misdiagnosed. The problem of pseudoseizures is well known by neurologists (King et al., 1982; Luther, McNamara, Carwile, Miller, & Hope, 1982), and the extent of the problem in persons with mental retardation is well documented (Holmes, McKeever, & Russman, 1983; Neill & Alvarez, 1986). When pseudoseizures are not recognized as such, the use of antiepileptic medication is rarely useful and is one of the leading causes of polypharmacy and subsequent intoxication.

Phenobarbital

Especially when first used, phenobarbital often leads to hyperactive behavior in children (Bacon, Cranage, Hierons, Rawlins, & Webb, 1981; Farwell et al., 1990). Most but not all affected children improve with the discontinuance of medication. The phenomenon is not related to the blood levels of phenobarbital, but it is correlated with prior history of behavior problems (Wolf et al., 1977; Wolf & Forsythe, 1978). Burd, Kerbeshian, and Fisher (1987) found that initiation of phenobarbital was followed by hyperactive behaviors in 16 out of 130 children with multiple handicaps and mental retardation. In some cases, the hyperactivity started abruptly after the initiation of therapy and lasted for months. There was improvement in all cases after the phenobarbital was discontinued, but a residual effect persisted in some patients. Ounsted (1955) and Ingram (1986) also found that phenobarbital exacerbated preexisting hyperactivity and aggressive tendencies.

Herranz et al. (1988) evaluated 392 children on long-term monotherapy with phenobarbital, primidone, phenytoin, carbamazepine, or valproic acid. The children were being treated for either epilepsy or febrile seizures. Increased frequencies of behavior problems were found with all antiepileptic medications but were much more frequent with phenobarbital. Phenobarbital was discontinued for as many as 4% of the children who were taking the drug.

Benzodiazepines

Benzodiazepines are also muscle relaxants. They are indicated in the treatment of spasticity, which has a relatively high incidence in people with mental retardation,

epilepsy, and the spastic form of cerebral palsy. In people needing a muscle relaxant who also have epilepsy, agents from the benzodiazepine group may serve a dual role (i.e., reduction of muscle spasms and seizures).

Carbamazepine

Some reports suggested that persons with developmental disabilities may experience an exacerbation of preexisting behavior problems when carbamazepine therapy is initiated. However, this is probably the exception more than the rule. The effects of carbamazepine are not related to the degree of mental retardation or the presence of brain damage, but since carbamazepine has both a low toxicity and minimal disruptive effects on cognition and behavior, it is widely used in persons with mental retardation.

Valproate

As noted earlier, coagulation problems may occur (rarely) with valproate, leading to hemorrhage or easy bruising. This may require excluding the drug in some patients with self-injury.

Lamotrigine

Little is known about the use of lamotrigine in persons with mental retardation, although one study reported a positive clinical experience in children attending a special residential school (Besag, 1992). Other studies are believed to have included patients with brain damage and mental retardation without reporting separate results for this population. For example, 62% of the children in the Schlumberger et al. (1994) study had mental retardation. Future researchers may find that lamotrigine is an important drug in the treatment of children and adults with brain damage or mental retardation. It has a wide spectrum of action, a good safety record, and encouraging results with persons with refractory seizures, especially in the Lennox-Gastaut syndrome (Oller, Russi, & Oller-Daurella, 1991; Timmings & Richens, 1992).

Polypharmacy

Several studies evaluated the reduction of anticonvulsants in patients with mental retardation receiving polypharmacy. Generally, the use of fewer drugs did not cause an increase in seizure frequency (Alvarez & Hazlett, 1983; Beghi et al., 1987; Coulter, 1988; Fischbacher, 1982; Wilkinson, Murphy, Georgeson, & D'souza, 1982). Improvements in behavior or cognition were reported by Mirza et al. (1993), Poindexter, Berglund, and Kolstoe (1993), and Theodore and Porter (1983). However, there were methodological limitations in some of these studies. For a more detailed account of indications, readers should consult Coulter (1993), Dodson and Pellock (1993), and Wyllie (1993).

CONCLUSIONS

The antiepileptic drugs are a heterogeneous group of medications whose common trait is their ability to suppress seizures. Depending upon the agent, the anticonvulsants are capable of causing a wide array of side effects that may vary in severity from having nuisance value to having life-threatening effects. The antiepileptic drugs have widely varying pharmacodynamic effects and are capable of interacting with one another and with a wide range of other drugs. Conversely, numerous other agents can influence the effects of the anticonvulsants. Physicians must have full knowledge of all agents being taken when treating a patient for epilepsy.

Antiepileptic drugs may have unintended effects on the person's cognitive, motor, or emotional state. This has been a difficult area of research because of methdological limitations. The available data suggest that phenobarbital may have mild adverse effects on memory and IQ. A smaller percentage of the studies suggest that phenytoin may have adverse cognitive-motor effects; furthermore, some studies suggest that valproate and carbamazepine may have harmful effects. However, individuals show considerable variations in these effects.

Phenobarbital is an effective drug in a variety of epileptic disorders. However, it is no longer considered a drug of first choice because of its possible behavioral and cognitive effects. Primidone also is a useful drug, but again, it is rarely indicated as a first choice because of its side effects and complex pharmacology. Phenytoin has long been a mainstay of therapy in epilepsy, but its use is giving way to newer agents. Many patients who were previously treated with phenobarbital, primidone, or phenytoin are successfully treated with carbamazepine. Carbamazepine generally gives equivalent seizure control but may cause fewer cognitive side effects. Carbamazepine also has a useful role in managing some patients with mood disorders. Oxcarbazepine, already approved in several countries but not in the U.S., is a promising antiepileptic drug.

Valproate is effective against many types of seizure disorders and can be helpful in manic disorder. The systemic side effects are significant but limited to a small number of individuals.

Gabapentin is a useful new arrival. Because of its safety and the absence of major interactions, gabapentin is an attractive medication for use with people with mental retardation. Initial clinical experiences suggest that vigabatrin may become an important drug for the treatment of severe epileptic disorders in both adults and children.

Finally, there are a number of special circumstances that need to be considered when these drugs are used with people with mental retardation. Foremost among these is the high prevalence of epilepsy in the population. Many people with mental retardation are likely to be receiving psychotropic agents, which heightens the need to be vigilant for drug interactions. History taking and monitoring of treatment may be much more difficult in people with mental retardation, and the prevalence of motor disorder (i.e., cerebral palsy) or self-injury may have implications for the choice of therapy.

REFERENCES

Aarli, J.A., & Tinder, O. (1975). Effects of antiepileptic drugs on serum and salivary IgA. *Scandinavian Journal of Immunology*, 4, 391–396.

Addy, D.P. (1990). Phenobarbitone and febrile seizures. *Archives of Disease in Childhood*, 65, 921.

Aldenkamp, A.P., Alpherts, W.C.J., Blennow, G., Elmqvist, D., Heijbel, J., Nilsson, H.L., Sandstedt, P., Tonnby, B., Wahlander, L., & Wosse, E. (1993). Withdrawal of antiepileptic medication in children—effects on cognitive function: The multicenter Holmfrid study. *Neurology*, 43, 41–50.

Aldenkamp, A.P., Alpherts, W.C.J., Moerland, M.C., Ottenvanger, N., & Van Parys, J.A.P. (1987). Controlled release carbamazepine: Cognitive side effects in patients with epilepsy. *Epilepsia*, 28, 507–514.

Alvarez, N., & Hazlett, J. (1983). Seizure management with minimal medication in institutionalized mentally retarded epileptics: A prospective study. First report after 4¹/₂ years of follow up. *Clinical Electroencephalography*, 14, 164–172.

Alvarez, N., & Sullivan, J. (1993). Successes in the EEG lab in obtaining EEGs. In D. Antanitus (Ed.), *Success stories in developmental disabilities* (Vol. 2, pp. 2–5). Balla Cynwyd, PA: Liberty Health Care.

Aman, M.G. (1984). Drugs and learning in mentally retarded persons. In G.D. Burrows & J.S. Werry (Eds.), *Advances in human psychopharmacology* (Vol. 3, pp. 121–163). Greenwich, CT: JAI Press.

Aman, M.G., Paxton, J.W., Field, C.J., & Foote, S.F. (1986). Prevalence of toxic anticonvulsant drug concentrations in mentally retarded persons with epilepsy. *American Journal of Mental Deficiency, 90,* 643–650.

Aman, M.G., Werry, J.S., Paxton, J.W., & Turbott, S.H. (1987). Effects of sodium valproate on psychomotor performance in children as a function of dose, fluctuations in concentration, and diagnosis. *Epilepsia, 28,* 115–128.

Aman, M.G., Werry, J.S., Paxton, J.W., & Turbott, S.H. (1994). Effects of phenytoin on cognitive-motor performance in children as a function of drug concentration, seizure type, and time of medication. *Epilepsia, 35,* 172–180.

Aman, M.G., Werry, J.S., Paxton, J.W., Turbott, S.H., & Stewart, A.W. (1990). The effects of carbamazepine on psychomotor performance in children as a function of drug concentration, seizure type, and time of medication. *Epilepsia, 31,* 51–60.

American Academy of Pediatrics Committee on Drugs. (1995). Behavioral and cognitive effects of anticonvulsant therapy. *Pediatrics, 96,* 538–540.

Andrewes, D.G., Bullen, J.G., Tomlinson, L., Elwes, R.D., & Reynolds, E.H. (1986). A comparative study of the effects of phenytoin and carbamazepine in new referrals with epilepsy. *Epilepsia, 27,* 128–134.

Anhut, H., Ashman, P., Feurstein, T.J., Sauerman, W., Saunders, M., Schmidt, B., & The International Gabapentin Group. (1994). Gabapentin (Neurontin) as add-on therapy in patients with partial seizures: A double-blind, placebo-controlled study. *Epilepsia, 35,* 795–801.

Bacon, C.J., Cranage, J.D., Hierons, A.M., Rawlins, M.D., & Webb, J.K.G. (1981). Behavioural effects of phenobarbital and phenytoin in small children. *Archives of Disease in Childhood, 56,* 836–840.

Barnes, S.E., & Bower, B.D. (1975). Sodium valproate in the treatment of intractable childhood epilepsy. *Developmental Medicine and Child Neurology, 17,* 175–181.

Beghi, E., Bollini, P., DiMascio, R.C., Cerisola, N., Merloni, T., & Manghi, E. (1987). Effects of rationalizing drug treatment of patients with epilepsy and mental retardation. *Developmental Medicine and Child Neurology, 29,* 363–369.

Berg, M.J., Finchman, R.W., Ebert, B.E., & Schottelius, D.D. (1988). Decrease of serum folates in healthy male volunteers taking phenytoin. *Epilepsia, 29,* 67–73.

Besag, F.C.M. (1992). Lamotrigine: Pediatric experience. In A. Richens (Ed.), *Clinical update on lamotrigine: A novel antiepileptic agent* (pp. 53–60). Turnbridge Wells: Wells Medical.

Bigler, D. (1985). Neurological sequelae after intoxication with sodium valproate. *Acta Neurologica Scandinavica, 72,* 351–352.

Boesen, F., Andersen, E.B., Jensen, E.K., &

Ladefoged, S.D. (1983). Cardiac conduction disturbances during carbamazepine therapy. *Acta Neurologica Scandinavica, 68,* 49–52.

Bohan, T.P., Roggers, P., & Roe, C.R. (1992). Valproate and carnitine. In L. Carter (Ed.), *Current concepts in carnitine research* (pp 19–26). Boca Raton: CRC Press.

Brodie, M.J., McPhail, E., MacPhee, G.J.A., & Gray, J.M.B. (1987). Psychomotor impairment and anticonvulsant therapy. *European Journal of Clinical Pharmacology, 31,* 655–660.

Brodie, M.J., Richens, A., & The U.K. Lamotrigine/Carbamazepine Monotherapy Trial Group. (1994). Lamotrigine versus carbamazepine: A double-blind comparative study in newly diagnosed epilepsy. *Epilepsia, 35*(Suppl. 8), 31.

Browne, T., & Penry, J. (1973). Benzodiazepines in the treatment of epilepsy. *Epilepsia, 14,* 277–310.

Browne, T.R. (1978). Clonazepam. *New England Journal of Medicine, 299,* 812–816.

Browne, T.R., Mattson, R.H., Penry, J.K., Smith, D.B., Treiman, D.M., Wilder, B.J., Ben-Menachem, E., McBride, R.G., & Sherry, K.M. (1991). Multicenter long-term safety and efficacy study of vigabatrin for refractory complex partial seizures: An update. *Neurology, 41,* 363–364.

Browne, T.R., Mattson, R.H., Penry, J.K., Smith, D.B., Treiman, D.M., Wilder, B.J., Ben-Menachem, E., Napoliello, M.J., Sherry, K.M., & Szabo, G.K. (1987). Vigabatrin for refractory complex partial seizures: Multicenter single-blind study with long-term follow-up. *Neurology, 37,* 184–189.

Burd, L., Kerbeshian, M.D., & Fisher, W. (1987). Does the use of phenobarbital as an anticonvulsant permanently exacerbate hyperactivity? *Canadian Journal of Psychiatry, 32,* 10–13.

Butlin, A.T., Danta, G., & Cook, M.L. (1984). Anticonvulsant effects on the memory performance of epileptics. *Clinical and Experimental Neurology, 20,* 27–35.

Calandre, E., Domingues-Granados, R., Gomez-Rubio, M., & Molina-Font, J.A. (1990). Cognitive effects of long term treatment with phenobarbital and valproic acid in school children. *Acta Neurologica Scandinavica, 81,* 504–506.

Camfield, C.S., Chaplin, S., Doyle, A.B., Shapiro, S.H., Cummings, C., & Camfield, P.R. (1979). Side effects of phenobarbital in toddlers: Behavioral and cognitive aspects. *Journal of Pediatrics, 95,* 361–365.

Camfield, P.R. (1979). Pancreatitis due to valproic acid. *Lancet, 1,* 1198–1199.

Cannon, D.J., Butler, W.H., Mumford, J.P., & Lewis, P.J. (1991). Neuropathological findings in patients receiving long-term vigabatrin therapy for chronic intractable epilepsy. *Journal of Child Neurology, 6*(Suppl. 2), 2S17–2S24.

Chadwick, D. (1993). The role of gabapentin in epilepsy management. In D. Chadwick (Ed.), *New trends in epilepsy management: The role of gabapentin* (pp. 59–65). London: Royal Society of Medicine Services.

Cloyd, J.C., & Kriel, R.L. (1981). Bioavailability of rectally administered valproic acid syrup. *Neurology, 31,* 1348–1352.

Cloyd, J.C., Kriel, R.L., Jones-Saete, C.M., Ong, B.Y., Jancik, J.T., & Remmel, R.P. (1992). Comparison of sprinkle versus syrup formulations of valproate for bioavailability, tolerance, and preference. *Journal of Pediatrics, 120,* 634–638.

Commission on Classification and Terminology of the International League Against Epilepsy. (1981). Proposal for revised clinical and electroencephalographic classification of epileptic seizures. *Epilepsia, 22,* 489–501.

Coulter, D. (1991). Carnitine, valproate and toxicity. *Journal of Child Neurology, 6,* 7–14.

Coulter, D., & Allen, R.J. (1980). Pancreatitis associated with valproic acid therapy. *Annals of Neurology, 7,* 92.

Coulter, D.L. (1988). Withdrawal of barbiturate anticonvulsant drugs: Prospective control study. *American Journal on Mental Retardation, 93,* 320–327.

Coulter, D.L. (1989). Withdrawal of sedative anticonvulsant drugs from mentally retarded persons: Development of guidelines. *Journal of Epilepsy, 1,* 67–70.

Coulter, D.L. (1993). Epilepsy and mental retardation: An overview. *American Journal on Mental Retardation, 98*(Suppl.), 1–11.

Crawford, P., Ghadualis, E., Lane, R., Blumhardt, L., & Catwalk, D. (1987). Gabapentin as an antiepileptic drug. *Journal of Neurology, Neurosurgery and Psychiatry, 50,* 682–686.

Dally, M.A. (1971). Antiepileptic and psychotropic effects of carbamazepine (Tegretol) in the treatment of psychomotor epilepsy. *Epilepsia, 12,* 325–334.

Dam, M. (1991). Vigabatrin in refractory epilepsy in adults and its application in children. *Journal of Child Neurology, 6*(Suppl. 2), 2S25–2S29.

Devinsky, O. (1995). Cognitive and behavioral effects of antiepileptic drugs. *Epilepsia, 36*(Suppl. 2), S46–S65.

Dinesen, H., Gram, L., Anderson, T., & Dam, M. (1984). Weight gain during treatment with valproate. *Acta Neurologica Scandinavica, 70,* 65–69.

Dodrill, C.B., & Wilensky, A. (1992). Neuropsychological abilities before and after 5 years of stable antiepileptic drug therapy. *Neurology, 2,* 327–334.

Dodson, E.W., & Pellock, J. M. (1993). *Pediatric epilepsy: Diagnosis and therapy.* New York: Demos.

Dreifuss, F.E. (1993). Classification of epilepsies in childhood. In E. Dodson & J.M. Pekock (Eds.), *Pediatric epilepsy:*

Diagnosis and therapy. New York: Demos.

Dreifuss, F.E., & Langer, D.H. (1988). Side effects of valproate. *The American Journal of Medicine, 84*(Suppl. Ia), 39–41.

Dreifuss, F.E., Langer, D.H., Moline, K.A., & Maxwell, J.E. (1989). Valproic acid hepatic fatalities: U.S. experience since 1984. *Neurology, 39*, 201–207.

Dreifuss, F.E., Santilli, N., Langer, D.H., Sweeney, K.P., Moline, K.A., & Menander, K.B. (1987). Valproic acid hepatic fatalities: A retrospective review. *Neurology, 37*, 379– 385.

Dren, A.T., Moore, E.L., & The U.S. Lamictal Protocol 05 Clinical Trial Group. (1991). Placebo-controlled, dose response evaluation of the efficacy and safety of lamotrigine (Lamictal) as add-on therapy in epileptic out-patients with partial seizures. *Epilepsia, 32*(Suppl. 3), 20.

Dulac, O., Chiron, C., Luna, D., Cusmai, R., Pajot, N., Beaumont, D., & Mondragon, S. (1991). Vigabatrin in childhood epilepsy. *Journal of Child Neurology, 6*(Suppl. 2), 2S30–2S37.

Eldridge, R., Iivanainen, M., Stern, R., Koerber, T., & Wilder, B.J. (1983). "Baltic" myoclonus epilepsy: Hereditary disorder of childhood made worse by phenytoin. *Lancet, 2*, 838–842.

Evans, R.W., & Gualtieri, C.T. (1985). Carbamazepine: A neuropsychological and psychiatric profile. *Clinical Neuropharmacology, 8*, 221–241.

Farwell, J., Young, J., Hartz, D., Sulzbacher, S., Ellenberg, J., & Nelson, K. (1990). Phenobarbital for febrile seizures: Effects on intelligence and on seizure recurrence. *New England Journal of Medicine, 322*, 364–369.

Feely, M., O'Callagan, M., Duggan, G., & Callaghan, N. (1980). Phenobarbital in previously untreated epilepsy. *Journal of Neurology, Neurosurgery and Psychiatry, 43*, 365–368.

Fischbacher, E. (1982). Effects of reduction anticonvulsants on well-being. *British Medical Journal, 285*, 423–424.

Fisher, J.H., Barr, A.N., Rogers, S.L., Fischer, P.A., & Trudeau, V. L. (1994). Lack of serious toxicity following gabapentin overdose. *Neurology, 44*, 982–983.

Fisher, R., & Blum, D. (1995). Clobazam, oxcarbazepine, tiagabine, topiramate, and other antiepileptic drugs. *Epilepsia, 36*(Suppl. 2), S105–S114.

Fishman, M.A. (1979). Commentary: Side effects of phenobarbital. *The Journal of Pediatrics, 95*, 403–404.

Forsythe, W.I., & Sills, M.A. (1984). One drug for childhood grand mal: Medical audit for three-year remissions. *Developmental Medicine and Child Neurology, 26*, 742–748.

Freeman, J.M. (1980). Febrile seizures: A consensus of their significance, evaluation, and treatment. *Pediatrics, 66*, 1009.

Friedman, D.L., Kastner, T., Plummer, A.T.,

Ruiz, M.Q., & Hanning, D. (1992). Adverse behavioral effects in individuals with mental retardation and mood disorders treated with carbamazepine. *American Journal on Mental Retardation, 96*, 541–546.

Friis, B., & Sardemann, H. (1977). Neonatal hypocalcaemia after intrauterine exposure to anticonvulsant drugs. *Archives of Disease in Childhood, 52*, 239–247.

Gaily, E. (1990). Distal phalangeal hypoplasia in children with prenatal phenytoin exposure: Results of a controlled anthropometric study. *American Journal of Medical Genetics, 35*, 574–578.

Gallassi, R., Morreale, A., Di Sarro, R., Marra, M., Lugaresi, E., & Baruzzi, A. (1992). Cognitive effects of antiepileptic drug discontinuation. *Epilepsia, 33* (Suppl. 6), S41–S44.

Gharib, H., & Munoz, J.M. (1974). Endocrine manifestations of diphenylhydantoin therapy. *Metabolism, 23*, 515–524.

Gillham, R.A., Williams, N., Wiedman, K.D., Butler, E., Larkin, J.G., & Brodie, M.J. (1990). Cognitive function in adult epileptic patients established on anticonvulsant monotherapy. *Epilepsy Research, 7*, 219–225.

Gilhus, N.E., & Aarli, J.A. (1981). Respiratory disease and nasal immunoglobulin concentrations in phenytoin-treated patients. *Acta Neurologica Scandinavica, 63*, 34–43.

Grant, S.M., & Heel, R.C. (1991). Vigabatrin. A review of its pharmacodynamic and pharmacokinetic properties, and therapeutic potential in epilepsy and disorders of motor control. *Drugs, 41*, 889–926.

Hahn, T.J. (1976). Bone complications of anticonvulsants. *Drugs, 12*, 201–211.

Hanna, D.R. (1992). Purple glove syndrome: A complication of intravenous phenytoin. *Journal of Neurosciences in Nursing, 24*, 340–345.

Hayes, A.G., & Chesney, T.M. (1993). Necrosis of the hand after extravasation of intravenously administered phenytoin. *Journal of the American Academy of Dermatology, 28*, 360–363.

Heller, A.J., Chesterman, R.D., Crawford, P., Chadwick, D., Johnson, A.L., & Reynolds, E.H. (1995). Phenobarbitone, phenytoin, carbamazepine, or sodium valproate for newly diagnosed adult epilepsy: A randomized comparative monotherapy trial. *Journal of Neurology, Neurosurgery, and Psychiatry, 58*, 44–50.

Herranz, J.L., Armijo, J.A., & Arteaga, R. (1988). Clinical side effects of phenobarbital, primidone, phenytoin, carbamazepine, and valproate during monotherapy in children. *Epilepsia, 29*, 794–804.

Holmes, G.L., McKeever, M., & Russman, B.S. (1983). Abnormal behavior or epilepsy? Use of long-term EEG and video monitoring with severely to profoundly men-

tally retarded patients with seizures. *American Journal of Mental Deficiency, 87*, 878–884.

Homan, R.W., & Rosenberg, H.C. (1993). Benzodiazepines. In E. Wyllie(Ed.), *The treatment of epilepsy: Principles and practice* (pp. 932–949). Philadelphia: Lea & Febiger.

Hug, G., McGraw, C.A., Bates, S.R., & Landrigan, E.A. (1991). Reduction of serum carnitine concentrations during anticonvulsant therapy with phenobarbital, valproic acid, phenytoin, and carbamazepine in children. *Journal of Pediatrics, 119*, 799–802.

Hutt, S.J., Jackson, P.M., Belsham, A., & Higgins, G. (1968). Perceptual-motor behavior in relation to blood phenobarbitone level: A preliminary report. *Developmental Medicine and Child Neurology, 10*, 626–632.

Hyuman, N.M., Dennis, P.D., & Sinclar, K.G. (1979). Tremor due to sodium valproate. *Neurology, 29*, 1177–1180.

Iivanainen, M., & Eldridge, R. (1987). Effect of phenytoin on the mental and physical function of patients with Baltic myoclonus epilepsy. *Italian Journal of Neurological Science, 8*, 313–317.

Iivanainen, M., & Himberg, J.J. (1982). Valproate and clonazepam in the treatment of severe progressive myoclonus epilepsy. *Archives of Neurology, 39*, 236–238.

Iivanainen, M., & Savolainen, H. (1983). Side effects of phenobarbital and phenytoin during long-term treatment of epilepsy. *Acta Neurologica Scandinavica, 68*(Suppl. 97), 49–67.

Iivanainen, M., Viukari, M., & Helle, E.P. (1977). Cerebellar atrophy in phenytoin-treated mentally retarded epileptics. *Epilepsia, 18*, 375–386.

Ingram, T.T.S. (1986). A characteristic form of overactive behaviour in brain damaged children. *Journal of Mental Science, 102*, 550–558.

Isojarvi, J.I.T., Laatikainen, T.J., Pakarinen, A.J., Juntunen, K.T.S., & Myllyla, V.V. (1993). Polycystic ovaries and hyperandrogenism in women taking valproate for epilepsy. *New England Journal of Medicine, 329*, 1383–1388.

Jaeken, J., van Goethem, C., Casaer, P., Devlieger, H., & Eggermont, E. (1979). Neutropenia during sodium valproate treatment. *Archives of Disease in Childhood, 54*, 985–986.

Jamerson, B.D., Dukes, G.E., Brouwer, K.L., Donn, K.H., Messenheimer, J.A., & Powell, J.R. (1994). Venous irritation related to intravenous administration of phenytoin versus fosphenytoin. *Pharmacotherapy, 14*, 47–52.

Jeavons, P.M., Bishop, A., & Harding, G. F. (1986). The prognosis of photosensitivity. *Epilepsia, 27*, S64–S65.

Jeavons, P.M., Clark, J.E., & Maheswari, M. (1977). Treatment of generalized epilepsies of childhood and adolescence with sodium valproate (Epilim). *Developmental Medicine and Child Neurology, 19,* 9–25.

Jones-Saete, C., Kriel, R.L., & Cloyd, J.C. (1992). External leakage from feeding gastrostomies in patients receiving valproate sprinkles. *Epilepsia, 33,* 692–695.

Kalff, R., Houtkooper, M.A., Meyer, J.W., Goeohart, D.M., Augusteijin, R., & Meinardi, H. (1984). Carbamazepine and serum sodium levels. *Epilepsia, 25,* 390–397.

Kalviainen, R., Partanen, J., Sivenius, J., Mumford, J., Saksa, M., & Riekkinen, P. J. (1991). Randomized controlled pilot study of vigabatrin versus carbamazepine monotherapy in newly diagnosed patients with epilepsy: An interim report. *Journal of Child Neurology, 6*(Suppl. 2), 2S60–2S69.

King, D.W., Gallagher, B.B., Marvin, A.J., Smith, D.B., Marcus, D.J., & Harlage, L.C. (1982). Pseudoseizures: Diagnostic evaluation. *Neurology, 32,* 18–23.

Konig, S.T.A., Siemes, H., Blaker, F., Boenigk, E., Grob-Selbeck, G., Hanefeld, F., Haas, N., Kohler, B., Koelfen, W., Korinthenberg, R., Kurek, E., Lenard, H.G., Penin, H., Penzien, J.M., Schunke, W., Schultze, C., Stephani, U., Stute, M., Traus, M., Weinmann, H.M., & Scheffner, D. (1994). Severe hepatotoxicity during valproate therapy: An update and report of eight new fatalities. *Epilepsia, 35,* 1005–1015.

Koskiniemi, M., & Hakamies, L. (1979). Valproic acid and coma. *Neurology, 29,* 1430.

Krishnamoorthy, K.S., Zaleraitis, E.L., Young, R.S.K., & Bermad, P.G. (1983). Phenytoin-induced choreoathetosis in infancy: Case report and a review. *Pediatrics, 72,* 831–834.

Kutt, H., Winters, W., Kokenge, R., & McDowell, E. (1964). Diphenylhydantoin metabolism: Blood levels and toxicity. *Archives of Neurology, 11,* 642–648.

Laub, C. M., Paetzke-Brunner, I., & Jaeger, G. (1986). Serum carnitine during valproic acid therapy. *Epilepsia, 21,* 559–562.

Leppik, I., & Wolff, D. (1993). Antiepileptic medication interactions. *Neurologic Clinics, 11,* 905–921.

Lerman, P., & Lerman-Sagie, T. (1995). Low-dose phenobarbital monotherapy in primary epilepsy: Long term follow-up study. *Epilepsia, 36*(Suppl. 3), S265–S266.

Levy, R.H., Pitlick, W.H., Troupin, A.S., Green, J.R., & Neal, J.M. (1975). Pharmacokinetics of carbamazepine in normal man. *Clinical Pharmacology and Therapeutics, 17,* 657–668.

Lifshitz, F., & Maclare, N.K. (1978). Vitamin D dependent rickets in institutionalized mentally retarded children receiving long term anticonvulsant therapy. I: A survey of 288 patients. *Journal of Pediatrics, 83,* 612.

Loiseau, P. (1981). Sodium platelet dysfunction and bleeding. *Epilepsia, 22,* 141–146.

Luther, J.S., McNamara, J.O., Carwile, S., Miller, P., & Hope, V. (1982). Pseudoepileptic seizures: Methods and video analysis to aid diagnosis. *Annals of Neurology, 32,* 18–23.

Maccario, M., & Lutsman, L. (1990). Paroxysmal nocturnal dystonia presenting as excessive daytime somnolence. *Archives of Neurology, 47,* 291–294.

Marchesi, G.F., Ladavas, E., Provinciali, L., Del Pesce, M., Fua, P., & Giuliani, G. (1980). Neuropsychological performances in patients treated with different antiepileptic drugs. *Monographs in Neural Sciences, 5,* 258–264.

Mathew, N.T., Saper, J.R., Silberstein, S.D., Rankin, L., Markley, H.G., Solomon, S., Rapoport, A.M., Silber, C.J., & Dalton, R. L. (1995). Migraine prophylaxis with divalproex. *Archives of Neurology, 52,* 281–286.

Matsuo, F., Bergen, D., Faught, E., Messenheimer, J.A., Dren, A.T., Rudd, G.D., & Lineberry, C.G. (1993). Placebo-controlled study of the efficacy and safety of lamotrigine in patients with partial seizures. *Neurology, 43,* 2284–2291.

Mattson, R.H., Cramer, J.A., Collins, J.F., Smith, D.B., Delgado-Escueta, A.V., Browne, T.R., Williamson, P.D., Trieman, D.M., McNamara, J.O., & McCutchen, C.B. (1985). Comparison of carbamazepine, phenobarbital, phenytoin, and primidone in partial and secondarily generalized tonic-clonic seizures. *New England Journal of Medicine, 313,* 145–151.

Mattson, R.H., Cramer, J.A., Williamson, P.D., & Novelly, R. (1978). Valproic acid in epilepsy: Clinical and pharmacological effects. *Annals of Neurology, 3,* 20–25.

Mattson, R.H., Petroff, O., Rothman, D., & Behar, K. (1994). Vigabatrin: Effects on human brain GABA levels by nuclear magnetic resonance spectroscopy. *Epilepsia, 35*(Suppl. 5), S29–S32.

McKauge, L., Tyrer, J.H., & Eadie, M.J. (1981). Factors influencing simultaneous concentrations of carbamazepine and its epoxide in plasma. *Therapeutic Drug Monitoring, 3,* 63–70.

McLean, M.J. (1994). Clinical pharmacokinetics of gabapentin. *Neurology, 44*(Suppl. 5), S17–S22.

McLean, M.J. (1995). Gabapentin. *Epilepsia, 36*(Suppl. 2), S73–S86.

Meador, K.J., Loring, D.W., Allen, M.E., Moore, E.E., Abney, B.A., & King, D.W. (1991). Comparative cognitive effects of carbamazepine and phenytoin in healthy adults. *Neurology, 41,* 1537–1540.

Meador, K.J., Loring, D.W., Huh, K., Gallagher, B.B., & King, D.W. (1990). Comparative cognitive effects of anticonvulsants. *Neurology, 40,* 391–394.

Meador, K.J., Loring, D.W., Moore, E.E., Thompson, W.O., Nichols, M.E.,

Oberzan, R.E., Durkin, M.W., Gallagher, B.B., & King, D. W. (1995). Comparative cognitive effects of phenobarbital, phenytoin, and valproate in healthy adults. *Neurology, 45,* 1494–1499.

Messenheimer, J.A. (1995). Lamotrigine. *Epilepsia, 36*(Suppl. 2), S87–S94.

Messenheimer, J.A., Ramsay, R.E., Willmore, L.J., Leroy, R.F., Zielinski, J.J., Mattson, R., Pellock, J.M., Valakas, A.M., Womble, G., & Risner, M. (1994). Lamotrigine therapy for partial seizures: A multicenter, placebo-controlled, double-blind, crossover trial. *Epilepsia, 35,* 113–121.

Mirza, W.U., Credeur, L.J., & Penry, J.K. (1993). Results of antiepileptic drug reduction in patients with multiple handicaps and epilepsy. *Drug Investigation, 5,* 320–326.

Mitchell, W.G., & Chavez, J. M. (1987). Carbamazepine versus phenobarbital for partial onset seizures in children. *Epilepsia, 28,* 56–60.

Monson, R.R., Rosenberg, L., Hartz, S.C., Shapiro, S., Heinonen, O.P., & Slone, D. (1973). Diphenylhydantoin and selected congenital malformations. *New England Journal of Medicine, 289,* 1049–1052.

Mumford, J.P., & Cannon, D. (1994). Vigabatrin. *Epilepsia, 35*(Suppl. 5), S25–S28.

Murphy, J.V., & Marquardt, K. M. (1982). Asymptomatic hyperammonemia in patients receiving valproic acid. *Archives of Neurology, 39,* 591–592.

Myers, W.C., & Carrera, F. (1989). Carbamazepine-induced mania with hypersexuality in a 9-year-old boy. *American Journal of Psychiatry, 146,* 400.

Neill, J.C., & Alvarez, N. (1986). Differential diagnosis of epileptic versus pseudoepileptic seizures in developmentally disabled persons. *Applied Research in Mental Retardation, 7,* 285–298.

Ney, G.C., Lantos, G., Barr, W.B., & Schaul, N. (1994). Cerebellar atrophy in patients with long-term phenytoin exposure and epilepsy. *Archives of Neurology, 51,* 767–771.

Oller, L.F.V., Russi, A., & Oller-Daurella, L. (1991). Lamotrigine in the Lennox-Gastaut syndrome. *Epilepsia, 32*(Suppl. 1), 58.

Ounsted, C. (1955). The hyperkinetic syndrome in epileptic children. *Lancet, 2,* 303–311.

Pakalnis, A., Drake, M.E., & Denio, L. (1989). Valproate associated encephalopathy. *Journal of Epilepsy, 2,* 41–44.

Pellock, J.M. (1987). Carbamazepine side effects in children and adults. *Epilepsia 28*(Suppl. 3), S64–S70.

Penry, J.K., Dean, J.C., & Riela, A.R. (1989). Juvenile myoclonic epilepsy: Long-term response. *Epilepsia, 30*(Suppl. 4), S19–S23.

Poindexter, A.R., Berglund, J.A., & Kolstoe, P.D. (1993). Changes in antiepileptic drug prescribing patterns in large institutions: Preliminary results of five-year experience. *American Journal on Mental Retardation, 98*, 24–40.

Pond, D. (1979). Epilepsy and mental retardation. In M. Craft (Ed.), *Tredgold's mental retardation* (pp. 331–345). London: Bailliére Tindall.

Porter, R.J., Penry, K.J., & Wolfe, A.A. (1976). Simultaneous documentation of clinical and electroencephalographic manifestations of epileptic seizures. In P. Kellaway & I. Peterson (Eds.), *Quantitative analytic studies in epilepsy* (pp. 253–268). New York: Raven Press.

Pulliainen, V., & Jokelainen, M. (1994). Effects of phenytoin and carbamazepine on cognitive functions in newly diagnosed epileptic patients. *Acta Neurologica Scandinavica, 89*, 81–86.

Ramsay, R.E.(1994). Clinical efficacy and safety of gabapentin. *Neurology, 44*(Suppl. 5), S23–S30.

Ramsay, R.E., Wilder, B.J., Berger, J.R., & Bruni, J. (1983). A double-blind study comparing carbamazepine with phenytoin as initial seizure therapy in adults. *Neurology, 33*, 904–910.

Reid, A.H., Naylor, G.J., & Kay, D.S. (1981). A double-blind, placebo controlled crossover trial of carbamazepine in overactive severely mentally handicapped patients. *Psychological Medicine, 11*, 109–113.

Reynolds, E.H. (1989). Phenytoin toxicity. In R. Levy, R. Mattson, B. Meldrum, J.K. Penry & F.E. Dreifuss (Eds.), *Antiepileptic drugs* (3rd ed., pp. 241–246). New York: Raven Press.

Richens, A. (1991). Pharmacology and clinical pharmacology of vigabatrin. *Journal of Child Neurology, 6*(Suppl. 2), 2S7-2S10.

Rodin, E.A., Rim, C.S., Kitano, H., Lewis, R., & Rennick, P.M. (1976). A comparison of the effectiveness of primidone versus carbamazepine in epileptic outpatients. *Journal of Nervous and Mental Disease, 163*, 41–46.

Rosenfeld, W.E., Leppik, I.E., Eates, J.R., & Mireles, R.E. (1987). Valproic acid loading during intense monitoring. *Archives of Neurology, 64*, 709–710.

Rushton, J.G., Stevens, J.C., & Miller, R.H. (1981). Glossopharyngeal (vagoglossopharyngeal) neuralgia: A study of 217 cases. *Archives of Neurology, 28*, 201–205.

Sackellares, J.C., Soo, I.L., & Dreifuss, F.E. (1979). Stupor followed by administration of valproic acid to patients receiving other anti-epileptic drugs. *Epilepsia, 20*, 697–703.

Sato, S., Penry, K.F., & Dreifuss, F.E. (1976). Electroencephalographic monitoring of generalized spike wave paroxysm in the hospital and at home. In P. Kellaway & I. Petersen (Eds.), *Quantitative analysis studies in epilepsy.* New York: Raven Press.

Savolainen, H., Iivanainen, M., Elovaara, E., & Tammisto, P. (1980). Distribution of 14C-phenytoin in rat Purkinje cells, cerebellar and cerebral neuronal tissue after a single intraperitoneal injection. *European Neurology, 19*, 115–120.

Schapel, G.J., Beran, T.G., Vadja, F.J.E., Berkovic, S.F., Mashford, M.L., Dunagan, F.M., Yuen, W.C., & Davies, G. (1993). Double-blind, placebo controlled, crossover study of lamotrigine in treatment-resistant partial epilepsy. *Journal of Neurology, Neurosurgery and Psychiatry, 56*, 448–453.

Schapiro, R.T. (1994). Symptom management in multiple sclerosis. *Annals of Neurology, 36*, S123–S129.

Schmidt, D., & Jacob, R. (1993). Clinical and laboratory monitoring of antiepileptic medication. In E. Wyllie (Ed.), *The treatment of epilepsy: Principles and practice* (pp.798–809). Philadelphia: Lea and Febiger.

Schmutz, M., Brugger, F., Gentsch, C., McLean, M.J., & Olpe, H.R. (1994). Oxcarbazepine: Preclinical anticonvulsant profile and putative mechanism of action. *Epilepsia, 35*(Suppl. 5), S47–S50.

Schlumberger, E., Chavez, F., Palacios, L., Rey, E., Pajot, N., & Dulac, O. (1994). Lamotrigine in treatment of 120 children with epilepsy. *Epilepsia, 35*, 359–367.

Shapiro, S., Hartz, S.C., Siskind, V., Mitchell, A.A., Slone, D., Rosenberg, L., Monson, R.R., & Heinonen, O.P. (1976). Anticonvulsants and parental epilepsy in the development of birth defects. *Lancet, 1*, 272–275.

Sherwin, A.L. (1993). Ethosuximide. In E. Wyllie (Ed.), *The treatment of epilepsy: Principles and practice* (pp. 923–931). Philadelphia: Lea & Febiger.

Shorvon, S., & Stefan, H. (1997). Overview of the safety of newer antiepileptic drugs. *Epilepsia, 38*(Suppl.), S45–S51.

Silverstein, F.S., Parrish, M.A., & Johnston, M.J. (1982). Adverse behavioral reactions in children treated with carbamazepine (Tegretol). *Journal of Pediatrics, 101*, 785–787.

Sintenie, J.B., Tuinebreijer, W.E., Kreis, R.W., & Breederveld, R.S. (1992). Digital gangrene after accidental intra-arterial injection of phenytoin (Epanutin). *European Journal of Surgery, 158*, 315–316.

Sivenius, J., Kalviainen, R., Mine, A., & Riekkinen, P. (1991). Double-blind study of gabapentin in the treatment of partial seizures. *Epilepsia, 32*, 539–542.

Smith, D.B. (1991). Cognitive effects of antiepileptic drugs. In D. Smith, D. Treiman, & M. Trimble (Eds.), *Advances in neurology* (Vol. 55, pp. 197–212). New York: Raven Press.

Smith, D.B., Mattson, R.H., Cramer, J.A., Collins, J.F., Novelly, R.A., Craft, B., & Veterans Administration Cooperative Study Group. (1987). Result of a nationwide Veterans Administration Cooper-

ative Study comparing the efficacy and toxicity of carbamazepine, phenobarbital, phenytoin, and primidone. *Epilepsia, 28*(Suppl. 3), S50–S58.

Snead, O.C. III., & Miles, M.V. (1985). Treatment of status epilepticus in children with rectal sodium valproate. *Journal of Pediatrics, 106*, 323–325.

Somerfeld-Ziskind, E., & Ziskind, E. (1940). Effect of phenobarbital on the mentality of epileptic patients. *Archives of Neurology and Psychiatry, 43*, 70–79.

Sordillo, P., Sagransky, D.M., Mercado, R., & Michelis, M.F. (1978). Carbamazepine-induced syndrome of inappropriate antidiuretic hormone secretion: Reversal by concomitant phenytoin therapy. *Archives of Internal Medicine, 138*, 299–301.

Soulayrol, R., & Roger, V. (1970). Effets psychiatriques defavorables des medications anti-epileptiques. *Revue de Neuropsychiatrie Infantile, 18*, 591–598.

Steiner, T.J., Silviera C., & Yuen, A.W.C. (1994). Comparison of lamotrigine (Lamictal) and phenytoin monotherapy in newly diagnosed epilepsy. *Epilepsia, 35*(Suppl. 7), 61.

Stinnet, E., Rodu, B., & Grizzle, W.E. (1987). New developments in understanding phenytoin-induced gingival hyperplasia. *Journal of the American Dental Association, 114*, 814–816.

Strandjord, R.E., & Johannessen, S.I. (1980). Single-drug therapy in patients with epilepsy: Serum levels and clinical effect. *Epilepsia, 21*, 655–662.

Sutula, T., Sackellares, J.C., Miller, J.O., & Dreifuss, M.B. (1981). Intensive monitoring in refractory epilepsy. *Neurology, 31*, 243–247.

Temkin, N.R., Dikmen, S.S., Wilensky, A.J., Keihm, J., Chabal, S., & Winn, H.R. (1990). A double blind study of phenytoin for the prevention of post-traumatic seizures. *New England Journal of Medicine, 323*, 497–502.

Theodore, W.H., & Porter, R.J. (1983). Removal of sedative hypnotic antiepileptic drugs from the regimens of patients with intractable epilepsy. *Annals of Neurology, 13*, 320–324.

Thompson, P., Huppert, F., & Trimble, M. (1980). Anticonvulsant drugs, cognitive function and memory. *Acta Neurologica Scandinavica 62*(Suppl. 80), 75–81.

Timmings, P.L., & Richens, A. (1992). Lamotrigine as an add-on drug in the management of Lennox-Gastaut syndrome. *European Neurology, 32*, 305–307.

Tomson, T., Svensson, J.O., & Hilton-Brown, P. (1989). Relationship of intraindividual dose to plasma concentration of carbamazepine: Indication of dose-dependent induction of metabolism. *Therapeutic Drug Monitoring, 11*, 533–539.

Trimble, M.R., & Corbett, J. (1980). Behavioral and cognitive disturbances in epileptic children. *Irish Medical Journal,*

73(Suppl.), 21–28.

Trimble, M.R., & Reynolds, E. (1976). Anticonvulsant drugs and mental symptoms. *Psychological Medicine*, 6, 169–178.

Trimble, M.R., & Thompson, P.J. (1986). Neuropsychological aspects of epilepsy. In I. Grant & K.M. Adams (Eds.), *Neuropsychological assessment of neuropsychiatric disorders* (pp. 321–346). New York: Oxford University Press.

U.K. Gabapentin Study Group. (1990). Gabapentin in partial epilepsy. *Lancet*, 335,1114–1117.

Uldall, P., Alving, J., Gram, L., & Beck, S. (1991). Vigabatrin in pediatric epilepsy— An open study. *Journal of Child Neurology*, 6(Suppl. 2), 2S38–2S44.

U.S. Gabapentin Study Group. (1994). The long-term safety and efficacy of gabapentin (Neurontin) as add-on therapy in drug-resistant partial epilepsy. *Epilepsy Research*, 18, 67–73.

U.S. Gabapentin Study Group No. 5. (1993). Gabapentin as add-on therapy in refractory partial epilepsy: A double-blind, placebo-controlled, parallel-group study. *Neurology*, 43, 2292–2298.

Verity, C.M., Hosking, G., & Easter, D.J. (1995). A multicentre comparative trial of sodium valproate and carbamazepine in pediatric epilepsy. *Developmental Medicine and Child Neurology*,7, 97–108.

Verma, N.P., Yusko, M.J., & Greiffenstein, M.F. (1993). Carbamazepine offers no psychotropic advantage over phenytoin in adult epileptic subjects. *Seizure, 2*, 53–56.

Vining, E.P., Carpenter, R.O., & Aman, M.G. (in press). Antiepileptics (Anticonvulsants). In J.S. Werry & M.G. Aman (Eds.), *Practitioner's guide to psychoactive drugs for children and adolescents* (2nd ed.). New York: Plenum Medical.

Vining, P.G., Mellis, D.E., Dorsen, M.M., Cataldo, S.P., Quaskey, S.A., Spielberg, S.P., & Freeman, J.M. (1987). Psychological and behavioral effects of antiepileptic drugs in children: A double blind comparison between phenobarbital and valproic acid. *Pediatrics*, 80, 165–174.

Wapner, I., Thurston, D.L., & Holowach, J. (1962). Phenobarbital: Its effect on learning in epileptic children. *Journal of the American Medical Association*, 182, 937.

White, S.H. (1997). Clinical significance of animal models and mechanism of action of potential antiepileptic drugs. *Epilepsia*, 38, S9–S17.

White, W.P., Plott, D., & Noton, J. (1966). Relative anticonvulsant potency of primidone: A double blind comparison. *Archives of Neurology*, 14, 31–35.

Wilkinson, I.A., Murphy, J.V., Georgeson, R., & D'souza, B. J. (1982). On site seizure clinic impact on the welfare of mentally retarded institutionalized patients. *Archives of Neurology*, 39, 41–43.

Williams, C.A., Tiefenbach, S., & McReynolds, J.W. (1984). Valproic acid-induced hyperammoniemia in mentally retarded adults. *Neurology*, 34, 550–553.

Willmore, L.J., Triggs, W.J., & Pellock, J.M. (1991). Valproate toxicity: Risk-screening strategies. *Journal of Child Neurology*, 6, 3–6.

Wolf, S.M., Carr, A., Davis, D.C., Davidson, S., Dale, P.E., Forsythe, A., Goldenberg, E.D., Hanson, R., Lulejian, G.A., Nelson, M., Treitman, P., & Weinsten, A. (1977). The value of phenobarbital in the child who has had a single febrile seizure: A controlled prospective study. *Pediatrics*, 59, 378–385.

Wolf, S.M., & Forsythe, A. (1978). Behavior disturbances, phenobarbital and febrile seizures. *Pediatrics*, 61, 728–731.

Wyllie, E. (Ed.). (1993). *The treatment of epilepsy: Principles and practice*. Philadelphia: Lea and Febiger.

Yerby, M.S. (1987). Problems and management of the pregnant woman with epilepsy. *Epilepsia*, 28(Suppl. 3), S29–S38.

Young, R.S., Alger, P.M., Bauer, L., & Lauderbaugh, D. (1986). A randomized, double-blind, crossover study of phenobarbital and mephobarbital. *Journal of Child Neurology*, 1, 361–363.

Antidepressant Drugs

Robert Sovner[1], Robert J. Pary[2], Anton Dosen[3], Angela Gedye[4],
Francisco J. Barrera[5], Dennis P. Cantwell[6], and Hans R. Huessy[7]

People with mental retardation and developmental disabilities have been treated with antidepressant drugs since these agents were introduced into clinical practice (Carter, 1966; Davies, 1961; Pilkington, 1962). Initially, patients were mostly selected on the basis of behavior problems and there was little attempt to diagnose and treat patients for specific psychiatric syndromes. Today, effort is made to diagnose a psychiatric syndrome, but especially with people with severe and profound mental retardation, this is often not possible. By 1970 these drugs had fallen out of favor for use with patients with mental retardation and developmental disabilities; however, renewed interest was stimulated by the introduction of selective serotonin reuptake inhibitors (SSRIs). Additionally, use has grown as a result of reports that people with mental retardation are vulnerable to the full spectrum of depressive disorders, obsessive-compulsive disorder (OCD), and impulse control disorders such as trichotillomania (see Reiss, 1994).

Currently antidepressants are used to treat people with depression and OCD and to a lesser extent, ritualistic behavior, self-injurious behavior (SIB), and aggression. Irreversible monoamine oxidase inhibitors (MAOIs) are only briefly discussed in this chapter because they are virtually never used with this population. This is because of the difficulty of maintaining a tyramine-free diet, which is needed with the MAOIs to avoid the risk of hypertensive crisis. Indications for the treatment of panic disorder and eating disorders (anorexia nervosa and bulimia nervosa) are not discussed because there has been little experience in diagnosing or treating these disorders in people with mental retardation and developmental disabilities (see Chapter 1).

PHARMACOLOGY

Antidepressants affect dopamine, norepinephrine, and serotonin (5-hydroxytryptamine) in the CNS. The effects are mediated in three ways: blockade of presynaptic neurotransmitter reuptake, direct agonist or antagonist activity, or the inhibition of neurotransmitter degradation (Preskorn, 1994). Antagonist effects at other neuroreceptor sites (e.g., acetylcholine, histamine) are not usually implicated in the drugs' therapeutic effects. The exact mechanisms of action for antidepressants remain unknown. It may be simplistic to assume that antidepressants act by increasing noradrenergic or serotonergic activity (Hyman, Arana, & Rosenbaum, 1995). The main argument against the mechanism being solely the blockade of reuptake is that such blockade can occur within hours, but often the antidepressant effect takes weeks to begin. This has led researchers to examine the effects of serotonin or monoaminergic activity on intraneuronal second messengers in post-synaptic cells (Janicak, Davis, Preskorn, & Ayd, 1993).

The pharmacological effects of the most commonly used heterocyclic agents are listed in Table 11-1. These drugs block the reuptake of serotonin or norepinephrine at presynaptic reuptake sites (Bolden-Watson & Richelson, 1993), but they differ from each other largely in their affinity for specific neurotransmitter systems. Heterocyclics are completely absorbed and undergo significant first-pass metabolism in the liver. Generally, all of these drugs can be prescribed on a once per day basis because of their long half-lives. Plasma heterocyclic levels can vary as much as 30-fold among individuals given the same dose of medications (Preskorn, 1993). The relationship of blood level to antidepressant response is strongest for nortriptyline, although established ranges for response also exist for imipramine, amitriptyline, and desipramine.

The SSRIs include fluoxetine, fluvoxamine, sertraline, and paroxetine and related drugs such as the triazolopyridines, nefazodone and trazodone, and venlafax-

1 Associate Professor of Psychiatry, Tufts University, Medford, MA
2 Associate Professor of Psychiatry, Southern Illinois University, Springfield, IL
3 President, European Association on Dual Diagnosis, Venray, The Netherlands
4 Private practice, Vancouver, British Columbia, Canada
5 Program Director, Southwestern (Ontario) Regional Center, Blenheim, Ontario, Canada
6 Joseph Campbell Professor of Child Psychiatry, University of California at Los Angeles, Los Angeles, CA
7 Professor Emeritus of Psychiatry, University of Vermont College of Medicine. Burlington, VT

Table 11-1. Heterocyclic Antidepressants

| Drug | Brand Names | Daily Dosage[a]/ Blood Level Range | Neurotransmitter Effects[f] | | | | | |
| | | | Reuptake Inhibition | | Direct Receptor Effects | | | |
			5-HT	NE	DA-2	ACH	HIS	-NE-1
amitriptyline[b]	Elavil	100-300 mg / 110-250 µg/L[c]	++[g]	++	0	---	---	---
amoxapine	Asendin	100-400 mg / 200-500 µg/L	+	+++	-	-	--	--
clomipramine[d]	Anafranil	100-250 mg / 80-100 µg/L	+++	++	-	--	--	--
desipramine	Norpramin	100-300 mg / 125-300 µg/L	+	+++	0	-	-	-
doxepin	Sinequan							
	Doxepin	100-300 mg / 100-200 µg/L[c]	+	++	0	--	---	---
imipramine[e]	Tofranil	100-300 mg / 200-350 µg/L[c]	++	++	0	--	--	--
maprotiline	Ludiomil	100-225 mg / 200-300 µg/L[c]	0	+	0	-	---	--
nortriptyline	Pamelor							
	Aventyl	50-150 mg / 50-150 µg/L	++[g]	+++	0	-	--	--
protriptyline	Vivactil	20-60 mg 100-200 µg/L	+	+++	0	---	--	-
trimipramine	Surmontil	100-300 mg / 180 µg/L	0	+	0	--	---	---

Note. Modified from Richelson (1994).

a Daily dose is for healthy adults. Children and the elderly will require lower doses.
b Metabolized into nortriptyline.
c Includes drug + active metabolite.
d Drug has a labeled indication for obsessive-compulsive disorder.
e Metabolized into desipramine.
f ACH = acetylcholine, DA = dopamine, 5-HT = 5-hydroxytryptamine (serotonin), HIS = histamine, NE = norepinephrine
g +++ = strong agonist activity, ++ = moderate agonist activity, + = weak agonist activity, 0 = none, - = weak antagonist activity, -- = moderate antagonist activity, --- = strong antagonist activity

Table 11-2. Selective Serotonin Reuptake Inhibitors, Related Drugs, and Bupropion

| Drug | Brand Names | Daily Dosage[a] | Neurotransmitter Effects[b] | | | | | | |
| | | | Reuptake Inhibition | | | Direct Receptor Effects[c] | | | |
			5-HT	NE	DA	DA	ACH	HIS	1-NE
fluoxetine	Prozac	20-80 mg	+++[c]	0	0	0	0	0	0
fluvoxamine	Luvox	50-300 mg	+++	+	0	-	0	0	0
paroxetine	Paxil	20-50 mg	+++	++	+	0	-	0	0
sertraline	Zoloft	50-200 mg	+++	+	0	0	0	0	0
trazodone	Desyrel	200-600 mg	+	+	0	0	0	-	--
nefazone	Serzone	100-600 mg	+	+	0	-	0	0	--
venlafaxine	Effexor	75-375 mg	++	+	0	0	0	0	0
bupropion	Wellbutrin	200-450 mg	0	0	+	0	0	0	0

Note. Adapted from Bolden-Watson & Richelson (1993) and Richelson (1994).

a Daily dose is for healthy adults. Children and the elderly will require lower doses.
b ACH = acetylcholine, DA = dopamine, 5-HT = 5-hydroxytryptamine (serotonin), HIS = histamine, NE = norepinephrine
c +++ = strong agonist activity, ++ = moderate agonist activity, + = weak agonist activity, 0 = none, - = weak antagonist activity, -- = moderate antagonist activity, --- = strong antagonist activity

ine. They are profiled in Table 11-2. At this time, evidence of differential efficacy is lacking. All of these drugs block the presynaptic reuptake of serotonin but differ with respect to potency and effects on other neurotransmitter systems (Bolden-Watson & Richelson, 1993) and on side effects. For example, nefazodone and trazodone are 5-HT2 receptor antagonists and are weaker SSRIs than other class members. Venlafaxine also is marketed as an inhibitor of norepinephrine reuptake. However, both nefazodone and paroxetine are more potent in inhibiting presynaptic norepinephrine reuptake than is venlafaxine (Bolden-Watson & Richelson, 1993). Clinically, trazodone seems to be less efficacious than other antidepressants for treating depression, but it is a useful hypnotic drug and may counteract migraine headaches precipitated by SSRIs (Dubovsky, 1994).

Bupropion is an aminoketone that blocks neuronal dopamine reuptake, but it is unknown if this is the mechanism of action for its therapeutic effects. Some people who have not responded to heterocyclics have responded to this drug. Bupropion is thought by some clinicians to be less likely to induce mania (Sachs et al., 1994).

SIDE EFFECTS

As is shown in Table 11-3, orthostatic hypotension is a common and potentially troublesome cardiovascular side effect that can occur with heterocyclic agents, even at subtherapeutic doses. It results in a precipitous fall in blood pressure when standing, possibly causing falls and fractures. People taking heterocyclics who complain of dizziness or who have falls, especially those taking medications that have significant α-1 receptor-blocking activity (e.g., amitriptyline), should have their blood pressure taken when both supine and standing. Imipramine, nortriptyline, and probably other heterocyclics can have a quinidine-like antiarrhythmic effect. These drugs slow cardiac conduction and, if there is a preexisting second- or third-degree bundle branch block, increase the risk of cardiac conduction complications (Roose & Glassman, 1989).

Heterocyclic agents block acetylcholine receptors and can cause dry mouth, blurred vision, urinary retention, and constipation. They also cause a central anticholinergic syndrome characterized by confusion, delirium, and possibly hallucinations. The risk of these reactions is increased if other anticholinergic agents, such as benztropine, antihistamines, or thioridazine, are coprescribed. Other adverse reactions include carbohydrate craving, vivid dreams, sexual dysfunction, and jitteriness (Nierenberg & Cole, 1991).

In a few cases, tardive dyskinesia was associated with antidepressants such as amitriptyline, imipramine, clomipramine, and doxepin. Usually, the individuals were older adults or had been exposed to neuroleptics or stimulants in the past. The tardive dyskinesia in these

Table 11-3. Heterocyclic Antidepressant Side Effects

Drug	Sedation	Orthostatic Hypotension	Constipation/ Dry Mouth	Cardio-toxicity	Insomnia	Weight Gain	Jitteriness	Seizures
amitriptyline	+++	+++	+++	+++	+	+++	0	++
amoxapine	+	++	+++	++	++	0/+	0/+	++
clomipramine	+++	++	+++	++	+	++	++	+++
desipramine	+	+	+	+++	+	+	++	+
doxepin	+++	++	+++	++	+	+++	+	+
imipramine	++	+++	++	+++	++	+++	+++	++
maprotiline	++	+	++	++	+	++	++	+++
nortriptyline	+	+	++	++	+	+	++	+
protriptyline	0/+	++	+++	++	+++	+	++	+
trimipramine	+++	++	++	++	+	++	+	+

Note. Adapted from Maxmen (1990) and Preskorn (1993).

a +++ = marked effects, ++ = moderate effects, + = weak effects, 0 = none reports may have been coincidental to the use of anti-depressants. Generally, antidepressants do not constitute a public health concern regarding tardive dyskinesia (Yassa, Camille, & Belize, 1987); it is highly unlikely that tardive dyskinesia is caused by exposure to antide-pressants alone. The one exception is amoxapine, which is metabolized into the neuroleptic, loxapine, which blocks dopamine receptors and can cause tardive dyski-nesia.

The most common side effects of SSRIs are headaches, dizziness, nausea, diarrhea, sedation, insomnia, sweating, tremor, dry mouth, anxiety, restlessness, and sexual dysfunction (see Table 11-4). Anxiety, tremor, and nausea are dose-related (Janicak et al., 1993). Except for an akathisia-like restlessness, severe diarrhea, and sexual dysfunction, the adverse effects of SSRIs seldom lead to discontinuation of drug therapy. The side effects of venlafaxine resemble those of the SSRIs (nausea, headache, nervousness, anorexia, sweating, dizziness, insomnia, somnolence, and sexual dysfunction). In contrast to the other drugs in this class, it may cause a sustained elevation of diastolic blood pressure, especially if the dose is above 300 mg/day (Anonymous, 1994).

The most common side effects with nefazodone and trazodone are sedation and cognitive slowing. Trazodone can also cause postural hypotension and priapism (invol-untary and persistent penile erection), and it reportedly aggravates arrhythmias in people with preexisting ventricular conduction abnormalities (Janicak et al., 1993). The side effects of bupropion resemble those of the SSRIs (nausea, restlessness, tremors, and insomnia), but there is a slightly increased rate of seizures (0.4%) with this drug compared to the heterocyclics and SSRIs. Risk factors for seizures include a daily dose greater than 450 mg/day and single doses of greater than 150 mg. The drug has few cardiovascular side effects (Wenger & Stern, 1983).

DRUG INTERACTIONS

A selective list of drug interactions with antidepressants appears in Table 11-5. The metabolism of tricyclic agents is inhibited by the SSRIs (e.g., fluoxetine, paroxetine, and sertraline) and phenothiazines (e.g., perphenazine and thioridazine). When heterocyclics are co-prescribed with either SSRIs or phenothiazines, signs of hetero-cyclic toxicity may develop. Because the heterocyclics have significant anticholinergic effects, using these drugs in combination with other agents that are anticholiner-gic (e.g., diphenhydramine or thioridazine) can result in delirium. Serious toxicity can result from overdose, including gradual accumulation caused by slow clearance (Preskorn & Burke, 1992).

The SSRIs are inhibitors of various cytochrome P-450 (CYP) enzymes (Preskorn, 1993) and may produce a marked increase in plasma concentrations of co-prescribed drugs such as carbamazepine (fluoxetine and fluvoxamine); heterocyclics including amitriptyline,

Table 11-4. Side Effects of Serotonin Selective Reuptake Inhibitors, Related Drugs, and Bupropion

Drug	Adverse Reactions[a]									
	Sedation	Orthostatic Hypotension	Constipation/ Dry Mouth	Cardio-toxicity	Insomnia	Nausea/ Vomiting	Diarrhea	Irritability	Head-aches	Seizures
fluoxetine	+	0	+	0/+	++	++	+	++	++	+
fluvoxamine	+	0	+	0/+	+	++	++	+	++	+
nefazodone	++	+	+	0/+	+	++	++	+	+	+
paroxetine	+	+	+	0/+	+	++	++	+	++	+
sertraline	++	0	+	0/+	+	++	++	+	++	+
trazodone	+++	++	+	0/+	0	++	++	+	+	+
venlafaxine	+	0	+	0/+	+	++	+	+	++	+
bupropion	++	0	+	0/+	++	+	+	++	++	+/++

Note. Adapted from Drug Facts and Comparisons (1995).

a +++ = marked effects, ++ = moderate effects, + = weak effects, 0 = none

Table 11-5. Selected Antidepressant Drug Interactions

Drug Class	Interacting With:	Comment
SSRIs[a]	cyproheptadine	Pharmacological reversal of antidepressant effects can result.
	monoamine oxidase inhibitors	Severe toxicity (characterized by elevated temperature, convulsions, cardiovascular collapse and death) can result.
fluoxetine	carbamazepine	Increase in carbamazepine plasma concentration can result in toxicity.
	clozapine	Increase in clozapine plasma concentration can result in toxicity.
	tricyclic antidepressants	Increase in tricyclic plasma concentration can result in toxicity.
nefazodone	triazolobenzodiazepines (alprazolam, triazolam)	Increase in triazolobenzodiazepine plasma concentration can result in toxicity.
paroxetine	cimetidine	Increase in cimetidine plasma concentation can result in toxicity.
	digoxin	Increase in digoxin plasma concentration can result in toxicity.
	phenobarbital	Decrease in phenobarbital and paroxetine plasma concentrations can result in loss of efficacy.
	phenytoin and related drugs	Increase in phenytoin and paroxetine plasma concentations can result in toxicity.
	warfarin	Increase in prothrombin time can result.
sertraline	diazepam	Increase in diazepam plasma concentration can result in toxicity.
	warfarin	Increase in warfarin plasma concentration can result in toxicity.
venlafaxine	cimetidine	Increase in venlafaxine plasma concentration can result in toxicity.
tricyclic agents	barbiturates	Decrease in tricyclic plasma concentration can result in a loss of efficacy.
	clonidine	Antagonism of antihypertensive effects of clonidine can result.
	methylphenidate	Increase in tricyclic plasma concentration can result in toxicity.
	monoamine oxidase inhibitors, irreversible type	Severe toxicity (characterized by hypertensive crisis or elevated temperature, convulsions, cardiovascular collapse and death) can result.
	phenothiazines	Increase in tricyclic plasma concentration can result in toxicity.
	SSRIs	Increase in tricyclic plasma concentration can result in toxicity.

Note. Adapted from Drug Facts and Comparisons (1995).

a The interaction effects of SSRIs are dependent on the specific cytochrome P450 enzymes that are involved in the metabolism of interacting agents. This is true for some tricyclic interactions as well.

desipramine, imipramine, and nortriptyline (fluoxetine, paroxetine); alprazolam; clonazepam; and triazolam (fluoxetine, fluvoxamine, and nefazodone). Generally, the SSRIs and related drugs rarely produce serious systemic toxicity and appear to be safer in overdose than heterocyclic antidepressants. There is a case report of an interaction between fluoxetine and a beta-blocker that resulted in the resting pulse dropping to 36 beats per minute (Walley, Pirmohamed, Proudlove, & Maxwell, 1993). The combination of fluoxetine and a beta-blocker could cause potentially serious bradycardia. Nefazodone inhibits the CYP 3A4 isoenzyme, potentially leading to increased plasma concentrations of nonsedating antihistamines such as terfenadine and astemizole, which has been associated rarely with serious arrhythmias and death (Anonymous, 1995). It is recommended that practitioners avoid prescribing nefazodone with either terfenadine or astemizole. Bupropion has very few clinically significant drug interactions. The safety level of bupropion during overdose is between that of the heterocyclics and the SSRIs (Janicak et al., 1993).

CLINICAL INDICATIONS EXCLUSIVE OF MENTAL RETARDATION

Affective Disorders and Obsessive-Compulsive Disorders (OCD)

All of the antidepressant drugs—cyclic compounds, SSRIs, and MAOIs—have an established role in managing major depressive disorders. According to Hyman et al. (1995), about 50% of patients with major depression will recover with an adequate trial of a single antidepressant medication, about 10% to 15% will show little improvement, and most of the remainder will show incomplete improvement. Because of their difficulty of use and potentially dangerous side effects, however, the MAOIs are usually reserved for only the most treatment-resistant patients who fail to respond to the SSRIs or cyclic compounds.

Antidepressants are also effective for managing atypical depression, depressive phases of bipolar disorder, and major depression with psychotic features. Although antidepressants can help to manage the depressive phases in bipolar disorder, they sometimes trigger manic phases or rapid cycling in patients with bipolar disorders. Some clinicians believe that patients with atypical depression (indicated by oversensitivity to rejection, unusual mood reactivity, extreme fatigue, oversleeping, and overeating) do not respond to cyclic compounds as well as to the MAOIs or SSRIs (Hyman et al., 1995). A major depressive disorder may also present in conjunction with psychotic features. When this occurs, combined antidepressants and neuroleptic therapy may provide more benefit overall than will either antidepressant or antipsychotic medication used alone (Hyman et al., 1995). Finally, some practitioners feel that there is a role for antidepressant drugs,

especially the SSRIs, in the treatment of dysthymic disorder (Hyman et al., 1995). Dysthymia is fundamentally similar to major depressive disorder, but the symptoms are less severe and of a chronic nature.

According to the American Psychiatric Association's (1993) *Practice Guidelines for Major Depressive Disorder in Adults*, currently accepted treatment of unipolar depression includes the following principles:

- Initiate treatment with one antidepressant at a time.
- Allow for a 4- to 6-week trial before ruling out the use of any particular antidepressant medication.
- Titrate to clinical response within the recommended maximum daily dose or plasma concentration for selected tricyclic antidepressants (TCAs).
- If no response has been achieved, consider augmentation therapy with an agent such as lithium or thyroid hormone.
- In treatment-refractory cases, consider combination therapy with an adrenergic and a serotonergic antidepressant.
- Once a remission has been achieved, continue treatment for at least 16 to 20 weeks before considering a drug-free trial.

OCD is indicated by the presence of intrusive thoughts that the patient finds very unpleasant and by the urge to perform rituals or repetitive actions to alleviate anxiety. Cognitive-behavioral treatment has been found to be effective for this disorder (van Blakom et al., 1994). Controlled clinical trials have demonstrated that clomipramine (Ananth, Pecknold, van den Steen, & Englesmann, 1981) and SSRIs such as fluoxetine (Wood, Tollefson, & Birkett, 1991) and fluvoxamine (Freeman, Trimble, Deakin, Stokes, & Ashford, 1994) have specific therapeutic effects for OCD. Trazodone also has been reported to be effective (Prasad, 1985). However, on the average, a smaller percentage of people with OCD than those with major depression respond favorably to appropriate antidepressants.

Attention-Deficit Hyperactivity Disorder

The use of TCAs to treat attention-deficit hyperactivity disorder (ADHD) in children is controversial, both with regard to efficacy and risk of cardiotoxic side effects. Nevertheless, this use is becoming more common (Biederman et al., 1989a, 1989b) because many patients do not respond favorably to stimulants or may show intolerable side effects.

Much of the research on the use of antidepressants for the treatment of ADHD has been focused on the use of imipramine. Several well-controlled studies with children showed that TCAs produced improvement in the symptoms of ADHD (Rapoport, Quinn, Bradbard, Riddle, & Brooks, 1974; Waizer, Hoffman, Polizos, & Englehardt, 1974; Werry, Aman, & Diamond, 1979; Winsberg, Bailer, Kupietz, & Tobias, 1972). Subsequently, results of several open (Gastfriend, Biederman, & Jellinek, 1984; Biederman et al., 1986) and controlled (Biederman et al., 1986, 1989a; Garfinkel, Wender, Sloman, & O'Neill, 1983) trials have supported the efficacy of desipramine and nortriptyline (Saul, 1985; Wilens, Biederman, Geist, Steingard, & Spencer, 1993). A smaller body of research has indicated a possible role for bupropion (Wender & Reimherr, 1990; Zametkin & Rapoport, 1987). Also the MAOIs, tranylcypromine and clorgyline, reduced disruptive behavior and enhanced performance on laboratory cognitive tests in small samples (Zametkin, Rapoport, Murphy, Linnoila, & Ismond, 1985). The effects of tranylcypromine and clorgyline on disruptive behavior in ADHD children were indistinguishable from those of dextroamphetamine, but the utility of MAOIs is limited by the risk of a tyramine-precipitated hypertensive crisis.

There are few studies on the effects of fluoxetine and other SSRIs in children with ADHD. In a preliminary trial, Barrickman, Noyes, Kuperman, Schumacher, and Verda(1991) investigated the effects of fluoxetine in 19 children and adolescents and found that 58% showed at least a moderate improvement in ADHD after six weeks on fluoxetine.

These data suggest that the TCAs are effective in ameliorating behavioral symptoms (e.g., overactivity and impulsiveness) in children with ADHD, although their effects on cognition and academic performance are probably limited. The drugs are regarded as a second-line treatment for ADHD (Pliszka, 1987). Other antidepressants have been less well-studied and constitute a third-line therapy. Stimulants appear to be superior to TCAs and remain the drugs of first choice in the treatment of ADHD. However, TCAs may be especially indicated for treating children with ADHD and coexisting mood or anxiety disorders (Rapoport et al., 1974) or with enuresis (Cox, 1982).

Treating children and adolescents, especially with daily doses of TCAs beyond 3.5 mg/kg, requires serum drug assays and EKG monitoring to reduce the risk of cardiovascular toxicity. The clinical response and any adverse effects should be carefully monitored after slowly titrating toward the lowest effective dose (Biederman et al., 1989b). Because TCAs are potentially cardiotoxic at high doses (Wilens et al., 1993), caution is warranted when they are prescribed to children, and their parents should be fully apprised of their adverse effects. TCAs may offer two advantages over stimulants in the treatment of ADHD. First, they have a longer half-life and allow for less frequent and more flexible drug dosage. Second, plasma levels can be measured to monitor compliance and toxicity to minimize the risk of abuse or dependence (Biederman et al., 1989a).

Nocturnal Enuresis

TCAs, particularly imipramine, have been used extensively in the pharmacological treatment of children with nocturnal enuresis (bed wetting). In 1960, MacLean first reported the efficacy of imipramine for nocturnal enuresis in children after observing that depressed adults who had been treated with imipramine described delayed micturition as a side effect. Since then, the anti-enuretic effect of TCAs, imipramine in particular, has been confirmed in a substantial number of double-blind studies. After extensive review, Blackwell and Currah (1973) concluded that TCAs are the only psychotropic drugs that have consistently proved to be more effective than placebo in the treatment of nocturnal enuresis in childhood. Conversely, several trials of TCAs with enuretic adults have yielded negative results (Dorison & Blackman, 1962; Hicks & Barnes, 1964). Although imipramine is considered to be the drug of first choice, desipramine and amitriptyline appear to be equally effective for the treatment of enuresis. Therefore, the choice among TCAs should be based on side effects and cost instead of efficacy. The efficacy of SSRIs is so far unknown.

When TCAs are effective, a therapeutic response is usually seen within the first week of treatment and sometimes after the first dose. The anti-enuretic effects of TCAs occur at lower oral dosages (i.e., 10 to 125 mg/day) than are required for a response to major depressive disorder. TCAs are generally not indicated for nocturnal enuresis in children under 6 years of age. Because tolerance to TCAs may develop, the anti-enuretic effect may diminish after two or three weeks of treatment (Furlanut et al., 1989; Rapoport et al., 1980). They are usually given for a 3-month period and then slowly tapered off to reduce the chances of a relapse. In case of a relapse, another 3-month course may be required. As was stated previously, cardiotoxicity is a serious concern in children treated with TCAs. Although TCAs are effective for treating enuresis and can rapidly reduce the frequency of wet nights at relatively low oral doses, behavioral techniques should be the first intervention in the treatment of enuresis. Psychopharmacotherapy should be reserved only for those who are nonresponsive to behavior modification.

The more established uses of antidepressants are for managing affective disorders, OCD, ADHD, and nocturnal enuresis. Antidepressants may also have efficacy in treating people with the following conditions (Hyman et al., 1995): panic disorder and other anxiety disorders, alcoholism comorbid with depression, bulimia, narcolepsy, migraine, chronic pain syndrome, and peptic ulcer. Some of these conditions, especially panic disorder (see McNally, 1994), respond well to cognitive-behavioral approaches separately or in combination with drug therapy.

CLINICAL INDICATIONS IN MENTAL RETARDATION

One important issue regarding the use of antidepressants with people with mental retardation and developmental disabilities is the relationship between depression and maladaptive behavior. Published reports have shown that a number of maladaptive behaviors can occur during a depressive illness, including aggression (Charlot, Doucette, & Mezzacappa, 1993; Laman & Reiss, 1987; Meins, 1993; Reiss & Rojahn, 1993), SIB (Charlot et al., 1993; Lowry & Sovner, 1992; Matin & Rundle, 1980; Pary, 1989), trichotillomania (Hamdan-Allen, 1991), and pica (Jawed, Krishnan, Prasher, & Corbett, 1993; Sovner, 1988). If an individual presents with SIB, for example, and also meets the criteria for major depression, antidepressant therapy should be considered for this individual.

Depression

Antidepressant therapy is the first-choice medication for any individual with mental retardation and developmental disabilities who meets the criteria for major depression and possibly for dysthymic disorder. The published reports on the use of antidepressant medications for the treatment of depression in adults with mental retardation are summarized in Table 11-6. With one exception (Aman, White, Vaithianathan, & Teehan, 1986), all of the reports were based on case histories or case series. Thus, there is a need for double-blind, placebo-controlled studies, especially since antidepessants are so widely used with this population.

As shown in Table 11-6, nine reports concerned the treatment of unipolar depression or depressive-like disorder. One was a placebo-controlled, crossover investigation of imipramine with 5 subjects in a mood disorder group and with 5 in an acting-out group (Aman et al., 1986). In this study, all of the subjects had profound mental retardation, and no benefit was found from imipramine in either group; deterioration was actually observed on scores on the Aberrant Behavior Checklist. The finding is subject to a variety of alternative explanations that merit additional research, including the possibility that initial doses of the drug may have been too high.

Mood disorders may also occur during childhood, at least in school-aged children and adolescents. Depression has been reported in children of preschool age, but there are disputes regarding its presentation and whether or not children with depression respond to antidepressant therapy (Johnston & Fruehling, 1994). Corbett (1979) stressed that there was "no doubt that depressive illness can be diagnosed in even profoundly retarded children where clearly defined changes in behavior occur with periods of withdrawal, misery, weeping, loss of appetite and weight, and change in sleeping pattern" (p. 13). Way (1983) reported dysthymic disorder in approximately 16% of the children referred to a psychiatric service, whereas psychotic depressive illness was diagnosed in approximately 2%. Benson (1985) reported that 15% of children and adolescents referred to an outpatient mental health clinic were suffering from a disorder characterized by depressed affect, low self-esteem, social withdrawal, and crying. Also, Dosen (1984) found that 16% of 194 children with mental retardation who were referred to a psychiatric clinic had a "depression-like" disorder, characterized in all by "affective hunger" and behavioral disturbances.

As is shown in Table 11-7, even fewer treatment studies have been reported for children with developmental disabilities. In total, three publications concern the uncontrolled treatment of 20 children. Some of these children were regarded as treatment responders, but anxiety and agitation occurred as side effects and no improvement was observed in OCD symptoms.

Antidepressant response in people with mental retardation and developmental disabilities typically has not been studied in clinical trials that meet scientific standards; that is, there are few double-blind studies with drug versus placebo conditions or drug versus drug cohorts. Short-term crossover studies in which subjects are their own controls may be problematic because antidepressant effects may last for extended periods after a drug is withdrawn. It is unclear whether the cognitive disabilities

Table 11-6. Reports of Antidepressant Therapy for Treatment of Depression in Adults with Mental Retardation

Authors	Diagnosis[a]	Subjects	Treatment[b]	Outcome
Davies (1961)	Possible MD	27 adults with Down syndrome.	NIA 30-150 mg/day.	19 (4 males and 15 females, age 6-40) who were "apathetic and listless" responded to treatment with "greater interest in surroundings."
Aman et al. (1986)	Depressive-like affective disorder	5 adults with depressive-like symptoms and with profound MR. 5 adolescents and adults with non-depressive disruptive behavior and profound MR.	Double-blind controlled comparison of IMI (3 mg/kg/day) and placebo, each given for 4 weeks with a 1-week washout.	Active drug caused worsening on Irritability, Social Withdrawal, and Hyperactivity subscales of the Aberrant Behavior Checklist regardless of diagnosis. Depressed group less active and disruptive group more active with medication during play.
Field et al. (1986)	Chronic MD	Woman with moderate MR, profound deafness and impaired vision secondary to congenital rubella. She had a 1-year history of "screaming outbursts," irritability, crying spells, 9 kg weight loss in 6-mos., and "irregular sleep pattern."	After placebo lead-in, there were 3 phases of IMI 100 mg/day administered for 3 wks., alternating with PLB for 2 wks.	IMI therapy compared to placebo resulted in consistent improvement in behavioral measures.
Pary (1989)	MD	Man with Down syndrome and moderate MR who had acute episode of sleep disturbance, decreased appetite, decreased interest, listlessness, depressed mood, work refusal, and severe self-injury.	NOR 100 mg/day (blood level 46 ng/ml).	Depressive symptoms remitted. No self-injury reported at followup.
Hamdan-Allen (1991)	MD	Man with autism, borderline intellectual function, depression, and trichotillomania. Trichotillomania began at age 16.	FLX (dosage not given) and followed for 8 months.	There was a complete remission of depression and trichotillomania.
Cook et al. (1992)	MD	A 17-year-old depressed woman was treated.	FLX 20 mg/day.	She had a "better mood," was "more considerate, and less lethargic."

Table 11-6 (Continued). Reports of Antidepressant Therapy for Treatment of Depression in Adults with Mental Retardation

Authors	Diagnosis[a]	Subjects	Treatment[b]	Outcome
Howland (1992)	MD = 3 AD = 3	6 adults who met DSM-III-R criteria for MD or AD. (One S had autism.)	Ss treated with FLX 20-40 mg/day and followed for 6-20 weeks.	Statistically significant decreases in Ham-D and CGI.
Ruedrich & Wilkinson (1992)	Chronic MD	Woman with mild MR with a history of SIB, anxiety, blunted affect, anhedonia, somatic preoccupation, and poor work performance.	AMO 150 mg/ unspecified length of followup.	She had a decrease in SIB, "brighter affect, better socialization, improved concentration, and less somatic preoccupation." She had failed to respond to FLV.
	Chronic MD	Woman with autism and severe MR, who at age 17 developed middle insomnia, crying, and severe SIB with persistent self-restraining.	AMO 300 mg/8 mos.	SIB "improved," middle insomnia remitted, frequency of crying spells decreased, and "virtually no self-restraints."
Sovner et al. (1993)	Chronic MD	Woman with severe MR living in a developmental center with SIB noted as early as age 16 and seasonal exacerbations of her symptoms.	FLX 20 mg/15 mos.	SIB was markedly improved with remission of symptoms of depression.
	Chronic MD	Adult with profound MR living in a developmental center with SIB noted at age 4.	FLX 20 mg/14 mos.	SIB and depressive symptoms remitted.

a AD = atypical depression, MD = major depression
b AMO = amoxapine, DMI = desipramine, FLX = fluoxetine, FLV = fluvoxamine, IMI = imipramine, NIA = nialamide, NOR = nortriptyline

associated with mental retardation affect antidepressant efficacy or merely represent a nonspecific factor that makes it difficult to assess treatment response. Another major issue is the difficulty in determining adverse reactions. Adverse reactions that produce physical or psychological distress can lead to the emergence of maladaptive behavior or to an increase in the frequency or severity of preexisting behavior.

Presently, all antidepressant medications appear to be about equally effective for treating depression in people with mental retardation and developmental disabiltiies. Because relative efficacy is not an issue, drug selection might be based partially on these factors: (a) whether or not a biological relative has a history of response to a specific drug, (b) the need to determine adequacy of response via drug blood-level assays, (c) side-effect profiles; (d) possible interactions with other drugs, and (e) history of previous response (when applicable). When there is no response to one class of antidepressants, changing to another sometimes can produce a positive response. For example, treatment with a heterocyclic agent can produce a therapeutic response for people who have failed adequate trials of SSRIs (Preskorn & Burke, 1992).

In treating adults with unipolar depression and developmental disabilities, some experienced clinicians initiate therapy with an SSRI—either fluoxetine, sertraline, or paroxetine. These drugs are generally well

Table 11-7. Reports of Antidepressant Therapy for Treatment of Depression in Children with Mental Retardation

Authors	Diagnosis[a]	Subjects	Treatment[b]	Outcome
Dosen (1982)	AD	12 children and adolescents.	IMI and AMI 2.5 mg/kg/day.	9/12 had a positive response.
Dosen (1990)	MD	4 children and adolescents.	IMI, 2 subjects; TRP + NIC, 2 subjects.	1/2 had a positive response. 2/2 had a positive response.
Ghaziuddin & Tsai (1991)	MD OCD	4 children with autism and MR.	FLX.	Depression improved, but no change in OCD. Anxiety and agitation reported as side effects.

a AD = atypical depression, MD = major depression, OCD = obsessive-compulsive disorder
b AMI = amitritipyline, DMI = desipramine, FLX = fluoxetine, IMI = imipramine, NIC = nicotinamide, TRP = tryptophan

tolerated, can be prescribed once per day, and have acceptable drug interactions. Clinical experience suggests that adverse behavioral reactions with fluoxetine have been a problem with some people with mental retardation, although fluoxetine has been widely prescribed. Alternative drugs are bupropion, nefazodone, trazodone, and venlafaxine. Bupropion is contraindicated in the presence of seizure disorder, which may limit its use with many people with mental retardation and developmental disabilities.

Tertiary amine TCAs (e.g., amitriptyline and imipramine) are not recommended as the treatment of first choice because of their side effects, especially anticholinergic effects. Nortriptyline, a secondary amine, is often better tolerated and may be considered as a possible first choice agent with people for whom blood level monitoring is an option. MAOIs are also not recommended because of the risk of consuming tyramine-containing foods, particularly aged cheese, which could precipitate a life-threatening hypertensive crisis. However, reversible monoamine oxidase inhibitors (RIMAs), such as moclobemide, do not cause this reaction (Hollister, 1994), and they warrant study for use with this population.

All antidepressants can induce mania (Wehr & Goodwin, 1987) and rapid cycling (Goodwin & Redfield Jamison, 1990, pp. 647-651; see also Sovner & Pary, 1993). The risk of mania is reduced when antidepressant therapy is administered in conjunction with a mood stabilizer such as lithium or valproate for the treatment of patients with bipolar disorder. Family members and caregivers should be warned about the

possibility of a dramatic and precipitous change in behavior, especially alterations in sleep and activity level.

There is disagreement on how to treat depression in childhood. Antidepressant therapy usually has not been demonstrated to be superior to placebo in controlled clinical trials with typically developing children (Jensen, Ryan, & Prien, 1992), although a recent trial of fluoxetine for children with depression was quite successful (Emslie et al., 1995). Since some children may respond to antidepressant therapy (Rosenberg, Holttum, & Gershon, 1994), some clinicians recommend treatment initiation with a heterocyclic agent such as desipramine or SSRI therapy.

Obsessive-Compulsive Disorder and Ritualistic Behavior

The classic forms of OCD—such as compulsive hoarding and checking—occur in people with mental retardation and developmental disabilities (see Reiss, 1994). Because these behaviors are anxiety-based, there is no controversy in diagnosing them as OCD, which, by definition, is an anxiety disorder. However, controversy exists regarding the extent to which ritualistic behavior, stereotypic behavior, or SIB is symptomatic of OCD (see Reiss, 1994). In order to be considered as OCD, these behaviors have to be performed to reduce anxiety and, according to DSM-IV criteria (American Psychiatric Association, 1994), intrusive thoughts must be present. With people with mental retardation, autism, or some other developmental disability, it is often difficult to determine whether the ritual is performed to reduce anxiety, to induce pleasure, or for some other reason; therefore, diagnoses of ritualistic and stereotypic behavior in this population can be controversial.

Although some authorities say that ritualistic behavior sometimes can be diagnosed as OCD (Vitello, Spreat, & Behar, 1989, see also Gedye, 1992), Reiss (1994, p. 79) has noted significant dissimilarities between OCD and the ritualistic behavior of people with developmental disabilities. For example, OCD is positively associated with IQ and usually treatable with cognitive-behavioral therapy, but ritualistic behavior in people with developmental disabilities is negatively correlated with IQ and is not treatable with cognitive-behavioral techniques. Even if SIB is not symptomatic of OCD, however, it may express an OCD-spectrum disorder. Moreover, Hollander (1993) has suggested that compulsive hair pulling (trichotillomania) may be relevant for conceptualizing certain types of repetitive behaviors.

SSRI therapy has been used to treat ritualistic behavior in individuals with developmental disabilities based on the use of these medications to treat OCD. The SSRIs may be used to treat aggression, stereotypies, and SIB. The published reports on the use of SSRIs and other antidepressants to treat OCD or ritualistic behavior in people with developmental disabilities are summarized in Table 11-8. Of the 11 published articles on this subject, 10 were based on single case reports or case series, and the majority of subjects were treated with fluoxetine. Gordon, Rapoport, Hamburger, State, & Mannheim (1992) published the results of a study involving 7 children and adolescents with autism and OCD symptoms. They were treated in a double-blind crossover trial with clomipramine and desipramine following a single-blind placebo lead-in. Clomipramine proved superior to desipramine with respect to change in OCD symptoms and also in factors related to autism.

Table 11-8 shows that only five definite cases of OCD treatment with antidepressants were reported—two by Cook, Terry, Heller, and Leventhal (1990), two by O'Dwyer, Holmes, and Collacott (1992), and one by Wiener and Lamberti (1993). The OCD symptoms treated were compulsions, anxiety, and fear. The subjects in the remainder of the reports listed in Table 11-8 are best characterized as displaying ritualistic behavior. These reports suggested variable degrees of reduction in problem behaviors, autistic symptoms, uncooperativeness, speech deviance, ordering behavior, and hyperactivity.

OCD is usually treated with a mixed reuptake inhibitor (e.g., clomipramine) and may only partially respond to pharmacotherapy (Jenike, 1993). A lack of response or poor response to one serotonergic agent suggests augmentation with another drug (such as lithium, buspirone, or clonidine) or the substitution of another agent (Jenike, 1993). When OCD is associated with tics, the co-administration of an SSRI and haloperidol may be more effective than an SSRI alone (Holzer et al., 1994).

Self-Injurious Behavior (SIB) and Aggression

For the treatment of conditions associated with poor impulse control, stereotypic behavior, or a pervasive developmental disorder, some clinicians experienced in treating people with develomental disabilities try an SSRI before a tricyclic agent or bupropion. Usual therapeutic doses are used. However, the use of pharmacotherapy for aggression and SIB is complicated by the fact that these behaviors may have multiple determinants (Davidson et al., 1994; Iwata et al., 1994; King, DeAntonio, McCracken, Forness, & Ackerland, 1994).

As is shown in Table 11-9, we identified seven reports on the treatment of aggression in the absence of other psychiatric disorders. Of the nine individuals in these reports, five were treated with fluoxetine and three were treated with trazodone. There were no clear-cut predictors of response. Subjects had a variety of developmental disorders including autism, Down syndrome, and Prader-Willi syndrome. None of the cases described the treatment of children. Aggression was reported to decrease in most of these cases, and improvements were also seen in managing tantrums, hoarding, SIB, and destructive behavior. It is difficult to make any general statements about the treatment of aggression based on these case reports. In only one case (Bernstein, 1992) was there a psychiatric diagnosis (organic personality disorder) for which aggression could be considered a primary symptom. In only two of the case reports was a controlled therapeutic trial conducted (Gedye, 1991a, 1991b), but a non-blind design was used.

Nine reports with 50 subjects (including 13 children) with SIB are summarized in Table 11-10. The subjects had a variety of developmental disorders, including pervasive developmental disorder, Cornelia de Lange syndrome, Prader-Willi syndrome, and Angleman syndrome. SIB was decreased in all of the reports, and variable improvements also occurred in explosive

Table 11-8. Reports of Antidepressant Therapy for Treatment of Obsessive-Compulsive Disorder (OCD) and Related Behaviors in Children and Adults with Mental Retardation

Authors	Diagnosis	Subjects	Treatment[a]	Outcome
Mehlinger (1989)	OCD + autism	Woman with ritualistic behavior — arranging objects in a special order, associated with aggression, when thwarted, and enuresis. She had a previous 2-week response to IMI.	FLX 20 mg every other day.	Treatment resulted in a reduction in ordering behavior and tantrums. Enuresis remitted.
Cook et al. (1990)	OCD	Woman with mild MR, compulsive phone calls to strangers, perseverative dishwashing, and a showering compulsion who had failed to respond to HAL, LOX, and TRF.	FLX 80 mg.	Response was measured using an adapted version of the Leyton Obsessional Inventory for Children. There was a clinically signficant decrease in compulsive behavior and she was more spontaneous.
	OCD	Man with borderline intellectual function with compulsive checking, preoccupation with order, and tactile defensiveness. He had failed to respond to THI. Authors wondered whether subject had an atypical pervasive developmental disorder.	FLX 80 mg.	Response was measured using an adapted version of the Leyton Obsessional Inventory for Children. There was a clinically significant decrease in compulsions.
McDougle et al. (1990)	OCD + autism	Woman with autism.	FLV 150 mg.	Missing outcome
Gordon et al. (1991)	"OCD symptoms" + autism	Children and adolescents with OCD symptoms assessed using a modified version of the obsessive-compulsive subscale of the Comprehensive Psychopathological Rating Scale (CPRS), NIMH Obsessive Compulsive Rating Scale , and the NIMH Global Obsessive-Compulsive and Anxiety Scales.	Treatment was administered in single-blind placebo lead-in with a double-blind crossover trial of DMI (mean dose at week 5, 111 mg/day vs. CLO 129 mg/day).	CLO was superior to DMI and placebo with respect to OCD symptoms and also to 4 factors of the CPRS: autism, anger/uncooperativeness, speech deviance, and hyperactivity.
Todd (1991)	OCD + autism	Man with borderline intellectual function who had a "marked perversion of grooming and writing activities" with frequent arm and hand flapping, and head swaying. When interrupted, he would become aggressive.	FLX 20 mg.	There was a 50% reduction in perseverative behavior and aggressive incidents within 4 weeks. Improvements continued for 14 months.

Table 11-8 (Continued). Reports of Antidepressant Therapy for Treatment of Obsessive-Compulsive Disorder (OCD) and Related Behaviors in Children and Adults with Mental Retardation

Authors	Diagnosis	Subjects	Treatment[a]	Outcome
Cook et al. (1992)	OCD	23 subjects with autism and 16 subjects with MR treated in an open trial. Three autistic boys with OCD and mild MR were treated. In addition, a woman with mild MR was treated.	Subjects treated with 10 to 40 mg FLX per day.	All 3 autistic boys had a decrease in OCD symptoms with a decrease in Clinical Global Impression Severity of Illness scale. The woman with MR did not respond.
McDougle et al. (1992)	OCD + autism	5 adolescents and adults who met criteria for autism and partial criteria for OCD. They had a variety of OCD features including hoarding, need for sameness, and touching/tapping. One subject had trichotillomania.	CLO, 50 to 250 mg/day.	All subjects had a good response to treatment as measured by the Aberrant Behavior Checklist.
O'Dwyer et al. (1992)	OCD + Down syndrome	Man with a 12-month history of the abrupt onset of checking and tidiness compulsions.	FLV 200 mg.	After 4 months of treatment, his compulsions remitted.
		Woman with a 9-year history of cleaning and orderliness compulsions following a sexual assault.	CLO 150 mg, FLX 40 mg.	Subject did not respond to treatment with either drug.
Bodfish & Madison (1993)	OCD	10 institutional residents with MR.	FLX 40 mg.	7/10 had a positive response.
Wiener & Lamberti (1993)	OCD	Woman with moderate MR, anxiety-related face rubbing, and compulsive telephone calls to her home to make sure that her family was all right.	SER 50 mg.	After 8 weeks, anxiety was reduced and she was "less distracted" by fears about the health of her family.

a CLO = clomipramine, DMI = desipramine, FLX = fluoxetine, FLV = fluvoxamine, IMI = imipramine, HAL = haloperidol, LOX = loxapine, SER = sertraline, THI = thioridazine, TRF = terfenadine.

outbursts, social behavior, eye contact, stereotypic behavior, food foraging, and (sometimes) aggression.

Brasic et al. (1994) prescribed clomipramine up to 200 mg at bedtime to treat five boys (age range 6-12 years). The boys had autism, severe mental retardation and movement disorders, and compulsions: two were aggressive and hyperactive, one had SIB and hyperactivity, and one was aggressive and had tantrums. With treatment, abnormal movements decreased significantly.

As was shown by a survey (Stein, Hollander, & Liebowitz, 1993), antidepressants (in particular the SSRIs) appear to be a relatively common clinical intervention for the treatment of compulsive-spectrum behavior in persons with Prader-Willi syndrome (PWS). Stein et al. designed a questionnaire to capture information on DSM-III-R psychopathology (American Psychiatric

Table 11-9. Reports of Antidepressant Therapy for Treatment of Aggression in Adults with Mental Retardation

Authors	Diagnosis	Subjects	Treatment[a]	Outcome
Dech & Budow (1991)	Prader-Willi syndrome	Young woman with mild MR, trichotillomania, trichophagia, and temper tantrums.	FLX 80 mg, 6 months.	Appetite diminished and weight stabilized. Tantrums and compulsive behavior slightly improved.
Gedye (1991a)	Alzheimer dementia in Down syndrome	Man with severe MR had a 2-year history of unprovoked aggression and occassional self-injury.	TRZ 200 mg/day.	Treatment administered in an open trial with an ABAB design (TRZ vs. no treatment). There was a 95% reduction in aggressive incidents during active treatment compared to baseline and drug-free trial.
Gedye (1991b)	Autism	Young man with severe MR and a history of severe overactivity, stereotypies, and aggression.	TRZ, 150 mg/day.	Treatment administered in an open trial with an ABAB design (TRZ vs. no treatment). There was a 70% and 75% reduction in target behavior during active treatment compared to baseline and drug-free trial.
Bernstein (1992)	Organic personality disorder	Man with mild MR and a 15-year history of impulsive aggression including assaults and wrist cutting.	TRZ, 6 weeks.	Treatment resulted in complete absence of aggression.
Singh (1993)	None stated	Man with mild MR and generalized tonic-clonic epilepsy with history of aggression, SIB, and compulsive toilet-blocking.	FLX 20 mg/day, CBZ 600 mg/day, 12-15 days.	All SIB and compulsive behavior remitted. Score on Violent and Destructive Behavior and Self-Abusive Behavior subscales of The Adaptive Behavior Scale (Nihira et al, 1975) decreased from 37 to 6. (Followup CBZ levels were not reported.)
	None stated	Woman with severe MR and generalized tonic-clonic epilepsy, with a history of temper outbursts and aggressive behavior.	FLX 40 mg/day, CBZ 800 mg/day, 6 weeks.	Violent and Destructive Behavior and Self-Abusive Behavior subscale scores decreased from 32 to 9.
	None stated	Adult with moderate MR and generalized tonic-clonic epilepsy, with a history of verbal and physical aggression, hair pulling, and SIB.	FLX 20 mg/day, CBZ 800 mg/day.	Violent and Destructive Behavior and Self-Abusive Behavior subscale scores decreased from 40 to 9.

Table 11-9 (Continued). Reports of Antidepressant Therapy for Treatment of Aggression in Adults with Mental Retardation

Authors	Diagnosis	Subjects	Treatment[a]	Outcome
Hellings & Warnock (1994)	Intermittent explosive disorder, Prader-Willi syndrome	Man with mild MR hoarding behavior	FLX 20 mg for 2 years.	Hoarding behavior significantly improved with relapse following drug discontinuation.
Jawed et al. (1994)	Pervasive developmental disorder, ocular albinism	Adolescent with severe MR with a 2-year history of aggression and SIB associated with overarousal.	FLV 50 mg/day.	After 2 weeks, he was more relaxed and SIB remitted. However, aggressive behavior increased in frequency.

a CBZ = carbamazepine, CLO = clomipramine, FLV = fluvoxamine, FLX = fluoxetine, THI = thioridazine, TRZ = trazodone

Association, 1987), behavioral problems, and drug history. In all, 349 questionnaires were returned, and Stein et al. found that 11.5% of the subjects were receiving an SSRI. For fluoxetine, the mean dose was 28.7 (± 14.7) mg with a mean duration of 14.7 (± 10.1) months.

Attention-Deficit Hyperactivity Disorder

Studies of the efficacy of TCAs for treating ADHD in children and adults with mental retardation and developmental disabilities are few and limited. Some authors have reported moderate or significant clinical improvements. Huessy and Ruoff (1984) reported that 9% of their patients in a state institution responded favorably to low doses (10 to 75 mg/day) of imipramine or amitriptyline. Improvements in attention span, mood, and sleep patterns and reduction of impulsivity, emotional lability, and SIB were seen. Hilton, Martin, Heffron, Hall, and Johnson (1991) described a 6-year-old boy with fragile X syndrome, who suffered from ADHD, nocturnal enuresis, and initial insomnia. The ADHD, nocturnal enuresis, and initial insomnia all responded to a trial of imipramine. The development of tolerance, however, required gradual increases in dosage from 0.8 to 2.4 mg/kg/day. Brown, Winsberg, Bialer, and Press (1973) reported good results with imipramine treatment for hyperactive-aggressive behavior disorders in three children with organic brain disease and mental retardation. However, all three developed seizures when their dosages were progressively increased to 150 to 225 mg per day. No prior history of seizures was mentioned, and two children maintained a seizure-free response after anticonvulsants were added.

Enuresis

The evidence to support the use of antidepressants to treat enuresis in people with mental retardation and developmental disabilities is quite limited (see Blackwell & Currah, 1973). Fisher, Murray, Walley, and Kiloh (1963) studied the efficacy of imipramine in a double-blind placebo controlled study among hospitalized patients aged 7 to 67 suffering from nocturnal enuresis. Imipramine in a daily dose of 25 to 50 mg was ineffective in controlling nocturnal enuresis. Drew (1967) compared the use of imipramine (50 and 100 mg/day), amitriptyline (100 mg/day), and placebo for men with severe mental retardation and observed no significant differences in the frequency of nocturnal enuresis. Similar null results were reported for TCAs used with adults without disabilities. In a double-blind placebo controlled study, Valentine and Maxwell (1968) investigated the effects of imipramine in 16 children, 3 to 11 years of age, with severe mental retardation and enuresis. The wetting frequency was similar after both imipramine (25 to 75 mg/day) and placebo. Conversely, Smith and Gonzales (1967) reported that 25 mg of nortriptyline significantly reduced the incidence of enuresis in 34 boys aged 8 to 18 who had IQs from 46 to 88. Twenty subjects showed a 50% improvement in wetting frequency after a 20-day period of medication. The majority of these subjects maintained continence after the medication was discontinued for 3 months. Possibly, the relatively weak results thus far are due to the age of the participants studied; most investigators appear to have used a large number of adults, which may have had an adverse effect on outcome.

Table 11-10. Reports of Antidepressant Therapy for Treatment of Self-Injury in Children and Adults with Mental Retardation

Authors	Diagnosis	Subjects	Treatment[a]	Outcome
O'Neill et al. (1986)	Cornelia de Lange syndrome	Man with temper tantrums, self-injury, aggression, disrupted sleep.	TRZ 200 mg QD + TRP 3 gm QD, 24 days	Marked improvement in aggression and SIB, sleep disturbance remitted. There was a fourfold reduction in tantrums. Whole blood 5-hydroxytryptamine increased from 55 ng/ml to 383 ng/ml.
Markowitz (1990)	SIB	8 adults with severe or profound MR were treated. All were receiving neuroleptic drug therapy.	FLX 20 mg/day (Increasing daily dose to 40 mg did not improve response.)	5/8 had a marked response, 2 had a moderate response, and 1 a mild response. Also self-stimulatory behaviors such as rocking and twirling improved.
Bass & Beltis (1991)	None given	Man with severe MR with a lifelong history of treatment-resistant SIB. He failed to respond to a double-blind, placebo-controlled trial of naltrexone.	FLX 20-50 mg, 2 years	Over course of the trial there was a 45% reduction in rates of SIB. FLX 40 mg/day was the optimal daily dose. Response was deemed to be clinically significant.
King (1991)	Pervasive developmental disorder	Man with cerebral palsy and moderate MR. Finger gnawing began at age 3 with progression to head hitting/banging during adolescence. Low frustration was a factor in precipitating SIB. He failed to respond to THI 600 mg/day.	FLX 40 mg, 70 days	FLX therapy produced a statistically significant decrease in SIB compared to baseline. Percentage of SIB-free days decreased from 8% during drug-free baseline to 66% during FLX treatment. Change was deemed clinically significant. Subject relapsed 70 days after FLX initiation.
Garber et al. (1992)	SIB and stereotypies	11 children and adolescents with moderate to profound MR.	CLO 3 mg/kg/day	Self-injury and stereotypies improved for 10/11 by at least 50%.
Markowitz (1992)	SIB	21 adults with severe to profound MR were treated. All 20 were receiving neuroleptic drug therapy, 6 were taking carbamazepine, 3 lithium, and 3 propranolol.	FLX 20-40 mg.	18/20 with SIB had a positive response. Restlessness, agitation, and self-stimulation responded in some cases when also present.

Table 11-10 (Continued). Reports of Antidepressant Therapy for Treatment of Self-Injury in Children and Adults with Mental Retardation

Authors	Diagnosis	Subjects	Treatment[a]	Outcome
Ricketts et al. (1993)	Organic mental syndrome, stereotypic habit disorder. 2 subjects manifested evidence of depression.	4 adults with self-injury.	FXT 40-60 mg, 12-28 weeks	Reduction in self-injury by 20% to 84%.
Hellings & Warnock (1994)	Stereotypy-habit disorder, dysthymic disorder, Prader-Willi syndrome	Woman with mild MR and skin picking.	FLX 40 mg & 60 mg on alternate days, 2 years	Skin picking remitted. Response of depressive symptoms not discussed.
	Stereotypy-habit disorder, Prader-Willi syndrome	Man with moderate MR, and non-insulin dependent diabetes mellitus, skin picking, and explosive outbursts.	FLX 20 mg/day, glybluride, 1 year	Less food foraging and fewer explosive outbursts reported. All skin lesions healed. He was more animated, talkative, and had increased energy. Relapse followed discontinuation of FLX to manage diarrhea.
Jawed et al. (1994)	Atypical pervasive developmental disorder	Adolescent boy with cerebral astrocytoma excised when he was 30-m.o. with features of a pervasive developmental disorder. SIB began at 9-y.o. He had a sleep initiation disturbance and was sensitive to loud noises.	FLV 50 mg/day (THI 100 mg/day was coprescribed), 9 months	Remission in SIB. Eye contact and "affectionate behavior" improved. THI was decreased to 50 mg/day.
	Pervasive developmental disorder, ocular albinism	Adolescent boy with severe MR with a 2-year history of aggression and SIB associated with overarousal.	FLV 50 mg/day	After 2 weeks, he was more relaxed and SIB remitted. However, aggressive behavior increased in frequency.

a CLO = clomipramine, FLV = fluvoamine, FLX = fluoxetine, THI = thioridazine, TRP = tryptophan, TRZ = trazodone

CONCLUSION

The cyclic compounds and SSRIs have an established role in managing major depressive disorder in people both with and without developmental disabilities. Antidepressant therapy is the first-choice medication for any individual with mental retardation who meets the criteria for major depression and possibly for dysthymic disorder. However, the evidence for such use is based mostly on extrapolation from the general population. Few well-controlled studies have been reported on the treatment of depression in people with mental retardation and developmental disabilities. Generally, the various antidepressant medications appear to be about equally effective. In treating unipolar depression in adults with developmental disabilities, however, some clinicians initiate therapy with an SSRI—either fluoxetine, sertraline, or paroxetine.

There is disagreement on how to treat depression in childhood. Antidepressant therapy usually has not been demonstrated to be superior to placebo in controlled clinical trials with typically developing children (Jensen et al., 1992), although a recent trial of fluoxetine for depressed children was quite successful (Emslie et al., 1995). Nevertheless, some children may respond to antidepressant therapy (Rosenberg et al., 1994), and when an antidepressant is considered, some clinicians recommend treatment initiation with a heterocyclic agent such as desipramine or SSRI therapy.

The antidepressants are used to treat a range of behav-ioral and psychiatric conditions in addition to depression. Based on extrapolation of effects for the general population, SSRIs are used to treat OCD in people with mental retardation. They also are used to treat ritualistic behavior, but there is controversy regarding the extent to which such ritualistic behaviors are symptoms of OCD. The SSRIs also are used to treat aggression, stereotypies, and SIB, although much research is needed to evaluate these indications more rigorously. Antidepressants, in particular the SSRIs, appear to be a relatively common clinical intervention for the treatment of compulsive-spectrum behavior. The evidence to support the use of antidepressants to treat enuresis in people with mental retardation is quite limited (see Blackwell & Currah, 1973).

REFERENCES

Aman, M.G., White, A.J., Vaithianathan, C., & Teehan, D.J. (1986). Preliminary study of imipramine in profoundly retarded residents. *Journal of Autism and Developmental Disorders, 16,* 263–273.

American Psychiatric Association. (1994). *Diagnostic and statistical manual of mental disorders* (4th ed.). Washington, DC: American Psychiatric Press.

American Psychiatric Association Work Group on Major Depressive Disorder.(1993). *Practice guidelines for major depressive disorder in adults.* Washington, DC: American Psychiatric Press.

Ananth, J., Pecknold, J.C., van den Steen, N., & Englesmann, F. (1981). Double-blind comparative study of clomipramine and amitriptyline in obsessive neurosis. *Progress in Neuropsychopharmacology and Biological Psychiatry, 5,* 257–262.

Anonymous. (1994). Venlafaxine: A new antidepressant. *The Medical Letter, 36,* 49–50.

Anonymous. (1995). Nefazodone for depression. *Medical Letter, 37,* 33–35.

Barrickman, L., Noyes, R., Kuperman, S., Schumacher, E., & Verda, M. (1991). Treatment of ADHD with fluoxetine: A preliminary trial. *Journal of the American Academy of Child and Adolescent Psychiatry, 30,* 762–767.

Bass, J.N., & Beltis, J. (1990). Therapeutic effect of fluoxetine on naltrexone-resistant self injurious behavior in an adolescent with mental retardation. *Journal of Child and Adolescent Psychopharmacology, 1,* 331–340.

Benson, B. (1985). Behavior disorder and mental retardation: Association with age, sex and level of functioning in an outpatient clinic sample. *Applied Research in Mental Retardation, 6,* 79–88.

Bernstein, L. (1992). Trazodone treatment of targeted aggression in mentally retarded man. *Journal of Neuropsychiatry, 4,* 348.

Biederman, J., Baldessarini, R.J., Wright, V., Knee, D., & Harmatz, J.S. (1989a). A double-blind placebo controlled study of desipramine in the treatment of ADD: I. Efficacy. *Journal of the American Academy of Child and Adolescent Psychiatry, 28,* 777–784.

Biederman, J., Baldessarini, R.J., Wright, V., Knee, D., Harmatz, J.S., & Goldblatt, A. (1989b). A double-blind placebo controlled study of desipramine in the treatment of ADD: II. Serum drug levels and cardiovascular findings. *Journal of the. American Academy of Child and Adolescent Psychiatry, 28,* 903–911.

Biederman, J., Gastfriend, D.R., & Jellinek, M.S. (1986). Desipramine in the treatment of children with attention deficit disorder. *Journal of Clinical Psychopharmacology, 6,* 359–363.

Blackwell, B., & Currah, J. (1973). The psychopharmacology of nocturnal enuresis. In I. Kalvin, R.C. Mackeith, & S.R. Meadow (Eds.), *Bladder control and enuresis* (pp. 213–257). London: Heinemann.

Bodfish, J.W., & Madison, J.T. (1993). Diagnosis and fluoxetine treatment of compulsive behavior disorder of adults with mental retardation. *American Journal on Mental Retardation, 98,* 360–367.

Bolden-Watson, C., & Richelson, E. (1993). Blockade by newly-developed antidepressants of biogenic amine uptake into rat brain synaptosomes. *Life Sciences, 52,* 1023–1029.

Brasic, J.R., Barnett, J.Y., Kaplan, D., Sheitman, B.B., Aisemberg, P., Lafarague, R.T., Kowalik, S., Clark, A., Tsaltas, M.O., & Young, J.G. (1994). Clomipramine ameliorates adventitious movements and compulsions in prepubertal boys with autistic disorder and severe mental retardation. *Neurology, 44,* 1309–1312.

Brown, D., Winsberg, B.G., Bialer, I., & Press, M. (1973). Imipramine therapy and seizures: Three children treated for hyperactive behavior disorders. *American Journal of Psychiatry, 130,* 210–221.

Carter, C.H. (1966). Nortriptyline HCl as a tranquilizer for disturbed mentally retarded patients: A controlled study. *American Journal of Medical Sciences, 251,* 465–467.

Charlot, L.R., Doucette, A.C., & Mezzacappa, E. (1993). Affective symptoms of institutionalized adults with mental retardation. *American Journal on Mental Retardation, 98,* 408–416.

Cook, E.H. Jr., Rowlett, R., Jaselskis, C., & Leventhal, B.L. (1992). Fluoxetine treatment of children and adults with autistic disorder and mental retardation. *Journal of the American Academy of Child and Adolescent Psychiatry, 31,* 739–745.

Cook, E.H. Jr., Terry, E.J., Heller, W., & Leventhal, B.L. (1990). Fluoxetine treatment of borderline mentally retarded adults with obsessive-compulsive disorder. *Journal of Clinical Psychopharmacology, 10,* 228–229.

Corbett, J.A. (1979). Psychiatric morbidity and mental retardation. In F.E. James & R.P. Snaith (Eds.), *Psychiatric illness and mental handicap* (pp. 11–25). London: Gaskell Press.

Cox, W.H. (1982). An indication for the use of imipramine in attention deficit disorder. *American Journal of Psychiatry, 139,* 1059–1060.

Davidson, P.W., Cain, N.N., Sloane-Reeves, J.E., Van Speybroech, A., Segel, J., Gutkin, J., Quijano, L.E., Kramer, B.M., Porter, B., Shoham, I., & Goldstein, E. (1994). Characteristics of community-based individuals with mental retardation and aggressive behavioral disorders. *American Journal on Mental Retardation, 98,* 704–716.

Davies, T.S. (1961). A monoamine oxidase inhibitor (Niamid) in the treatment of the mentally subnormal. *Journal of Mental Science, 107,* 115–118.

Dech, D., & Budow, L. (1991). The use of fluoxetine in an adolescent with Prader-Willi syndrome. *Journal of the American Academy of Child and Adolescent Psychiatry, 30,* 298–302.

Dorison, E.E., & Blackman, S. (1962). Imipramine in the treatment of adult enuretics. *American Journal of Psychiatry, 119,* 474.

Dosen, A. (1982). Ervaringen met psychofarmaca bij zwakzinnige kinderen. *Tijschrifft Kindergeneeskunde, 50,* 10–19.

Dosen, A. (1984). Depressive conditions in mentally retarded children. *Acta Paedopsychiatrica, 50,* 29–40.

Dosen, A. (1990). *Psychische en gedragsstoornissen bij zwaksinnigen.* Amsterdam, Mepple: Boom.

Drew, L.R.H. (1967). Drug control of incontinence in adult mental defectives. *Medical Journal of Australia, 2,* 206–207.

Facts and Comparisons. (1995). *Drug interaction facts.* (1995). St. Louis, MO: Authors.

Dubovsky, S.L. (1994). Beyond the serotonin reuptake inhibitors: Rationales for the development of new serotonergic agents. *Journal of Clinical Psychiatry, 55(Suppl. 2),* 34–44.

Emslie, G.J., Wleinberg, W.A., Kowatch, R.A., Hughes, C.W., Carmody, T.J., & Rush, A.J. (1995). *Fluoxetine treatment of depression in children and adolescents.* Paper presented at the 35th annual meeting of the New Clinical Drug.

Field, C.J., Aman, M.G., White, A.J., & Vaithianathan, C. (1986). A single-subject study of imipramine in a mentally retarded woman with depressive symptoms. *Journal of Mental Deficiency Research, 30,* 191–198.

Fisher, G.W., Murray, F., Walley, M.R., & Kiloh, L.G. (1963). A controlled trial of imipramine in the treatment of nocturnal enuresis in mentally subnormal patients. *American Journal of Mental Deficiency, 67,* 536–538.

Freeman, C.P.L., Trimble, M.R., Deakin, J.F.W., Stokes, T.M., & Ashford, J.J. (1994). Fluvoxamine versus clomipramine in the treatment of obsessive compulsive disorder: A multicenter, randomized, double-blind, parallel group comparison. *Journal of Clinical Psychiatry, 55,* 301–305.

Furlanut, M., Montanari, G., Benetello, P., Bonin, P., Schiaulini, P., & Pellegrino, P.A. (1989). Steady-state serum concentrations of imipramine, its main metabolites and clinical response in primary enuresis. *Pharmacology Research, 21,* 561–566.

Garber J.H., McGonigle, J.J., Slomka, T.T., & Monteverde, E. (1992). Clomipramine treatment of stereotypic behaviors and

self-injury in patients with developmental disabilities. *Journal of the American Academy of Child and Adolescent Psychiatry, 31,* 1157–1160.

Garfinkel, B.D., Wender, P.H., Sloman, L., & O'Neill, I. (1983). Tricyclic antidepressants and methylphenidate treatment of attention deficit disorder in children. *Journal of the American Academy of Child and Adolescent Psychiatry, 22,* 343–348.

Gastfriend, D.R., Biederman, J., & Jellinek, M.S. (1984). Desipramine in the treatment of adolescents with attention-deficit disorder. *American Journal of Psychiatry, 141,* 906–908.

Gedye, A. (1991a). Serotonergic treatment for aggression in a Down's syndrome adult showing signs of Alzheimer's disease. *Journal of Mental Deficiency Research, 35,* 247–258.

Gedye, A. (1991b). Trazodone reduced aggressive and self-injurious movements in a mentally handicapped male patient with autism. *Journal of Clinical Psychopharmacology, 11,* 275–276.

Gedye, A. (1992). Recognizing obsessive-compulsive disorder in clients with developmental disabilities. *The Habilitative Mental Healthcare Newsletter, 11,* 73–77.

Ghaziuddin, M., & Tsai, L. (1991). Depression in autistic disorder. *British Journal of Psychiatry, 159,* 721–723.

Goodwin, F.J., & Redfield Jamison, K. (1990). *Manic-depressive illness.* New York: Oxford University Press.

Gordon, C.T., Rapoport, J.L., Hamburger, S.D., State, R.C., & Mannheim, G.B. (1992). Differential response of seven subjects with autistic disorder to clomipramine and dispramine. *American Journal of Psychiatry, 149,* 363–366.

Hamdan-Allen, G. (1991). Brief report: Trichotillomania in an autistic male. *Journal of Autism and Developmental Disorders, 21,* 79–82.

Hellings, J.A., & Warnock, J.K. (1994). Self-injurious behavior and serotonin in Prader-Willi syndrome. *Psychopharmacology Bulletin, 30,* 245–250.

Hicks, W.R., & Barnes, E.H. (1964). A double-blind study of the effect of imipramine on enuresis in 100 naval recruits. *American Journal of Psychiatry, 120,* 812.

Hilton, D.K., Martin, C.A., Heffron, W.M., Hall, B., & Johnson, G.L. (1991). Imipramine treatment of ADHD in a fragile X child. *Journal of the American Academy of Child and Adolescent Psychiatry, 30,* 831–834.

Hollander, E. (1993). Obsessive-compulsive spectrum disorders: An overview. *Psychiatric Annals, 23,* 355–358.

Hollister, L. (1994). New psychotherapeutic drugs. *Journal of Clinical Psychopharmacology, 14,* 50–63.

Holzer, J.C., Goodman, W.K., McDougle, C.J., Baer, L., Boyarksy, B.K., Leckman, J.F., & Price, L.H. (1994). Obsessive-com-

pulsive disorder with and without a chronic tic disorder. *British Journal of Psychiatry, 164,* 469–473.

Howland, R.H. (1992). Fluoxetine treatment of depression in mentally retarded adults. *Journal of Nervous and Mental Disease, 180,* 202–205.

Huessy, H.R., & Ruoff, P.A. (1984). Towards a rational drug usage in a state institution for retarded individuals. *Psychiatric Journal of the University of Ottawa, 9,* 56–58.

Hyman, S.E., & Arana, G.W. (1995). Antidepressant Drugs. In *Handbook of Psychiatric Drug Therapy* (pp. 43–92). Boston: Little, Brown and Co.

Iwata, B.A., Pace, G.M., Dorsey, M.F., Zarcone, J.R., Vollmer, T.R., Smith, R.G., Rodgers, T.A., Lerman, D.C., Shore, B.A., Mazaleski, J.L., Goh, H.L., Edwards Cowdery, G., Kalsher, M.J., McCosh, K.C., & Willis, K.D. (1994). The functions of self-injurious behavior: An experimental-epidemiological analysis. *Journal of Applied Behavior Analysis, 27,* 215–240.

Jacobs, B.L. (1991). Serotonin and behavior: Emphasis on motor control. *Journal of Clinical Psychiatry, 52(Suppl. 12),* 17–23.

Janicak, P.G., Davis, J.M., Preskorn, S.H., & Ayd, F.J. Jr. (1993). Treatment with antidepressants. In P.G. Janiacak (Ed.), *Principles and practice of psychopharmacotherapy* (pp. 209–292). Baltimore: Williams & Wilkins.

Jawed, S.H., Krishnan, V.H.R., & Cassidy, G. (1994). Self-injurious behaviour and the serotonin link: Two case illustrations and theoretic overview. *Irish Journal of Psychological Medicine, 11,* 165–168.

Jawed, S.H., Krishnan, V.H.R., Prasher, V.P., & Corbett, J. (1993). Worsening of pica as a symptom of depressive illness in a person with severe mental handicap. *British Journal of Psychiatry, 162,* 835–837.

Jenike, M.A. (1993). Augmentation strategies for treatment-resistant obsessive-compulsive disorder. *Harvard Review of Psychiatry, 1,* 17–26.

Jensen, P.S., Ryan, N.D., & Prien, R. (1992). Psychopharmacology of child and adolescent major depression: Present status and future directions. *Journal of Child and Adolescent Psychopharmacology, 2,* 11–22.

Johnston, H.F., & Fruehling, J.J. (1994). Using antidepressant medication in depressed children: An algorithm. *Psychiatric Annals, 24,* 348–356.

King, B.H. (1991). Fluoxetine reduced self-injurious behavior in an adolescent with mental retardation. *Journal of Child and Adolescent Psychopharmacology, 1,* 321–329.

King, B.H., DeAntonio, C., McCracken, J.T., Forness, S.R., & Ackerland, V. (1994). Psychiatric consultation in severe and profound mental retardation. *American Journal of Psychiatry, 151,* 1802–1808.

Laman, D.L., & Reiss, S. (1987). Social skills deficiencies associated with depressed mood in mentally retarded adults. *American Journal of Mental Deficiency, 92,* 224–229.

Lowry, M.A., & Sovner, R. (1992). Severe behavior problems associated with rapid cycling bipolar disorder in two adults with profound mental retardation. *Journal of Mental Deficiency Research, 36,* 269–281.

MacLean, R.E.G. (1960). Imipramine hydrochloride and enuresis. *American Journal of Psychiatry, 117,* 551.

Markowitz, P.I. (1990). Fluoxetine treatment of self-injurious behavior in mentally retarded patients. *Journal of Clinical Psychopharmacology, 10,* 299–300.

Markowitz, P.I. (1992). Effect of fluoxetine on self-injurious behavior in the developmentally disabled: A preliminary study. *Journal of Clinical Psychopharmacology, 12,* 27–31.

Matin, M.A., & Rundle, A.T. (1980). Physiological and psychiatric investigations into a group of mentally handicapped subjects with self-injurious behaviour. *Journal of Mental Deficiency Research, 24,* 77–85.

McDougle, C.J., Price, L.H., & Goodman, W.K. (1990). Fluvoxamine treatment of coincident autistic disorder and obsessive compulsive disorder: A case report. *Journal of Autism and Developmental Disorders, 20,* 537–543.

McDougle, C.J., Price, L.H., Volkmar, F.R., Goodman, W.K., Ward-O'Brien, D., Nielsen, J., Bregman, J., & Cohen, D.J. (1992). Clomipramine and autism: Preliminary evidence of efficacy. *Journal of the American Academy of Child and Adolescent Psychiatry, 31,* 746–750.

McNally, R.J. (1994). *Panic disorder.* New York: Guilford Press.

Meins, W. (1995). Assessment of depression in mentally retarded adults: Reliability and validity of the Children's Depression Inventory (CDI). *Research in Developmental Disabilities, 14,* 299–312.

Nierenberg, A.A., & Cole, J.O. (1991). Antidepressant adverse drug reactions. *Journal of Clinical Psychiatry, 52*(Suppl. 6), 40–47.

O'Dwyer, J., Holmes, J., & Collacott, R.A. (1992). Two cases of obsessive-compulsive disorder in individuals with Down's syndrome. *Journal of Nervous and Mental Disorders, 180,* 603–604.

O'Neill, M., Page, N., Adkins, W.N., & Eichelman, B. (1986). Tryptophan-trazodone treatment of aggressive behavior. *Lancet, 2,* 859–856.

Pary, R.J. (1989). Pretreatment systolic orthostatic blood pressure depression in Down's syndrome. *Journal of Clinical Psychopharmacology, 9,* 146–147.

Pilkington, T.L. (1962). A report on "Tofranil" in mental deficiency. *American Journal of Mental Deficiency, 66,* 729–732.

Pliszka, S.R. (1987). Tricyclic antidepressants in the treatment of children with attention deficit disorder. *Journal of the American Academy of Child and Adolescent Psychiatry, 26,* 127–132.

Prasad, A. (1985). Efficacy of trazodone as an anti-obsessional agent. *Pharmacology Biochemistry and Behavior, 22,* 347–348.

Preskorn, S.H. (1993). Pharmacokinetics of antidepressants: Why and how they are relevant to treatment. *Journal of Clinical Psychiatry, 54 (Suppl. 9),* 14–34.

Preskorn, S.H. (1994). Antidepressant drug selection: Criteria and options. *Journal of Clinical Psychiatry, 55 (Suppl. 9),* 6–22.

Preskorn, S.H., & Burke, M. (1992). Somatic therapy for major depressive disorder: Selection of an antidepressant. *Journal of Clinical Psychiatry, 53 (Suppl. 9),* 5–18.

Rapoport, J. (1965). Childhood behavior and learning problems treated with imipramine. *International Journal of Neuropsychiatry, 1,* 635–642.

Rapoport, J.L., Mikkelsen, E.J., Zavadil, A., Nee, L., Gruenan, C., Mendleson, W., & Gellen, J.C. (1980). Childhood enuresis. II: Psychopathology, tricyclic concentration in plasma and antienuretic effect. *Archives of General Psychiatry, 37,* 1146–1152.

Rapoport, J., Quinn, P.O., Bradbard, G., Riddle, K.D., & Brooks, E. (1974). Imipramine and methylphenidate treatments of hyperactive boys. *Archives of General Psychiatry, 30,* 789–793.

Reiss, S. (1994). *Handbook of challenging behavior: Mental health aspects of mental retardation.* Worthington, OH: IDS Publishing Corporation.

Reiss, S., & Rojahn, J. (1993). Joint occurrence of depression and aggression in children and adults with mental retardation. *Journal of Intellectual Disability Research, 37,* 287–294.

Richelson, E. (1994). Pharmacology of antidepressants: characteristics of the ideal drug. *Mayo Clinic Proceedings, 69,* 1069–1081.

Ricketts, R.W., Goza, A.B., Ellis, C.R., Singh, Y.N., Singh, N.N., & Cooke, J.C., III. (1993). Fluoxetine treatment of severe self-injury in young adults with mental retardation. *Journal of the American Academy of Child and Adolescent Psychiatry, 32,* 865–869.

Roose, S.P., & Glassman, A.H. (1989). Cardiovascular effects of tricyclic antidepressants in depressed patients. *Journal of Clinical Psychiatry Monograph Series, 7,* 1–18.

Rosenberg, D.R., Holttum, J., & Gershon, S. (1994) *Text of pharmacotherapy for child and adolescent psychiatric disorders* (pp. 55–103). New York: Brunner/Mazel.

Ruedrich, S.L., & Wilkinson, L. (1992). Atypical unipolar depression in mentally retarded patients: Amoxapine treatment. *Journal of Nervous and Mental Disease, 180,* 206–207.

Sacks B., & Smith, S. (1989). People with Down's syndrome can be distinguished on the basis of cholinergic dysfunction. *Journal of Neurology, Neurosurgery and Psychiatry, 52,* 1294–1295.

Sachs, G.S., Lafer, B., Stoll, A.L., Banov, M., Thibault, A.B., Tohen, M., & Bernstein, J.F. (1994). A double-blind trial of bupropion versus desipramine for bipolar depression. *Journal of Clinical Psychiatry, 55,* 391–393.

Saul, R.C. (1985). Nortriptyline in attention-deficit disorder. *Clinical Neuropharmacology, 8,* 382–384.

Singh, A.N. (1993). Case report 2: Fluoxetine treatment of self-injurious behaviour in mental retardation and its interaction with carbamazepine. *Journal of Drug Development, 6,* 23–24.

Smith, E.H., & Gonzales, R. (1967). Nortriptyline hydrochloride in the treatment of enuresis in mentally retarded boys. *American Journal of Mental Deficiency, 71,* 825–827.

Sovner, R. (1988). Behavioral psychopharmacology. In J. Stark, J. F.J. Menolascino, M. Albarelli, & V. Gray (Eds.), *Mental retardation and mental health: classification, diagnosis, treatment, services* (pp. 229–242). New York: Springer-Verlag.

Sovner, R., Fox, C.J., Lowry, M.J., & Lowry, M.A. (1993). Fluoxetine treatment of depression and associated self-injury in two adults with mental retardation. *Journal of Intellectual Disability Research, 37,* 301–311.

Sovner, R., & Pary, R.J. (1993). Affective disorders in developmentally disabled persons. In J.L. Matson & R.P. Barrett (Eds.), *Psychopathology in the mentally retarded* (pp. 87–147). Needham Heights, MA: Allyn and Bacon.

Stein, D.J., Hollander, E., & Liebowitz, M.R. (1993). Neurobiology of impulsivity and the impulse control disorders. *Journal of Neuropsychiatry and Clinical Neurosciences, 5,* 9–17.

Todd, R.D. (1991). Fluoxetine in autism. *American Journal of Psychiatry, 148,* 1089.

Valentine, A.A., & Maxwell, C. (1968). Enuresis in severely subnormal children: A clinical trial of imipramine. *Journal of Mental Subnormality, 14,* 84–90.

van Blakom, A.J.L.M., van Oppen, P., Vermeulen, A.W.A., Van Dyck, R., Navta, M.C.E., & Vorst, H.C.M. (1994). A meta-analysis on the treatment of obsessive-compulsive disorder: A comparison of antidepressant, behavior, and cognitive therapy. *Clinical Psychology Review, 14,* 359.381.

Vitello, B., Spreat, S., & Behar, D. (1989). Obsessive-compulsive disorder in mentally retarded patients. *Journal of Nervous and Mental Disorders, 177,* 232–236.

Waizer, J., Hoffman, S.P., Polizos, P., & Englehardt, D. (1974). Outpatient treatment of hyperactive children with imipramine. *American Journal of Psychiatry, 131,* 587–591.

Walley, T., Pirmohamed, M., Proudlove, C., & Maxwell, D. (1993). Interaction of fluoxetine and metoprolol. *Lancet, 341,* 967–968.

Way, M.C. (1983). *The symptoms of affective disorder in severely retarded children.* Paper presented at the meeting of the International Association for the Scientific Study of Mental Deficiency Congress, Toronto.

Wehr, T.A., & Goodwin, F.K. (1987). Can antidepressants cause mania and worsen the course of affective illness? *American Journal of Psychiatry, 144,* 1403–1411.

Wiener, K., & Lamberti, J.S. (1993). Sertraline and mental retardation with obsessive-compulsive disorder. *American Journal of Psychiatry, 150,* 1270.

Wender, P.H., & Reimherr, F.W. (1990). Bupropion treatment of attention-deficit hyperactivity disorders in adults. *American Journal of Psychiatry, 147,* 1018–1020.

Wenger, T.L., & Stern, W.C. (1983). The cardiovascular profile of bupropion. *Journal of Clinical Psychiatry, 44,* 176–182.

Werry, J.S., Aman, M.G., & Diamond, E. (1979). Imipramine and methylphenidate in hyperactive children. *Journal of Child Psychology and Psychiatry, 21,* 27–35.

Wilens, T.E., Biederman, J., Geist, D.E., Steingard, R., & Spencer, T. (1993). Nortriptyline in the treatment of ADHD: A chart review of 58 cases. *Journal of the American Academy of Child and Adolescent Psychiatry, 32,* 343–349.

Winsberg, B.G., Bailer, I., Kupietz, S., & Tobias, J. (1972). Effects of imipramine and dextroamphetamine on behavior of neuropsychiatrically impaired children. *American Journal of Psychiatry, 128,* 1424–1431.

Wood, A., Tollefson, G.D., & Birkett, M. (1991). Pharmacotherapy of obsessive compulsive disorder: Experience with fluoxetine. *International Clinical Psychopharmacology, 8,* 301–306.

Yassa, R., Camille, Y., & Belize, L. (1987). Tardive dyskinesia in the course of antidepressant therapy: A prevalence study and review of the literature. *Journal of Clinical Psychopharmacology, 7,* 243–246.

Zametkin, A., & Rapoport, J.L. (1987). Noradrenergic hypothesis of attention deficit disorder with hyperactivity: A critical review. In H.Y. Meltzer (Ed.), *Psychopharmacology: The third generation of progress* (pp. 837–842). New York: Raven Press.

Zametkin, A., Rapoport, J.L., Murphy, D., Linnoila, M., Ismond, D. (1985). Treatment of hyperactive children with monoamine oxidase inhibitors: I. Clinical efficacy. *Archives of General Psychiatry, 42,* 962–966.

Anxiolytics and Sedatives

John S. Werry[1]

The term *anxiolytic* (or anti-anxiety) medication is restricted here to drugs whose primary use is to relieve anxiety arising in normal life or in nonpsychotic psychiatric disorders. This definition distinguishes anxiolytics from other anti-anxiety agents used primarily in the treatment of psychosis or severe mood disorders. That is, the anxiolytics are distinguished from antipsychotic and antidepressant medications.

Historically, the term *sedation* refers to a reduction of the level of arousal by chemical means. Because this can now be achieved in a variety of neurochemical ways with correspondingly different clinical pictures, the term lacks precise meaning. The term *sedative* refers to drugs used primarily to induce sleep. This term is being replaced by modern terms like *hypnotic,* which means sleep-inducing.

Anxiolytic and sedative drugs have been around for more than 100 years and the more modern ones, like the benzodiazepines, for over 30 years (American Psychiatric Association [APA], 1990; Gelenberg, Bassuk, & Schoonover, 1991; Gilman, Rall, Nies, & Taylor, 1990; Greenblatt & Shader, 1974). There are three main groups of these drugs: (1) central nervous system (CNS) depressants, (2) antihistaminic and anticholinergic sedatives, and (3) atypical, a relatively new group. Opiates and some analgesics also have anxiolytic or sedative properties, but they will not be discussed here because they are not used in the treatment of anxiety. The main classes, subgroups, and examples of anxiolytics and sedatives are set out in Table 12–1.

With the exception of the use of antihistamines for very young children, benzodiazepines have displaced all other traditional anxiolytic and sedative drugs such as barbiturates, meprobamate (Equanil), chloral hydrate, and paraldehyde. This is because benzodiazepines and their analogs offer a high level of safety and a wide variety of duration of effect: from 2 to 4 hours with triazolam (Halcion) to days with chlordiazepoxide (Librium). Most of the newer medications such as zopiclone (Imovane), although not benzodiazepines, are similar to selective depressants and offer no real advance. However, there are a few new atypical anxiolytics such as buspirone (Buspar) that are truly different. Because there is little similarity among the three classes of anxiolytic drugs, they will be discussed separately.

CNS DEPRESSANTS

This group of drugs has the common property of effecting a progressive depression of brain function. The traditional sedatives such as alcohol, barbiturates, paraldehyde, and chloral hydrate are subclassified as the

---

Table 12-1
Anxiolytic and Sedative Substances

General CNS Depressants
  Alcohol
  Anesthetic Agents and Gases
  Anticonvulsants (older types—phenobarbital,
    phenytoin, primidone, etc.)
  Sedatives (older types—e.g., barbiturates,
    chloral hydrate, paraldehyde, meprobamate)
  Volatile Solvents and Gasoline

Partial or Selective CNS Depressants
  Benzodiazepines, Zopiclone

Atypical Anxiolytics
  Buspirone

Anticholinergics and Antihistamines
  Hyoscine and Belladonna Derivatives
  Antihistamines

Analgesics
  Opiates
  Other Analgesics

---

1 Emeritus Professor of Psychiatry, University of Auckland, New Zealand

Table 12-2. Benzodiazepines

Class & Drug (Brand Names)	Daily Dose* (mg/kg)	Active Metabolites**
I. Long half-life (>13 hrs)/high mg potency		
Clonazepam (Klonopin, Rivotril)	0.007-0.05	No
II. Long half-life (>13 hrs)/low mg potency		
Chlordiazepoxide (Librium)	0.2-0.5	Yes
Diazepam (Valium)	0.07-0.5	Yes
Clorazepate (Tranxene)	0.2-0.8	Yes
Flurazepam (Dalmane)	0.2-0.4	Yes
Nitrazepam (Mogadon)	0.06-0.14	No
III. Short half-life (<13 hrs)/high mg potency		
Lorazepam (Ativan)	0.014-0.08	No
Alprazolam (Xanax)	0.014-0.08 ***	No
Triazolam (Halcion)	0.0017-0.007	No
IV. Short half-life(<13 hrs)/low mg potency		
Oxazepam (Serax, Serapax)	0.14-1.7	No
Temazepam (Restoril, Euhypnos)	0.2-0.4	No

Note.   * Doses are for adults converted to mg/kg by dividing by 70. Doses and indications have not been established in children or adolescents.
    ** Clinical action may be longer than elimination half-life where active metabolites are produced.
    *** Upper range of alprazolam is for panic disorder only.

general CNS depressants because of their widespread, indiscriminate action (Baldessarini, 1990). Most of the drugs developed since the mid 1960s are selective or partial CNS depressants and consist almost exclusively of benzodiazepines and cogenors like zopiclone. The selective CNS depressants have displaced the general CNS depressants except for use in anesthesiology and in the management of epilepsy. The more important benzodiazepines are detailed in Table 12–2.

Pharmacodynamics

CNS depressants belong to a large class of organic, mostly highly lipid-soluble gases, liquids, and solids used medically, industrially, socially, and illicitly. Their common action is related to their capacity to slow neuronal excitability by interfering with ionic flows (especially of chloride) across membranes (Baldessarini, 1990), which results in increased resistance to induction and passage of the nerve impulse. Effects are achieved in one of the following two ways.

1. Because of their high lipid solubility, CNS depressants may have a direct effect on the membrane, which produces an effect on all nervous (and other) tissue (Kennedy & Longnecker, 1990). These depressants fall under the class name of general CNS depressants (Baldessarini, 1990). Alcohol is the prototypic drug in this class. Recent work suggests that this general effect may be mediated through widely distributed glutamine and aspartate receptors rather than directly on the membrane as was originally believed (Tsai, Gastfriend, & Coyle, 1995).

2. Selective CNS depressants are so-called because they have an effect on specific receptors such as GABA, which produces a limited effect (Baldessarini, 1990). These drugs are known popularly as minor tranquilizers.

Benzodiazepine drugs are typical of this group.

Although the mechanism of action is different, both selective and general depressants produce a reduction in ionic flux, raising the threshold to excitation (Kutcher, Reiter, Gardner, & Klein, 1992; Rall, 1990). In clinical practice, the difference between general and selective depressants in therapeutic dosage is not as great as is commonly supposed. Their basic pharmacological similarity is suggested by their cross-tolerance or their ability to serve as substitutes for one another in terms of dependence and withdrawal (APA, 1990). However, in overdose, the selective depressants are clinically distinctive. The action of selective depressants is limited in its effect when the target receptors become saturated, but the action of general depressants continues to increase, through coma to death, in a dose-dependent way. Thus the therapeutic ratio is very high for selective depressants, whereas that of the general depressants is usually low, which makes the general depressants much more dangerous drugs.

Although it is customary to distinguish between the general and the selective CNS depressants, there is merit in identifying all of these substances as belonging to one class having similar basic effects and differing only in their toxicology, pharmacokinetics, and clinical indications. The use of these drugs is determined largely by their pharmacokinetics, or speed of onset and duration of action. Gaseous or highly volatile substances are employed in anesthesia because, once inhaled, they enter directly into pulmonary circulation and reach the brain in a few seconds. This effect will disappear quickly as the substance is taken up by lipid tissues throughout the rest of the body. These drugs also are abused by adolescents who seek a quick "buzz." Inhaled substances will not be discussed further here because they have limited use in psychopharmacology.

Types, Potencies, and Pharmacokinetics

As is shown in Table 12–2, there are considerable differences among the various benzodiazepines in potency. For example, a normal adult dose of triazolam (Halcion) is about 0.125 mg, whereas that of diazepam (Valium) is 50 to 100 times higher. The various benzodiazepines also show important pharmacokinetic differences; however, there is little difference in action or efficacy. The uses for these drugs often reflect the physician's personal preferences rather than pharmacological differences.

Most benzodiazepines are quickly and sufficiently absorbed, and peak blood concentrations occur in about 30 minutes (Baldessarini, 1990). Some drugs such as oxazepam and clonazepam are only slowly absorbed; therefore, their peak concentrations in the blood may take several hours to build up. With the possible exception of lorazepam (Gelenberg et al., 1991), intramuscular dosage is irregularly absorbed and should be used only when essential oral medication is refused. Intravenous use is potentially dangerous because it can lead to rapid, very high brain concentrations. Taking this risk is unjustifiable except in certain situations, such as status epilepticus.

After absorption, the pharmacokinetics become rather complex (APA, 1990; Baldessarini, 1990). Distribution is rapid into highly perfused lipid tissues like the brain. After a single dose, effects may disappear quickly because other, less vascular tissues such as fat stores absorb the drug more slowly. Also, some drugs such as diazepam show a secondary peak after about 6 to 12 hours, suggestive of enterohepatic recirculation.

Inactivation occurs in the liver, and a pharmacodynamic equilibrium will ultimately be achieved as expected after about 4 to 5 half-lives. However, this time span may not reflect the timeframe of actual clinical actions because some drugs produce active metabolites such as diazepam to nordiazepam to oxazepam, which may prolong detectable effects for up to 100 hours. Much of the original data on duration of action was misleading, because they were based on a single dose given before lipid stores became saturated or active metabolites were produced. The drugs that produce no or only trivial active metabolites are lorazepam, oxazepam, temazepam, alprazolam, triazolam, and nitrazepam (APA, 1990; Greenblatt & Shader, 1974). Actions of benzodiazepines are thought to reflect the actual momentary concentrations of the drug or its active metabolites at receptor sites, and these actions are thought to be rapidly reversible.

CNS and Other System Effects

All but insignificant clinical effects of the benzodiazepines stem from their effect on the brain, which is to depress excitability of nerve tissue (Kutcher et al., 1992; Rall, 1990). Consequently, all produce a dose-dependent progressive depression of brain function. With selective depressants, however, this effect reaches a plateau in deep sleep, well short of fatal coma. This stopping of the progressive effect is caused by receptor saturation in the brain.

Neurophysiologically, CNS depression blocks brain stem activating system stimulation. This has a number of consequences, including depression of spinal reflexes, raised seizure threshold, depression of after-discharges in the limbic system, mild depression of REM sleep, and suppression of Stage 4 sleep with prolongation of total sleep time (Baldessarini, 1990). The production of any significant degree of muscle relaxation is debatable, despite a widespread clinical assumption that this is the case (Baldessarini, 1990).

Behaviorally, the depression of brain function is seen as a dose-dependent reduction in the level of arousal. As with alcohol consumption, the effects begin with the most advanced functions of intellect and progress to include social judgment, inhibition, and motor coordination. Only in higher doses or in particular individuals will true intoxication occur. Intoxication is a sign that dosage is excessive, and it should be an unusual occurrence with benzodiazepines. Unlike alcohol, benzodiazepines do not cause dangerous vomiting, and unconsciousness supervenes because they do not produce gastric irritation and the neurotoxic metabolite acetaldehyde. Fortunately, overdoses are rarely life-threatening; it is almost impossible to kill oneself with benzodiazepines if they are taken orally and without any other drugs.

The effects of benzodiazepines and other sedatives are influenced by the social setting and the person's mood. In relaxed people, sleep is likely to intervene at a low dose; in anxious people, higher doses are required to induce sleep. In group situations, bonhomie is likely to prevail, but when conflict arises, this can change quickly to aggression or panic. The benzodiazepines are used to achieve anxiolysis without sedation. However, the gap between anxiolysis and sedation is quite narrow as measured by blood levels (Baldessarini, 1990).

Research with both experimental subjects and psychiatric patients indicates that these drugs may impair cognition and performance in most people; however, in people who are highly anxious, there may be some improvement. According to the American Psychiatric Association Task Force on Benzodiazepine Dependence, these impairments usually occur in memory, psychomotor speed, motor coordination, and sustained attention (APA, 1990, pp. 42-48). There are two possible effects on memory: (a) impairment of consolidation or delayed recall, which may occur even when there is no sedation or other psychomotor impairment, and (b) anterograde amnesia (blackouts), which usually occurs after acute, higher intravenous dosage but also in association with alcohol and with high potency short-acting drugs like triazolam. Conversely, discontinuation may be associated with improved function, as has been indicated by self-reports and appropriate laboratory tests. Benzodiazepines generally do not affect well-learned habits.

Very little research has been reported on psychomotor effects for certain special populations. Two studies with anxious children and adolescents revealed mild improvement in psychomotor functioning (Aman & Werry, 1982; Simeon et al., 1992). There have been few systematic studies of the psychomotor effects of benzodiazepines and other sedative drugs in people with mental retardation (Aman & Werry, 1982; Simeon et al., 1992). Very little is known about the effects of therapeutic doses on cognition and speed of performance in people with mental retardation. However, there is no plausible reason to assume that people with mental retardation are less vulnerable to the well-documented impairments of cognition and speed of performance seen in other populations.

When used in therapeutic dosages, the benzodiazepines have almost no important effects on other body systems (Rall, 1990). There is some mild depression of function in the respiratory and cardiovascular systems, but these are of little clinical significance. As was previously noted, there is no clinically significant effect on muscle tone (Baldessarini, 1990).

Side Effects, Toxic Effects, and Interactions

The adverse effects of benzodiazepines and their analogs are behavioral disinhibition, hyperactivity, irritability, aggressiveness, and sedation. Sedation is a particularly common side effect. These drugs also produce intoxication similar to that produced by alcohol. The drugs may impair memory, other cognitive functions, and motor coordination, and they may slow psychomotor function. The drugs are subject to abuse and produce dependence. Withdrawal symptoms include anxiety, insomnia, tremor, restlessness, irritability, muscle tension, sweating, nausea, and seizures (APA, 1990). Rebound symptoms, which consist of exacerbation of original symptoms appearing rapidly after discontinuance, are now recognized as potential problems with these drugs. Benzodiazepine side effects are most likely to occur (a) with the high-potency or short-acting drugs, (b) at high dosages such as those used for panic disorder, (c) after continuous use of four months or more, (d) after abrupt rather than graduated discontinuance, and (e) with abuse of other drugs, especially alcohol.

The most important interactions of both general and selective CNS depressants are with other psychotropic drugs depressing brain function, independent of the mechanism by which this is achieved. For example, the action of CNS depressants is augmented by neuroleptics, anticholinergics, antihistaminics, and many other antidepressants. Although the selective CNS depressants like the benzodiazepines are not fatal in overdose if taken alone, they can become lethal if taken in combination with most other psychotropic drugs. The general CNS depressants have a number of other serious drug interactions, notably with the anticoagulants and anticonvulsants. Benzodiazepines have very few of these interactions, although they do affect blood levels of phenytoin and digoxin, and they can be affected themselves by antacids, disulfiram, and cimetidine (see Baldessarini, 1990; Gelenberg et al. 1991).

Clinical Indications Exclusive of Mental Retardation

Anxiety is a universal and normal experience important for survival and adaptation. It is usually harmless. However, anxiety is maladaptive when it is persistent, durable, or disruptive. There are three situations in which therapeutic interventions for anxiety may be attempted:

- when a person is reacting strongly to a stressful event, for example, when a person experiences an unusually strong bereavement following loss of a loved one;

- when anxiety is so severe, persistent, or pervasive that it significantly interferes with the overall adaptation and functioning of the person affected; and

- when anxiety is associated with a psychopathological state such as dementia or schizophrenia.

In addition to being used as anti-anxiety agents, these drugs may be used for the induction of sleep, induction of anesthesia, control of excited behavior, control of epilepsy, and stabilization of mood. The latter two will not be discussed here because they are covered in other chapters. Anxiolytics may be prescribed to treat symptoms,

symptom complexes, or disorders. Interventions are rarely curative and usually symptomatic in effect.

The indications for use in psychiatric disorders are shown in Table 12–3; these are based on literature reviews and expert authorities (APA, 1990; Baldessarini, 1990; McNally 1994; Roy-Byrne & Wingerson, 1992). Some of the indications are better established than others. Although the literature is large, much of it is difficult to interpret, because it addresses symptoms such as anxiety rather than modern discrete, DSM-IV disorders (APA, 1994). There are few sound studies that address specific categories of psychiatric disorder.

Adjustment Disorders and v Codes. Anxiolytics may be used to treat adjustment disorders, which are stress-related and begin within three months of the onset of the stressor and extend not more than six months beyond its cessation (APA, 1994). Bereavement has a separate diagnostic category, although it is a kind of adjustment disorder. The majority of people with stress-related disorders are seen by generic physicians rather than by psychiatrists, behavior pediatricians, and other mental health specialists. These physicians account for most of the prescriptions for anxiolytics. Clinically, these drugs are held to be most useful in the management of acute anxiety for people who are without personality disorders (Baldessarini, 1990). Some authorities believe that the clinical indications for use with people diagnosed with adjustment disorders and v codes should be restricted to acute cases, to people who have no other psychiatric or personality disorder, and to people for whom other common nonpharmacological measures have failed.

Sleep Disorders. Because CNS depressants are highly effective in inducing sleep, they may be used in the treatment of various sleep disorders, although now only with benzodiazepines and their analogs. However, the dose required often produces a degree of diurnal sedation, and the quality of sleep is often inferior. Because benzodi-

---

Table 12-3. Indications for the Use of CNS Depressant Type Anxiolytic Drugs in Psychiatric Disorders in Adults

Established Indications	Probable Indications	Possible Indications
Panic Disorder	Adjustment Disorder with Anxiety	Akathisia
Generalized Anxiety Disorder	Acute Stress-related Insomnia	Tourette Disorder
Social Phobia	Circadian Rhythm Disturbances	Severely Excited States (emergencies)
Mania/Excited Schizophrenia		

Note. Ordinarily, these indications are for short term (<4 months) only.

azepines are effective and safe only when used for short periods, physicians face a difficult question when evaluating possible use for sleep disorders. It is much easier to start patients on these drugs than it is to terminate use. There is, however, a general consensus that they can be indicated for temporary insomnia caused by external circumstances that cause distress to the person afflicted, but that they should be given in the lowest dose possible and for only a very few days with proper medical follow-up (Rall, 1990).

Panic Disorder. Panic attacks are acute episodes of anxiety that occur without warning. They may be associated with agoraphobia, in which a person becomes afraid to venture out of the house and away from resources that might bring assistance should another panic attack occur. Evidence has been obtained for both the efficacy of pharmacological treatment and cognitive-behavioral therapy (McNally, 1994), with different people responding to the two therapies. Many authorities believe that combined medication and cognitive-behavioral therapy is the best approach for achieving long-term benefits (McNally, 1994).

The antidepressants, especially imipramine, are the preferred pharmacological treatment for panic disorder (McNally, 1994). However, benzodiazepines have been used with success and safety with those who do not respond to antidepressants, which is about 20% of cases. These drugs also are indicated when immediate relief is important. Unlike the antidepressants, the effect of benzodiazepines occur within a week or so, although it takes four to eight weeks for the effect to peak (Roy-Byrne & Wingerson, 1992). Alprazolam in doses of 2 to 4 mg/day in four divided doses (sometimes up to 6 mg and rarely up to 10 mg) has been shown to be effective. Clonazepam in lower doses and lorazepam in higher doses are also used for panic disorder, although they are less well studied. The use of benzodiazepines in the treatment of panic disorder is probably best restricted to non-responders to antidepressants or to those for whom immediate relief is imperative. The drugs may also be used as an adjunct to beginning behavioral treatment.

Generalized Anxiety Disorder (GAD) and Social Phobia. GAD is indicated by frequent worry and pervasive anxiety. In DSM-IV (APA, 1994), GAD includes what used to be called overanxious disorder of childhood in the DSM-III. The benzodiazepines seem useful for the treatment of GAD. Pharmacological management is similar to that for panic disorder, except that the doses are generally about half as much. Because of the recurrent nature of the GAD, medication use may become chronic, and buspirone is preferable in the first instance.

Benzodiazepines have also been used to treat social phobia, which is associated with a fear of rejection, but scientific research has been minimal.

Excited/aggressive states. The use of long-acting benzodiazepines in combination with antipsychotic medication is a matter of some concern. The combination acts synergistically to enhance CNS depression. When high doses are needed, which is likely to be the case in treating excited states, these two types of drugs together may cause toxicity. Additionally, as with the older CNS depressants (Hanzel, Kalachnik, & Harder, 1992), with benzodiazepines there is always the possibility of effecting disinhibition or actually making some patients more rather than less excited. These effects have been demonstrated to occur in children (Graae, Milner, Rizzotto, & Klein, 1994).

Nevertheless, long-acting benzodiazepines like diazepam or clonazepam have been used in adults with some success for treating excited states associated with mania and schizophrenia. In studies by Gelenberg et al. (1991) and by McClellan and Werry (1992), a reduction in the amount of antipsychotic medication needed to control behavior was reported.

Other indications. Benzodiazepines may be helpful in the treatment of akathisia, or restless legs, which is an often overlooked complication of neuroleptic medication (Baldessarini, 1990; Gross, Hull, Lytton, Hill, & Pienel, 1993). They have also been used to treat Tourette syndrome both for adults and children and as an adjunct to clonidine treatment of Tourette syndrome (Steingard, Goldberg, Lee, & DeMaso, 1994). The studies evaluating these uses were poorly controlled, however (Werry & Aman, in press). Also, there is likely to be an interaction between clonidine and benzodiazepines, both of which have sedation as their most common side effect (Werry & Aman, in press).

Special Considerations for Children and Adolescents. Several researchers have reviewed clinical studies of the use of anxiolytics for children (Bernstein & Borchardt, 1991; Coffey, 1990; Kutcher et al., 1992, Werry & Aman, in press). All concluded that, although there is strong evidence attesting to the value of benzodiazepines in the treatment of adults with anxiety disorders, there are very few reliable data on children or adolescents. Some studies suggest a beneficial effect (Aman & Werry, 1982; Bernstein & Borchardt, 1991; Coffey, 1990; Simeon et al., 1992), but most are at least 10 to 15 years old or methodologically unsound (Bernstein & Borchardt, 1991; Kutcher et al., 1992). In one of the few properly controlled studies, Simeon et al. (1992) showed that although alprazolam was associated with improvement in children with overanxious disorder (now GAD) or avoidant disorder, it was little better than placebo. A controlled study of clonazepam (in doses up to 2 mg daily) in childhood anxiety disorders also failed to produce evidence of efficacy (Graae et al., 1994).

Much better data are needed evaluating effects in children and adolescents. Extrapolation of results from studies of adults is problematic for the following reasons. Anxiety disorders in children and adolescents are developmentally distinct from those in adults, and the two may not be continuous (Bernstein & Borchardt, 1991; Werry, 1991). Benzodiazepines are not indicated for the adult disorders seen most commonly in children and adolescents, such as simple phobic disorders and obsessive-compulsive disorder, because other types of drugs or behavior therapy are more effective (Brown, Hertz, & Barlow, 1992; Werry & Wollersheim, 1989). The benzodiazepines may pose greater risks for children and adolescents by exposing them to the chemical way of dealing with anxiety or to potentially dependency-producing drugs (APA, 1990). Although the benzodiazepines and other sedatives are used widely for children and adolescents with sleep disorders (Dahl, 1992; Richman, Douglas, Hunt, Landsdown, & Levere, 1985), authorities differ in their views of the agents' efficacy and safety for this population. Whereas one authority has drawn favorable conclusions (Coffey, 1990), others are more skeptical or prefer alternative treatments (Dahl, 1992; Horne, 1992; Richman et al., 1985).

Indications in Mental Retardation

Anxiolytic drugs have been used in a small but significant minority of people with mental retardation, including those residing in community programs and in institutions (Aman, Sarphare, & Burrow, 1995; Aman & Singh, 1988; Lipman, DiMascio, Reatig, & Kirson, 1978; Sprague & Werry, 1971). Estimates of possible prevalence range up to 5%. Most of the clinical use of anxiolytics has been for the control of disruptive behavior (Aman et al., 1995; Intagliata & Rinck, 1985).

Much of the research on benzodiazepines and mental retardation has involved only children. LaVeck and Buckley (1961) examined a variety of drugs used for children attending a training school. In one study, meprobamate (an older, non-benzodiazepine anxiolytic) was given in combination with promazine (a neuroleptic) and tested in 54 children who had mental retardation, spasticity, and unspecified psychopathology. Although more children in the treatment group were judged to be improved

(11 of 27 subjects; 41%) than in the control group (4 of 27; 15%), the difference was not statistically significant. These same authors compared chlordiazepoxide (30 to 75 mg/day) with placebo in 28 children who had mental retardation and unspecified behavior problems. A crossover design was used, whereby each child eventually received both treatments. Chlordiazepoxide produced a nonsignificant increase in undesirable behavior and resulted in less continuous play, more toy changes, and more hyperactivity in a standard playroom situation. This was a relatively sophisticated study for its time.

In an uncontrolled trial, Krakowski (1963) assessed chlordiazepoxide in 51 children having a variety of emotional and behavioral problems, including 12 children with moderate or severe mental retardation. Overall, 67% of the group (and 50% of those with mental retardation) were thought to respond favorably. Symptoms regarded most responsive in treatment were insomnia (88% of those with the symptom), phobias (78%), crying spells (78%), and anxiety (76%), whereas disobedience (52%), impulsiveness (53%), and lying (55%) were regarded as less responsive. Kraft, Ardali, Duffy, Hart, and Pearce (1965) described 130 children treated with chlordiazepoxide (30 to 130 mg/day). In this uncontrolled study, there were small subgroups with brain damage and with mental retardation. Only 3 of 14 and 0 of 5 participants, respectively, were thought to have a good or excellent response to treatment.

Walters, Singh, and Beale (1977) assessed the effects of three doses (3.0 to 4.5 mg; thrice daily) of lorazepam (Ativan) prescribed for seven institutionalized children diagnosed as hyperactive. This was a placebo-controlled crossover study, but dose was confounded with time (i.e., the same sequence of doses occurred for all children). Lorazepam produced significant increases in hyperactive behavior, assessed by direct observations in the classroom. Side effects recorded in the subjects' medical records included anorexia, lethargy, aggression, and irritability, which coincided with the two larger lorazepam doses, but not with placebo. In a more recent case study, Bond, Mandos, and Kurtz (1989) found that midazolam, an ultra short-acting benzodiazepine used primarily as anesthesia, was useful in controlling recurrent aggression in three persons with mental retardation who were 14, 17, and 26 years old. The drug was given by intramuscular injection in doses of 5 to 10 mg and appeared to be useful in crisis situations. According to another report, clorazepate and alprazolam were found to be helpful for people with mental retardation (Gross et al., 1993).

Finally, three studies by the Costa Mesa group need to be mentioned before concluding this review, even though the drugs assessed appear not to have included the benzodiazepine group. Barron and Sandman (1983) classified 100 residents in terms of whether they exhibited self-injury or stereotypic behavior. The subjects were also classified in terms of whether or not they showed a "paradoxical" response to sedative-hypnotic drugs, which were defined as any chemical substance that exerts a nonselective general depressant action upon the CNS (chloral hydrate, secobarbital, and chlorpromazine were given as examples of sedative-hypnotics). A paradoxical response was defined as maintained wakefulness and resistive, combative, restless, uncooperative, or abusive behavior following large doses of sedative-hypnotics. Barron and Sandman reported that the presence of self-injury and stereotypy, especially in combination, were associated with a paradoxical response. For example, in the first study, Barron and Sandman (1983) found that 69% of participants with both self-injury and stereotypy exhibited a paradoxical response as compared with none of the participants with no self-injury or stereotypy. In their second study, Barron and Sandman (1985) found that both the presence of self-injury and lower IQ were associated with a paradoxical response to sedative-hypnotic drugs. In 1992, Sandman and Barron reported on a group of 648 residents and found once again that self-injury and stereotypy were associated with a paradoxical response to sedative-hypnotics.

In summary, most of the therapeutic research on benzodiazepines and mental retardation has focused on children and adolescents. The studies in which children with anxiety and internalizing symptoms were studied were poorly controlled, but symptoms reflecting high-anxious behaviors appeared to be more responsive to treatment than were disruptive behaviors (e.g., Krakowski, 1963). In the better controlled studies, researchers assessed the effects of benzodiazepines on children with disruptive and hyperactive behavior (e.g., Graae et al., 1994; LaVeck & Buckley, 1961; Walters et al., 1977) and found, if anything, that the anxiolytics actually worsened the behavior. One finding with older subjects (14 to 26 years) did appear to show some degree of control over aggression (Bond et al., 1989). The clinical response to benzodiazepines may also be atypical in people with high levels of self-injury and stereotypy. It is possible that self-injury and stereotypy may be proxy variables (i.e. stand-ins for low functional levels), because their prevalence increases as functional level declines.

It is clear that there is a need for more research, especially studies involving adults, to look at the efficacy of the benzodiazepines for people with mental retardation.

We need studies that assess these agents in conditions known or believed to be benefited in the general population, namely in adjustment disorders, sleep disorders, GAD, and possibly akathisia. In view of the Barron and Sandman studies, people with severe or profound mental retardation and those with self-injury or stereotypic behavior should be evaluated for paradoxical effects. In this way, we can see if these markers portend an adverse response. In the meantime, the benzodiazepines might be assumed to be equally effective for treating the same disorders both in people with mental retardation and in the general population. Clinicians should be especially vigilant about detecting unusual effects at lower functional levels or where self-injury or stereotypic behavior is evident. As they are for children in general, benzodiazepines are probably contraindicated for use with children with mental retardation and attention-deficit/hyperactivity disorder (ADHD) and other disruptive behaviors.

Prescribing Guidelines

The majority of people who use anxiolytics and sedatives do so safely and for short durations (APA, 1990). Nevertheless, these drugs have acquired bad press primarily because they reputedly are overused and abused and foster dependency. The following are some guidelines to follow when prescribing anxiolytics for people with mental retardation:

- The anxiety or insomnia should be a recent change in function, apparent to observers, and disabling.

- Either the indication or diagnosis should conform to one of the established indications for adults, or the relief sought should be probably accomplishable promptly and without adverse effects. It will be possible to discontinue use within a short period, say a maximum of two months.

- There is a favorable risk/benefit analysis compared with alternative approaches, such as behavior therapy.

- The effects of the drug treatment can be monitored carefully for therapeutic benefit and possible adverse effects.

Except in emergencies, benzodiazepines should be given orally. Except with lorazepam and midazolam, intramuscular absorption is poor and slower than with oral dosing (Baldessarini, 1990; Gelenberg et al., 1991). Intravenous use should be reserved for medical emergencies, and proper resuscitation equipment should be at hand.

Generally, low-potency, long-acting drugs like diazepam (Valium) should be preferred, because their adverse effects have been far better researched (APA, 1990). These are the only anxiolytics currently accepted by the U.S. Food and Drug Administration for use with children under 12 years (Coffey, 1990). Also, the high-potency and short-acting drugs are suspected of presenting dependence, rebound, and withdrawal problems (APA, 1990). In the case of sleep disturbances, however, a short-acting drug may be preferable, particularly if it is to be given for only a very few days.

Dosage and duration have not been established for people with mental retardation. Generally, physicians should begin with a low dose and increment slowly over intervals of about five days to a week, except in emergencies or anticipated short-term use. Care is needed in using these drugs with any other sedating agent.

If a drug is given at intervals about equal to the half-life (approximately 24 hours for long-acting drugs), then peak and trough blood levels will vary by 50%. Because there is a narrow relationship between anxiolytic action and sedative blood levels (about 1:2), it is desirable to give benzodiazepines in smaller divided doses: two (for long-acting agents) to four (short-acting agents) times daily to prevent these surges in blood level (Baldessarini, 1990). In the case of sleep disorders, the drug is prescribed once per day.

ANTIHISTAMINES AND ANTICHOLINERGICS

For more than 40 years, antihistamines have been preferred over other drugs for dealing with sleep disorders and fussiness in infants and young children. Nevertheless, the action and clinical utility of antihistamines in the treatment of sleep disorders has been poorly studied (Werry & Carlielle, 1982). The most popular drugs are hydroxyzine (Atarax, Vistaril), diphenhydramine (Benadryl), promethazine (Phenergan), and trimeprazine (Vallergan). However, because most antihistamines are not subject to regulation by prescription, they are also a common component of over-the-counter hypnotics (Garrison, 1990).

Diphenhydramine was one of the first antihistamines to be synthesized and used clinically. Promethazine and trimeprazine are phenothiazines, structurally very similar to chlorpromazine except in the shortened/branched side chain. The accidental discovery of the antipsychotic action of chlorpromazine arose primarily from the search for better antihistamines in the late 1940s, by which time the use of antihistamines as sedating and anesthetic adjuncts was well-established.

Pharmacodynamics and Pharmacokinetics

The precise cause of the sedating effect of antihistamines is unknown (Werry, 1980). Most are powerful muscarinic anticholinergics, which are also sedating. Their sedating effects may partly explain their CNS effects, because acetylcholine is an important transmitter in arousal and sleep systems (Werry, 1980). However, histamine is probably also involved as a central neurotransmitter in the arousal system; histamine may have a sedating effect in its own right. Blockade of both these neurotransmitters may also have stimulating actions, although this may be more akin to delirium or cognitive disruption than true stimulation (Garrison, 1990).

Diphenhydramine and the phenothiazine antihistamines have an effective duration of action of 4 to 6 hours. The phenothiazines can produce active metabolites and have longer durations of action with repeated use. Hydroxyzine has an action that may last anywhere from 6 to 24 hours. More research is needed on the pharmacokinetics of these drugs.

System/Physical Effects

Most of the system effects of antihistamines stem from their anticholinergic properties. Cardiovascular effects include increased heart rate. There may be some degree of vasodilatation in high doses, causing a fall in blood pressure. Other anticholinergic actions reflect down-regulation of the parasympathetic autonomic nervous system, which affect primary secretion of saliva and sweat, gastrointestinal and bladder contractility, and accommodation of the lens in the eye.

The primary effect in the CNS is sedation, which differs qualitatively from that produced by CNS depressants (Werry, 1980). The effect lacks the dose-dependent systematic and progressive CNS depression of brain function. The action is selective and does not produce the pleasant sensations associated with anxiolysis. The drugs specifically address certain phases of sleep rather than a general flattening out of sleep phases. Because of the central role that acetylcholine plays in memory, cognition can be disrupted. In higher dosage, these drugs can produce delirium.

Table 12-4. Risks and Side Effects Associated with Anxiolytics

Risk Factors	Side Effects		
	CNS Depressants	Anticholinergics	Atypical
Dose	"Intoxication"	Excitement	Dysphoria
Duration	Coma/Death	Delirium	Dizziness
Age (extremes)	Aggression	Cognitive Impairment	Insomnia
Developmental Level	Cognitive Impairment	Parasympathetic	Nausea
Brain Damage	Depression	(reduced activity)	
Personality	Dependence	Synergism	
Social Ambience	Withdrawal		
Familial	Synergism		
Drug Interactions			
Coexistent Disease			
Idiosyncratic			

Side Effects, Toxic Effects, and Interactions

The common side effects of these drugs are dry skin, dry mouth, blurred vision, constipation, bladder problems, and tachycardia. In the CNS, restlessness, irritability, excitement, insomnia, dizziness (Garrison, 1990), and even delirium can occur, especially with higher doses (See Table 12-4). The classical atropinic delirium seen with belladonna poisoning is accompanied by hot, dry skin and widely dilated pupils. Theoretically, delirium may be more common in those with already compromised brain function (e.g., people with old age or severe mental retardation). However, it is unclear how common these side effects are in clinical practice. Even though their action is quite different from those of other sedating drugs, the antihistamines augment the action of all CNS depressants. They also will augment the parasympatholytic action of anticholinergic drugs, such as the anti-Parkinsonian drugs, low-potency neuroleptics, and tricyclic antidepressants.

Clinical Indications Exclusive of Mental Retardation

The primary medical use of these drugs is for allergies. They are commonly found in over-the-counter remedies for coughs and colds, and this can be important when other drugs are prescribed. As was noted already, these drugs are used primarily for sleep disturbances and, in small children and infants, for fussiness (Richman, 1985; Werry & Carlielle, 1982). In the past, diphenhydramine and hydroxyzine were used for disruptive behavior in younger children (Fish & Shapiro, 1965), but these uses seem to have waned.

Because there have been few systematic studies, much of what is assumed about these drugs is based on clinical experience. The short-acting drugs like diphenhydramine may show little prolongation of duration of sleep. The longer-acting hydroxyzine may continue to act throughout most of the waking day. With repeated dosing, these drugs are likely to show loss of sedative effect.

These drugs do not usually eliminate night-waking entirely, and the problem recurs when the drugs are discontinued, unlike behavioral methods that produce more enduring improvement (Horne, 1992; Richman et al., 1985). Doses reported are 1 mg/kg for diphenhydramine (Benadryl) and 30 to 60 mg of trimeprazine in infants and toddlers (Richman, 1985).

Some have advocated the use of anti-motion sickness medication for treating children with specific learning disabilities (e.g., Frank & Levinson, 1976-1977, 1977). Most of the anti-motion sickness drugs are antihistamines with marked anticholinergic properties. In a thorough review of the data on the use of anti-motion sickness drugs as a treatment for learning disabilities, Aman and Rojahn (1992) concluded that there was not a likely role for their use, and they speculated that these drugs may be positively harmful for these children, especially for youngsters with inattention and overactivity.

Antihistamines are from time to time considered for managing disruptive behavior, although there are few data to support the practice. In one of the few studies to assess their use in this context, Zametkin, Reeves, Webster, and Werry (1986) compared the effects of promethazine with a no-drug baseline and with methylphenidate on children with ADHD. Promethazine failed to improve behavior for the group as a whole, and it caused significant deterioration in several children.

Indications in Mental Retardation

Most of the studies on antihistamines and mental retardation were done some time ago. Craft (1957) reported the results of a crossover study of placebo and hydroxyzine (Atarax) for 10 adults and 13 children with aggressive and destructive behavior. All participants were residents of a large institution, and most had profound mental retardation. Both drug conditions were implemented for one month, and behavior was rated by nursing staff on a standardized scale that was constructed to assess activity level, aggression, and social behavior with other residents. No significant changes were observed.

Segal and Tansley (1957) conducted a parallel groups study with children having mild mental retardation who attended a residential school. The children were described as being maladjusted, and 16 each were assigned to the hydroxyzine (20 mg/day) and the placebo group. All children were rated by their teachers on global 5-point scales for activity level, application during class, and progress in school. No differences occurred between the treatments. The teachers were also asked to indicate how certain they were that the children were on medication. They correctly classified 14 of 16 experimental subjects as being in the hydroxyzine group and 12 of 16 control subjects as being in the placebo group. This, of course, may simply indicate that the teachers were able to identify side effects, such as drowsiness.

Craft (1959) conducted a study of promethazine (Phenergan) use for 18 patients (16 adults and 2 children) with IQs below 38 and with hyperactive, destructive, or aggressive behavior. Up to 150 mg/day of the drug was used, and change was measured on three global scales said to address activity, aggression, and antisocial behavior. No significant changes were observed, and the statistical test used was not specified. The drug caused sedation and staggering gait in some participants.

The findings offer little support for the use of antihistamines to manage acting-out or hyperactive behavior in children with mental retardation. Because they are useful for treating infants and young children with sleep disturbances and fussiness, future research may show a similar indication for children with mental retardation. For people with mental retardation, the available data are mostly from studies of children; furthermore, all of the available data are based on treatment of individuals with disruptive behavior.

ATYPICAL ANXIOLYTICS

Buspirone (Buspar) is the most important member of this group. Its receptor profile is quite different from the benzodiazepines in that it is without any effect on GABA receptors but acts primarily at presynaptic dopamine and post-synaptic and 5HT1A (serotonergic) receptors (Baldessarini, 1990; Kutcher et al., 1992). Like carbamazepine (Tegretol), it also increases firing in the brain stem adrenergic (arousal) system (Coffey, 1990), which may explain its lack of sedative effects. It is said to be free of cognitive depression effects and has little potential to produce dependency (Baldessarini, 1990; Coffey, 1990; Kutcher et al., 1992). The source of its anxiolytic action is unknown. It has a short half-life (2-11 hours) with no active metabolites (Coffey, 1990; Kutcher et al., 1992). Hence, it must be given three times daily to be effective clinically.

Clinical Indications Exclusive of Mental Retardation

In adults, buspirone is used to treat generalized, anticipatory, and situational anxiety. In children it might be helpful in overanxious disorder, avoidant behavior, phobic disorders, obsessive-compulsive disorder, and ADHD (Coffey, 1990; Kutcher et al., 1992). It also is used to treat aggressive behavior associated with autism and for head injury. However, there are only a very few case reports and open studies of use with children and adolescents (see Mandoki, 1994); therefore, doses and indications are not yet firmly established for these populations. Buspirone's anxiolytic properties take up to four weeks to emerge, which is much longer than that for the benzodiazepines (Baldessarini, 1990; Coffey, 1990; Kutcher et al., 1992).

For children, doses can be derived by dividing the adult dosage (10 to 60 mg/day) by 70 to convert them to mg/kg. The suggested doses are approximately 0.2 to 0.8 mg/kg per day. These doses are on the conservative side; in some studies doses have averaged around 18 mg/day (Werry & Aman, in press). This dose is further subdivided for twice to thrice daily administration. Because buspirone is relatively new, it cannot at this stage be recommended for other than experimental use for children and adolescents (Coffey, 1990; Kutcher et al., 1992; Werry & Aman, in press), although it lacks side effects of the type that cause concern about the benzodiazepines. Further study is indicated. Care is needed if used with monoamine oxidase inhibitors (MAOIs), because hypertension has been reported as an interaction effect (Coffey, 1990).

Indications in Mental Retardation

Realmuto, August, and Garfinkel (1989) conducted an open trial with four children having autism. All children were observed for a two-week baseline period (in which no medication was given), followed by a four-week buspirone phase, followed by four weeks of either methylphenidate or fenfluramine treatment. Two or three children with marked hyperactivity showed substantial improvements on standardized behavior rating scales; another child showed significant reductions in stereotypic behavior with buspirone.

Ratey, Sovner, Mikkelsen, and Chmielinski (1989) described their experiences in managing 14 adults, aged 23 to 63 years, with buspirone. Three of these patients had autism, most were given a diagnosis of GAD, and most of them also presented with anxiety and aggressive or self-injurious behavior. Nine of the 14 patients were said to respond favorably, often to smaller than usual doses of 5 to 20 mg (Werry & Aman, in press).

There is only one controlled study of the use of buspirone in this population. In a study with a multiple baseline design, Ratey, Sovner, Parks, and Rogentine (1991) compared the use of placebo and buspirone for six adults who presented with both anxiety disorders and at least one aggressive or self-injurious incident per week. Five of the six subjects showed drug-related decreases in aggression (between 26% and 63%), whereas anxiety was rated by staff as increased in four subjects and decreased in two. The authors concluded that the study demonstrated that buspirone is useful in decreasing aggression and (rather incongruously, given the results) that buspirone had no clear anxiety-reducing properties for these subjects.

Finally, Ricketts et al. (1994) studied five residents who were treated with either buspirone alone (two subjects) or with buspirone as an adjunct to thioridazine (Mellaril). The individuals were monitored with direct observations during a baseline period and with several doses of buspirone, which were given in open fashion. All five subjects showed some reduction in self-injury, with the amount of reduction ranging from 13% to 72%. The degree of reduction was dependent, in part, on dosage, with the most effective dose being 30 mg/day for three subjects and 52.5 mg/day for two subjects.

Hence there is some reason to believe that buspirone may prove to be beneficial for some individuals with developmental disabilities, although it is not clear at this stage what characteristics are likely to forecast a favorable response. In the only controlled study (Ratey et al., 1991), anxiety itself was found not to improve although comorbid aggression did. In the uncontrolled case report by Ratey et al. (1989), both anxiety and disruptive behaviors (e.g., aggression and self-injury) were considered to be responsive. Ricketts et al. (1994) found meaningful reductions in self-injury, but it was not clear whether or not the improved behaviors were related to anxiety disorder. Finally, in contrast to the data with the benzodiazepines, the Realmuto et al. (1989) trial suggested a possible role for buspirone in managing hyperactivity in autism.

Buspirone might be used for treating symptoms associated with elevated anxiety, but it is not necessarily easy to discern anxiety in people with more severe degrees of mental retardation. Where it appears that high anxiety is involved in a serious disorder (e.g., when self-injury is associated with periods of known stress in a person having severe or profound mental retardation), a trial of buspirone might be considered.

As with other anxiolytics, much of the use of buspirone in people with mental retardation has been for the treatment of aggressive behavior. This use appears promising, particularly because buspirone may be relatively free of side effects such as disinhibition or sedation. Most of the evidence of efficacy comes from uncontrolled studies with patients with brain injury, autism, and mental retardation (e.g., Gedye, 1991; Mandoki, 1994; Werry & Aman, in press).

CONCLUSIONS

Anxiolytic drugs are widely used to treat adults for acute insomnia, acute anxiety, panic, and GAD. There are also reports of efficacy in the control of excited psychotic states, akathisia, and Tourette syndrome. The selective CNS depressants (benzodiazepines and analogs such as zopiclone) have replaced the general CNS depressants (e.g., barbiturates, paraldehyde, and chloral hydrate) because of their safety. However, these newer drugs can have a number of important adverse and hangover effects, which include sedation, irritability, depression, paradoxical excitement, dependence, impairment of latency of responding, impairment of memory, and impairment of motor coordination. Their role in facilitating or impairing concurrent psychosocial treatments is unestablished. Most adverse effects are dose- and duration-dependent; they more commonly occur with high-potency, short-acting benzodiazepines. In many cases, these adverse effects can be avoided if the drugs are used less than four months (APA, 1990).

There are few studies on the efficacy and safety of anxiolytics with people with mental retardation. However, there is concern about possible adverse effects on cognition. It is important that anxiolytics are used only to relieve distress in the patient, not to reduce excessive behavior that is annoying to caretakers. Prescribers should be particularly alert in using depressant anxiolytics for people with self-injurious or stereotypic behavior (especially in those with both) because of the possibility of a paradoxical response.

Buspirone may have a role in the management of aggression and anxiety in people with mental retardation. It seems to lack most of the side effects of the depressant anxiolytics. However, there are reasons to suspect that its real role may have little to do with anxiety but instead with excited states. Properly controlled studies are needed.

Because of the absence of methodologically sound scientific research on the efficacy and safety of anxiolytics in people with mental retardation, these drugs should be used cautiously and carefully monitored for benefit and side effects.

- The use of anxiolytics may be considered when (a) a psychiatric disorder is diagnosed and (b) an anxiolytic drug is indicated for that disorder for people who do not have mental retardation.

- The use of antihistaminic/anticholinergic medications for sedation of infants and small children, especially those with sleep disorders, is supported by clinical observations; however, scientific studies are needed.

- The use of anxiolytic drugs in the control of other conditions (such as acutely disturbed behavior, Tourette syndrome, and akathisia) requires proper investigation. Use is not recommended at this time, apart from treating acute psychotic states.

REFERENCES

Aman, M.G., & Rojahn, J. (1992). Pharmacological intervention. In N.N. Singh & I. L. Beale (Eds.), *Learning disabilities: Nature, theory, and treatment* (pp. 478–525). New York: Springer-Verlag.

Aman, M.G., Sarphare, G., & Burrow, W.A. (1995). Psychotropic drugs in group homes: Prevalence and relation to demographic/psychiatric variables. *American Journal on Mental Retardation, 99,* 500–509.

Aman, M.G., & Singh, N.N. (1988). Patterns of drug use, methodological considerations, measurement techniques, and future trends. In M.G. Aman & N.N. Singh (Eds.), *Psychopharmacology of the developmental disabilities* (pp. 1–28). New York: Springer-Verlag.

Aman, M.G., & Werry, J.S. (1982). Methylphenidate and diazepam in severe reading retardation. *Journal of the American Academy of Child Psychiatry, 21,* 31–37.

American Psychiatric Association. (1990). *Benzodiazepine dependence, toxicity, and abuse: A task force report.* Washington DC: American Psychiatric Press.

American Psychiatric Association. (1994). *Diagnostic and statistical manual of mental disorders* (4th ed.). Washington, DC: American Psychiatric Press.

Baldessarini R.J. (1990). Drugs and the treatment of psychiatric disorders. In A.G. Gilman, T.W. Rall, A.S. Nies, & P. Taylor (Eds.), *Goodman and Gilman's the pharmacological basis of therapeutics* (8th ed., pp. 383–435). New York: Pergamon Press.

Barron, J., & Sandman, C.A. (1983). Relationship of sedative-hypnotic response to self-injurious behavior and stereotypy by mentally retarded clients. *American Journal of Mental Deficiency, 88,* 177–186.

Barron, J., & Sandman, C.A. (1985). Paradoxical excitement to sedative-hypnotic drugs in mentally retarded clients. *American Journal of Mental Deficiency, 90,* 124–129.

Bernstein, G.A., & Borchardt, C.M. (1991). Anxiety disorders of childhood and adolescence: A critical review. *Journal of the American Academy of Child and Adolescent Psychiatry, 30,* 519–532.

Bond, S., Mandos, L., & Kurtz, M.B. (1989). Midazolam for aggressivity and violence in three mentally retarded patients. *American Journal of Psychiatry, 146,* 925–926.

Brown, T.A., Hertz, R.M., & Barlow, D.H. (1992). New developments in cognitive-behavioral treatment of anxiety disorders. In A. Tasman & M.B. Riba (Eds.), *Review of psychiatry* (Vol. 11, pp. 260–284). Washington, DC: American Psychiatric Press.

Coffey, B.J. (1990). Anxiolytics for children and adolescents: Traditional and new drugs. *Journal of Child and Adolescent Psychopharmacology, 1,* 57–86.

Craft, M.J. (1957). Tranquillizers in mental deficiency: Hydroxyzine. *Journal of Mental Science, 103,* 855–857.

Craft, M.J. (1959). Mental disorders in the defective: The use of tranquillizers. *American Journal of Mental Deficiency, 64,* 63–71.

Dahl, R.E. (1992). The pharmacologic treatment of sleep disorders. *Psychiatric Clinics of North America, 15,* 161–178.

Fish, B., & Shapiro, T. (1965). A typology of children's psychiatric disorders its application to a controlled evaluation of treatment. *Journal of the American Academy of Child Psychiatry, 4,* 32–52.

Frank, J., & Levinson, H.N. (1976–1977). Seasickness mechanisms and medications in dysmetric dyslexia and dyspraxia. *Academic Therapy, 11,* 133–143.

Frank, J., & Levinson, H.N. (1977). Antimotion sickness medications in dysmetric dyslexia and dyspraxia. *Academic Therapy, 12,* 411–424.

Garrison, J.C. (1990). Histamine, bradykinin, 5-hydroxytryptamine, and their antagonists. In A.G. Gilman, T.W. Rall, A.S. Nies, & P. Taylor (Eds.), *Goodman and Gilman's the pharmacological basis of therapeutics* (8th ed., pp. 575–599). New York: Pergamon Press.

Gedye, A. (1991). Buspirone alone or with serotonergic diet reduced aggression in a developmentally disabled adult. *Biological Psychiatry, 30,* 88–91.

Gelenberg A.J., Bassuk, E.L., & Schoonover, S.C. (1991). *The practitioner's guide to psychoactive drugs* (3rd ed.). New York: Plenum Press.

Gilman, A.G., Rall, T.W., Nies, A.S., & Taylor, P. (Eds.). (1990). *Goodman and Gilman's the pharmacological basis of therapeutics* (8th ed.). New York: Pergamon Press.

Graae, F., Milner, J., Rizzotto, L., & Klein, R.G. (1994). Clonazepam in childhood anxiety disorders. *Journal of the American Academy of Child and Adolescent Psychiatry, 33*, 372–376.

Greenblatt, D.J., & Shader, R.I. (1974). *Benzodiazepines in clinical practice.* New York: Raven Press.

Gross, E.J., Hull, H.B., Lytton, G.J., Hill, J.A., & Pienel, W.C. (1993). Case study of neuroleptic-induced akathisia: Important implications for people with mental retardation. *American Journal on Mental Retardation, 98*, 156–164.

Hanzel, T.E., Kalachnik, J.E., & Harder, S.R. (1992). A case of phenobarbital exacerbation of preexisting maladaptive behavior partially suppressed by chlorpromazine and misinterpreted as chlorpromazine efficacy. *Research in Developmental Disabilities, 13*, 381–392.

Horne, J. (1992). Sleep and its disorders in children. *Journal of Child Psychology and Psychiatry, 33*, 473–487.

Intagliata, J., & Rinck, C. (1985). Psychoactive drug use in public and community facilities for mentally retarded persons. *Psychopharmacology Bulletin, 21*, 268–278.

Kennedy, S.I.L., & Longnecker, D.E. (1990). History and principles of anesthesiology. In A.G. Gilman, T.W. Rall, A.S. Nies, & P. Taylor (Eds.), *Goodman and Gilman's the pharmacological basis of therapeutics* (8th ed., pp. 269–284). New York: Pergamon Press.

Kraft, A., Ardali, C., Duffy, J., Hart, J., & Pearce, P.R. (1965). A clinical study of chlordiazepoxide used in psychiatric disorders of children. *International Journal of Neuropsychology, 1*, 433–437.

Krakowski, A.J. (1963). Chlordiazepoxide in treatment of children with emotional disturbances. *New York State Journal of Medicine, 63*, 3388–3392.

Kutcher, S.P., Reiter, S., Gardner, D.M., & Klein, R. (1992). The pharmacotherapy of anxiety disorders in children and adolescents. *Psychiatric Clinics of North America, 15*, 41–45.

LaVeck, G.D., & Buckley, P. (1961). The use of psychopharmacological agents in retarded children with behavior disorders. *Journal of Chronic Diseases, 13*, 174–183.

Lipman, R.S., DiMascio, A., Reatig, N., & Kirson, T. (1978). Psychotropic drugs and mentally retarded children. In M.A. Lipton, A. DiMascio, & K.F. Killam (Eds.), *Psychopharmacology: A generation of progress* (pp. 1437–1449). New York: Raven Press.

Mandoki, M. (1994). Buspirone treatment of traumatic brain injury in a child who is highly sensitive to adverse effects of psychotropic medications. *Journal of Child and Adolescent Psychopharmacology, 4*, 129–139.

McClellan, J.M., & Werry, J.S. (1992). Schizophrenia. *Psychiatric Clinics of North America, 15*, 131–148.

McNally, R.J. (1994). *Panic disorder: A critical analysis* (pp. 81–104). New York: Guilford Press.

Rall, T.W. (1990). Hypnotics and sedatives; ethanol. In A.G. Gilman, T.W. Rall, A.S. Nies, & P. Taylor. (Eds.), *Goodman and Gilman's the pharmacological basis of therapeutics* (8th ed., pp. 345–382). New York: Pergamon Press.

Ratey, J.J., Sovner, R., Mikkelsen, E., & Chmielinski, H.E. (1989). Buspirone therapy for maladaptive behavior and anxiety in developmentally disabled persons. *Journal of Clinical Psychiatry, 50*, 382–384.

Ratey, J., Sovner, R., Parks, A., & Rogentine, K. (1991). Buspirone treatment of aggression and anxiety in mentally retarded patients: A multiple baseline, placebo lead-in study. *Journal of Clinical Psychiatry, 52*, 159–162.

Realmuto, G.M., August, G.J., & Garfinkel, B.D. (1989). Clinical effect of buspirone in autistic children. *Journal of Clinical Psychopharmacology, 9*, 122–125.

Richman, N. (1985). A double-blind drug trial of treatment in young children with waking problems. *Journal of Child Psychology and Psychiatry, 26*, 591–598

Richman, N., Douglas, J., Hunt, H., Landsdown, R., & Levere, R. (1985). Behavioural methods in the treatment of sleep disorders: A pilot study. *Journal of Child Psychology and Psychiatry, 26*, 581–590.

Ricketts, R.W., Goza, A.B., Ellis, C.R., Singh, Y.N., Chambers, L.V.N., Singh, N.N., & Cooke, J.C. (1994). Clinical effects of buspirone on intractable self-injury in adults with mental retardation. *Journal of the American Academy of Child and Adolescent Psychiatry, 33*, 270–276.

Roy-Byrne, P.P., & Wingerson, D. (1992). Pharmacotherapy of anxiety disorders. In A. Tasman & M.B. Riba (Eds.), *Review of psychiatry* (Vol 11, pp.360–384). Washington DC: American Psychiatric Press.

Sandman, C.A., & Barron, J.L. (1992). Paradoxical response to sedative/hypnotics in patients with self-injurious behavior and stereotypy. *Journal of Developmental and Physical Disabilities, 4*, 307–316.

Segal, L.J., & Tansley, A.E. (1957). A clinical trial with hydroxyzine (Atarax) on a group of maladjusted educationally subnormal children. *Journal of Mental Retardation, 103*, 677–681.

Simeon, J.G., Ferguson, H.B., Knott, V., Roberts, N., Ganthier, B., DuBoise, C., & Wiggins, D. (1992). Clinical, cognitive, and neurophysiological effects of alprazolam in children and adolescents with overanxious and avoidant disorders. *Journal of the American Academy of Child and Adolescent Psychiatry, 31*, 29–33.

Sprague, R.L., & Werry J.S. (1971). Methodology of psychopharmacological studies in the retarded. In N.R. Ellis (Ed.), *International review of mental retardation* (Vol. 5, pp. 147–219). New York: Academic Press.

Steingard, R.J., Goldberg, M., Lee, D., & DeMaso, D.R. (1994). Adjunctive use of clonazepam treatment of tic symptoms in children with comorbid tic disorders and ADHD. *Journal of the American Academy of Child and Adolescent Psychiatry, 33*, 394–399.

Tsai, G., Gastfriend, D.R., & Coyle, J.T. (1995). The glutamatergic basis of human alcoholism. *American Journal of Psychiatry, 152*, 332–340.

Walters, A., Singh, N.N., & Beale, I.L. (1977). Effects of lorazepam on hyperactivity in retarded children. *New Zealand Medical Journal, 86*, 473–475.

Werry, J.S. (1980). Anticholinergic sedatives. In G.D. Burrow & J.S. Werry (Eds.), *Advances in human psychopharmacology* (Vol. 1, pp. 19–42). Greenwich, CT: JAI Press.

Werry, J.S. (1991). Overanxious disorder: A review of its taxonomic properties. *Journal of the American Academy of Child and Adolescent Psychiatry, 30*, 533–544.

Werry, J.S., & Aman, M.G. (in press). Anxiolytics and miscellaneous drugs. In J.S. Werry & M.G. Aman (Eds.), *A practitioner's guide to psychoactive drugs for children and adolescents* (2nd ed). New York: Plenum Press.

Werry, J.S., & Carlielle, J. (1982). The nuclear family, suburban neurosis, and iatrogenesis in Auckland mothers of young children. *Journal of the American Academy of Child and Adolescent Psychiatry, 22*, 172–179.

Werry, J.S., & Wollersheim, J.P. (1989). Behavior therapy with children and adolescents: A twenty-year overview. *Journal of the American Academy of Child and Adolescent Psychiatry, 28*, 1–18.

Zametkin, A.J., Reeves, J.C., Webster, L., & Werry, J.S. (1986). Promethazine treatment of children with attention deficit disorder with hyperactivity—ineffective and unpleasant. *Journal of the American Academy of Child Psychiatry, 25*, 854–856.

Mood Stabilizers

Ann R. Poindexter[1], Nancy Cain[2], David J. Clarke[3],
Edwin H. Cook, Jr.[4], John A. Corbett[5], Andrew Levitas[6]

The term *mood stabilizer* was applied to lithium salts when it became clear that these compounds were effective in the treatment of patients with bipolar disorders. Both lithium carbonate and lithium citrate are used therapeutically throughout the world (Baldessarini, 1990). Available therapeutic preparations range in strength from 300 mg to 400 mg lithium carbonate. Additionally, a number of anticonvulsant drugs—such as carbamazepine, valproic acid, and clonazepam—also have been found to be effective as mood stabilizers in some patients with bipolar or schizoaffective disorders (Schatzberg & Cole, 1991). A list of proprietary and generic drugs for the United States is provided in Table 13-1. Although all facets of lithium's pharmacology are discussed in this chapter, those anticonvulsants that are also mood stabilizers (i.e., carbamazepine, valproic acid, and clonazepam) are discussed here only in terms of their clinical effects. The pharmacology, systems effects, and interactions of the antiepileptic mood stabilizers are discussed in Chapter 10.

PHARMACOLOGY

Pharmacodynamics

Lithium, the lightest of the alkali metals, shares some characteristics with sodium and potassium. It is abundant in some alkaline mineral-spring waters. Lithium affects the neurotransmitters serotonin and norepinephrine at nerve terminals and receptors, and on various membranes. It may inhibit some intracellular messenger systems, especially in regard to the roles played by a compound called phosphatidylinositor 4, by 5-biphosphate (PIP2), and by inositol. It attenuates G-protein (Manji, 1992), which is present in higher amounts in the brains of people with manic depressive illness. Its action may affect the complex regulation of functional properties of multiple proteins in multiple neuronal cell types (Hyman & Nestler, 1993; Kofman & Belmaker,

1993). However, much remains unknown about its mechanism of action in the brain.

Although the biochemical and physiological mechanisms for the psychotropic effects of carbamazepine have not been fully explained, these mechanisms may differ from those responsible for its anti-epileptic effects (McElroy & Keck, 1995; Post, 1988a, 1988b). This possibility is suggested by the different lengths of time required for therapeutic effectiveness. The onset of therapeutic effectiveness is rapid in the treatment of seizures and paroxysmal pain disorders but not in the treatment of mania.

Pharmacokinetics

Lithium is absorbed readily and almost completely from the gastrointestinal tract. Complete absorption occurs in about eight hours, with peak concentrations in blood plasma occurring two to four hours after an oral dose. Slow-release preparations of lithium carbonate minimize early peaks, but absorption is more variable.

Lithium's passage across the blood-brain barrier is slow, and when a steady rate is achieved, the concentration in the cerebrospinal fluid is about 40% to 50% of the concentration in plasma. Concentrations in the brain are comparable to those in plasma, but the peak concentration in the brain is reached up to 24 hours later than in plasma. This difference can result in a delayed occurrence of neurotoxic effects after an overdose, even when the plasma concentration has already peaked and is declining (Price & Heninger, 1994). Lithium does not bind to plasma proteins.

The elimination half-life of lithium averages 20 to 24

---

1 Consultant Physician, Conway, AR
2 Clinical Associate Professor of Psychiatry, University of Rochester School of Medicine and Dentistry, Rochester, NY
3 Senior Lecturer in Developmental Psychiatry, University of Birmingham, Birmingham, United Kingdom
4 Director, Laboratory of Developmental Neurochemistry, University of Chicago, Chicago, IL
5 Professor of Developmental Psychiatry, University of Birmingham, Birmingham, United Kingdom
6 Assistant Professor of Clinical Psychiatry, University of Medicine and Dentistry of New Jersey, Stratford, NJ

Table 13-1. Mood Stabilizer Drugs Available in the United States and the United Kingdom

Trade Name	Manufacturer	Preparation Available
LITHIUM		
Cibalith-S	Ciba Pharmaceutical	syrup, 8mEq lithium/5 mL (300 mg lithium carbonate equivalent)
Eskalith	SmithKline Beecham	300 mg lithium carbonate (capsules and tablets)
Eskalith Controlled Release	SmithKline Beecham	450 mg lithium carbonate
lithium carbonate	Roxane	300 mg lithium carbonate (capsules, tablets, and lithium citrate syrup)
Lithonate Capsules and Lithotabs	Solvay	300 mg lithium carbonate
Camcolit 250 & 400	Norgine Limited	250 mg and 400 mg lithium carbonate
Liskonum	SmithKline	450 mg/12.2 mmol lithium carbonate (controlled release)
Phasal	Lagap Pharmaceuticals	300 mg lithium carbonate
Priadel 200 & 400	Delandale Laboratories	200 mg and 400 mg lithium carbonate (controlled release)
CARBAMAZEPINE		
Atretol Tablets	Athena	200 mg carbamazepine
Tegretol Chewable	CibaGeneva	100 mg carbamazepine
Tegretol Suspension	CibaGeneva	100 mg/5 mL carbamazepine
Tegretol Tablets	CibaGeneva	200 mg carbamazepine
carbamazepine	Warner Chilcott	100 mg carbamazepine (chewable)
VALPROIC ACID/SODIUM VALPROATE		
Depakene Capsules	Abbott	250 mg valproic acid
Depakene Syrup	Abbott	250 mg/5 mL valproic acid
Depakene Tablets	Abbott	125 mg divalproex sodium 250 mg divalproex sodium 500 mg divalproex sodium (delayed release)
Depakene Sprinkle	Abbott	125 mg divalproex sodium (delayed release particles in capsules)

Note. Adapted from Medical Economics Data Production Co. (1996).

hours. About 95% of a single dose of lithium is eliminated in the urine. About one-third to two-thirds of a dose is excreted within 6 to 12 hours; the remainder is excreted slowly over 10 to 14 days. With repeated administration, lithium excretion increases during the first 5 to 6 days, until steady-state is reached between ingestion and excretion (Baldessarini, 1990).

SYSTEM/PHYSICAL EFFECTS

Lithium at therapeutic concentration has very little psychotropic effect in healthy individuals. It is not thought to cause sedation, depression, or euphoria (Baldessarini, 1990), but weak to moderate declines in cognitive-motor performance have been reported (see the next section). Lithium increases the number of white cells in the blood stream, up to about one and a half times the normal range. The actual number is not correlated with the blood lithium concentration (Ozdemir et al., 1994).

Individuals treated with lithium often have small changes in thyroid functioning, which is probably due to slight interference with the synthesis of thyroid hormone. Lithium also may have effects on the metabolism of water, which results in decreased reabsorption of water by the kidney (Baldessarini, 1990). Prolonged use of lithium causes a benign and reversible depression of the T-wave on an electrocardiogram. The cause of this depression is unknown, but it is not due to depletion of sodium or potassium.

SIDE EFFECTS/TOXIC EFFECTS

Acute intoxication is characterized by vomiting, severe diarrhea, coarse tremor, ataxia, coma, and convulsions (Baldessarini, 1990). Because lithium has a low therapeutic index—perhaps as low as 2 or 3 (Baldessarini, 1990)—there is a higher than usual risk of toxicity; however, the risk of fatality is low. Of 4,560 incidents of toxic exposure to lithium reported to poison control centers in 1993, only three individuals died, all from suicide (Litovitz, Clark, & Soloway, 1994).

Lithium dosage is adjusted to achieve both therapeutic response and sub-toxic blood levels. Generally, trough levels of about 0.7 to 1.0 mEq/L are appropriate for maintenance therapy in the treatment of mania or psychotic excitement. Levels of up to 1.5 mEq/L are sometimes needed in acute mania (Schatzberg & Cole, 1991). Blood levels should be obtained about 12 hours after the last dose, because therapeutic standards are based on measurements performed at this time interval. Blood samples obtained after shorter intervals are likely to yield values in the toxic range (even when the dose is nontoxic), whereas those obtained after longer periods yield values that appear subtherapeutic (Price & Heninger, 1994). In practice, drug levels are usually drawn before the first morning dose, at which time a relatively steady state has been achieved.

Up to 75% of patients treated with lithium experience some side effects (American Psychiatric Association [APA], 1994). People with mental retardation appear to experience side effects with lithium at about the same rate as does the general population (Pary, 1991a). As compared with other groups, African Americans have decreased sodium-lithium transport in the kidneys and higher red blood cell to plasma lithium ratios. They often need a lower lithium dose than do Caucasians (Strickland et al., 1991). Additionally, nearly 25% of African Americans develop hypertension, and several parts of the treatment regimen for hypertension can significantly affect lithium plasma levels and the risk for toxicity (Strickland, Lawson, & Lin, 1993).

The most common side effect is tremor, usually noticed in the fingers. This tremor is similar in appearance to an intention, coffee-induced, or familial tremor. It is faster than the pseudo-Parkinsonian tremor frequently seen as a result of neuroleptic therapy. Tremor and other side effects are often worse at peak lithium blood levels and often can be decreased by rearrangement of dosage intervals. Propranolol at doses from 30 to 160 mg a day can be used to reduce tremors. At very high lithium concentrations, gross tremulousness and ataxia (loss of coordination) with dysarthria (difficulty speaking) occur, and the affected individual shows gross neurological disorder, confusion, or, less often, delirium (Schatzberg & Cole, 1991).

Bell, Cole, Eccleston, and Ferrier (1993) reported four cases of lithium-induced neurotoxicity at normal therapeutic levels and reviewed the literature for similar events. They identified several risk factors for neurotoxicity, including rapid dosage regimens, concomitant neuroleptic treatment, preexisting electroencephalogram (EEG) abnormalities, undetected cerebral pathology, organic impairment, and genetic susceptibility. Adverse effects of therapeutic serum lithium levels on cognition and memory in normal volunteers have also been reported (Hill & Stoudemire, 1993; Judd, Squire, Butters, Salmon, & Paller, 1987; Weingartner, Rudorfer, &

Linnoila, 1985). Studies of healthy adults using double-blind randomized designs have found mild cognitive dysfunctions, ranging from decreased concentration and performance speed to memory impairment (Kocsis et al., 1993). Studies with patient populations differ among themselves.

Chronic nausea and watery diarrhea can occur together or separately as signs of lithium toxicity. If irritation of the stomach lining is causing nausea after each dose, a sustained-release preparation might be tried in an effort to reduce the irritation. If diarrhea is a problem and is not due to a high serum lithium level, then a liquid lithium preparation might be tried for faster absorption in the upper gastrointestinal tract. Generally, any side effect that usually occurs one or two hours after each oral dose of the standard preparation might be minimized by switching to a sustained-release form.

Some people gain weight progressively after starting lithium therapy and may lose several pounds rapidly when lithium therapy is stopped. Some people have an increased appetite with resultant weight gain. Another possible side effect is edema (body fluid accumulation). Many people show a transitory decrease in thyroid hormone levels early in lithium therapy. A rare complication is goiter. Persistent hypothyroidism may also be caused by lithium, and although researchers have found this to be rare (Schatzberg & Cole, 1991), some clinicians feel that it occurs far more commonly than is generally reported in the literature (R. Pary & A. Levitas, personal communication, June, 1995).

Lithium causes noticeable polyuria (increased urine production), with secondary increased thirst, in approximately 20% of people. In a few individuals polyuria may become severe, with urine volume increasing up to 8 liters a day, leading to difficulty in concentrating urine and maintaining adequate lithium serum levels. If polyuria is distressing and if lithium therapy is clearly necessary, a thiazide diuretic may be very cautiously added. (Chlorothiazide at a dose of 500 mg/day decreases lithium clearance by about half. Therefore, if 500 mg of chlorothiazide per day is added, lithium dosage should be decreased by 50% and then carefully adjusted according to measured serum levels.)

Individuals with mental retardation who receive lithium may be unable to access fluids without assistance, so that they may receive either too little or too much water (A. Levitas, personal communication, December, 1994). These people should be monitored closely during lithium therapy. Daisley, Barton, and Williams (1990) reported a case of acute, fatal lithium toxicity in a man after five days of religious fasting, during which he drank only one glass of milk and ate only one teacup of porridge a day. He had previously been on a self-imposed, no-salt, vegetarian diet.

Major renal impairment due to lithium is said to be quite rare, but it may occur on occasion (Schatzberg & Cole, 1991). Gitlin (1993) stated that up to 5% of people treated with lithium may develop signs of renal insufficiency, but he failed to compare this number with rates of renal insufficiency in the general population or in patients with untreated bipolar disorders. A few cases have been reported in which a cardiac condition called "sick sinus node" syndrome has resulted from lithium therapy, but this also seems to be rare.

A variety of rashes have been reported to be associated with lithium therapy. Some allergic rashes may occur in reaction to ingredients other than lithium in a particular lithium preparation; these rashes may disappear if a different preparation is substituted. Alopecia (hair loss) can occur, but it often resolves spontaneously, even if the lithium is continued (Schatzberg & Cole, 1991). A number of reviewers have mentioned the increased risk of congenital abnormalities, particularly Ebstein's anomaly of the heart, in infants whose mothers received lithium during pregnancy. Cohen, Friedman, Jefferson, Johnson, and Weiner (1994) recently reevaluated the risks to infants exposed to lithium in the first trimester. Their analysis of epidemiologic data indicated that the risk of anomalies is lower than was previously suggested but still higher than for the general population. Schou (1993) evaluated available information and concluded that there appears to be no lithium withdrawal syndrome. He noted, however, a risk of relapse of the original symptoms if medication is withdrawn.

DRUG INTERACTIONS

Drug interactions of lithium are shown in Table 8-2. Lithium interacts with thiazide diuretics, metronidazole (Flagyl), spectinomycin (Trobicin), and tetracycline to produce toxic effects. Decreased renal lithium clearance is associated with aspirin, diclofenac (Voltaren), ibuprofen, indomethacin, naproxen, phenylbutazone, sulindac (Clinoril), and other nonsteroidal anti-inflammatory drugs. Increased lithium toxicity resulting from sodium depletion is associated with furosemide (Lasix). Increased lithium levels are associated with clonazepam (Klonopin), diltiazem, and methyldopa (Watsky & Salzman, 1991). Increased risk of neurotoxicity has been reported with carbamazepine and verapamil.

Some years ago, a number of reports suggested that lithium and haloperidol (Haldol) might interact to produce permanent neurological defects. Tupin and Schuller (1978) critically reviewed these cases and concluded that lithium intoxication alone could explain each of them. They also noted, as did Baldessarini (1990), that lithium and haloperidol have been used in combination extensively and safely for a number of years. The combined drugs are considered to be very useful in controlling many instances of severe manic behavior. Substances that decrease lithium levels via increased renal clearance include acetazolamide (Diamox), aminophylline, caffeine, theophylline, mannitol, sodium bicarbonate, sodium chloride, and urea. Other substances that decrease lithium levels are verapamil and sulfamethoxazole-trimethoprim (Septra, Bactrim) (Watsky & Salzman, 1991).

CLINICAL INDICATIONS FOR PEOPLE WITHOUT MENTAL RETARDATION

Lithium

Mania. Cade, the individual who first reported possible therapeutic effects of lithium, observed in 1949 that waters of certain wells in Britain were said to have special virtue in the treatment of mental illness. Cade suspected that their efficacy might be related to the lithium content in the waters. He reported cases of dramatic improvement in mania with lithium therapy. Since these anecdotal reports, the efficacy of lithium in the treatment of mania has been demonstrated in numerous research studies (APA, 1994). Lithium has been used extensively in the United States since 1970.

Bowden et al. (1994) reported a placebo-controlled, parallel group study of lithium for patients with acute mania. They found that lithium and divalproex were significantly more effective than placebo. Marked improvement occurred in 49% of the lithium group versus only 25% of the placebo group. A history of previous lithium response was a strong predictor of response to lithium.

There is some evidence that people with mania who respond poorly to lithium are anxious and depressed (Abou-Saleh, 1993; Swann et al., 1986). According to the APA (1994), lithium is about equally effective in preventing both episodes of mania and major episodes of depression. Lithium decreases the intensity of manic episodes and reduces mood variations between episodes.

Major Depression. Lithium was reported to have some value in augmentation of antidepressant therapy for people with resistant major depression (Manning & Connor, 1994). Fava et al. (1994) recently found that high-dose fluoxetine and fluoxetine plus lithium were the most effective treatments for individuals who had failed to respond to eight weeks of treatment with 20 mg fluoxetine alone.

Brain Injury. Glenn et al. (1989) prescribed lithium for ten brain-injured patients with severe, unremitting aggression, self-destructive behavior, or both, or severe affective instability. Five had a dramatic response marked by a significant increase in participation in rehabilitation activities. One had a moderate response, and one had a dramatic initial response that disappeared after seven weeks. Three had neurotoxic side effects that prevented further use of lithium. Two of these were also taking neuroleptics. Actual efficacy of lithium treatment may have been difficult to assess in some of these individuals because three patients received phenobarbital, which has reported side effects of aggression and refusal (Hanzel, Kalachnik, & Harder, 1992; Poindexter, Berglund, & Kolstoe, 1993). Two of the five individuals with marked improvement were receiving phenobarbital at the onset of lithium treatment, but one had phenobarbital discontinued during the lithium trial. One of the individuals with neurotoxicity was receiving phenobarbital. The authors concluded that lithium can be a useful treatment for aggressive behavior and affective instability after brain injury but has a significant potential for neurotoxicity in this population, particularly when used with neuroleptics. Cardenas and McLean (1992) suggested that lithium is more effective than carbamazepine in the treatment of people with traumatic brain injury but that the principal use for these individuals is for manic, cyclothymic, or explosive behavior.

Aggression. Lithium reduces aggression in many people at serum concentrations equivalent to those that are used for affective disorders (Peet & Pratt, 1993). Eichelman (1988) noted that lithium decreases aggressive behavior in fish and rodents, and he attributed this effect to lithium's ability to decrease the functional availability of norepinephrine. Sheard, Marini, Bridges, and Wagner (1976) reported a double-blind placebo-controlled study of the effect of lithium on aggressive behavior, utilizing data on 66 inmates, aged 16 to 24, in a medium-security prison. All individuals studied were healthy and nonpsychotic and had a history of chronic impulsive aggressive behavior. None had organic brain disease, and all were able to comprehend the written material used in the study. The lithium-treated group had a significant decrease in violent behavior. Tupin (1978) suggested that lithium is most effective when aggressive behavior is associated with extreme stimulus sensitivity ("hair trigger") and extreme impulsivity (inability to reflect on the meaning or intent of the stimulus).

Based on a literature review, Corrigan, Yudofsky, and Silver (1993) suggested that lithium significantly decreases aggressive acts in people with mental retardation, children with behavioral disorders, head-injured adults, prison inmates, schizophrenic adults, and adults with personality disorders. However, lithium may increase the frequency of aggressive behavior in patients with complex partial seizures. The reviewers noted that many reports had methodological flaws and imprecise outcome measures. Lenox and Manji (1995) reached similar conclusions, adding that most studies were conducted in large institutional settings and that little research was reported on the anti-aggressive effects of lithium in an outpatient setting. They suggested that additional studies of lithium for the treatment of aggression are warranted, not only to define the range of clinically responsive conditions but also to study the neurobiological mechanisms underlying its efficacy.

Use in Children. In a recent literature review, Alessi, Naylor, Ghaziuddin, and Zubieta (1994) found that lithium was being used with increasing frequency to treat children and adolescents who have psychiatric disorders, including adolescent bipolar disorder, childhood aggression, and behavior disorders associated with mental retardation and developmental disabilities. Campbell et al. (1972) reported results of a controlled crossover study in which lithium and chlorpromazine treatment of hyperactive, severely disturbed young children were compared. They found no statistically significant difference between the two drugs and no statistically significant change from baseline to therapy with either drug.

DeLong (1978) described 12 children with severe, chronic behavior problems who benefited from lithium therapy. A double-blind placebo-controlled crossover study of 4 of these children supported a specific behavioral effect of lithium. IQ was at least 90 in 11 of the children. Four had abnormal EEGs. McDaniel (1986) suggested that lithium was not effective in children with attention-deficit disorder with hyperactivity and was only minimally effective in children with conduct disorders with hyperactivity and aggressiveness. He noted that many earlier investigators had shown that lithium provided significant benefit to children with symptoms consistent with manic depressive illness.

Carlson, Rapport, Pataki, and Kelly (1992) treated 11 children hospitalized in a psychiatric facility who were considered good candidates for lithium therapy. All had full-scale IQ scores on the WISC-R between 81 and 129. While on lithium treatment, the children had weekly behavioral evaluations and showed improvement in the areas of self-control, aggression, and irritability. Results were stronger after 8 weeks than after 4 weeks. Seven of these children were studied through a double-blind crossover comparison. The investigators found that only three of the children improved enough to be discharged. They suggested that lithium is worth a try with children with treatment-refractory behavior disorders.

Carbamazepine

Mania. Carbamazepine was developed in the late 1950s in Switzerland. Its efficacy in treating people with epilepsy and paroxysmal pain syndromes was first demonstrated in Europe in the early 1960s (McElroy & Keck, 1995). Post (1988a) reviewed both uncontrolled studies and double-blind controlled studies that support the efficacy of carbamazepine for treating people with acute mania. In these studies, carbamazepine exerted its acute antimanic effect without untoward sedation, extrapyramidal side effects, or other unpleasant subjective side effects described by people treated with neuroleptics. Significant improvement in sleep occurred during the first week of treatment. Excited-hyperactive symptoms tended to improve more rapidly than did psychotic symptoms.

Post (1988a) noted that the joint use of carbamazepine and lithium is tolerated well by most patients. He suggested that the two drugs may be started simultaneously in the management of the acute episodes of severe mania. Carbamazepine may help control the extreme elements of excitation and aggression prior to the onset of an adequate response to lithium. Conversely, Bowden (1995) advocated changing only one drug or dosage level at a time, with very careful documentation of response.

Major Depression. Post, Uhde, Roy-Byrne, and Joffe (1988) reported results of a double-blind study of the antidepressant effects of carbamazepine, which seemed to indicate that this drug had some acute antidepressant efficacy in addition to its acute antimanic and longer-term prophylactic efficacy in both phases of manic depressive illness. Prior to that report, only in three controlled studies had the efficacy of carbamazepine for the treatment of individuals with unipolar or bipolar major depression been examined (McElroy & Keck, 1995), but each study showed a significant antidepressant effect of carbamazepine.

Bipolar Disorders. Ballenger (1988) has concluded that carbamazepine is effective in both acute treatment and long-term management of patients with affective illnesses. Schatzberg and Cole (1991) suggested that, despite the absence of U.S. Food and Drug Administration (FDA) approval for the use of carbamazepine in the treatment of affective illnesses, the available clinical evidence supports such use for treatment-resistant patients with bipolar disorders. They expect that 25% to 50% of these patients will show clear clinical benefit.

Mielke (1994) suggested that anticonvulsants, such as carbamazepine and valproate, are highly effective for treatment of bipolar disorders, with treatment results similar to those of lithium, and that anticonvulsants decrease the frequency or severity of mood cycles and the number of hospitalizations. Post, Altshuler, Ketter, Denicoff, and Weiss (1991) argued that, from a clinical perspective, carbamazepine and valproate now provide a treatment alternative or adjunct to lithium for patients with refractory bipolar disorder. They concluded that there are considerable data on carbamazepine that strongly support its psychotropic properties for individuals with epilepsy, independent of its efficacy in improving seizure control.

Aggression. Barratt (1993) described three kinds of aggression: medically related, premeditated or planned, and impulsive or hair trigger response. He evaluated the use of carbamazepine in an outpatient population. His preliminary results suggested that the medication was effective in decreasing impulsive aggressive acts, although the number of subjects was too small for statistical significance.

Personality Disorders. In a discussion of pharmacotherapy for people with borderline personality disorder, Cowdry and Gardner (1988) described a double-blind crossover trial of placebo and four medications, one of which was carbamazepine. The individuals on carbamazepine demonstrated a marked decrease in the severity of behavioral dyscontrol.

Sodium Valproate

Mania. Valproic acid was first synthesized in the United States in late 19th century and was used as an organic solvent. Its antiepileptic properties were discovered accidentally in 1963 in France. The first report of valproate having therapeutic effects for people with bipolar disorders appeared in France in 1966. A number of uncontrolled

studies and six controlled trials have provided evidence of valproate's effectiveness in the treatment of acute mania (McElroy & Keck, 1995). Preliminary results of an ongoing multicenter community-based open trial of valproate treatment for affective disorders showed that the drug is frequently effective and has a favorable side effect profile (Brown, 1989). The U.S. FDA recently approved manic episodes of bipolar disorder as a new indication for valproate prescription ("Manic Episodes," 1995).

Mixed Affective Disorders. McElroy and Keck (1993) suggested that for individuals with bipolar or schizoaffective disorders who are inadequately responsive to or unable to tolerate standard therapies, valproate is an acute and prophylactic treatment option, either as a single agent or with lithium, neuroleptic, carbamazepine, antidepressant, or thyroid hormone therapy. Schaff, Fawcett, and Zajecka (1993) gave valproate to 63 patients with a variety of affective disorders that had proved refractory to conventional pharmacotherapy with lithium or carbamazepine. Forty-seven persons (74.6%) had a positive response. The positive response was found for 84% of the lithium failures, 69% of the carbamazepine failures, and 81% of the rapid cyclers. Fourteen percent had drug side effects serious enough to indicate drug withdrawal. Twelve individuals had recurrent, major bipolar depression; these individuals were considered to be "covert cyclers." They responded to valproate, sometimes in combination with antidepressant therapy.

Unipolar and Bipolar Depression. We could find no controlled studies on the use of valproate for treatment of acute unipolar or bipolar major depression. Open studies suggest that valproate is less effective in treatment of acute depression than in acute mania (McElroy & Keck, 1995). Kemp (1992) found no published data on the issue but reported one case of a person with treatment-resistant depression who appeared to respond well to valproate.

Dementia. Lott, McElroy, and Keys (1995) treated 10 nursing home patients, aged 71 to 94 years and who had dementia and behavioral agitation, with open-label valproate over periods of time ranging from 4 to 34 weeks. Change in behavioral agitation was rated by nursing home staff members. Eight of the 10 patients showed a 50% or greater reduction in the frequency of episodes of behavioral agitation. Response was maintained for all patients, and side effects were minimal.

Clonazepam

Mania. Clonazepam is a high-potency benzodiazepine that has been used as an anticonvulsant. Chouinard reviewed the English language literature in 1987 and concluded that clonazepam was useful for agitation, pressured speech, and increased motor activity for people with mania or manic-spectrum disorders. Chouinard (1988) later reported a prospective double-blind study of 12 individuals with acute mania. Individuals were randomly chosen to receive either lithium or clonazepam for 10 days and then were switched to the other drug. He noted a trend toward clonazepam being more effective than lithium for overactivity and pressured speech.

Keck, McElroy, and Nemeroff (1992) reviewed the literature and commented that benzodiazepines, including clonazepam, might have mostly a sedative rather than an antimanic effect. They drew this conclusion even though they considered these drugs to be helpful in the early tranquilization of patients with acute mania. They also noted that most reports on benzodiazepines were based on only a few patients and did not include long-term evaluations.

In a retrospective study, Sachs, Rosenbaum, and Jones (1990) evaluated 20 persons who initially were receiving lithium and a neuroleptic. When clonazepam was added, neuroleptics were discontinued successfully for 6 patients, and the dosage was reduced for 7 other patients. In a follow-up study, Sachs, Weilberg, and Rosenbaum (1990) observed an additional 20 individuals who received lithium and neuroleptic medications. One randomized group was maintained on the initial regimen while another received clonazepam associated with a slow taper of neuroleptic medication. No new episodes occurred in the clonazepam group, whereas two occurred in the control group.

Bipolar Disorders. Two reports suggested that clonazepam may be helpful for some individuals with bipolar depression. In an open prospective study, Kishimoto et al. (1988) found that clonazepam was as effective as antidepressants as an adjunct to lithium. Zetin and Freedman (1986) described two women who were cousins, one of whom developed mania on imipramine and became "zombie-like" on lithium. Her cousin had depression with intermittent hypomania. Both women improved with the addition of small doses of clonazepam.

Aronson, Shukla, and Hirschowitz (1989) reported the results of an open study of five patients with bipolar disorders who were lithium resistant. All of these individuals had a history of psychotic episodes and were receiving neuroleptics. A trial of clonazepam therapy was begun in which neuroleptics were tapered off in the first three weeks. There were three persons with mania and two with delusional depression. All five relapsed within 15 weeks of medication changes. Chouinard (1989) suggested that these results may have been due to the rapid neuroleptic taper.

Psychotic and Schizoaffective Symptoms. Freinhar and Alvarez (1985) reported two cases in which people with symptoms of mania but not of psychosis responded to clonazepam. Although clonazepam caused improvements in symptoms such as pressured speech, flight of ideas, tangentiality, hyperactivity, distractibility, and sleeplessness, it had no effect on symptoms such as grandiosity or ideas of reference. Victor, Link, Binder, and Bell (1984) reported on three patients with schizoaffective disorder and mania who were treated with clonazepam after they showed little or no response to neuroleptic medication. Clonazepam decreased agitation and anxiety in all three people, and it diminished intrusiveness and increased tolerance of social interactions in two. Two became cooperative in therapy.

CLINICAL INDICATIONS FOR PEOPLE WITH MENTAL RETARDATION

Indications Based on Established Data

A number of researchers have evaluated the frequency of usage and effects of lithium in people with mental retardation who resided in institutional and community settings (Burd et al., 1991; Hancock, Weber, Kaza, & Her, 1991; Pary, 1993; Poindexter, 1989; Tu, 1979). Prescription frequencies were relatively low in each study, varying from 0.6% to 5.4%. In a literature review, Yudofsky, Silver, and Schneider (1987) found several reports of cases in which lithium was effective with some aggressive adolescents with mental retardation. Of the two double-blind, placebo-controlled studies, one showed significant improvement in aggressive behavior in 17 of 25 individuals with mental retardation, and the other showed a decrease in aggressive behavior in only 2 of 8 persons.

Naylor, Donald, LePoidevin, and Reid (1974) reported equivocal results from a double-blind trial of long-term lithium treatment of 14 institutionalized adults with mental retardation, ranging in age from 19 to 58. Mental retardation levels ranged from borderline to severe; 9 had manic depression, 2 were suspected of having manic depression, and 3 had epileptic psychosis, catatonia, or residual schizophrenia. Each person

received 1 year of lithium treatment and 1 year of placebo. Blood levels, measured 21 hours after the last dose
of long-action lithium, ranged from 0.6 to 1.0 mEq/L.
The number of weeks ill during the year on lithium was
significantly less than the number of weeks ill during the
year on placebo. The number of individual episodes was
about the same for each year, with the number of
episodes somewhat higher during the year on placebo.
The differences were not statistically significant. The
authors stressed the importance of making a diagnosis of
manic depressive illness in affected individuals with
mental retardation, because this disorder is potentially
treatable.

Worrall, Moody, and Naylor (1975) treated 8 aggressive non-manic depressive women with mental retardation with lithium in a double-blind, placebo-controlled
study. They found that aggression was reduced in 3 individuals, increased in 1, and unchanged in 2. Treatment
for 2 people had to be discontinued because they apparently developed neurotoxicity. In a double-blind trial
lasting four months for 42 individuals with mental retardation, Craft et al. (1987) assessed the effect of lithium
on aggression as compared to placebo. They excluded
anyone with cyclic behavior. Seventy-three percent of
people in the lithium-treated group showed a reduction
in aggression, as was indicated by measures of both
frequency and severity.

Luchins and Dojka (1989) completed a retrospective
chart study of individuals with mental retardation, a
history of aggression, and self-injurious behavior. Six
received propranolol and 11 received lithium.
Comparison of frequency of behavior 3 months prior to
treatment with the first 3-month period at therapeutic
lithium levels or maximal propranolol dose showed that
these drugs were essentially equal in the reduction of
both index behaviors.

In Smith and Perry's (1992) literature review of
nonneuroleptic treatment of disruptive behavior for
people with organic mental syndromes, all of the lithium studies included individuals with mental retardation.
In the open, prospective group, 19 of 23 persons (83%)
improved; in the double-blind, placebo-controlled group,
36 of 53 persons (68%) improved. One study showed a
positive placebo response in 6 of 21 individuals (30%).
These authors suggested that a 2- to 6-week trial of lithium carbonate in adequate dosage is a reasonable clinical approach to treat behavior disorders for people with
mental retardation.

Langee (1990) reported results of a 10-year retrospective study of 74 institutionalized persons with severe
or profound mental retardation who received lithium

carbonate for various behavior disorders unresponsive to
other medications or treatments. Behavioral data were
recorded regularly and coordinated with medication use.
Thirty-one individuals (42%) demonstrated sustained
major reduction or elimination of behavioral symptoms.
For 16 of these, symptoms recurred after medication was
withdrawn one or more times, and symptoms improved
when medication was restarted. Characteristics that indicated greater likelihood of response to lithium included
older age and presenting symptoms of psychosis,
although all characteristics studied were seen in both the
responder and nonresponder groups.

Indications Based on Clinical Observation or Hypothesis

A number of investigators have reported anecdotal data
related to the effects of lithium on individuals with
mental retardation. In 1974 Micev and Lynch reported
the results of treatment of 10 individuals with severe
mental retardation for a period of 12 weeks. They found
that 5 of the 9 who had aggressive tendencies showed
substantial improvement, 3 improved slightly, and 1
showed no change. Outbursts of aggressive behavior
became less frequent and easier to control. Improvement
was more obvious in people with self-mutilating behavior, in that the behavior ceased in 6 of 8 persons.

Sovner and Hurley (1981) reviewed the literature and
presented two cases. They concluded that the available
data supported the use of lithium to manage behavior
disorders in people with mental retardation and a history of lifelong hyperactivity, aggressiveness, or self-mutilation. They recommended conducting drug-free trials
after a therapeutic effect was obtained to assess the need
for continued treatment. Singh and Millichamp (1985)
noted that uncontrolled investigations and several case
studies suggested that lithium might be effective in
controlling self-injurious behavior in people with mental
retardation. Although Winchel and Stanley (1991)
pointed out that the weight of evidence supported the
use of lithium and carbamazepine to treat self-injury in
individuals with mental retardation, substantiating
evidence is not available to indicate that carbamazepine
alone is useful for the treatment of self-injury.

Case reports of successful treatment with lithium for
individuals with autism and bipolar symptomatology
were made by Kerbeshian, Burd, and Fisher (1987) and
by Steingard and Biederman (1987). Additionally,
Clarke, Littlejohns, Corbett, and Joseph (1989) reported on four individuals with pervasive developmental

disorder associated with psychosis in adulthood. One of these, with moderate mental retardation and psychotic disorder not otherwise specified, responded well to electroconvulsive therapy and lithium. A second, diagnosed with schizophrenia, was treated with antipsychotics and lithium and experienced a complete remission after about 15 months of treatment. A third person, diagnosed with autistic disorder and major depressive episode, eventually responded to amitriptyline and chlorpromazine, but stabilized on lithium. The fourth person showed no change (D.J. Clarke, personal communication, October, 1994).

Glue (1989) reported results of an open-treatment trial of lithium or lithium and carbamazepine with 10 individuals with mental retardation who met DSM-III criteria for rapid cycling affective disorder and who were hospitalized in New Zealand. These individuals had mild to severe mental retardation, ranged in age from 26 to 59 years, and had family histories of high rates of mental illness, including affective disorders. Five of these persons improved after treatment, two of whom completely recovered for at least six months. The 2 who recovered completely responded to a combination of lithium and carbamazepine. Three others had decreased frequency and severity of mood swings, either on lithium monotherapy or on lithium and carbamazepine. Providing additional anecdotal indication of the efficacy of lithium for individuals with mental retardation, Steven King (personal communication, June, 1995) reported relatively successful treatment of more than 30 institutionalized adults in Ohio. Functional levels varied from mild to profound mental retardation; target symptoms primarily were self-injurious behavior, hyperactivity, and sleep abnormalities.

Lapierre and Reesal (1986) suspected that the side-effect profile is the same for individuals with mental retardation as for others, but Ruedrich, Grush, and Wilson (1990) feared that neurotoxic effects of lithium, even when administered in the accepted therapeutic range, may be more prevalent in people with mental retardation. One problem in assessing the results of any lithium therapy is determining whether or not a clinical trial has been adequate. Pary (1991b) reviewed articles on establishing guidelines for optimal clinical trials of lithium for people with mental retardation and major affective illness. He recommended that a serum concentration of at least 0.5 mEq/L to 1.0 mEq/L be achieved, unless the individual responds or trial-ending side effects appear. He also suggested that the treatment be maintained at this level for six to eight weeks before concluding that the individual would not respond.

Sovner (1989) reported on 5 adults with bipolar disorders and mental retardation who were treated with valproate. Four of these individuals had marked improvement with valproate, and one had a moderate response. Kastner, Finesmith, and Walsh (1993) reported results of an open trial of valproate for affective symptoms for people with mental retardation. From a group of 209 individuals serially referred to a tertiary-care medical center for evaluation of behavioral symptoms, they selected a study group of 21, with ages ranging from 8 to 40 years. The selection criteria were irritability, sleep disturbance, aggression or self-injurious behavior, and behavioral cycling. To be included, individuals had to have at least three of these symptoms. The group was studied prospectively for two years. Two were lost to follow-up, and one had side effects necessitating drug discontinuation. Of the 18 who completed the study, 14 (78%) responded favorably. Psychotropic medication prescribed at the time of enrollment was usually discontinued. Nine of 10 receiving neuroleptics and all 3 receiving phenobarbital had those medications withdrawn. History of epilepsy or suspicion of seizures was strongly associated with a favorable response to valproate. Data on improvement are difficult to interpret, however, because the fact that phenobarbital was discontinued during the course of valproate treatment may have had a confounding effect. This discontinuance alone would be expected to decrease irritability and aggression (Poindexter et al., 1993).

We could find only one published report on the use of clonazepam with individuals with mental retardation. Freinhar (1985) described a 19-year-old woman with an IQ of 64 who was agitated and displayed violent, assaultive behavior. Clonazepam produced a calming effect at low dosages; temper tantrums and aggression were eliminated when the dosage was raised. No lethargy associated with treatment was observed.

Cain and her associates at the University of Rochester (N. Cain, personal communication, June, 1995) treated five individuals with mental retardation with clonazepam, and clinical improvement was noted in three. Three of the treated group had a bipolar disorder, supported by family history in two cases. One of these individuals could no longer receive neuroleptic medication because of significant tardive dyskinesia. Her excess motor activity and intrusiveness interfered with her community placement. Both symptoms were greatly reduced with clonazepam. Another individual with a schizoaffective disorder could not tolerate increases in neuroleptic dosage but had significant anxiety and remnants of delusions. Used as an adjunct medication, clonazepam reduced anxiety and eliminated delusions. Another individual who was nonverbal and was treated with neuroleptic medication for a psychotic disorder required neuroleptic withdrawal because of a general medical condition. She subsequently developed anxiety and excessive motor activity, which appeared to respond well to clonazepam therapy.

We could not find any studies in which the effects of lithium on learning or cognition for individuals with mental retardation were evaluated. Apparently very few individuals with mental retardation and aggression have been treated systematically with lithium or with anticonvulsant medication. In the absence of psychosis, use of lithium, carbamazepine, or valproate probably should be considered before use of neuroleptic medications for aggressive individuals. This is partially because of the dangers of tardive dyskinesia and other side effects of neuroleptic treatment.

CONCLUSIONS

Lithium preparations are relatively simple chemical compounds used in the United States since 1970, primarily for mood disorders and for treatment of aggression that is refractory to other treatments. The primary target for lithium in the brain is unknown, as is the mechanism of action, but some believe that lithium's antimanic and antidepressant effects probably involve inhibition of specific steps in the cycle of development of "second messengers" within the brain nerve cells themselves.

Lithium is readily absorbed when taken orally. Its therapeutic index, the ratio of the median fatal dose to the median therapeutic dose, is relatively low (narrow), indicating a need to monitor lithium blood levels carefully. Lithium blood levels should be obtained before the first morning dose is received. Many side effects can be minimized with adjustment of dosage and with changes in types of lithium preparations. Lithium has particularly significant drug interactions with thiazide diuretics.

Although the efficacy of carbamazepine for treatment of epilepsy and paroxysmal pain syndromes has been clearly demonstrated since the early 1960s, more recent studies indicate its efficacy for some individuals with acuta mania and other affective disorders. Additional studies suggest some therapeutic effects for people with aggression and behavioral dyscontrol.

The first report of valproate having therapeutic effects in bipolar disorder was published in 1966. The results of a number of studies since then confirmed its effectiveness in acute mania, mixed affective disorders, and dementia.

Clonazepam, a high-potency benzodiazepine drug used as an anticonvulsant, also is reported to have some efficacy as a treatment for mania or manic-spectrum disorders.

The clearest psychiatric indications for lithium, carbamazepine, valproate, and clonazepam are for treating mood disorders. The drugs are used to treat mania and also as adjunct medication in the treatment of depression. Lithium, carbamazepine, and valproate have an anti-aggressive effect apart from their effects on specific psychiatric syndromes. For this reason, a carefully conducted clinical trial with any of these preparations may be of great value to some individuals with traumatic brain injury or with mental retardation, particularly those who have failed to respond to a variety of behavioral treatment programs and other medications.

REFERENCES

Abou-Saleh, M.T. (1993). Who responds to prophylactic lithium therapy? British Journal of Psychiatry, 163(Suppl. #2), 20–16.

Alessi, N., Naylor, M.W., Ghaziuddin, M., & Zubieta, J.K. (1994). Update on lithium carbonate therapy in children and adolescents. Journal of the Academy of Child and Adolescent Psychiatry, 33, 291–304.

American Psychiatric Association. (1994). Practice guideline for the treatment of patients with bipolar disorder. American Journal of Psychiatry, 151(Suppl.), 1–36.

Aronson, T.A., Shukla, S., & Hirschowitz, J. (1989). Clonazepam treatment of five lithium-refractory patients with bipolar disorder. American Journal of Psychiatry, 146, 77–80.

Baldessarini, R.J. (1990). Drugs and the treatment of psychiatric disorders. In A.G. Gilman, T. W. Rall, A.S. Nies, & P. Taylor (Eds.), Goodman and Gilman's the pharmacological basis of therapeutics (8th ed., pp. 383–435). New York: Pergamon Press.

Ballenger, J.C. (1988). The clinical use of carbamazepine in affective disorders. Journal of Clinical Psychiatry, 49(Suppl. 4), 13–19.

Barratt, E.S. (1993). The use of anticonvulsants in aggression and violence. Psychopharmacology Bulletin, 29, 75–81.

Bell, A.J., Cole, A., Eccleston, D., & Ferrier, I.N. (1993). Lithium neurotoxicity at normal therapeutic levels. British Journal of Psychiatry, 162, 689–692.

Bowden, C.L. (1995). Treatment of bipolar disorder. In A.F. Schatzberg & C.B. Nemeroff (Eds.), The American Psychiatric Press textbook of psychopharmacology (pp. 603–614). Washington, DC: American Psychiatric Press.

Bowden, C.L., Brugger, A.M., Swann, A.C., Calabrese, J.R., Janicak, P.G., Petty, F., Dilsaver, S.C., Davis, J.M., Rush, A.J., Small, J.G., Garza-Trevino, E.S., Risch, S.C., Goodnik, P.J., & Morris, D.D. (1994). Efficacy of divalproex vs. lithium and placebo in the treatment of mania. Journal of the American Medical Association, 271, 918-924.

Brown, R. (1989). U.S. experience with valproate in manic depressive illness: A multicenter trial. Journal of Clinical Psychiatry, 50(Suppl.), 13–16.

Burd, L., Fisher, W., Vesely, B.N., Williams, M., Kerbeshian, J., & Leech, C. (1991). Prevalence of psychoactive drug use among

North Dakota group home residents. *American Journal on Mental Retardation, 96,* 119–126.

Cade, J.F.J. (1949). Lithium salts in the treatment of psychotic excitement. *Medical Journal of Australia, 36,* 349–352.

Campbell, M., Fish, B., Korein, J., Shapiro, T., Collins, P., & Koh, C. (1972). Lithium and chlorpromazine: A controlled crossover study of hyperactive severely disturbed young children. *Journal of Autism and Childhood Schizophrenia. 2,* 234–263.

Cardenas, D.D., & McLean, A. (1992). Psychopharmacologic management of traumatic brain injury. *Physical Medicine and Rehabilitation Clinics of North America, 3,* 273–290.

Carlson, G.A., Rapport, M.D., Pataki, C.S., & Kelly, K.L. (1992). Lithium in hospitalized children at 4 and 8 weeks: Mood, behavior, and cognitive effects. *Journal of Child Psychology and Psychiatry, 33,* 411–425.

Chouinard, G. (1987). Clonazepam in acute and maintenance treatment of bipolar affective disorder. *Journal of Clinical Psychiatry, 48*(Suppl.), 29–36.

Chouinard, G. (1988). The use of benzodiazepines in the treatment of manic-depressive illness. *Journal of Clinical Psychiatry, 49*(Suppl.), 15–19.

Chouinard, G. (1989). Clonazepam in treatment of bipolar psychotic patients after discontinuation of neuroleptics [Letter to the editor]. *American Journal of Psychiatry, 146,* 1642.

Clarke, D.J., Littlejohns, C.S., Corbett, J.A., & Joseph, S. (1989). Pervasive developmental disorders and psychoses in adult life. *British Journal of Psychiatry, 155,* 692–699.

Cohen, L.S., Friedman, J.M., Jefferson, J.W., Johnson, E.M., & Weiner, M.L. (1994). A reevaluation of risk of in utero exposure to lithium. *Journal of the American Medical Association, 271,* 146–150.

Corrigan, P.W., Yudofsky, S.C., & Silver, J.M. (1993). Pharmacological and behavioral treatment for aggressive psychiatric inpatients. *Hospital and Community Psychiatry, 44,* 125–133.

Cowdry, R. W., & Gardner, D. L. (1988). Pharmacotherapy of borderline personality disorder. *Archives of General Psychiatry, 45,* 111–119.

Craft, M., Ismail, I.A., Krishnamurti, D., Matthews, J., Regan, A., Seth, R.V., & North, P.M. (1987). Lithium in the treatment of aggression in mentally handicapped patients: A double-blind trial. *British Journal of Psychiatry, 150,* 685–689.

Daisley, H., Barton, E.N., & Williams, C.T. (1990). Fatal lithium toxicity during a religious fast [Letter to the editor]. *Southern Medical Journal, 83,* 364.

DeLong, G.R. (1978). Lithium carbonate treatment of select behavior disorders in children suggesting manic-depressive illness.

Journal of Pediatrics, 93, 689–694.

Eichelman, B. (1988). Toward a rational pharmacotherapy for aggressive and violent behavior. *Hospital and Community Psychiatry, 39,* 31–39.

Fava, M., Rosenbaum, J. F., McGrath, P.J., Stewart, J.W., Amsterdam, J.D., & Quitkin, F.M. (1994). Lithium and tricyclic augmentation of fluoxetine treatment for resistant major depression: A double-blind, controlled study. *American Journal of Psychiatry, 151,* 1372–1374.

Freinhar, J.P. (1985). Clonazepam treatment of a mentally retarded woman [Letter to the editor]. *American Journal of Psychiatry, 142,* 1513.

Freinhar, J.P., & Alvarez, W.H. (1985). Use of clonazepam in two cases of acute mania. *Journal of Clinical Psychiatry, 46,* 29–30.

Gitlin, M.J. (1993). Lithium-induced renal insufficiency. *Journal of Clinical Psychopharmacology, 13,* 276–279.

Glenn, M.B., Wroblewski, B., Parziale, J., Levine, L., Whyte, J., & Rosenthal, M. (1989). Lithium carbonate for aggressive behavior or affective instability in ten brain-injured patients. *American Journal of Physical Medicine and Rehabilitation, 68,* 221–226.

Glue, P. (1989). Rapid cycling affective disorders in the mentally retarded. *Biological Psychiatry, 26,* 250–256.

Hancock, R.D., Weber, S.L., Kaza, R., & Her, K. S. (1991). Changes in psychotropic drug use in long-term residents of an ICF/MR facility. *American Journal on Mental Retardation, 96,* 137–141.

Hanzel, T.E., Kalachnik, J.E., & Harder, S.R. (1992). A case of phenobarbital exacerbation of preexisting maladaptive behavior partially suppressed by chlorpromazine and misinterpreted as chlorpromazine efficacy. *Research in Developmental Disabilities, 13,* 381–392.

Hill, C.D., & Stoudemire, A. (1993). Diagnostic and treatment complications of memory dysfunction in mood disorders. In J.M. Oldham, M. Riba, & A. Tasman (Eds.), *Review of psychiatry* (Vol. 12, pp. 783–804). Washington, DC: American Psychiatric Press.

Hyman, S.E., & Nestler, E.J. (1993). *The molecular foundations of psychiatry* (pp. 138–140). Washington, DC: American Psychiatric Press.

Judd, L.L., Squire, L.R., Butters, N., Salmon, D.P., & Paller, K.A. (1987). Effects of psychotropic drugs on cognition and memory in normal humans and animals. In H.Y. Meltzer (Ed.), *The third generation of progress* (pp. 1457–1466). New York: Raven Press.

Kastner, T., Finesmith, R., & Walsh, K. (1993). Long-term administration of valproic acid in the treatment of affective symptoms in people with mental retardation. *Journal of Clinical Psychopharmacology, 13,* 448–451.

Keck, P.E., McElroy, S.L., & Nemeroff, C.B. (1992). Anticonvulsants in the treatment of bipolar disorder. *Journal of Neuropsychiatry and Clinical Neurosciences, 4,* 395–405.

Kemp, L.E. (1992). Sodium valproate as an antidepressant. *British Journal of Psychiatry, 160,* 121–123.

Kerbeshian, J., Burd, L., & Fisher, W. (1987). Lithium carbonate in the treatment of two patients with infantile autism and atypical bipolar symptomatology. *Journal of Clinical Psychopharmacology, 7,* 401–405.

Kishimoto, A., Kamata, K., Sugihara, T., Ishiguro, S., Hazama, H., Mizukawa, R., & Kunimoto, N. (1988). Treatment of depression with clonazepam. *Acta Psychiatrica Scandanavica, 77,* 81–86.

Kocsis, J.H., Shaw, E.D., Stokes, P.E., Wilner, P., Elliot, A.S., Sikes, C., Myers, B., Manevitz, A., & Parides, M. (1993). Neuropsychologic effects of lithium discontinuation. *Journal of Clinical Psychopharmacology, 13,* 268–276.

Kofman, O., & Belmaker, R.H. (1993). Biochemical, behavioral, and clinical studies of the role of inositol in lithium treatment and depression. *Biological Psychiatry, 34,* 839–852.

Langee, H.R. (1990). Retrospective study of lithium use for institutionalized mentally retarded individuals with behavior disorders. *American Journal on Mental Retardation, 94,* 448–452.

Lapierre, Y.D., & Reesal, R. (1986). Pharmacologic management of aggressivity and self-mutilation in the mentally retarded. *Psychiatric Clinics of North America, 9,* 745–754.

Lenox, R.H., & Manji, H.K. (1995). Lithium. In A.F. Schatzberg & C.B. Nemeroff (Eds.), *The American Psychiatric Press textbook of psychopharmacology* (p. 322). Washington, DC: American Psychiatric Press.

Litovitz, T.L., Clark, L.R., & Soloway, R.A. (1994). 1993 annual report of the American Association of Poison Control Centers Toxic Exposure Surveillance System. *American Journal of Emergency Medicine, 12,* 546–555.

Lott, A.D., McElroy, S.L., & Keys, M.A. (1995). Valproate in the treatment of behavioral agitation in elderly patients with dementia. *Journal of Neuropsychiatry and Clinical Neurosciences, 7,* 314–319.

Luchins, D.J., & Dojka, D. (1989). Lithium and propranolol in aggression and self-injurious behavior in the mentally retarded. *Psychopharmacology Bulletin, 25,* 372–375.

Manic episodes can be treated with Depakote. (1995, September 7). *Medical Tribune,* p. 11.

Manji, H.K. (1992). G Proteins: Implications for psychiatry. *American Journal of Psychiatry, 149,* 746–760.

Manning, J.S., & Connor, P.D. (1994). Antidepressant augmentation with lithium.

Journal of Family Practice, 39, 379–383.

McDaniel, K.D. (1986). Pharmacologic treatment of psychiatric and neurodevelopmental disorders in children and adolescents. Clinical Pediatrics, 25, 198–204.

McElroy, S.L., & Keck, P.E. (1993). Treatment guidelines for valproate in bipolar disorder and schizoaffective disorder. Canadian Journal of Psychiatry, 39(Suppl. 2), S62–S66.

McElroy, S.L., & Keck, P.E. (1995). Antiepileptic drugs. In A.F. Schatzberg & C.B. Nemeroff (Eds.), The American Psychiatric Press textbook of psychopharmacology (pp. 351–375). Washington, DC: American Psychiatric Press.

Medical Economics Data Production Co. (1996). Physicians' desk reference (50th ed.). Montvale, NJ: author.

Micev, V., & Lynch, D.M. (1974). Effect of lithium on disturbed severely mentally retarded patients. British Journal of Psychiatry, 125, 110.

Mielke, D.H. (1994). Anticonvulsant therapy for mood disorder. Southern Medical Journal, 87, 685–688.

Naylor, G.J., Donald, J.M., LePoidevin, D., & Reid, A.H. (1974). A double-blind trial of long-term lithium therapy in mental defectives. British Journal of Psychiatry, 124, 52–57.

Ozdemir, M.A., Sofuoglu, S., Tanrikulu, G., Aldanmy, F., Esel, E., & Dundar, S. (1994). Lithium-induced hematologic changes in patients with bipolar affective disorders. Biological Psychiatry, 35, 210–213.

Pary, R. (1991a). Side effects during lithium treatment for psychiatric disorders in adults with mental retardation. American Journal on Mental Retardation, 96, 269–273.

Pary, R. (1991b). Towards defining adequate lithium trials for individuals with mental retardation and mental illness. American Journal on Mental Retardation, 95, 681–691.

Pary, R. (1993). Psychoactive drugs used with adults and elderly adults who have mental retardation. American Journal on Mental Retardation, 98, 121–127.

Peet, M., & Pratt, J.P. (1993). Lithium: Current status in psychiatric disorders. Drugs, 46, 7–17.

Poindexter, A.R. (1989). Psychotropic drug patterns in a large ICF/MR facility: A ten-year experience. American Journal on Mental Retardation, 93, 624–626.

Poindexter, A.R., Berglund, J.A., & Kolstoe, P.D. (1993). Changes in antiepileptic drug prescribing patterns in large institutions: Preliminary results of a five-year experience. American Journal on Mental Retardation, 98(Suppl.), 34–40.

Post, R.M. (1988a). Effectiveness of carbamazepine in the treatment of bipolar affective disorder. In S. McElroy & H.G. Pope, Jr. (Eds.), Use of anticonvulsants in psychiatry (pp. 1–23). Clifton, NJ: Oxford Health Care.

Post, R.M. (1988b). Time course of clinical effects of carbamazepine: Implications for mechanisms of action. Journal of Clinical Psychiatry, 49(Suppl. 4), 13–19.

Post, R.M., Altshuler, L.L., Ketter, T.A., Denicoff, K., & Weiss, S.R.B. (1991). Antiepileptic drugs in affective illness: Clinical and theoretical implications. In D.B. Smith, D.M. Treiman, & M.R. Trimple (Eds.), Advances in neurology: Vol. 55. Neurobehavioral problems in epilepsy (pp. 239–277). New York: Raven Press.

Post, R.M., Uhde, T.W., Roy-Byrne, P.P., & Joffe, R.T. (1988). Antidepressant effects of carbamazepine. In S. McElroy & H.G. Pope, Jr. (Eds.), Use of anticonvulsants in psychiatry (pp. 29–34). Clifton, NJ: Oxford Health Care.

Price, L.H., & Heninger, G.R. (1994). Lithium in the treatment of mood disorders. New England Journal of Medicine, 331, 591–598.

Ruedrich, S.L., Grush, L., & Wilson, J. (1990). Beta adrenergic blocking medications for aggressive or self-injurious mentally retarded persons. American Journal on Mental Retardation, 95, 110–119.

Sachs, G.S., Rosenbaum, J.F., & Jones, L. (1990). Adjunctive clonazepam for maintenance treatment of bipolar affective disorder. Journal of Clinical Psychopharmacology, 10, 42–47.

Sachs, G.S., Weilburg, J.B., & Rosenbaum, J.F. (1990). Free communications: Treatment of mood disorders. Clonazepam vs. neuroleptics as adjuncts to lithium maintenance. Psychopharmacology Bulletin, 26, 137–143.

Schaff, M.R., Fawcett, J., & Zajecka, J.M. (1993). Divalproex sodium in the treatment of refractory affective disorders. Journal of Clinical Psychiatry, 54, 380–384.

Schatzberg, A.F., & Cole, J.O. (1991). Manual of clinical psychopharmacology (2nd. ed., pp. 145–166). Washington, DC: American Psychiatric Press.

Schou, M. (1993). Is there a lithium withdrawal syndrome? British Journal of Psychiatry, 163, 514–518.

Sheard, M.H., Marini, J.L., Bridges, C.I., & Wagner, E. (1976). The effect of lithium on impulsive aggressive behavior in man. American Journal of Psychiatry, 133, 1409–1413.

Singh, N.N., & Millichamp, C.J. (1985). Pharmacological treatment of self-injurious behavior in mentally retarded persons. Journal of Autism and Developmental Disorders, 15, 257–267.

Smith, D.A., & Perry, P.J. (1992). Nonneuroleptic treatment of disruptive behavior in organic mental syndromes. Annals of Pharmacotherapy, 26, 1400–1408.

Sovner, R. (1989). The use of valproate in the treatment of mentally retarded persons with typical and atypical bipolar disorders. Journal of Clinical Psychiatry, 50(Suppl.), 40–43.

Sovner, R., & Hurley, A. (1981). The management of chronic behavior disorders in mentally retarded adults with lithium carbonate. Journal of Nervous and Mental Disease, 169, 191–195.

Steingard, R., & Biederman, J. (1987). Lithium responsive manic-like symptoms in two individuals with autism and mental retardation. Journal of the American Academy of Child and Adolescent Psychiatry, 26, 932–935.

Strickland, T.L., Lawson, W., & Lin, K.M. (1993). Interethnic variation in response to lithium therapy among African-American and Asian-American populations. In K.M. Lin, R.E. Poland, & G. Nakasaki (Eds.), Psychopharmacology and psychobiology of ethnicity (pp. 107–121). Washington, DC: American Psychiatric Press.

Strickland, T.L., Raganath, V., Lin, K.M., Poland, R.E., Mendoza, R., & Smith, M.W. (1991). Psychopharmacologic considerations in the treatment of Black American populations. Psychopharmacology Bulletin, 127, 441–448.

Swann, A.C., Secunda, S.K., Katz, M.M., Koslow, S.H., Maas, J.W., Chang, S., & Robbins, E. (1986). Lithium treatment of mania: Clinical characteristics, specificity of symptom change, and outcome. Psychiatry Research, 18, 127–141.

Tu, J.B. (1979). A survey of psychotropic medication in mental retardation facilities. Journal of Clinical Psychiatry, 40, 125–128.

Tupin, J.P. (1978). Usefulness of lithium for aggressiveness. American Journal of Psychiatry, 135, 1118.

Tupin, J.P., & Schuller, A.B. (1978). Lithium and haloperidol incompatibility reviewed. Psychiatric Journal of the University of Ottawa, 3, 245–251.

Victor, B.S., Link, N.A., Binder, R.L., & Bell, I.R. (1984). Use of clonazepam in mania and schizoaffective disorders. American Journal of Psychiatry, 141, 1111–1112.

Watsky, E.J., & Salzman, C. (1991). Psychotropic drug interactions. Hospital and Community Psychiatry, 42, 247–256.

Weingartner, H., Rudorfer, M.V., & Linnoila, M. (1985). Cognitive effects of lithium treatment in normal volunteers. Psychopharmacology, 86, 472–474.

Winchel, R.M., & Stanley, M. (1991). Self-injurious behavior: A review of the behavior and biology of self-mutilation. American Journal of Psychiatry, 148, 306–317.

Worrall, E.P., Moody, J.P., & Naylor, G.J. (1975). Lithium in non-manic depressives: Antiaggressive effect and red blood cell lithium values. British Journal of Psychiatry, 126, 464–468.

Yudofsky, S.C., Silver, J.M., & Schneider, S.E. (1987). Pharmacologic treatment of aggression. Psychiatric Annals, 17, 397–407.

Zetin, M., & Freedman, M.J. (1986). Clonazepam in bipolar affective disorder [Letter to the editor]. American Journal of Psychiatry, 143, 1055.

Stimulants

L. Eugene Arnold[1], Kenneth Gadow[2], Deborah A. Pearson[3], and Christopher K. Varley[4]

Some of the most commonly prescribed psychotropic drugs for children, including those with mental retardation, are the stimulants. This drug class includes methylphenidate hydrochloride (Ritalin), dextroamphetamine sulfate (Dexedrine), magnesium pemoline (Cylert), racemic amphetamine sulfate (Benzedrine, which is no longer available), Adderall (a mix of various salts of dextroamphetamine and racemic amphetamine), methamphetamine (Desoxyn), and deanol (Deaner). The latter, a precursor of acetylcholine, is the only one that would not be considered a sympathomimetic stimulant. Other stimulants, not generally used therapeutically, include cocaine. Nicotine (a cholinergic stimulant) is currently being studied for possible therapeutic application, but is still considered experimental at this writing. Caffeine is both a drug and a food component; at times it has been claimed to be therapeutic for attention-deficit hyperactivity disorder (ADHD), and individual children may anecdotally benefit, but controlled studies have not substantiated efficacy at a generalizable group level (e.g., Arnold, Christopher, Huestis, & Smeltzer, 1978; Huestis, Arnold, & Smeltzer, 1975). Fenfluramine (Pondimin) is an amphetamine analogue whose main effect is on the serotonergic system. At usual doses, it may produce more CNS depression than stimulation (Pinder, Brogden, Sawyer, Speight, & Avery, 1975). Fenfluramine is covered separately in chapter 18.

PHARMACOLOGY[5]

Pharmacodynamics

The primary mode of action of dextroamphetamine is believed to be that of enhancing catecholamine activity in the CNS, probably by increasing the availability of norepinephrine and dopamine at the synaptic cleft. The precise mechanism is still poorly understood, but probably involves both release from prsynaptic vesicles and inhibition of reuptake. Its specific mode of action is even less clearly understood. Methylphenidate may have a greater effect on dopamine activity than on other neurotransmitters, but this remains speculative at present. Pemoline is similar in function to these two, although it has minimal sympathomimetic effects and is structurally dissimilar. Its specific mechanism of action is poorly understood.

Catecholaminergic (especially noradrenergic) receptors are widely distributed throughout the brain. Partly because of this wide distribution, the actual site of action of the stimulants within the CNS remains speculative. Early investigators conjectured that brain stem activation was the primary locus, but lately the midbrain or frontal cortex have been implicated more. Some studies of cerebral blood flow have suggested that activity in the area of the striatum and the connections between the orbitofrontal and limbic regions are enhanced during stimulant treatment (Lou, Henriksen, & Bruhn, 1984; Lou, Henriksen, Bruhn, Børner, & Nielsen, 1989). Moreover, using positron-emission tomography (PET) scans, Zametkin et al. (1990) have demonstrated increased brain metabolic activity in the bilateral orbitofrontal area and in the left sensorimotor and parietal areas following a single dose of methylphenidate given to seven adults with ADHD. Surprisingly, a suppression of activity was noted in the left temporal region following stimulant administration, but because the brain is complex, changes in one area of the brain may be consequences of those in other areas. Gualtieri, Hicks, and Mayo (1983) have hypothesized that the

---

1 Special Expert, Child and Adolescent Disorders Research Branch, National Institute of Mental Health, Now Emeritus Professor of Psychiatry, Ohio State University, Columbus, OH
2 Professor of Child and Adolescent Psychiatry, State University of New York at Stony Brook, Stony Brook, NY
3 Associate Professor of Psychiatry and Behavioral Science, University of Texas Medical School, Houston, TX
4 Associate Professor of Psychiatry, University of Washington, Seattle, WA
5 The sections on pharmacology and physical effects are based on "Stimulants" by R. A. Barkley, G. J. DuPaul, and A. Costello, 1993, in J. S. Werry and M. G. Aman (Eds.), *Practitioner's Guide to Psychoactive Drugs for Children and Adolescents* (pp. 205-237), New York, Plenum Medical Book Company.

stimulants act to "canalize" or decrease fluctuation and variability in arousal, attention, and CNS reactivity, thereby enhancing the persistence of responding and increasing cortical inhibition. Others (e.g., Haenlein & Caul, 1987) have proposed that the stimulants decrease the threshold for reinforcement through enhancement of the arousal of the CNS behavioral activation (reward) system, thereby creating a persistence of responding to tasks or activities, that is, events in which the organism engages are now more reinforcing, resulting in prolonged responding to them.

Pharmacokinetics

Stimulants are almost always given orally, are swiftly absorbed from the gastrointestinal tract, cross the blood-brain barrier quickly and easily, and are rapidly eliminated from the body within 24 hours (Diener, 1991). Dextroamphetamine reaches peak plasma levels in children within 2 to 3 hours, with a plasma half-life between 4 and 6 hours (but with substantial inter-individual variability). The breakdown of dextroamphetamine occurs mainly in the liver, where deamination and p-hydroxylation transform it mainly to benzoic acid. A significant proportion is excreted in the urine, ranging from 2% in very alkaline urine to as high as 80% in very acidic urine, so that high gastric activity and some treatments for urinary infections may affect concentration substantially (Brown, Hunt, Ebert, Bunney, & Kopin, 1979). Behavioral effects are noticeable within 30 to 60 minutes, appear to peak between 1 and 2 hours post-ingestion, and usually dissipate within 4 to 6 hours (Dulcan, 1990).

Methylphenidate reaches peak plasma levels within 1.5 to 2.5 hours after ingestion. The plasma half-life is usually between 2 and 3 hours, and the drug is entirely metabolized within 12 to 24 hours with almost none of the drug appearing in the urine (Diener, 1991; Wargin et al., 1983). The metabolic pathway for its decomposition and elimination seems to be via de-esterification to ritalinic acid, to a lesser degree via hydroxylation to p-hydroxymethylphenidate, and the remainder to oxoritalinic acid and oxomethylphenidate, all of which are pharmacologically inactive (Cantwell & Carlson, 1978). As with dextroamphetamine, behavioral effects occur within 30 to 60 minutes, peak within 1 to 3 hours, and are dissipated within 3 to 5 hours after ingestion in most children. The plasma half-life of so-called sustained-release methylphenidate has been found to be essentially similar: between 2 and 6 hours, with a peak plasma

level reached within 1 to 4 hours. Behavioral effects of this preparation appear to occur within 1 to 2 hours, peak within 3 to 5 hours, and slowly diminish until approximately 8 hours post-ingestion. It is important to note, however, that considerable inter-individual variability exists with respect to these parameters, and that there are clinical implications for the frequency of dosage. The plasma level does appear to be dose-related (Patrick, Mueller, Gualtieri, & Breese, 1987), but dose level has not been shown to correlate with clinical effect.

Pemoline appears to have a shorter half-life with children (7 to 8 hours) than with adults (11 to 13 hours) and reaches peak plasma levels 2 to 4 hours post-ingestion (Sallee, Stiller, Perel, & Bates, 1985). Within 24 hours, 50% to 75% of the dose seems to be excreted in the urine. The time course and response characteristics of its behavioral effects were not documented until recently. Whereas it was once thought that clinical effects were not fully evident for 2 to 3 weeks after starting medication, Pelham, Swanson, Furman, Wilson, and Schwindt (1995) recently reported that pemoline is fully effective on the first day of the effective dose. The half-life of pemoline possibly increases with chronic use, which may lead to a build-up in plasma levels. This may explain the earlier impression of delayed behavioral effects (up to 3 to 4 weeks) reported by some investigators (e.g., Dulcan, 1990).

Peak or absolute blood levels are less useful for predicting behavioral effects than is dosage level (Kupietz, 1991; Swanson, 1988). Peak behavioral changes often seem to lag behind peak blood levels by as much as an hour. Performance on learning tasks, however, may correspond more closely to blood levels (Kupietz, 1991; Swanson, Kinsbourne, Roberts, & Zucker, 1978), although the data are sparse. Consequently, when behavioral change is the goal of treatment, blood levels appear to have no clinical utility in establishing the therapeutic range or response for any individual case. When changes in learning performance are targeted, blood levels may eventually provide more promising information about establishing a therapeutic range, although here again inter- and intra-individual variability are quite high (Kupietz, 1991). Drawing blood to guide therapeutic adjustments to patients' stimulant medication is not recommended (Shaywitz & Shaywitz, 1991; Swanson, 1988) except possibly in resistant cases.

Tolerance to these drugs has not been established in research, but clinical anecdotes suggest decreased efficacy of the drugs in some cases over prolonged administration. Dulcan (1990) suggested that this finding may stem from hepatic autoinduction, behavioral noncompliance with the prescribed regimen, growth (outgrowing the dose), or contextual factors such as stress (e.g., a move, divorce, or change in school classroom) or altered expectations of caregivers. It is also possible, given the inherent complexity of dopamine receptors, that compensatory changes in the number of receptor sites may occur.

PHYSICAL EFFECTS

Both methylphenidate and d-amphetamine produce acute growth hormone release and suppress prolactin in both children and adults, which could lead to alterations in cortisol beta-endorphins. However, as Reeve and Garfinkel (1991) noted, long-term effects on the hypothalamic-pituitary-growth hormone axis have not been demonstrated. Despite some evidence of initial growth inhibition by these drugs, effects on eventual adult height or skeletal stature are often clinically insignificant (Klein & Mannuzza, 1988). Effects on weight are also frequently minimal, resulting in a loss of 1 to 2 pounds during the initial year of treatment and often showing a rebound in growth by the second or later years of treatment (Dulcan, 1990; Gittelman, Landa, Mattes, & Klein, 1988; Reeve & Garfinkel, 1991). All of the stimulants seem to reduce appetite to some degree, although this is temporary and mainly limited to the time of peak effects (Cantwell & Carlson, 1978).

A large albeit inconclusive literature exists on the physiological effects of the stimulants (Barkley, 1977, 1990; Brown et al, 1979; Cantwell & Carlson, 1978; Diener, 1991; Dulcan, 1990; Elia & Rapoport, 1991; Gittelman et al., 1988; Gualtieri et al, 1983; Haenlein & Caul, 1987; Hastings & Barkley, 1978; Klein & Mannuzza, 1988; Kupietz, 1991; Lou et al., 1984, 1989; Patrick et al., 1987; Redman & Zametkin, 1991; Reeve & Garfinkel, 1991; Rosenthal & Allen, 1978; Sallee et al., 1985; Shaywitz & Shaywitz, 1991; Swanson, 1988; Swanson et al., 1978; Taylor, 1986; Wargin et al., 1983). Heart rate, as well as systolic and diastolic blood pressure, may be increased by these medications; however, these effects appear to be small and moderated by a number of factors. For instance, higher dosages of stimulants are linearly related to increasing levels of heart rate, and these effects are dependent on both the premedication heart rate and the time course of the medication (Kelly, Rapport, & DuPaul, 1988). The

changes in cardiovascular functioning that do occur are often mild (about 6-15 beats per minute in heart rate, about 5-10 mm Hg in blood pressure), are clearly dose-dependent, and are often outweighed by other normal daily physiologic stresses such as digestion (Aman & Werry, 1975; Hastings & Barkley, 1978). Pemoline may be less likely to produce these effects on heart rate and blood pressure (Knights & Viets, 1975). Heart rate variability is reduced by methylphenidate, as is heart rate deceleration to a reaction time task. The latter result is consistent with changes in cognitive functions, such as attention span and concentration. In all studies, cardiovascular effects of stimulants are subject to tremendous intra- and inter-individual variability. Notably, African-American adolescents may have a greater risk for developing an increase in diastolic blood pressure (Brown & Sexson, 1989).

Effects of stimulants on autonomic nervous system functioning have been noted in the literature for several decades. Skin conductance is often increased, primarily at doses of methylphenidate over 15 mg/day (Hastings & Barkley, 1978), whereas effects on both nonspecific and specific galvanic skin responses are equivocal (Barkley & Jackson, 1977; Satterfield & Dawson, 1971).

Background electrical activity of the CNS is sometimes increased by the stimulants, usually noted in reduced alpha or slow-wave activity, and CNS sensitivity to stimulation may also be heightened as measured by EEGs and audio- and visual-evoked potentials (Barkley & Jackson, 1977; Brown & Sexson, 1989; Coons, Klorman, & Borgstedt, 1987; Hastings & Barkley, 1978; Kelly et al., 1988; Knights & Viets, 1975; Peloquin & Klorman, 1986; Rosenthal & Allen, 1978; Satterfield & Dawson, 1971; Taylor, 1986). Consequently, cerebral blood flow and brain metabolic activity may be increased. These effects seem selective, however, being concentrated primarily in the anterior frontal regions bilaterally as documented in recent studies, including some using cerebral blood flow and PET (Barkley, 1977; Barkley & Jackson, 1977; Brown et al., 1979; Brown & Sexson, 1989; Cantwell & Carlson, 1978; Coons et al., 1987; Diener, 1991; Dulcan, 1990; Elia & Rapoport, 1991; Gittelman et al., 1988; Gualtieri et al., 1983; Haenlein & Caul, 1987; Hastings & Barkley, 1978; Kelly et al., 1988; Klein & Mannuzza, 1988; Knights & Viets, 1975; Kupietz, 1991; Lou et al., 1986; Patrick et al., 1987; Peloquin & Klorman, 1986; Redman & Zametkin, 1991; Reeve & Garfinkel, 1991; Rosenthal & Allen, 1978; Sallee et al., 1985; Satterfield & Dawson, 1971; Shaywitz & Shaywitz, 1991; Swanson,

1988; Swanson et al., 1978; Taylor, 1986; Wargin et al., 1983; Zametkin et al., 1990). Effects on the reticular activating system may also be noted, probably leading to the increases in heart rate, blood pressure, and in a few cases, respiration. Effects on various aspects of sleep seem insignificant other than a mild delay in sleep onset, or insomnia, experienced by the majority of patients who take stimulants after noon. Some evidence points to a temporary reduction in REM sleep that often returns to normal within several months (Hastings & Barkley, 1978). In summary, the stimulants appear to have minor effects on physical systems. What effects are seen involve increases in certain aspects of both autonomic and central nervous system activity, typically small and relatively insignificant clinically.

TOXIC EFFECTS AND SIDE EFFECTS[6]

At clinical doses, stimulants do not have toxicity in the sense of threatening life or causing permanent harm, and death from overdose by ingestion is so rare that it is unknown to clinicians who have years of prescribing experience. However, there have been a few recent deaths from recreational parenteral administration. Stimulants have a very wide safety margin compared to most other psychotropic drugs and to most prescription drugs in general. At moderate doses, they produce few serious side effects, but some common nuisance ones. The adverse drug reactions observed in children and adolescents with mental retardation appear to be similar to those reported for youngsters with hyperactivity without mental retardation (e.g., Gadow, 1982), but comparison studies have not been conducted.

At the onset of drug treatment, the two most common side effects are insomnia and anorexia (loss of appetite). Insomnia is typically not a problem if medication is administered only in the morning, and for children with normal IQ usually not even if administered at noon. If a late dose is necessary, the physician may prescribe an additional drug in the evening (e.g., diphenhydramine) to induce sleep (Arnold, 1973). Anorexia usually can be managed by taking the pill just before meals and eating before it takes effect. Other minor side effects are also possible. These include headache, stomachache, nausea, irritability, and increased talkativeness. Children typically develop a tolerance for these reactions, but the dose may have to be reduced and then increased more gradually to lessen the degree of discomfort.

Perhaps the most distressing adverse reactions for care providers are changes in appearance and mood and the suppression of spontaneity. Laufer, Denhoff, and Riverside (1957) described the change of appearance in some children and adolescents as the "amphetamine look" (1957): "A pale, pinched, serious facial expression with dark hollows under the eyes. It is of no serious consequence but the parents must be prepared for adverse comment concerning the child's appearance" (p. 471). They also reported a marked decrease in activity: "Sometimes, if too high a dosage (of Dexedrine) is given, the counteraction of the syndrome may go to the extreme of 'freezing' the patient or fixating him to what he is doing, and may even put him to sleep" (p. 470).

Changes in activity level are not always appreciated if they are extreme. Parents sometimes comment that their child is "overly quiet," "stares into space," or "has a stillness about him that I don't like" (Gadow, 1977, p. 35). These changes in activity level and mood prompt teachers and parents to describe some children treated with stimulants as looking like zombies (Sprague & Gadow, 1976). In their study of boys who had no diagnosis at all (no mental retardation and no mental illness), Rapoport et al. (1978) found that dextroamphetamine made them appear "unusually inactive, not simply less restless" (p. 562).

In children, changes in mood may give the appearance of depression. Schain and Reynard (1975) reported that 6.4% of the 6- to 12-year-old children in their study became withdrawn, lethargic, and apathetic when taking methylphenidate. The prevalance of these reactions appears to be higher among preschool-age children. Other changes in mood include weepiness, irritability, euphoria, and fearfulness. Drowsiness, a side effect one would not ordinarily associate with stimulants, is sometimes reported by parents and teachers of young children (Gadow, 1982). This effect of stimulants also appears in older children as well as in adults (Montagu & Swarbrick, 1975; Tecce & Cole, 1974).

The cognitive side effects of stimulant drugs have been demonstrated most clearly on tasks that require paired-associate learning (Swanson et al., 1978) and flexibility in thinking (Robbins & Sahakian, 1979). There are at least three types of reactions. Some children do more poorly on cognitive tasks regardless of the dose of stimulant medication. Others do not benefit from treatment when the dosage of medication is too high. It appears as if they get too much of a good thing. Medication

---

6 This section is based on *Pharmacotherapy and Mental Retardation* by K. D. Gadow and A. D. Poling, 1988, Boston: Little, Brown.

improves attention span to the point that the child is overfocused. On tasks that require problem-solving ability, the child exhibits perseverative errors, making the same mistake over and over (Dyme, Sahakian, Golinko, & Rabe, 1982). Because these reactions are difficult to diagnose without the aid of an actual laboratory task, clinicians have generally recommended more conservative dosages in their suggested guidelines for treatment. A third type of reaction occurs in children who show a favorable response to lower doses. When given a dose that is too high, they do less well on some types of tasks than if they were not taking medication at all. In other words, the favorable response noted on the lower dose is reversed, and children actually perform less well than they would without medication.

Although there is little evidence that these drugs can impair classroom academic activities, the findings from two studies suggest that higher doses of medication may suppress academic productivity in some children (Rapport et al., 1982; Sulzbacher, 1972). Tannock et al. (1995) found higher doses to be associated with a decrement in performance from optimal dose, although still better than periods without medication. Numerous other researchers failed to find cognitive impairment with increasing dose (e.g., Pelham, Bender, Caddell, Booth, & Moorer, 1985); the most likely explanation is specificity of effect, confined to certain functions tapped by only certain tests. Academic impairment does not appear to be a serious risk for most children, especially at low to moderate dosages of medication.

Other possible side effects of stimulant medication do not occur very often but still need to be monitored. Involuntary movements of muscles may occur. These include a variety of actions such as protrusion of the mouth, grimacing, facial tics (spasm or twitching of the facial muscles), choreoathetoid (jerking and writhing) movements of arms or legs, and twisting of the head and neck (e.g., Denckla, Bemporad, & MacKay, 1976; Gadow, 1982; Husain, Chapel, & Malek, 1980; Mattson & Calverley, 1968; Robbins & Sahakian, 1979). These drugs can cause stereotypies such as nail biting or lead to an increase in the frequency of stereotypies or tics in children who already have these problems prior to treatment (e.g., Robbins & Sahakian, 1979; Wulbert & Dries, 1977). In some cases, these side effects will abate with reduced dosage. In others, treatment may have to be discontinued or the child switched to a different medication.

There have been reports of stimulant-induced hallucinations (Lucas & Weiss, 1971) and psychosis (Greenberg, Deem, & McMahon, 1972), but these are rare. Children who experience such a reaction may complain about seeing or hearing things or feeling that their skin is crawling. Discontinuation or substantial dosage reduction is recommended.

It is reported that methylphenidate can cause seizures in children who are brain-damaged, have abnormal EEGs, or are prone to develop a seizure disorder (e.g., Millichap, 1968, 1969, 1973). Nevertheless, the risk of a seizure disorder subsequent to stimulant drug therapy seems rare (Gadow, 1982). In a controlled study of 10 children with both seizures and ADHD, Feldman, Crumrine, Handen, Alvin, and Teodori (1989) found no difference between methylphenidate and placebo in number or type of seizures or concentrations of concurrent anticonvulsive medication, but they did find significant behavioral improvement with methylphenidate. Some clinicians believe that amphetamine may be safer than methylphenidate for patients with a previous seizure history who are not currently taking anticonvulsants.

Stimulant drugs also have an effect on the cardiovascular system. Methylphenidate, for example, has been shown to increase both blood pressure and heart rate (Ballard, Boileau, Sleator, Massey, & Sprague, 1976). Although there is considerable variability across children in terms of the magnitude of the effect, in general, the higher the dose of methylphenidate the greater the need to evaluate this potential reaction. At lower dosages (0.3 to 0.5 mg/kg), these side effects are usually negligible and do not appear to have any adverse effect on the child even after long-term treatment (Hechtman, Weiss, & Perlman, 1984; Satterfield, Schell, & Barb, 1980).

Care providers are often concerned about the long-term consequences of stimulant drug use. Although the benign, short-term side effects of methylphenidate and dextroamphetamine are well documented, only a few researchers have investigated potential long-term adverse drug reactions. There are a number of problems inherent in conducting well-controlled follow-up studies, problems not peculiar to the area of stimulants and hyperactive children. The only side effects associated with long-term stimulant drug therapy that have been reported so far are clinically trivial but statistically significant reductions in height and weight gain (Safer & Allen, 1973). That is, children who received dextroamphetamine or fairly high doses of methylphenidate (e.g., Mattes & Gittelman, 1983), gained less height and weight than would have been expected had they not been placed on medication. When drug treatment is stopped, children usually show a growth rebound, an increase in growth rate that compensates for the slower rate they experience while medicated (Safer & Allen, 1973). In contrast, well-controlled studies of children receiving low and moderate doses of methylphenidate, with breaks from treatment whenever clinically feasible, have failed to demonstrate growth suppression (Kalachnik, Sprague, Sleator, Cohen, & Ullmann, 1982; McNutt, Boileau, Cohen, Sprague, & von Neumann, 1977).

The Pediatric Advisory Panel of the U.S. Food and Drug Administration reviewed the available literature about stimulants and growth suppression (Roche, Lipman, Overall, & Hung, 1979) and concluded that "stimulant drugs, particularly in the 'high normal' dose range, moderately suppress growth and weight...(but) early growth suppression during treatment is no longer evident in adulthood" (p. 849). A recent study of adults who were treated with stimulants when younger showed no adverse effect on either weight or height (Hechtman et al., 1984). Nevertheless, because some children may be affected to a greater degree than others, treatment should be carefully monitored with regular height and weight checks. At present there is no evidence that long-term treatment with methylphenidate in low doses (approximately 0.25 mg/kg twice a day) adversely affects the functioning of the liver, the endocrine glands, or the cardiovascular system (Satterfield et al., 1980).

DRUG INTERACTIONS

Stimulants are compatible with most other drugs. The main interactions of concern occur with antidepressants and anticonvulsants. Stimulants inhibit the liver enzymes that metabolize antidepressants and some anticonvulsants (e.g., carbamazepine), so that concomitant administration elevates the plasma level obtained from a given dose of tricyclic antidepressant or anticonvulsant. This situation can be managed through prescribing lower doses of tricyclics and checking plasma levels. Of greater concern is the interaction with monoamine oxidase inhibitors (MAOIs), which inhibit the neuronal enzymes that catabolize the catecholamine neurotransmitters (dopamine and norepinephrine). Stimulants release catecholamines into the synaptic cleft and prevent their presynaptic reuptake; MAOI inhibition of catecholamine catabolism contributes to an accumulation that becomes excessive, commonly resulting in hypertension and other adrenergic-excess symptoms. Generally, therefore, stimulants and MAOIs should not be used concomitantly, though newer reversible MAOIs may prevent this interaction. Over-the-counter decongestant-antihistamine compounds used as cold and allergy remedies can occasionally either interfere with the beneficial action of stimulants or add to their effect, but they do not pose any known danger in customary doses.

Recent reports of three deaths (two in the United States) of children taking the combination of methylphenidate and clonidine have caused concern. All three cases were complicated by physical comorbidity (preexisting cardiac fibrosis, seizure disorder, and abnormal anesthetic reaction). Additional risk factors appeared to be multiple additional medications and inconsistent compliance with the dosage regimen (Swanson et al., 1995; see also Chapter 15 for a more detailed discussion of these cases). Although the risk appears low relative to the large number of children taking this combination, the risk factors may be more common in patients with mental retardation. It should be noted for patients already taking this combination that *abrupt interruption of chronic clonidine is more dangerous than continuation.*

CLINICAL INDICATIONS EXCLUSIVE OF MENTAL RETARDATION

Stimulants are used mainly for the treatment of ADHD (see Table 14-1 for a complete list of diagnostic criteria); as many as 3% of school-age children have taken them for this reason. Stimulants have also been shown to be effective for many adults with ADHD (Wender, Reimherr, Wood, & Ward, 1985; Wender, Wood, & Reimherr, 1991). From 1990 to 1994, the prescription rate for adults grew proportionately more than for children, although it remains well below 1%. The short-term efficacy of stimulants for treating people who have ADHD is as well documented as is any treatment in psychiatry. However, long-term efficacy has not been well established scientifically and is currently the object of study. The clinical use of stimulants is controversial in some quarters, because the U. S. Drug Enforcement Administration classified the amphetamines and methylphenidate as controlled substances. Nevertheless, many practitioners regard stimulants as the treatment of choice for ADHD. Ninety percent or more of people properly diagnosed as having ADHD (combined and hyperactive-impulsive subtypes) respond favorably to treatment with stimulants if two or more are tried in

Table 14-1. Diagnostic Criteria for Attention-Deficit/Hyperactivity Disorder

A. Either (1) or (2):

(1) six (or more) of the following symptoms of **inattention** have persisted for at least 6 months to a degree that is maladaptive and inconsistent with developmental level:

Inattention
(a) often fails to give close attention to details or makes careless mistakes in schoolwork, work, or other activities
(b) often has difficulty sustaining attention in tasks or play activities
(c) often does not seem to listen when spoken to directly
(d) often does not follow through on instructions and fails to finish schoolwork, chores, or duties in the workplace (not due to oppositional behavior or failure to understand instructions)
(e) often has difficulty organizing tasks and activities
(f) often avoids, dislikes, or is reluctant to engage in tasks that require sustained mental effort (such as schoolwork or homework)
(g) often loses things necessary for tasks or activities (e.g., toys, school assignments, pencils, books, or tools)
(h) is often easily distracted by extraneous stimuli
(i) is often forgetful in daily activities

(2) six (or more) of the following symptoms of **hyperactivity-impulsivity** have persisted for at least 6 months to a degree that is maladaptive and inconsistent with developmental level:

Hyperactivity
(a) often fidgets with hands or feet or squirms in seat
(b) often leaves seat in classroom or in other situations in which remaining seated is expected
(c) often runs about or climbs excessively in situations in which it is inappropriate (in adolescents or adults, may be limited to subjective feelings of restlessness)
(d) often has difficulty playing or engaging in leisure activities quietly
(e) is often "on the go" or often acts as if "driven by a motor"
(f) often talks excessively

Impulsivity
(g) often blurts out answers before questions have been completed
(h) often has difficulty awaiting turn
(i) often interrupts or intrudes on others (e.g., butts into conversations or games)

B. Some hyperactive-impulsive or inattentive symptoms that caused impairment were present before age 7 years.

C. Some impairment from the symptoms is present in two or more settings (e.g., at school [or work] and at home).

D. There must be clear evidence of clinically signifcant impairment in social, academic, or occupational functioning.

E. The symptoms do not occur exclusively during the course of a Pervasive Developmental Disorder, Schizophrenia, or other Psychotic Disorder and are not better accounted for by another mental disorder (e.g., Mood Disorder, Anxiety Disorder, Dissociative Disorder, or a Personality Disorder).

Code based on type:
314.01 Attention-Deficit/Hyperactivity Disorder, Combined Type: if both Criteria A1 and A2 are met for the past 6 months
314.00 Attention-Deficit/Hyperactivity Disorder, Predominantly Inattentive Type: if Criterion A1 is met but Criterion A2 is not met for the past 6 months
314.01 Attention-Deficit/Hyperactivity Disorder, Predominantly Hyperactive-Impulsive Type: if Criterion A2 is met but Criterion A1 is not met for the past 6 months
Coding note: For individuals (especially adolescents and adults) who currently have symptoms that no longer meet full criteria, "In Partial Remission" should be specified.

Reproduced with permission of American Psychiatric Association from *Diagnostic and Statistical Manual of Mental Disorders*, 4th ed., Washington, DC: American Psychiatric Association, 1994, pp. 84-85.

succession. Stimulants usually help all three primary symptoms of ADHD: inattention, hyperactivity, and impulsivity. They increase on-task behavior, task completion, and behavioral self-control. They reduce distractibility, restlessness, motor overactivity, and impulsive recklessness.

Stimulants are also indicated for treating narcolepsy (irrespective of age), depression in the elderly, neutralization of drug-induced sedation, and potentiation of non-MAOI antidepressants. Amphetamine has a mild anticonvulsant effect in slow-wave epilepsy and has been known to potentiate anticonvulsant treatment in otherwise intractable cases. Although once used for weight loss in obesity, stimulants are no longer recommended for this purpose because the effect is transient and there is a mild danger of addiction.

CLINICAL INDICATIONS IN MENTAL RETARDATION AND PERVASIVE DEVELOPMENTAL DISORDER

Table 14-2 summarizes Sprague and Werry's (1971) review of research published between 1937 and 1970 on stimulant use for patients. In Table 14-3, we summarize research published from 1971 to 1996. In reviewing this research, we devised scales to rate (a) the quality of study design and (b) the degree to which treatment with stimulants was found to be beneficial (see column 4). In the remainder of this section, we summarize the conclusions that can be drawn from this research regarding the primary treatments for which stimulants are indicated for use with people with mental retardation and pervasive developmental disorders.

Importance of Diagnosis

One conclusion readily gleaned from Tables 14-2 and 14-3 is that stimulants seem to ameliorate the symptoms of ADHD, but not those for most other targeted conditions. For people with ADHD without mental retardation, stimulants have been shown to ameliorate inattention, hyperactivity, and impulsivity. In some cases, related cognitive functions, such as memory or perceptual ability, have also been shown to improve. Drug effects on IQ and on behavior unrelated to ADHD have been negligible. For example, stereotyped behavior

seemed unaffected in the large majority of patients treated with stimulants. Stimulants are usually not helpful in the treatment of people who internalize problems. On the other hand, Aman, Kern, McGhee, and Arnold (1993a) found that methylphenidate suppressed enuresis and encopresis compared to placebo for a sample in which many children had taken methylphenidate for a while before entering the study.

The usefulness of stimulants for the treatment of learning and behavior symptoms in children with pervasive developmental disorder (PDD), including autism, is unclear. Campbell et al. (1972), for example, found that dextroamphetamine (Dexedrine) often exacerbated symptoms of autism by increasing social withdrawal and stereotypies, and even made some youngsters more hyperactive and irritable. Their sample, however, was confined to preschoolers, known to be overly sensitive to such adverse effects (Ounsted, 1955). Other investigators reported favorable treatment outcomes (reduction of hyperactivity symptoms and aggression) for elementary school-aged children with autism receiving dextroamphetamine (Geller, Guttmacher, & Bleeg, 1981) and methylphenidate (Birmaher, Quintana, & Greenhill, 1988; Strayhorn, Rapp, Donina, & Strain, 1988; Vitriol & Farber, 1981). Therefore, it seems appropriate for clinicians to consider low doses of this drug for empirical trials with school-age children with PDD who have symptoms of ADHD.

Thus, the primary clinical indications for stimulants with people with mental retardation appears to be the same for children and adults without mental retardation—namely, treatment of symptoms of ADHD. The efficacy of stimulants for treating other problems, such as aggression or narcolepsy, in the presence of mental retardation has been little studied, however. The value of stimulants for children with PDD and ADHD symptoms is uncertain at this time: Although it is clear that the core symptoms of autism are not improved, the symptoms of hyperactivity and inattentiveness may be improved.

Sensitivity, Side Effects, and Time of Action

Research strongly suggests that patients with mental retardation are more sensitive to stimulants than average children. They may require lower doses, develop more side effects, and metabolize the drugs more slowly. For example, Handen et al. (1991) reported more adverse effects than are usually encountered in patients of normal IQ with ADHD. Aman, Marks, Turbott,

Wilsher, and Merry (1991a) and Aman et al. (1993a) reported effects on sleep and found significant benefit with a single morning dose, in contrast to the usual twice and even thrice daily dosing in patients of normal IQ.

Modulation by IQ or MA

Some research has also suggested that patients with severe and profound mental retardation do not respond well to the catecholaminergic stimulants. Samples consisting entirely of patients in these categories generally did not show benefit. Furthermore, two studies showed benefits significantly greater for people with IQs above 45 compared to people with IQs below 45 (Aman et al., 1991a, 1993a). At the lower IQ level, fenfluramine showed an advantageous trend (Aman et al., 1993a). Mayes, Crites, Bixler, Humphrey, and Mattison (1994) found nonsignificant trends supporting a lower response rate in children with mental retardation, but they also found some response with youngsters having an IQ as low as 23.

Quality of response may be related somewhat to mental age (MA) and cognitive maturity (Aman, 1996), because preschoolers of average IQ have sometimes been noted clinically not to respond well to methylphenidate but then to respond later during school age. This phenomenon seems to be more of a threshold effect rather than a linear relationship (Arnold, 1993). Conversely, Mayes et al. (1994), although finding a nonsignificant association of response with age for children with mental retardation, found a significant inverse relationship of response with age for children with ADHD alone (without mental retardation), including a good response in four preschoolers.

CLINICAL CONSIDERATIONS

Diagnosis

The diagnosis of ADHD should be made mainly on the basis of caretakers' observations of the symptoms cited in the DSM-IV. Patients should be examined to rule out mimicking conditions, such as anxiety or mood disorders, which may be more likely in adults than in children. Mania or depression as a cause of agitation and restlessness can often be distinguished by their episodic nature (not chronic and not predating an age

of 7 years). Family history may also be helpful. A precipitating event suggests that anxiety or mood disorder, rather than ADHD, may be the correct diagnosis. However, the symptoms of ADHD can also be exacerbated by stress. According to the DSM-IV, ADHD symptoms should be assessed with respect to mental age to avoid false positive diagnoses. The proportion of children with mental retardation who have ADHD has been estimated in one survey at about 15% to 20% (Epstein, Cullinan, & Gadow, 1986), about three times the general population risk, and the proportion with prominent ADHD symptoms (not necessarily at the diagnostic threshold) has been estimated as high as 50% in clinical samples.

Dosage

The dosage of stimulants for children has been the subject of considerable research. For patients with and without mental retardation, the dosage requirements vary widely among individuals. Since researchers have not established an optimal dosage schedule for patients with mental retardation, the standard practice for patients without mental retardation is used. Physicians should start with a low dose (e.g., 5 mg of methylphenidate or amphetamine in the morning) and titrate gradually up (every few days or weekly) against side effects and clinical benefit, going to b.i.d. or t.i.d. dosage or sustained release forms when needed. There is no absolute cap (side effects limit the dose), but it is rare to find additional net benefit (benefit minus side effects) from pushing doses beyond 60 to 70 mg methylphenidate per day or 30 to 40 mg dextroamphetamine per day for patients without mental retardation (most respond at much lower doses), and there is some reason to believe that patients with mental retardation, and especially those with PDD, may require lower doses. The range of dosage reported in the literature for children with ADHD and mental retardation is as follows: For methylphenidate, dosage ranged from 2.5 to 50 mg per day and from 0.3 mg/kg to 1.0 mg/kg. For dextroamphetamine, the range was 5 to 20 mg per day and from 0.2 mg/kg to 0.8 mg/kg. Adults may tolerate higher total milligrams than do children, but not in proportion to body mass.

Sustained Release Preparations

There is no literature on the effects of sustained release

methylphenidate on patients with mental retardation and little on the effects of sustained release forms of amphetamine. There is little persuasive evidence of differences in side effects in sustained release compared with the standard forms. For methylphenidate, some studies of cognitively average children have shown little or no advantage of the sustained-release form over regular medication. The sustained release medication produces a more variable absorption rate and less predictable blood levels.

Dose-response Curve and Learning

A series of studies of average-ability children suggested that the optimal dose for learning may be lower than the best dose for behavioral improvement (Sprague & Sleator, 1973, 1975, 1977). Although this dose-response curve is not accepted by all authorities, if correct it may be especially relevant for patients with mental retardation. The lesson may be summed up in the well-drilling expression, "Don't drill past water." Some authors report that the optimal dose for academic performance is about half to a third that for optimal behavioral benefit. Thus the target symptoms (inattention and academic performance vs. externalizing hyperactivity, disruptiveness, or aggression) may determine the optimal dosage range for a given patient.

Variable Efficacy

If the first stimulant tried does not work, another one may work; at least two should be tried before giving up, and three trials are advisable. However, with individual exceptions, the younger the child (below age 5) or the lower the IQ (below 45), the less effective the usual catecholamine stimulants may be. Below IQ 50, other agents such as thioridazine, guanfacine, or clonidine may work better. However, the effectiveness of these agents is not as well supported by scientific data, and they may have more serious side effects.

Age Considerations

Recommendations about age must depend mainly on research with patients of average IQ. Some authors and clinicians have noted less benefit and more side effects in preschoolers than in older children. Side effects with preschoolers may include depression. A child who fails

to respond as a preschooler may respond at a later age, so a second trial with the same drug several years later may be useful if symptoms persist. There is very little clinical experience with prescribing stimulants for adults who have mental retardation and ADHD, but adults with mental retardation are vulnerable for persistent ADHD, and, therefore, they may be candidates for stimulants. Cautious individual empiricism must therefore guide the clinician.

Preference for Monotherapy

Polypharmacy for ADHD has become more popular in recent years, but it is possible to manage most patients with ADHD satisfactorily with a single stimulant. There is no reason to believe that the presence of mental retardation invalidates this principle. When a stimulant does not work, other drugs, such as tricyclic antidepressants (imipramine, nortriptyline), bupropion, or clonidine (more recently guanfacine) may be tried alone. As a last resort, combinations of medications may be tried, but safety is an unsettled question with most combinations.

Comorbidity

The presence of comorbidity such as with depression, anxiety, or tics may suggest that a nonstimulant drug be used to treat both disorders. However, even with comorbidity, a stimulant may provide satisfactory relief. The presence of obsessive-compulsive symptoms may suggest use of a serotonin-reuptake inhibitor.

Relative Safety

Compared to other psychoactive drugs and anticonvulsants, stimulants are relatively safe. For example, they can be used in the presence of cardiac disease, a consideration with many adult patients with mental retardation. In fact, if it were not for their abuse potential, they would probably be candidates for over-the-counter availability. However, polymorphic metabolism with genetic differences may be more of an issue for people with mental retardation. Because stimulants show almost immediate results if the given dose is effective, a trial can be done rather quickly and usually with minimal discomfort, even if the patient is a nonresponder. These are important points for educating consumers and caretakers, who may be frightened by media coverage challenging the use of stimulants or suggesting that their use leads to drug abuse.

Rating Scales

Traditionally, clinicians and researchers working with children with ADHD have relied heavily on behavior rating scales, both to confirm a diagnosis of ADHD and to measure the impact of treatment. Perhaps the most popular of the scales is the Conners series, available in both extended and abbreviated (10-item) forms. However, the relevance of these scales with children having other than mild mental retardation is unknown. Other scales have been developed for patients with mental retardation and may be more useful for this population. Some authorities have recommended correcting for developmental level by choosing norms based on the patient's mental age. Pearson and Aman (1994) presented data suggesting that such a correction may not be necessary.

Pill Swallowing

Many children with mental retardation, especially Down syndrome, have difficulty swallowing pills or tablets. For such children, a behavior-shaping program using increasing sizes of cake decors can often train pill swallowing. Alternately, the medicine can be crushed and put in applesauce, yogurt, ice cream, or mashed potatoes. The use of specialized cups that deliver medication in such a way that the patient does not see it coming should be considered only as a last resort; the use of unseen pills cause choking or jeopardize trust in care providers. Crushing cannot be used for sustained release forms, but the beads in Dexedrine spansules can be poured out of the capsule and handled the same as a crushed tablet, as long as they are not chewed.

Long-term Use

There is no evidence of serious deleterious side effects from either short- or long-term use of stimulants. Nevertheless, most experts advise annual reassessments of the need for stimulant medication, which can easily be done by tapering the dose and monitoring for any deterioration in behavior.

CONCLUSION

Stimulants appear to benefit many individuals with both ADHD and mental retardation. Several cautionary points are worth consideration. There exist comparatively few studies of this topic, especially studies of high quality. The few well-controlled studies showing efficacy concerned people with mild and moderate mental retardation; efficacy in those with profound or severe mental retardation has not been well documented and may be much lower. It can be difficult to diagnose ADHD in people with mental retardation or other developmental disability, especially in people with low IQs. Given that side effects may be more frequent and that people with mental retardation often have difficulty describing their feelings and behavior, special attention should be given to documenting safety and efficacy. In no study has the course of disorder, duration of treatment effect, development of tolerance, or long-term side effects in this population been examined. In patients who appear to respond to stimulant medications, ongoing monitoring of benefits and costs is essential.

REFERENCES

Alexandris, A., & Lundell, F.W. (1968). Effect of thioridazine, amphetamine, and placebo on the hyperkinetic syndrome and cognitive area in mentally deficient children. *Canadian Medical Association Journal*, 98, 92–96.

Aman, M.G. (1982). Stimulant drug effects in developmental disorders and hyperactivity—toward a resolution of disparate findings. *Journal of Autism and Developmental Disorders*, 12, 385–398.

Aman, M.G. (1996). Stimulants in the developmental disabilities revisited. *Journal of Developmental and Physical Disabilities*, 8, 347–365.

Aman, M.G., Kern, R.A., Arnold, L.E., & McGhee, D.E. (1991). Fenfluramine and mental retardation. *Journal of the American Academy of Child and Adolescent Psychiatry*, 30, 507–508.

Aman, M.G., Kern, R.A., McGhee, D.E., & Arnold, L.E. (1993a). Fenfluramine and methylphenidate in children with mental retardation and ADHD: Clinical and side effects. *Journal of the American Academy of Child and Adolescent Psychiatry*, 32, 851–859.

Aman, M.G., Kern, R.A., McGhee, D.E., & Arnold, L.E. (1993b). Fenfluramine and methylphenidate in children with mental retardation and ADHD: Laboratory effects. *Journal of Autism and Developmental Disorders*, 23, 491–505.

Aman, M.G., Marks, R.E., Turbott, S.H., Wilsher, C.P., & Merry, S.N. (1991a). Clinical effects of methylphenidate and thioridazine in intellectually subaverage children. *Journal of the American Academy of Child and Adolescent Psychiatry*, 30, 246–256.

Aman, M.G., Marks, M.B., Turbott, S.H., Wilsher, C.P., & Merry, S.N. (1991b). Methylphenidate and thioridazine in the treatment of intellectually subaverage children: Effects on cognitive-motor performance. *Journal of the American Academy of Child and Adolescent Psychiatry, 30,* 816–824.

Aman, M.G., & Singh, N.N. (1982). Methylphenidate in severely retarded residents and the clinical significance of stereotypic behavior. *Applied Research in Mental Retardation, 3,* 345–358.

Aman, M.G., & Werry, J.S. (1975). The effects of methylphenidate and haloperidol on the heart rate and blood pressure of hyperactive children with special reference to time of action. *Psychopharmacology, 43,* 163–168.

American Psychiatric Association. (1994). *Diagnostic and statistical manual of mental disorders* (4th ed.). Washington, DC: American Psychiatric Press.

Anton, A.H., & Greer, M. (1969). Dextroamphetamine, catecholamines, and behavior. *Archives of Neurology, 21,* 248–252.

Arnold, L.E. (1973). The art of medicating hyperkinetic children. *Clinical Pediatrics, 12,* 35–41.

Arnold, L.E., Christopher, J., Huestis, R. & Smeltzer, D.J. (1978). Methylphenidate vs. d-amphetamine vs. caffeine in MBD: Controlled comparison by placebo washout design with Bayes analysis. *Archives of General Psychiatry, 35,* 463–473.

Arnold, L.E. (1993). Clinical pharmacological issues in treating psychiatric disorders of patients with mental retardation. *Annals of Clinical Psychiatry, 5,* 189–197.

Ballard, J.E., Boileau, R.A., Sleator, E.K., Massey, B.H., & Sprague, R.L. (1976). Cardiovascular responses of hyperactive children to methylphenidate. *Journal of the American Medical Association, 236,* 2870–2874.

Barkley, R.A. (1977). A review of stimulant drug research with hyperactive children. *Journal of Child Psychology and Psychiatry and Allied Disciplines, 18,* 137–165.

Barkley, R.A. (1990). *Attention-deficit hyperactivity disorder: A handbook for diagnosis and treatment.* New York: Guilford Press.

Barkley, R.A., & Jackson, T., Jr. (1977). Hyperkinesis, autonomic nervous system activity, and stimulant drug effects. *Journal of Child Psychology and Psychiatry and Allied Disciplines, 18,* 347–357.

Bell, A., & Zubek, J.P. (1961). Effects of deanol on the intellectual performance of mental defectives. *Canadian Journal of Psychology, 15,* 172–175.

Berkson, G. (1965). Stereotyped movements of mental defectives: VI. No effect of amphetamine or a barbiturate. *Perceptual and Motor Skills, 21,* 698.

Birmaher, B., Quintana, H., & Greenhill, L.L. (1988). Methylphenidate treatment of hyperactive autistic children. *Journal of the American Academy of Child and Adolescent Psychiatry, 27,* 248–251.

Blacklidge, V., & Ekblad, R. (1971). The effectiveness of methylphenidate hydrochloride (ritalin) on learning and behavior in public school educable mentally retarded children. *Pediatrics, 47,* 923–926.

Blue, A.W., Lytton, G.J., & Miller, O.W. (1960). The effect of methylphenidate on intellectually handicapped children [Abstract]. *American Psychologist, 15,* 393.

Breitmeyer, J.M. (1969). *Effects of thioridazine and methylphenidate on learning and retention in retardates.* Unpublished master's thesis, University of Illinois, Urbana-Champaign, IL.

Brown, G.L., Hunt, R.D., Ebert, M.H., Bunney, W.E., & Kopin, I.J. (1979). Plasma levels of d-amphetamine in hyperactive children. *Psychopharmacology, 62,* 133–140.

Brown, R.T., & Sexson, S.B. (1989). Effects of methylphenidate on cardiovascular responses in attention-deficit hyperactivity disordered adolescents. *Journal of Adolescent Health Care, 10,* 179–183.

Burgio, L.D., Page, T.J., & Capriotti, R.M. (1985). Clinical behavioral pharmacology: Methods for evaluating medications and contingency management. *Journal of Applied Behavior Analysis, 18,* 45–59.

Campbell, M., Fish, B., David, R., Shapiro, T., Collins, P., & Koh, C. (1972). Response to tri-iodothyronine and dextroamphetamine: A study of preschool schizophrenic children. *Journal of Autism and Childhood Schizophrenia, 2,* 343–358.

Campbell, M., Small, A.M., Collins, P.J., Friedman, E., David, R., & Genieser, N. (1976). Levodopa and levoamphetamine: A crossover study in young schizophrenic children. *Current Therapeutic Research, 19,* 70–86.

Cantwell, D., & Carlson, G. (1978). Stimulants. In J. Werry (Ed.), *Pediatric psychopharmacology* (pp. 171–207). New York: Brunner/Mazel.

Carter, C.H. (1956). The effects of reserpine and methylphenidate (ritalin) in mental defectives, spastics, and epileptics. *Psychiatric Research Reports, 4,* 44–48.

Carter, C.H., & Maley, M.C. (1957). Parental [sic] use of methylphenidate (ritalin). *Diseases of the Nervous System, 18,* 146–148.

Christensen, D.E. (1975). Effects of combining methylphenidate and a classroom token system in modifying hyperactive behavior. *American Journal of Mental Deficiency, 80,* 266–276.

Coons, H.W., Klorman, R., & Borgstedt, A.D. (1987). Effects of methylphenidate on adolescents with a childhood history of attention deficit disorder: II. Information processing. *Journal of the American Academy of Child and Adolescent Psychiatry, 26,* 368–374.

Craft, M. (1959). Mental disorder in the defective: The use of tranquilizers. *American Journal of Mental Deficiency, 64,* 63–71.

Cutler, M., Little, J.W., & Strauss, A.A. (1940). The effect of Benzedrine on mentally deficient children. *American Journal of Mental Deficiency, 45,* 59–65.

Davis, K.V. (1971). The effect of drugs on stereotyped and nonstereotyped operant behavior in retardates. *Psychopharmacologia, 22,* 195–213.

Davis, K.V., Sprague, R.L., & Werry, J.S. (1969). Stereotyped behavior and activity level in severe retardates: The effect of drugs. *American Journal of Mental Deficiency, 73,* 721–727.

Denckla, M.B., Bemporad, J.R., & MacKay, M.C. (1976). Tics following methylphenidate administration. *Journal of the American Medical Association, 235,* 1349–1351.

Diener, R.M. (1991). Toxicology of ritalin. In L.L. Greenhill & B.B. Osmon (Eds.), *Ritalin: Theory and patient management* (pp. 34–43). New York: Mary Ann Liebert.

Dulcan, M.K. (1990). Using psychostimulants to treat behavioral disorders of children and adolescents. *Journal of Child and Adolescent Psychopharmacology, 1,* 7–20.

Dyme, I.Z., Sahakian, B.J., Golinko, B.E., & Rabe, E.F. (1982). Perseveration induced by methylphenidate in children. *Progress in Neuropsychopharmacology, 6,* 269–273.

Elia, J., & Rapoport, J.L. (1991). Ritalin versus dextroamphetamine in ADHD: Both should be tried. In L.L. Greenhill & B.B. Osmon (Eds.), *Ritalin: Theory and patient management* (pp. 69–74). New York: Mary Ann Liebert.

Epstein, M.H., Cullinan, D., & Gadow, K.D. (1986). Teacher ratings of hyperactivity in learning-disabled, emotionally disturbed, and mentally retarded children. *Journal of Special Education, 20,* 219–229.

Fehr, F., & Sprague, R. (1969, October). *The effects of methylphenidate on two flash thresholds and physiological arousal of behavioral problem children as a function of rest and distraction conditions.* Paper presented at the meeting of the Society for Psychophysiological Research, Monterey, CA.

Feldman, H., Crumrine, P., Handen, B. L., Alvin, R., & Teodori, J. (1989). Methylphenidate in children with seizures and attention-deficit disorder. *American Journal of Diseases of Children, 143,* 1081–1086.

Fish, C.H., & Bowling, E. (1962). Effect of amphetamine on speech defects in the mentally retarded. *California Medicine, 94,* 109–111.

Gadow, K.D. (1977). *Psychotropic and antiepileptic drug treatment with children in early childhood special education* Champaign, IL: University of Illinois, Institute for Child Behavior and Development. (ERIC Document Reproduction Service No. ED 162 494).

Gadow, K. D. (1982). School involvement in pharmacotherapy for behavior disorders.

Journal of Special Education, 16, 385–399.

Gadow, K.D., & Pomeroy, J.C. (1990). A controlled case study of methylphenidate and fenfluramine in a young mentally retarded, hyperactive child. Australia and New Zealand Journal of Developmental Disabilities, 16, 323–334.

Gadow, K.D., Pomeroy, J.C., & Nolan, E.E. (1992). A procedure for monitoring stimulant medication in hyperactive mentally retarded school children. Journal of Child and Adolescent Psychopharmacology 2, 131–143.

Geller, B., Guttmacher, L.B., & Bleeg, M. (1981). Coexistence of childhood onset pervasive developmental disorder and attention-deficit disorder with hyperactivity. American Journal of Psychiatry, 138, 388–389.

Gittelman, R., Landa, B., Mattes, J.A., & Klein, D.F. (1988). Methylphenidate and growth in hyperactive children. Archives of General Psychiatry, 45, 1127–1130.

Gualtieri, C.T., Hicks, R.E., & Mayo, J.P. (1983). Hyperactivity and homeostasis. Journal of the American Academy of Child and Adolescent Psychiatry, 22, 382–384.

Haenlein, M., & Caul, W.F. (1987). Attention-deficit disorder with hyperactivity: A specific hypothesis of reward dysfunction. Journal of the American Academy of Child and Adolescent Psychiatry, 26, 356–362.

Hagerman, R.J., Jackson, C., Amiri, K., Silverman, A.C., O'Connor, R., & Sobesky, W. (1992). Girls with fragile X syndrome: Physical and neurocognitive status and outcome. Pediatrics, 89, 395–400.

Hagerman, R.J., Murphy, M.A., & Wittenberger, M.D. (1988). A controlled trial of stimulant medication in children with the fragile X syndrome. American Journal of Medical Genetics, 30, 377–393.

Handen, B.L., Breaux, A.M., Gosling, A., Ploof, D.L., & Feldman, H. (1990). Efficacy of methylphenidate among mentally retarded children with attention-deficit hyperactivity disorder. Pediatrics, 86, 922–930.

Handen, B.L., Breaux, A.M., Janosky, J., McAuliffe, S., Feldman, H., & Gosling, A. (1992). Effects and noneffects of methylphenidate in children with mental retardation and ADHD. Journal of the American Academy of Child and Adolescent Psychiatry, 31, 455–461.

Handen, B.L., Feldman, H., Gosling, A., Breaux, A.M., & McAuliffe, S. (1991). Adverse side effects of methylphenidate among mentally retarded children with ADHD. Journal of the American Academy of Child and Adolescent Psychiatry, 30, 241–245.

Handen, B.L., Janosky, J., McAuliffe, S., Breaux, A.M., & Feldman, H. (1994). Prediction of response to methylphenidate among children with ADHD and mental retardation. Journal of the American Academy of Child and Adolescent Psychiatry, 33, 1185–1193.

Handen, B.L., McAuliffe, S., Janosky, J., Feldman, H., & Breaux, A.M. (1995). Methylphenidate in children with mental retardation and ADHD: Effects on independent play and academic functioning. Journal of Developmental and Physical Disabilities, 7, 91–103.

Hastings, J.E., & Barkley, R.A. (1978). A review of psychopharmacological research with hyperactive children. Journal of Abnormal Child Psychology, 7, 413–447.

Hechtman, L., Weiss, G., & Perlman, T. (1984). Young adult outcome of hyperactive children who received long-term stimulant treatment. Journal of the American Academy of Child Psychiatry, 23, 261–269.

Helsel, W.J., Hersen, M., & Lubetsky, J.J. (1988). Stimulant drug in children and adolescents with mental retardation: A review. Journal of the Multihandicapped Person, 1, 251–269.

Helsel, W.J., Hersen, M., & Lubetsky, J.J. (1989). Stimulant medication and the retarded. Journal of the American Academy of Child and Adolescent Psychiatry, 28, 138–139.

Helsel, W.J., Hersen, M., Lubetsky, J.J., Fultz, S.A., Sisson, L., & Harlovic, C. H. (1989). Stimulant drug treatment of four multihandicapped children using a randomized single-case design. Journal of the Multihandicapped Person, 2, 139–154.

Hilton, D.K., Martin, C.A., Heffron, W.M., Hall, B.D., & Johnson, G.L. (1991). Imipramine treatment of ADHD in a fragile X child. Journal of the American Academy of Child and Adolescent Psychiatry, 30, 831–834.

Huestis, R.D., Arnold, L.E. & Smeltzer, D. (1975). Caffeine vs. methylphenidate and d-amphetamine in minimal brain dysfunction: A double-blind comparison. American Journal of Psychiatry, 132, 868–871.

Husain, A., Chapel, J., & Malek, A.P. (1980). Methylphenidate, neuroleptics and dyskinesia-dystonia. Canadian Journal of Psychiatry, 25, 254–258.

Johnson, C.R., Handen, B.L., Lubetsky, M.J., & Sacco, K.A. (1994). Efficacy of methylphenidate and behavioral intervention on classroom behavior in children with ADHD and mental retardation. Behavior Modification, 18, 470–487.

Kalachnik, J.E., Sprague, R.L., Sleator, E.K., Cohen, M.N., & Ullmann, R.K. (1982). Effect of methylphenidate on stature in hyperactive children. Developmental Medicine and Child Neurology, 25, 586–595.

Kelly, K.L., Rapport, M.D., & DuPaul, G.J. (1988). Attention-deficit disorder and methylphenidate: A multi-step analysis of dose response effects on children's cardiovascular functioning. International Clinical Psychopharmacology, 3, 167–181.

Klein, R.G., & Mannuzza, S. (1988). Hyperactive boys almost grown up: III. Methylphenidate effects on ultimate height. Archives of General Psychiatry, 45, 1131–1134.

Knights, R.M., & Viets, A. (1975). Effects of pemoline on hyperactive boys. Pharmacological Biochemistry and Behavior, 3, 1107–1114.

Kupietz, S.S. (1991). Ritalin blood levels and their correlations with measures of learning. In L.L. Greenhill & B.B. Osmon (Eds.), Ritalin: Theory and patient management (pp. 247–256). New York: Mary Ann Liebert.

Laufer, M.W., Denhoff, E., & Riverside, R.I. (1957). Hyperkinetic behavior syndrome in children. Journal of Pediatrics, 50, 463–474.

Levy, J.M., Jones, B.E., & Croley, H.T. (1957). Effects of methylphenidate (ritalin) on drug-induced drowsiness in mentally retarded patients. American Journal of Mental Deficiency, 62, 284–287.

Lobb, H. (1968). Trace GSR conditioning with Benzedrine in mentally defective and normal adults. American Journal of Mental Deficiency, 73, 239–246.

Lou, H.C., Henriksen, L., & Bruhn, P. (1984). Focal cerebral hypoperfusion in children with dysphasia and/or attention-deficit disorder. Archives of Neurology, 41, 825–829.

Lou, H.C., Henriksen, L., Bruhn, P., Børner, H., & Nielson, J.B. (1989). Striatal dysfunction in attention-deficit and hyperkinetic disorder. Archives of Neurology, 46, 48–52.

Lucas, A., & Weiss, M. (1971). Methylphenidate hallucinosis. Journal of the American Medical Association, 217, 1079–1081.

Mattes, J.A., & Gittelman, R. (1983). Growth of hyperactive children on maintenance regimen of methylphenidate. Archives of General Psychiatry, 40, 317–321.

Mattson, R.H., & Calverley, J.R. (1968). Dextroamphetamine-sulfate-induced dyskinesias. Journal of the American Medical Association, 204, 400–402.

Mayes, S.D., Crites, D.L., Bixler, E.O., Humphrey, F.J., Jr., & Mattison, R.E. (1994). Methylphenidate and ADHD: Influence of age, IQ, and neurodevelopmental status. Developmental Medicine and Child Neurology, 36, 1099–1107.

McConnell, T.R., Cromwell, R.L., Bialer, I., & Son, C.D. (1964). Studies in activity level: VII. Effects of amphetamine drug administration on the activity level of retarded children. American Journal of Mental Deficiency, 68, 647–651.

McNutt, B.A., Boileau, R.A., Cohen, M.N., Sprague, R.L., & von Neumann, A. (1977). Effects of long-term stimulant medication on the growth and body composition of children: II. Report on two years. *Psychopharmacology Bulletin, 13,* 36–38.

Millichap, J.G. (1968). Drugs in management of hyperkinetic and perceptually handicapped children. *Journal of the American Medical Association, 206,* 1527–1530.

Millichap, J.G. (1969). Management of hyperkinetic behavior in children with epilepsy. *Modern Treatment, 6,* 1233–1246.

Millichap, J.G. (1973). Drugs in management of minimal brain dysfunction. *Annals of the New York Academy of Sciences, 205,* 321–334.

Molitch, M., & Eccles, J.P. (1937). Effect of Benzedrine sulfate on the intelligence scores of children. *American Journal of Psychiatry, 94,* 587–590.

Molitch, M., & Sullivan, J.P. (1937). Effect of Benzedrine sulfate on children taking New Stanford Achievement Test. *American Journal of Orthopsychiatry, 7,* 519–522.

Montagu, J.D., & Swarbrick, L. (1975). Effect of amphetamines in hyperkinetic children: Stimulant or sedative. *Developmental Medicine and Child Neurology, 17,* 293–298.

Morris, J.V., MacGillivary, R.C., & Mathieson, C.M. (1955). The results of the experimental administration of amphetamine sulfate in oligophrenia. *Journal of Mental Science/British Journal of Psychiatry, 101,* 131–140.

Moskowitz, H. (1941). Benzedrine therapy for the mentally handicapped. *American Journal of Mental Deficiency, 45,* 540–543.

Ounsted, C. (1955). The hyperkinetic syndrome in epileptic children. *Lancet, 2,* 303–311.

Patrick, K.S., Mueller, R.A., Gualtieri, C.T., & Breese, G.R. (1987). Pharmacokinetics and actions of methylphenidate. In H.Y. Meltzer (Ed.), *Psychopharmacology: The third generation of progress.* New York: Raven Press.

Payton, J.B., Burkhart, J.E., Hersen, M., & Helsel, W. J. (1989). Treatment of ADHD in mentally retarded children: A preliminary study. *Journal of the American Academy of Child and Adolescent Psychiatry, 28,* 761–767.

Pearson, D.A. & Aman, M.G. (1994). Ratings of hyperactivity and developmental indices: Should clinicians correct for developmental level? *Journal of Autism and Developmental Disorders, 24,* 395–411.

Pelham, W.E., Bender, M.E., Caddell, J., Booth, S., & Moorer, S.H. (1985). Methylphenidate and children with attention-deficit disorder: Dose effects on classroom academic and social behavior. *Archives of General Psychiatry, 42,* 941–952.

Pelham, W.E., Swanson, J.M., Furman, M.B., & Schwindt, H. (1995). Pemoline effects on children with ADHD: A time-response by dose-response analysis on classroom measures. *Journal of the American Academy of Child and Adolescent Psychiatry, 34,* 1504–1513.

Peloquin, L.J., & Klorman, R. (1986). Effects of methylphenidate on normal children's mood, event-related potentials, and performance in memory scanning and vigilance. *Journal of Abnormal Psychology, 95,* 88–98.

Pinder, R.M., Brogden, R.D., Sawyer, P.R., Speight, T.M., & Avery, G.S. (1975). Fenfluramine: A review of its pharmacological properties and therapeutic efficacy in obesity. *Drugs, 10,* 241–323.

Rapoport, J.L., Buschbaum, M.S., Zahn, T.P., Weingartner, H., Ludlow, C., & Mikkelsen, E.J. (1978). Dextroamphetamine: Cognitive and behavioral effects in normal prepubertal boys. *Science, 199,* 560–563.

Rapport, M.D., Murphy, H.A., & Bailey, J.S. (1982). Ritalin vs. response cost in the control of hyperactive children: A within-subject comparison. *Journal of Applied Behavior Analysis, 15,* 215–216.

Realmuto, G.M., August, G.J., & Garfinkel, B.D. (1989). Clinical effect of buspirone in autistic children. *Journal of Clinical Psychopharmacology, 9,* 122–125.

Redman, C.A., & Zametkin, A.J. (1991). Ritalin and brain metabolism. In L.L. Greenhill & B.B. Osmon (Eds.), *Ritalin: Theory and patient management* (pp. 301–309). New York: Mary Ann Liebert.

Reeve, E., & Garfinkel, B. (1991). Neuroendocrine and growth regulation: The role of sympathomimetic medication. In L.L. Greenhill & B.B. Osmon (Eds.), *Ritalin: Theory and patient management* (pp. 289–300). New York: Mary Ann Liebert.

Robbins, T.W., & Sahakian, B.J. (1979). "Paradoxical" effects of psychomotor stimulant drugs in hyperactive children from the standpoint of behavioral pharmacology. *Neuropharmacology, 18,* 931–950.

Roche, A.F., Lipman, R.S., Overall, J.E., & Hung, W. (1979). The effects of stimulant medication on the growth of hyperkinetic children. *Pediatrics, 63,* 847–850.

Rosenthal, R.H., & Allen, T.W. (1978). An examination of attention, arousal, and learning dysfunction of hyperkinetic children. *Psychological Bulletin, 85,* 689–715.

Safer, D.J., & Allen, R.P. (1973). Factors influencing the suppressant effects of two stimulant drugs on the growth of hyperactive children. *Pediatrics, 5l,* 660–667.

Sallee, F., Stiller, R., Perel, J., & Bates, T. (1985). Oral pemoline kinetics in hyperactive children. *Clinical Pharmacology and Therapeutics, 37,* 606–609.

Satterfield, J.H., & Dawson, M.E. (1971). Electrodermal correlates of hyperactivity in children. *Psychophysiology, 8,* 191–197.

Satterfield, J.H., Schell, A.M., & Barb, S.D. (1980). Potential risk of prolonged administration of stimulant medication for
hyperactive children. *Developmental and Behavioral Pediatrics, 1,* 102–107.

Schain, R.J., & Reynard, C.L. (1975). Observations on effects of central stimulant drug (methylphenidate) in children with hyperactive behavior. *Pediatrics, 55,* 709–716.

Schell, R.M., Pelham, W.E., Bender, M.E., Andree, J.A., Law, T., & Robbins, F. R. (1986). The concurrent assessment of behavioral and psychostimulant interventions: A controlled case study. *Behavioral Assessment, 8,* 373–384.

Schickedanz, D.I. (1967). *Effects of thioridazine and methylphenidate on performance of a motor task and concurrent motor activity in retarded boys.* Unpublished bachelor's thesis, University of Illinois at Urbana-Champaign.

Schmidt, K. (1982). The effect of stimulant medication in childhood-onset pervasive developmental disorder: A case report. *Journal of Developmental and Behavioral Pediatrics, 3,* 244–246.

Shafto, F., & Sulzbacher, S. (1977). Comparing treatment tactics with a hyperactive preschool child: Stimulant medication and programmed teacher intervention. *Journal of Applied Behavior Analysis, 10,* 13–20.

Shaywitz, S.E., & Shaywitz, B.A. (1991). Attention-deficit disorder: Diagnosis and role of ritalin in management. In L.L. Greenhill & B.B. Osmon (Eds.), *Ritalin: Theory and patient management* (pp. 45–68). New York: Mary Ann Liebert.

Sporn, A., & Pinsker, H. (1981). Use of stimulant medication in treating pervasive developmental disorder. *American Journal of Psychiatry, 138,* 997.

Sprague, R., Barnes, K., & Werry, J. (1970). Methylphenidate and thioridazine: Learning, reaction time, activity and classroom behavior in emotionally disturbed children. *American Journal of Orthopsychiatry, 40,* 615–628.

Sprague, R.L., & Gadow, K.D. (1976). The role of the teacher in drug treatment. *School Review, 85,* 109–140.

Sprague, R.L., & Sleator, E.K. (1973). Effects of psychopharmacologic agents on learning disorders. *Pediatric Clinics of North America, 20,* 719–735.

Sprague, R.L., & Sleator, E.K. (1975). What is the proper dose of stimulant drugs in children? *International Journal of Mental Health, 4,* 75–118.

Sprague, R.L., & Sleator, E.K. (1977). Methylphenidate in hyperkinetic children: Differences in dose effects on learning and social behavior. *Science, 198,* 1274–1276.

Sprague, R.L., & Werry, J.S. (1971). Methodology of psychopharmacological studies with the retarded. In N. R. Ellis (Ed.), *International review of research in mental retardation* (Vol 5, pp. 147–219). New York: Academic Press.

Sprague, R.L., Werry, J.S., Greenwold, W.E.,

& Jones, H. (1969, November). *Dosage effects of methylphenidate on learning of children*. Paper presented at the meeting of the Psychonomic Society, St. Louis, MO.

Sprague, R.L., Werry, J.S., & Scott, K.G. (1967, May). *Effects of dextroamphetamine on activity level and learning in retarded children*. Paper presented at the meeting of the Midwestern Psychological Association, Chicago, IL.

Strayhorn, J.M., Rapp, N., Donina, W., & Strain, P.S. (1988). Randomized trial of methylphenidate for an autistic child. *Journal of the American Academy of Child and Adolescent Psychiatry, 27*, 244–247.

Sulzbacher, S.I. (1972). Behavior analysis of drug effects in the classroom. In G. Semb (Ed.), *Behavior analysis and education* (pp. 37–52). Lawrence: University of Kansas.

Swanson, J., Kinsbourne, M., Roberts, W., & Zucker, K. (1978). Time-response of the effect of stimulant medication on the learning ability of children referred for hyperactivity. *Pediatrics, 61*, 21–29.

Swanson, J. M. (1988). Measurement of serum concentrations and behavioral response in ADHD children to acute doses of methylphenidate. In L. B. Bloomindale (Ed.), *Attention-deficit disorder: New research in attention, treatment, and psychopharmacology*. New York: Pergamon Press.

Swanson, J.M., Flockhart, D., Udrea, D., Cantwell, D., Connor, D., & Williams, L. (1995). Clonidine in the treatment of ADHD: Questions about safety and efficacy. *Journal Child and Adolescent Psychopharmacology, 5*, 301–304.

Tannock, R., Schacar, R., Logan, E. (1995). Methylphenide and cognitive flexibility: Dissociated dose effects in hyperactive children. *Journal of Abnormal Child Psychology, 23*, 235–266.

Taylor, E.A. (1986). *The overactive child*. Philadephia: Lippincott.

Tecce, J.J., & Cole, J.O. (1974). Amphetamine effects in man: Paradoxical drowsiness and lowered electrical brain activity (CNV). *Science, 185*, 451–453.

Triantafillou, M. (1972). Pemoline in overactive mentally handicapped children. *British Journal of Psychiatry, 121*, 577.

Varley, C.K., & Trupin, E.W. (1982). Double-blind administration of methylphenidate to mentally retarded children with attention-deficit disorder: A preliminary study. *American Journal of Mental Deficiency, 86*, 560–566.

Vitriol, C., & Farber, B. (1981). Stimulant medication in certain childhood disorders. *American Journal of Psychiatry, 138*, 1517–1518.

Volkmar, F., Hoder, E.L., & Cohen, D.J. (1985). Inappropriate uses of stimulant medications. *Clinical Pediatrics, 24*, 127–130.

Wargin, W., Patrick, K., Kilts, C., Gualtieri, C.T., Ellington, K., Mueller, R. A., Kraemer, G., & Breese, G.R. (1983). Pharmacokinetics of methylphenidate in man, rat, and monkey. *Journal of Pharmacological Experimental Therapy, 226*, 382–386.

Wender, P.H., Reimherr, F.W., Wood, D., & Ward, M. (1985). A controlled study of methylphenidate in the treatment of attention-deficit disorder, residual type, in adults. *American Journal of Psychiatry, 142*, 547–552.

Wender, P.H., Wood, D.R., & Reimherr, F.W. (1991). Pharmacological treatment of attention-deficit disorder, residual type (ADD–RT) in adults. In L.L. Greenhill & B.B. Osman (Eds.), *Ritalin: Theory and patient management* (pp. 25–33). New York: Mary Ann Liebert.

Wulbert, M., & Dries, R. (1977). The relative efficacy of methylphenidate (ritalin) and behavior-modification techniques in the treatment of a hyperactive child. *Journal of Applied Behavior Analysis, 10*, 21–31.

Zametkin, A., Nordahl, T., Gross, M., King, A.C., Semple, W.E., Rumsey, J., Hamburger, S., & Cohen, R.M. (1990). Cerebral glucose metabolism in adults with hyperactivity of childhood onset. *New England Journal of Medicine, 323*, 1361–1366.

Zimmerman, F.T., & Burgemeister, B.B. (1958). Action of methylphenidylacetate (ritalin) and reserpine in behavior disorders in children and adults. *American Journal of Psychiatry, 115*, 323–328.

Zrull, J.P., Westman, J. C., Arthur, B., & Bell, W.A. (1963). A comparison of chlordiazepoxide, d-amphetamine and placebo in the treatment of hyperkinetic syndrome in children. *American Journal of Psychiatry, 120*, 590–591.

Table 14-2. Summary of Research on Stimulant

Drug	Date	N	Placebo (Yes) No-Drug (ND) None (No)	Random assignment	Double blind
Amphetamine (Benzedrine)					
1. Alexandris and Lundell	1968	21	Yes	Yes	Yes
2. Craft	1959	18	Yes	Yes, Latin square	Yes
3. Cutler et al.	1940	(?)	ND	"Matched"	No
4. Lobb	1968	160	Yes	Yes	Yes
5. Molitch and Eccles	1937	93	Yes	No	Yes
6. Molitch and Sullivan	1937	96	Yes	No	Yes
7. Morris et al.	1955	50	Yes	No	No
8. Moskowitz	1941	23	No	No	No
d-Amphetamine (Dexedrine)					
1. Anton and Greer	1969	6	ND	No	No
2. Bell and Zubek	1961	75	Yes	"Matched"	Yes
3. Berkson	1965	4	Yes	Yes, cross-over	Yes
4. Fish and Bowling	1962	106	Yes	No	Yes
5. McConnel et al.	1964	57	Yes	Yes, cross-over	Yes
6. Sprague et al.	1967	8	Yes	No, cross-over	Yes
7. Zrull et al.	1963	16	Yes	No, cross-over	Yes
Methylphenidate (Ritalin)					
1. Blue et al.	1960	60	Yes	(?)	(?)
2. Breitmeyer	1969	16	Yes	Yes, cross-over	Yes
3. Carter	1956	49	No	No	No
4. Carter and Maley	1957	130	No	No	No
5. Davis	1971	10	Yes	Yes, cross-over	Yes
6. Davis et al.	1969	9	Yes	Yes, cross-over	Yes
7. Fehr and Sprague	1969	8	Yes	Yes, cross-over	Yes
8. Levy et al.	1957	61	Yes	Yes	Yes
9. Schickedanz	1967	24	Yes	Yes, cross-over	Yes
10. Sprague et al.	1970	12	Yes	Yes, cross-over	Yes
11. Sprague et al.	1969	16	Yes	Yes, cross-over	Yes
12. Zimmerman and Burgemeister	1958	108	No	"Matched"	No

Reproduced with permission from R.L. Sprague and J.S. Werry (1971).

Use For Patients with Mental Retardation 1937–1970

Dosage	Standardized evaluations	Statistics and interpretations
7.5-75 mg	Developed scale (?) WISC	42 one-tail t tests, F tests, significant F test
30 mg	Malamud Scale	Test not specified, not significant
5-7.5 mg	Developed questionnaire (?) Binet	Summary data, some gains on form boards
2 mg/kg	Galvanic skin response	F tests, significant
10, 20, 30 mg	Kent EGY, formboards	Change scores
10 mg	Stanford Achievement	Gain scores
5, 10, 15 mg	Paired associates, Binet	24 t tests, 2 significant
Varied	No	Case histories
10 mg	Urine samples for catechols	F test, significant
10 mg	Fergus Falls Scale, WAIS	18 t tests on gains, 3 significant
10 mg, 15 mg/100 lb.	Berkson Scale	Test not specified, not significant
15 mg	No	% Improvement
7.5, 15 mg	Developed scale r = .86, activity	Test not specified, not significant
10 mg	Learning and activity	3 F tests, 2 significant
10 mg	Developed checklist (?) WISC	% Improvement
?	CTMM	Summary statement
0.4 mg/kg	Learning, activity	F tests, significant
10-30 mg	No	% Improvement
20-55 mg. I.M.	No	Summary statement
0.5 mg/kg	Learning, actity	F tests, significant
0.4 mg/kg	Berkson & Davenport modified r = .61 to .88	F tests, significant
0.3 mg/kg	Flicker fusion, GSR	28 t tests, 16 significant
30-60 mg	Developed scale (?)	5 inappropriate X^2, 5 significant, 1 significant
0.44 mg/kg	Marble dropping	F test, significant
0.25 mg/kg, 0.35 mg/kg	Learning, activity	F tests, significant
0.10, 0.20, 0.30, 0.40 mg/kg	Learning, activity	F tests, significant
10-40 mg	WAIS	No statistics, data curves

Table 14-3. Summary of Research on Stimulant Use For Patients with

Study	Design[1]	N[2]	Quality of Study/ Quality of Outcome[3]	Age in years/ Mean age in years	IQ/ Mean IQ	Diagnosis/ Target Symptoms	Setting[4]	Drug[5]/Dose[6]
Blacklidge & Ekblad (1971)	C DB	19 (M) 12 (F)	2/+1	9-14/11.9	51-80/70	No disruptive behavior diagnosis: all in classes for mild MR	PS	MPH 10 mg at 8 am & noon
Davis (1971)	C DB	10 (M)	2/0	12-21/18.4	Severe and moderate MR	Stereotypies	I	MPH 0.5mg/kg
Campbell et al. (1972)	NDC NB	13 (M) 3 (F)	2/-2	3-6/4.3	28-96	Schizophrenia (10), Autism (2), OBS (2), ADHD (1)	I	DEX 1.25-10 mg/d (mean 4.8 mg)
Sulzbacher (1972)	C DB	1 (M)	2/+3	8	60	Minimal brain damage, overactive	PS	DEX 5mg & 10mg
Triantafillou (1972)	NB NDC	9	1/-1	12-16	Severely subnormal	Overactive	I	PEM 20 mg tds
Christensen (1975)	C DB *	10 (M) 6 (F)	3/+1	9-15/11.8	3-68/51	Hyperactive	I	MPH 0.3 mg/kg 1.5 h before class
Campbell et al. (1976)	C DB	10 (M) 1 (F)	5/0	3-6/5.4	36-90	Childhood schizophrenia	I	LEV 3.5-42 mg/d (mean 13.4 mg)
Shafto & Sulzbacher (1977)	DB NDC *	1 (M)	2/+1	4	Mental retard-ation, language delay	Non-compliant, emotionally disturbed, echolalia, overactive	PS	MPH 5 mg & 15 mg (.33 mg/kg, 1.0 mg/kg)
Geller et al. (1981)	NDC NB	2 (M)	1/+4	9/12	68/92	PDD, ADD, aggressive PDD, ADD	AH HR	DEX 5 mg/d DEX 10 mg/d
Sporn & Pinsker (1981)	NB NDC	1 (F)	1/-2	26	?	Atypical adult disorders (Hx of MBD)	I	MPH (dose n/a)

Mental Retardation or Pervasive Developmental Disorder 1971–1996

Rating Instruments and Effects Rated[7]

Disruptive Behavior	Attention/ Cognition	Other Target Symptoms	Adverse Effects
Burk's Behavior Rating Scale (RS) by teacher (+) and by parent (-)	Arithmetic scale of WRAT (ST) (0) Grays Oral Reading Paragraphs, Form A (ST) (0) Porteus Mazes, Vineland Revision (ST) (0) Teacher's Report (CL) (+)	None	No comment
Not noted	Not noted	Stereotypies (L) (+/-)	No comment
Clinical Global Impression (RS) (-) Symptom Severity (RS) (Fish) (-)	Inattention on Symptom Severity (RS) (Fish) (0)	Stereotypic, autistic symptoms (RS) (Fish)	Irritability, hyperactivity, appetite loss very frequent
Talking out in class (DO) (+tend) Getting out of seat in class (DO) (+tend)	Academic Performance (DO) Speed Error Rate Math (0) (-tend) Writing (+tend) (0) Reading (0) (-tend)	None	No comment
Hyperactivity aggressiveness destructiveness antisocial (CL) (+/-tend) 4 marked deterioration; 3 improved	Not assessed	None	4/9 showed a marked deterioration in all aspects of their behavior
Out of seat activity (L) (0) Conners, short and long forms (RS) (0) Modified Werry Quay time sampled observations (DO) (+)	Academic performance (DO) (0) Conners, short and long form (RS) (0)	None	No comment
Global improvement scale (CL) (0), Symptom severity scale (CL) (0)			Loss of appetite, loss of weight, exacerbation of preexisting stereotypies
Washington Social Code (DO) hyperactivity (+tend) at higher dose	Washington Social Code (DO) (+tend)	Intelligibility of speech and social interaction from the Washington Social Code (DO) (-)	Insomnia at higher dose
Anecdotal reports of hyperactivity (+tend), aggression (+tend), PDD (0)			
			Fragmented thinking (DO) (-) Delusional ideas (DO) (-) Lethargy (DO) (-) Enuresis or encopresis (not specified) (DO) (-)

Table 14-3 (Continued). Summary of Research on Stimulant Use For Patients with

Study	Design[1]	N[2]	Quality of Study/ Quality of Outcome[3]	Age in years/ Mean age in years	IQ/ Mean IQ	Diagnosis/ Target Symptoms	Setting[4]	Drug[5]/Dose[6]
Vitriol & Farber (1981)	NB	1	1/+3	8	?	Autism, ADHD	HR	MPH 10 mg/d
Aman (1982)	Review							
Aman & Singh (1982)	DB C 1 wk. each	28	5/0	13.6-26.4	4-34	(MR): Behavior, instruction-following, physiology	I	MPH 0.3 & 0.6 mg/kg/d placebo
Schmidt (1982)	NDC NB	1 (M)	1/+3	7	?	PDD, hyperactive	PS	MPH 40 mg/d 50 mg/d
Varley & Trupin (1982)	C DB	7 (M) 3 (F)	4/+3	4-15	48-77	ADHD	PS	MPH .3 & .6 mg/kg/d (median 15) & 25 mg/d, split 8am & noon
Burgio et al. (1985)	NDC NB	3 (M)	2/+2	11-21	0-35	Aggressive, hyperactive, stereotypies	PS	DEX 10-20 mg/d THI 100-400 mg/d
Volkmar et al. (1985)	NB CR	6 (M) 2 PDD No MR	1/-2	6–7/8	most>70	PDD (2), TS (2), P-C prob, ODD	HR	MPH 2.5-25 DEX 7.5 mg PEM 37.5 mg/d
Schell et al. (1986)	C DB	1 (M)	2/+4	5	60	Hyperactive	PS	MPH 6 mg (0.3 mg/kg)
Birmaher et al. (1988)	NDC	8 (M) 1 (F)	2/+2	4-16	?	Autism	PS	MPH 10-50 mg/d (mean 25 mg b.i.d.)
Hagerman et al. (1988)	C DB	13 (M) 2 (F)	4/+3	3-11/7	29-77/58	fragile X, ADD	PS	MPH 0.3 mg/kg b.i.d. DEX 0.2 mg/kg (spansule)
Helsel et al. (1988)	Review Article							
Strayhorn et al. (1988)	SC SB C	1 (M)	2/+3	6	50	Autism	MR	Placebo 0.5 mg/kg MPH

Mental Retardation or Pervasive Developmental Disorder 1971–1996

Rating Instruments and Effects Rated[7]

Disruptive Behavior	Attention/ Cognition	Other Target Symptoms	Adverse Effects
Clin. impression: hyperactivity (+tend)	Clinical impression: Attention & concentration (+tend)	Clinical impression: Speech, social behav., relatedness (+tend)	No adverse effect reported
Review Article			
No differences (0) on behavior rating (RS), Adaptive Behavior Scale, ward & mealtime behavior (DO)	No differences (NS) on instruction-following (ST, DO), Adaptive Behavior Scale	No difference (NS) on Adaptive Behavior Scale and ward & mealtime behavior except less food eaten with MPH (DO)	Reduced food (-) consumption (anorexia?). No other physiological differences (0) (DO)
Anecdotal reports of ADD symptoms (+ tend) with 40 mg/day; months later anecdotal reports of ADD symptoms (-tend) 50 mg/day			
Conners Abbreviated Parent and Teacher Rating Scales (R) 5 of 10 improved in higher dose condition (+)	As measured by Conners RS (+)	None	No significant side effects
Aggression (DO) (+tend) and disruption (DO) (+tend) decreased in one S, self stimulation (DO) (-tend) and attention (DO) (-tend) in two Ss			Appropriate social decreased in one subject; self stimulation increased in one subject
No benefit (Ss selected for adverse effects)			Stereotypy, tics, hallucinations, agitation, aggression (Ss selected for adverse effects)
Compliance (DO) (+tend)	Word identification (L) (+tend)		
Conners P & T (RS) (+) Children's Psychiatric (RS) (+)	Conners P & T (RS) (+) Children's Psychiatric (RS) (+)	Autistic (RS) (0)	AIMS (RS) (0) 2/9 mild initial insomnia
MPH resulted in improvement in teacher ratings of attention (RS) (+), socialization skills (RS) (+), but not statistically significant for DEX (+NS)			Significant side effects for DEX but not MPH
Hyperactivity (CL) (+) Destructiveness (CL) (+) Disobedience (CL) (+)	Concentration (CL) (+)	Stereotypies (CL) (+) Appropriate verbal behavior (DO) (+)	Sadness (CL) (+) Temper tantrums (CL) (+)

Table 14-3 (Continued). Summary of Research on Stimulant Use For Patients with

Study	Design[1]	N[2]	Quality of Study/ Quality of Outcome[3]	Age in years/ Mean age in years	IQ/ Mean IQ	Diagnosis/ Target Symptoms	Setting[4]	Drug[5]/Dose[6]
Feldman et al. (1989)	DB C	8 (M) 2 (F)	5/+4	6.8-10.8	No IQs: 2 Ss in MR class, 1 in "Brain-damaged" class, 2 in LD, 1 in ED, 4 in mainstream (Majority of Ss non-MR)	ADHD & epilep. seizures (w/o seizures at time of study-on epileptic drug)	HR	0.3 mg/kg b.i.d. MPH placebo (b.i.d.)
Helsel, Hersen, & Lubetsky (1989)	DB C	13	?	5-15	39-80	ADHD	AH	Stimulants
Helsel, Hersen, Lubetsky et al. (1989	SC DB	2 (M) 2 (F)	3/+3	4.9-7.9	39-80	ADHD	AH	Placebo; MPH 0.3, 0.45, 0.6 mg/kg (b.i.d.) One also received 0.75 & 0.9 mg/kg
Payton et al. (1989)	SC C DB	3 (M)	2/+3	6-7.8	61, 66, NS	ADHD symptoms (movement, on-task)	AH	Placebo S1: DEX .22 & .44 mg/kg S2: MPH .4 & .6 mg/kg S3: MPH .28, .55, .83, 1.1 mg/kg (all b.i.d.)
Realmuto et al. (1989)	NDC NB	2 (M)	1/-2	9	50	Autistic disorder	?	MPH 10 mg b.i.d.
Gadow & Pomeroy (1990)	C DB	1 (M)	2/+4	4	45	Hyperactive	PS	MPH 2.5– 15 mg b.i.d. FEN 20 or 30 mg/d
Gadow et al. (1992)	C DB	1 (M) 1 (F)	2/+4	10 12	50 66	ADD plus H	PS	MPH 0.3, 0.6 mg/kg placebo

Mental Retardation or Pervasive Developmental Disorder 1971–1996

Rating Instruments and Effects Rated[7]

Disruptive Behavior	Attention/ Cognition	Other Target Symptoms	Adverse Effects
CPRS (RS): CD (0), Imp-HA (0), HA Index (0) CTRS (RS): HA, HA Index (+), CD (0)	Attn/Imm. Memory on WISC-R Digit Span (ST) (0) Impulsivity, MFFT (ST) (0) Attention-"Discriminant Reaction Time Test" (L)(0) CPRS (RS): Learning Problem (0)	Neuromotor Output/Finger Tapping (L) (+) EEG (0) Epileptiform Features (0) CPRS (RS): Psychosomatic, anxiety (0)	
Decrease in "Social Behavior" (DO) (went from interactive to isolative (-tend)			"Idiosyncratic Response" to dose level
IOWA Conner (RS): Aggression (0) Abbrev. CTRS (RS) (+/-tend) Affective ratings (based on anecdotal staff reports taken retrospectively from charts (+/0, tend)	Time on Task (DO) (+tend) Task Accuracy (DO) (+tend) Duration of Task Completion (DO) (+/0, tend)	Play Activity (DO)(+tend)	One child went from euphoric (actually silly & disruptive) during placebo condition to dysphoric (withdrawn & noninteractive) at .6 mg/kg
Decrease in excessive movement (DO) with DEX and MPH (+tend) Abbrev. CTRS (RS) with DEX, MPH (+tend)	Increased on-task behavior (DO) with DEX, MPH (+tend)		Some dyskinetic movements of mouth, head, & shoulders with .83 mg/kg & 1.1 mg/kg doses of MPH in Subj. 3
Hyperactivity (CL) (0/-)			Increased stereotypies (CL) in one subject (-) Increased hyperactivity (CL) in one subject (-)
Initially, MPH resulted in improvement of teacher ratings of ADHD behaviors (RS) (+tend); months later MPH exacerbated ADHD behaviors (RS) (-tend); fenfluramine improved ADHD behaviors (RS) (+tend)			Irritability on higher dose of MPH
ADD and aggressive behaviors (DO) (+); ADD and aggressive behaviors (CL) (+)			

Table 14-3 (Continued). Summary of Research on Stimulant Use For Patients with

Study	Design[1]	N[2]	Quality of Study/ Quality of Outcome[3]	Age in years/ Mean age in years	IQ/ Mean IQ	Diagnosis/ Target Symptoms	Setting[4]	Drug[5]/Dose[6]
Handen et al. (1990)	DB C	11 (M) 1 (F)	5/+3	6–9	50-74	ADHD	HR	MPH 0.3 & 0.6 mg/kg placebo (b.i.d.)
Handen, et al. (1991)	DB C	22 (M) 5 (F)	4/+3	6.7-12.1	48-74	ADHD	HR	MPH 0.3 & 0.6 mg/kg placebo (b.i.d.)
Aman et al. (1991)	DB C	20 (M)	5/+2	5–13	Up to 78	ADHD	HR PS	MPH 0.4 mg/kg/q AM FEN 0.75 mg/kg b.i.d. placebo b.i.d.
Aman et al. (1991a)	DB C	25 (M) 5 (F)	5/+3	4.1-16.5/10	Untestable to 90, mean of 29 testable $Ss = 52.3\pm20.4$ 27 Ss≤76	ADHD (24), ADD sans (4), and/or CD (3), PDD (1)	HR PS	MPH 0.4 mg/kg/q AM TDZ 0.85 mg/kg b.i.d. placebo b.i.d.
Aman et al. (1991b)	DB C	25 (M) 5 (F)	5/+3	4.1–16.5/10	Mean of 29 testable $Ss= 52.3\pm20.4$ 27 Ss≤76	ADHD (24), ADD sans (4), and/or CD (3), PDD (1)	HR PS	MPH 0.4 mg/kg/q AM TDZ 0.85 mg/kg b.i.d. placebo b.i.d.
Hilton et al. (1991)	NDC	1 (M)	1/-2	6	58	fragile X, ADHD	AH	IMI 10 mg b.i.d., t.i.d. MPH 7.5 mg/d
Hagerman et al. (1992)	NDC	9 (F)	1/+4	<18	?	fragile X, ADHD	PS	MPH DEX

Mental Retardation or Pervasive Developmental Disorder 1971–1996

Rating Instruments and Effects Rated[7]

Disruptive Behavior	Attention/ Cognition	Other Target Symptoms	Adverse Effects
CTRS (RS): CD (+), HA (+), HA Index (+) CAP (RS): Overactivity (+)	Work Output (DO)(+) Work Accuracy (DO) (0) Sustained Atten-CPT(L)(+) Learning, PAL (L) (0) CTRS (RS): Inattention (+) CAP (RS): Inattention (+)	Social Interaction/Play (DO) (+/-)	Increase in staring (R) in 6/12 Ss (-) Increase in drowsiness (R) in 4/12 Ss (-) Social withdrawal (R) in 1/12 (-)
Decrease in High Activity Rate (DO) (+) Motor Movements (DO) (0)		Appetite (CL) (0) Decreased Anxiety (CL) (+) Decreased Irritability (CL) (+) Dizziness (CL) (0) Drowsiness (CL) (0) Headache (CL) (0) Moodiness (CL) (0) Sadness (CL) (0) Social Withdrawal (CL) (0) Somatic Complaints (CL) (0) Staring (CL) (0) Stomachache (CL) (0)	Motor tics (CL) in 3/27 Subjects at 0.6 mg/kg MPH dosage Severe social withdrawal in 2/27 Ss at .3 mg/kg 6 Ss had/med d/c'ed due to side effects *Please note:* This study consisted of examining symptoms of "side effects" (as assessed by a symptom checklist).
Fenfluramine reduced motor behavior more than MPH (RS) (+)		Enuresis and encopresis lower with MPH than with placebo or fenfluramine (CL) (+NS)	1 case halitosis & body odor with FEN (-NS). FEN more drowsiness than MPH or placebo (RS). FEN lower pulse & blood pressure than MPH. FEN 1.8 lbs.<placebo 4 cases stereotypy (CL) (-NS)
MPH best (+) on CTRS & HA, CD factors, teacher global (RS). MPH signif. better compliance (+) (psychologist rating). Parent ratings (+NS). MPH response w. IQ>45, MA>4.5 (ST), unconstricted attn (L)	MPH best (+) on teacher inattention factor of CTRS, trend (+NS) on parent RBPC Attention Problem factor (RS). MPH response (+) with IQ>45, MA>4.5 (ST), unconstricted attn (L)	Instruction-following (ST, DO), anxiety-withdrawal, detachment, isolation (RS) all unremarkable (0, NS)	NS effects on P, BP, wt. (-NS) Depression (-tend): 11 MPH, 7 placebo, 4 thior. Insomnia (-): 9 MPH, 3 placebo, 4 TDZ Anorexia: MPH>TDZ (-) (RS) No diff. seizures (DO)
MPH reduced seat movements during tasks (L)	MPH improved accuracy on matching to sample, omission errors on CPT (L) (+). Trend of MPH reducing error time on graduated holes (L) (+NS). IQ (ST) (0); MFF (ST) (+NS)	MPH lengthened delay (+) on matching-to-sample task (ST), trend of shortening response time on short-term memory (L) (+NS)	NS adverse effects on 7 cognitive lab tests by either drug (L, ST) (0)
Improvement in ratings of ADHD behaviors (RS) (+tend) Worsening in ratings of ADHD behaviors (RS) (-tend)		Improved sleep (+tend), decrease in enuresis (+tend)	Increased heart rate, tolerance for therapeutic response
Anecdotal reports of behaviorial improvement (+tend)			

Table 14-3 (Continued). Summary of Research on Stimulant Use For Patients with

Study	Design[1]	N[2]	Quality of Study/ Quality of Outcome[3]	Age in years/ Mean age in years	IQ/ Mean IQ	Diagnosis/ Target Symptoms	Setting[4]	Drug[5]/Dose[6]
Handen et al. (1992)	DB C	10 (M) 4 (F)	5/+4	6-12	48-74	ADHD	HR	MPH 0.3, 0.6 mg/kg placebo
Aman et al. (1993a)	DB C	20 (M) 8 (F)	5/+3	5-13/8.8	Untestable to 78. Mean of 26 testable Ss = 61	ADHD Nonautistic	HR	MPH 0.4 mg/kg/q AM FEN 0.75 mg/kg b.i.d. placebo b.i.d.
Aman et al. (1993b)	DB C	20 (M) 8 (F)	5/+3	5-13/8.8	Untestable to 78. Mean of 26 testable Ss = 61	ADHD, Nonautistic	HR	MPH 0.4 mg/kg/q AM FEN 0.75 mg/kg b.i.d. placebo b.i.d.
Handen et al. (1994)	DB C	31 (FM) 16 (F)	5/+4	6.1-12.5	48-77	ADHD	HR	MPH 0.3 mg/kg to 0.6 mg/kg placebo
Johnson et al.[9] (1994)	SC DB C	3	2/+2	6.4–7.1	62–69	ADHD, ODD	HR	MPH 0.3 mg/kg to 0.6 mg/kg placebo

Mental Retardation or Pervasive Developmental Disorder 1971–1996

Rating Instruments and Effects Rated[7]

Disruptive Behavior	Attention/ Cognition	Other Target Symptoms	Adverse Effects
Restlessness (DO) (+) In-seat behavior (DO) (0) Activity (DO) (+/-) Gross Motor (DO) (0) Aggressiveness (DO) (0) CTRS (RS): CD (+), HA (+), HA Index (+) CAP (RS): Overactivity (+)	Work Output (DO) (+) (NS) Sustained Attn-CPT (L) (+) Learning (L) (0) Auditory Memory, Buschke Selective Reminding (ST) (0) On-task behavior (DO) (+/-) CTRS (RS): Inattention (+) CAP (RS): Inattention (+)	Play Intensity (DO) (0) # Toy Changes (DO) (0) Prosocial Behavior (DO) (0)	
Both drugs better than plac, (RS) (+) on teacher & parent ratings of conduct, HA, & motor excess, teacher irritability, parent global rating. Fenflur. better (+) on parent irritability (RS), Conners Abbrev. Questionnaire	MPH better than placebo (+) on teacher rating of attn	Both drugs better than placebo (+) on sensory response of Real Life Rating Scale. Fenfluramine better (+) than MPH on inappropriate speech (RS). NS effect (+NS) on stereotypy, tension/anxiety, lethargy/withdrawal (RS)	(RS) (-): Insominia: FEN>plac Drowsiness:FEN>plac=MPH Anorexia: FEN=MPH>pl (DO) (-): P: MPH>plac>FEN sys BP: MPH=plac>FEN dias BP: MPH>plac=FEN Wt: plac=MPH>fFEN.
Borh drugs improved hyperactivity (RS) (+) by blind examiner ratings. MPH reduced seat movement by lab test (L) (+)	FEN better than placebo (+) on memory task, increased response time (ST, L). MPH reduced: commission errors on CPT (L) (+), response time (L) (+). Both improved attn (RS) (+) by examr ratings, not by L test (L) (+NS).	Both drugs improved mood (+) by blind examiner ratings (RS)	Not reported
Higher baseline ratings on CPRS (RS)-Imp/HA related to decrease on CTRS (RS) Inattention, CD, and Attention CPT (L) with MPH (+) Higher baseline ratings on CPRS (RS): CD asso. with increased work output (DO), improved CPT (L) responses on MPH (+) Higher baseline ratings on CTRS (RS) HA Index assoc. with greater gains in on-task behavior, increased attention, and decreased scores on CTRS (RS)-HA Index ratings with MPH (+)	Lower IQ associated with greater improvement in work output on MPH (+) Higher MA associated with greater gains in work accuracy with MPH (+)	Gender-males had greater decreases in CPRS (RS)-CD with MPH (+) Race–Subjects from Caucasian familes had greater increases in attention span with MPH (+) Higher SES (socio-economic status) with more gains in CPT (L) performance (+)	
Decreased Fidgetiness (DO) (+tend) for 2/3 Ss	Increases in On-task Behavior (DO) (+tend) for 2/3 Ss Improved Task Accuracy (DO) (+tend) for 2/3 Ss		

Table 14-3 (Continued). Summary of Research on Stimulant Use For Patients with

Study	Design[1]	N[2]	Quality of Study/ Quality of Outcome[3]	Age in years/ Mean age in years	IQ/ Mean IQ	Diagnosis/ Target Symptoms	Setting[4]	Drug[5]/Dose[6]
Mayes et al. (1994)	DB C	58 (M) 11 (F)	3/+4	1.8–13/7.1	23–136/86	ADHD symptoms, autism, CP, multiple neurological diagnoses	HR	MPH titrated individually, starting at 0.3 mg/kg t.i.d. range 2.5–10 mg t.i.d.
Handen et al. (1995)	DB C	22	5/+4	6–12	50–77	ADHD	HR	MPH 0.6 mg/kg placebo 0.3 mg/kg

*Behavior modification treatment also being provided simultaneously with medication.

1 G = parallel group design (drug vs. placebo), C = crossover design, NDC = drug vs. no drug comparison, DB = double blind, SG = single blind, NB = nonblind, SC = single case, CR = case report.

2 M = male, F = female.

3 Methodological rigor rating.
   Scale: 1 to 5
      1 Report of clinical experience, no controlled medication administrations, no use of reliable and valid dependent measures, no statistical test of efficacy
      2 Significant limitations, but some use of controls and methodology, e.g., rigorous protocol but 3 or fewer subjects; adequate number of subjects but symptoms poorly defined or unlikely to change on meds (e.g., stereotypies)
      3 Moderate limitations in study (e.g., diagnosis and symptom not precise; 4-9 subjects: confounding effects of behavioral or other pharmacologic treatment)
      4 Generally well done but minor limitations in study (e.g., adequate numbers, well-defined population, but use of single rating scale)
      5 Model study; controlled trial, using double blind procedures and reliable/valid dependent measures, clear symptoms and diagnosis of sample, adequate sample size (at least 10)
   Outcome rating: -5 to +5, where -5 is marked deterioration; -3 is moderate deterioration; 0 is no change; +3 moderate improvement; +5 marked improvement.

4 I = institution, PS = public school, HR = home reared, AH = acute hospital, SF = special facility.

5 MPH = methylphenidate, DEX = dextroamphetamine, AMP = racemic amphetamine, PEM = pemoline, LEV = levoamphetamine, TDZ = thioridazine, FEN= fenfluramine, IMI = imipramine.

6 Unit dose and number of times daily (mean and/or range).

7 RS = rating scale, L = laboratory analog device, DO = direct observation, ST=standardized test, CL = Checklist, (+) = improved performance/decreased symptoms, (-) decreased performance/increased symptoms, (0) = no change, (+/-) = mixed findings, +tend = favorable tendency without statistical test, +NS = favorable tendency found not significant (missing statistical significance).

8 This study explored the best predictors of drug response rather than evaluate effects *per se.*

9 This study compared medication to medication and behavior modification. Only effect of medication is reported.

Mental Retardation or Pervasive Developmental Disorder 1971–1996

Rating Instruments and Effects Rated[7]

Disruptive Behavior	Attention/ Cognition	Other Target Symptoms	Adverse Effects
For MR/DD Ss: Conners HA Index (RS) (+) by parents teachers, inpt staff.			SE N.S. related to Dx, age, IQ SE = irritability, anorexia, lethargy, insomnia, stomachache, nausea/vomiting Stereotypy in 7 MR/DD Ss, 1 other
Decreased Movement (DO) (0) Decreased Out of Seat Behavior (DO) (+)	Increases in On-task behavior (DO) (+)	Play Intensity (DO) (+) Vocalizations (DO) (+) Toy Pickups (DO) (+) Toy Leaves (DO) (+) Toy Touches (DO) (+)	

Clonidine

Randi Hagerman[1], Joel D. Bregman[2], Emanuel Tirosh[3,4]

Clonidine hydrochloride is a centrally acting agent that has been prescribed primarily as an antihypertensive agent. Although clonidine was initially developed in 1967 as a vasoconstricting nasal decongestant, its capacity to lower blood pressure from a central action led to broader use. Clonidine has a number of uses in the treatment of behavioral and mental disorders. For example, it has been used to treat people with attention-deficit hyperactivity disorder (ADHD; Hunt, Minderaa, & Cohen, 1986), Tourette syndrome (Leckman et al., 1991), and autism (Fankhauser, Karumanchi, German, Yates, & Karumanchi, 1992).

Clonidine is the generic name; Catapres is a trade name. The drug is available in pill form for oral administration and in cutaneous patch form for transdermal application (Catapres-TTS). Clonidine hydrochloride tablets are available in the following strengths: 0.1 mg, 0.2 mg, and 0.3 mg. The clonidine transdermal patch is available in 3 sizes (3.5 cm^2, 7.0 cm^2, and 10.5 cm^2) designed to deliver 0.1 mg (TTS-1), 0.2 mg (TTS-2), and 0.3 mg (TTS-3) of clonidine per day for approximately one week (somewhat less time in children). Chemically, clonidine is a derivative of imidazoline. The chemical name of the oral preparation is 2-(2,6-dichlorophenylamino)-2-imidazoline hydrochloride ($C_9H_9Cl_2N_3 \cdot HCl$) and the chemical name of the transdermal preparation is 2,6-dichloro-N-2-imidazolidinylidenebenzenamine.

PHARMACODYNAMICS AND PHARMACOKINETICS

Clonidine acts as an agonist at presynaptic alpha$_2$-adrenergic receptors within the brain stem. Specific sites of action include the locus coeruleus and the ventrolateral medulla, where clonidine reduces firing and reduces the release of norepinephrine (Quintin, Ghigone, & Pujol, 1987). Clonidine suppresses central catecholamine metabolism, resulting in a reduction in sympathetic outflow. Studies in rats indicate that clonidine suppresses the catecholamine response to hemorrhage, controlled hypotension, and stress-induced immobilization. These effects are dose-dependent (Gillon, Quintin, Ghigone, & Pujol, 1987; Quintin et al., 1986, 1987). Clonidine also prevents withdrawal-induced hyperactivity and diarrhea in diazepam-dependent rats (Kunchandy & Kulkarni, 1986). Stimulation of the alpha$_2$-receptor is implicated, because this response is blocked by pretreatment with the alpha$_2$-adrenergic antagonist, yohimbine. Clonidine also stimulates parasympathetic outflow, which slows the heart because of increased vagal tone (Goodman & Gilman, 1990).

Recently, a natural substance was purified from calf brain that displaces clonidine binding to the alpha$_2$-receptors. This substance, agmatine, is decarboxylated arginine (Li et al., 1994). Arginine decarbonlase synthesizes agmatine, which in turn stimulates imidazoline receptors and centrally inhibits sympathetic responses. Agmatine is nature's clonidine, an endogenous hormone with a neurotransmitter effect.

Following oral administration, clonidine is absorbed rapidly and reduces blood pressure within 30 to 60 minutes. Maximal reductions in blood pressure occur 2 to 4 hours after an oral dose. Peak plasma levels are achieved in 3 to 5 hours. The usual plasma half-life is 8 to 12 hours in children and 12 to 16 hours in adults, although this can increase to 40 hours in individuals with significant renal impairment. About 40% to 60% of an oral dose is excreted unchanged in the urine within 24 hours, whereas most of the remainder is metabolized by the liver. The transdermal patch is designed to release clonidine at a constant rate for approximately one week. Therapeutic plasma levels are reached 2 to 3 days following application of the patch. Removal of the

1 Professor of Pediatrics, University of Colorado Health Science Center, Child Development Unit, The Children's Hospital, Denver, CO

2 Associate Professor of Psychiatry, Emory Autism Research Center, Emory University School of Medicine, Atlanta, GA

3 Pediatrician, Hannah Khoushi Child Development Center, Haifa Medical Center, Haifa, Israel

4 Other committee members included Edwin Cook Jr., M.D., Howard Demb, M.D., Margaret Klitzke, D.O., Mauri Mattila, M.D., James McCracken, M.D., Stephen Schroeder, Ph.D., Luke Tsai, M.D., Rameshwari Tumuluru, M.D., and Christopher Varley, M.D.

patch results in stable plasma levels for about 8 hours, after which there is a gradual decline in plasma levels. The standard oral dose for treating Tourette syndrome is 3-4 μg/kg/day, and for treating ADHD the dose is 3-6 μg/kg/day (Hunt, Capper, & O'Connell, 1990). The oral dose is usually started at bedtime or twice a day and gradually increased to 3 or 4 times a day (at meals and at bedtime).

Treatment with clonidine results in decreases in peripheral and renal vascular resistance, blood pressure, and heart rate. Cardiac output may decrease by 15% to 20% acutely, with a return to baseline following chronic treatment. Orthostatic hypotension may rarely occur because of a reduction in venous return with systemic venodilatation. Postural reflexes, cardiovascular responses to exercise, renal blood flow, and glomerular filtration rates remain essentially unchanged. Retention of salt and water may occur in the kidney and in the intestine.

Clonidine stimulates the release of growth hormone in both children and adults. However, this effect occurs following acute but not chronic administration. Limited evidence supports a growth-promoting effect of clonidine. The effect has been significant in controlled studies, but it has not been as significant as growth hormone replacement (Volta et al., 1991). Studies in rats have not revealed carcinogenic potential. In rabbits, teratogenic effects have not been found. However, studies with rats have indicated increased resorption when clonidine was administered very early in gestation. Well-controlled studies of the teratogenic potential of clonidine in humans have not been conducted. A preliminary report of 22 young school-age children who were exposed to clonidine prenatally showed no evidence of major neurological or behavioral effects in comparison to control subjects (Huisjes, Hadders-Algra, & Touwen, 1986), although a possible increase in hyperactivity and sleep difficulties was indicated. A relationship with the severity of maternal hypertension during pregnancy could not be ruled out.

SIDE EFFECTS AND TOXIC EFFECTS

The most common side effects of clonidine include dry mouth, drowsiness, dizziness, constipation, and sedation. Sedation is the main problem in the pediatric population and has led to the use of very small doses (1/4 tablet or 1/2 of a 0.1 mg tablet per dose), particularly for young children. Sedation occurs in more than 50% of patients, but it usually abates after the first two to four weeks of therapy. It may also abate with the use of the transdermal patch, because its peak dosage levels are lower; the patch may also be cut to lower the dose (the TTS-1 patch is designed to give 0.1 mg total dose over the day). The patch, however, may cause a contact dermatitis in approximately 20% to 40% of patients. This problem occurs more commonly in fair-skinned people and can be treated with hydrocortisone cream when the patch is removed. For more severe irritation, Decadron spray or a Vancenase AQ spray is used. These sprays have an aqueous base and dry quickly on the skin prior to placing the patch and often will dramatically decrease skin irritation (personal communication, W. McMahon & S. Stiefel, June 15, 1995).

Other possible side effects include nausea and vomiting, anorexia, malaise, fatigue, weakness, transient elevations in liver enzymes, weight gain, anxiety, agitation, dysphoria, headache, sleep disturbance, orthostatic symptoms, palpitations, tachycardia, bradycardia, arrhythmias (rarely), impotence, loss of libido, and nocturia (bed wetting). Clonidine may induce or exacerbate depression in 5% of children or adolescents who have a prior history of depression or a family history of mood disorders (Hunt et al., 1990). A number of other possible adverse reactions have been reported; however, they are very rare or not clearly related to clonidine. Guanfacine (Tenex) is an alternative drug to clonidine. It is also a presynaptic-alpha$_2$ receptor agonist, but it is less sedating and causes less hypotension than clonidine (Kugler, Seus, Krauskopf, Brecht, & Raschig, 1990) because it is a more selective alpha$_{2A}$-adrenergic receptor agonist (Uhlen & Wikberg, 1991).

Abrupt withdrawal of clonidine has been associated with hypertension, agitation, nervousness, and headache. After high dose or long-term treatment, sudden withdrawal may cause dangerous elevations in blood pressure in addition to a fast or irregular pulse and chest pain. The simultaneous use of beta blockers may worsen rebound hypertension. *Patients and their families must be warned about suddenly stopping the medication.* When discontinuing clonidine, gradual dosage reductions should occur over several days. This is not necessary with the clonidine patch, because skin reserves will provide such a taper when the patch is removed.

Toxic effects of clonidine from an overdose include pallor and hypotension, bradycardia, respiratory depression, and drowsiness progressing to coma and miosis (Wiley, Wiley, Torrey, & Henretig, 1990). Symptoms may develop rapidly, but they usually resolve within 24 hours. Clonidine intoxication has been more common with increased use of the medication for a variety of problems including ADHD (Wasserman, 1989). Naloxone may be an important antidote, showing effectiveness in 80% of cases, but the response is variable and often only one or two signs are reversed by naloxone (Wasserman, 1989). Hypotension is commonly not relieved by naloxone, but does respond to intravenous fluids. Severe toxicity has been reported in young children even after relatively small doses of clonidine. Wedin, Richardson, and Wallace (1990) reported that a 3-year-old child who ingested one 0.2 mg clonidine tablet developed coma, respiratory depression, and hypotension. This is the lowest toxic dose reported for a child. Hypothermia, seizures, and arrhythmias have also been reported from an overdose of clonidine (Conner & Watanabe, 1979). One case of overdose with clonidine occurred when a young child pulled off his patch and chewed it. Parents must be warned about the dangers of an overdose.

Clonidine lowers cardiac output by 20% to 25% through lowering heart rate and decreasing sympathetic tone (Kallio, Saraste, Scheinin, Hartiala, & Scheinin, 1990). In a study of healthy individuals (ages 22 to 83 years), systolic blood pressure fell 23%, sinus rate decreased 8%, sinus automatic activity decreased 15%, and there was a 4% to 6% slowing in nodal conduction (which positively correlated with age) when clonidine was given intravenously (Clementy, Castagné, Wicker, Dallocchio, & Bricaud, 1986). Previously, arrhythmias have been reported only in patients with cardiac disease, particularly those receiving digoxin or on extremely high doses of clonidine (Kibler & Gazes, 1977). Long-term (10-year) use of clonidine with 128 patients with hypertension was associated with improvement in EKG findings as hypertension improved, yielding an overall good safety profile for clonidine (Fender, Inserra, & Medina, 1987).

Two case reports of children have prompted questions as to whether EKG monitoring is necessary in clonidine therapy. Dawson, VanderZanden, Werkman, Washington, and Tyma (1989) reported that a 10-year-old boy with intermittent explosive disorder who received clonidine just after propranolol was tapered and discontinued promptly developed bradycardia (46 beats/minute) and first-degree heart block. Chandran (1994) described three children who were taking clonidine with other medications, including two with tricyclics and one with thioridazine. One patient had bradycardia (55 beats/minute) and supraventricular premature complexes, and the two patients also on tricyclics had nonspecific

intraventricular conduction delays, T-wave abnormalities, and possible anterior ischemia by EKG (the patients were not symptomatic). These abnormalities disappeared when clonidine was discontinued.

Jaffe, Livshits, and Bursztyn (1994) reported the development of an atrioventricular (AV) block in two older adult patients who were treated with verapamil to which a minimal dose of clonidine was added. The AV block resolved in both cases after the medications were discontinued. The authors hypothesized that both of these antihypertensive medications can work synergistically to slow conduction dramatically at the AV node and that their combination should be avoided.

Swanson, Flockhart, Udrea, and Cantwell (1995) reported three cases of sudden death associated with the use of clonidine and methylphenidate, two in the United States and one in Australia. A 9-year-old boy who had fetal alcohol syndrome, Tourette syndrome, and seizures was on an excessively high dose of clonidine (0.8 mg/day), in addition to 60 mg/day of methylphenidate. He apparently had acutely overdosed on fluoxetine (Prozac) and promethazine; he died in the midst of a grand mal seizure. The second case was a 7-year-old boy who was born prematurely with extensive fibrotic scarring of the heart, consistent with severe perinatal hypoxic injury. The extensive fibrotic scarring included the mitral capillary muscles and extensive areas of the left ventricle. The cause of death was considered to be cardiac. In Australia an 8-year-old girl was taking 0.2 mg of clonidine/day and methylphenidate. She had undergone two general anesthesias, 4 weeks and 1 week prior to death, and the second anesthesia was associated with prolonged vomiting from which she recovered. On the day of death, she awoke with vomiting and subsequently had circulatory collapse and died. Blood work was negative for any detectable clonidine or methylphenidate. Although these deaths may be unrelated to clonidine or its use with methylphenidate, it is uncertain whether clonidine could have added to the complications in these cases.

These cases of sudden death in children and adolescents have been widely discussed and are reviewed in detail elsewhere (Fenichel, 1995; Popper, 1995; Swanson et al., 1995). The recent reports of death, plus the rare cases of dysrhythmias, suggest a need for more caution in the use of clonidine, particularly for patients with cardiac problems or in those who are using other medications that impact the heart. A routine EKG should be done when clonidine is combined with other medications or for patients who have symptoms of bradycardia, dizziness, or a history of cardiac disease.

DRUG INTERACTIONS

Adverse drug interactions are rare with clonidine. Sedation is increased when clonidine is combined with alcohol, barbiturates, or other sedatives. Large doses of clonidine added to alcoholic drinks cause a prompt knock-out effect. Clonidine has been used by robbers for this purpose in some European countries. Clonidine may also exacerbate the anticholinergic effects (dryness of mouth, constipation, and urinary retention) of other medications including antidepressants and anticholinergics (Hunt et al., 1990). Diuretics will further decrease blood pressure and are often therapeutically combined with clonidine to treat hypertension. Tricyclic antidepressants (TCAs) may inhibit the effects of clonidine, perhaps because of their adrenergic blocking effects.

Sudden withdrawal of a TCA, which was given to a hypertensive patient who was stabilized with clonidine, resulted in serious hypotension (Cocco & Ague, 1977). Therefore, the combined use of TCAs and clonidine should be monitored carefully, and TCAs should not be withdrawn precipitously (Chapman, 1994; Wilens & Biederman, 1994). An interactive effect was found when clonidine was added to mianserin, a tetracyclic antidepressant (Elliott, Whiting, & Reid, 1983). Fluphenazine decanoate combined with clonidine produced delirium in one patient. Another patient died following combined treatment with a diuretic, clonidine, and thioridazine. Yet another experienced insulin-induced hypoglycemia following clonidine administration (Hedland, Dymbling, & Humbelt, 1972).

Monoamine oxidase inhibitors (MAOIs), sympathomimetic amines, levodopa, tolazoline, and general anesthetics may decrease the antihypertensive effect of clonidine. The antihypertensive effect of clonidine is enhanced by atenolol or by other beta-blockers and diuretics. Guanethidine, propranolol, digitalis, and digitalis glycosides should be used cautiously in combination with clonidine because of possible additive effects on heart rate resulting in severe bradycardia. Paradoxical hypertension has been reported with the concomitant use of clonidine and propranolol; this is a special concern if clonidine is abruptly discontinued. The pressor response to ephedrine may increase in patients treated with clonidine. The anti-Parkinson effect of levodopa may decrease if clonidine is added. The dose of fentanyl or other pre-anesthetic agents should be reduced in patients who receive clonidine. The combination of verapamil and clonidine should be avoided.

CLINICAL INDICATIONS EXCLUSIVE OF MENTAL RETARDATION

Multiple Tic Disorders

Although neuroleptics, specifically haloperidol or pimozide, are the most effective agents for treating severe tics, they are also associated with significant side effects including tardive dyskinesia. Many physicians use clonidine instead of neuroleptics because the side effects are not as serious (Borison, Arg, Hamilton, Diamond, & David, 1983; Cohen, Riddle, & Leckman, 1992; Cohen, Young, Nathanson, & Shaywitz, 1979; Leckman et al., 1985).

Cohen, Detlor, Young, and Shaywitz (1980) reported that 70% of patients with Tourette syndrome responded to clonidine. Initially patients felt a sense of calm with a decrease in anger, a decrease in irritability, and a feeling of mellowness. As the dose was increased to 3 to 4 μg/kg/day (0.15 mg/day), improvements in compulsive behavior and a reduction in phonic and motor tics occurred within 2 to 4 weeks. By the third month, there was a plateau of benefit with some waxing and waning of symptoms. By 5 months, a fourth phase occurred when the dose was increased to 4 to 6 μg/kg/day to sustain clinical improvement.

The long-term benefit in tic reduction has been questioned (Goetz, Tanner, et al., 1987). Some patients develop a resistance to treatment. Some investigators have suggested that clonidine may reduce prominent obsessive-compulsive symptomatology in some cases (Goetz, Shannon, Carroll, Tanner, & Weingarten, 1987). A beneficial effect on symptoms also was reported by Hewlett, Vinogradov, and Agras (1992). Transient exacerbation of tics following initial treatment with clonidine has been reported (Huk, 1989); however, this adverse effect appears to be very uncommon. Clonidine may also be effective in blocking neuroleptic withdrawal-induced symptoms (Max & Rasmunsen, 1986).

Clonidine was more effective than placebo in improving motor tics, vocal tics, impulsivity, and hyperactivity in a recent double-blind, 12-week clinical trial with 47 patients with Tourette syndrome, aged 7 to 48 (Leckman et al., 1991). Most side effects were mild and were limited to the first six weeks. At a dose of 3 to 5 μg/kg/day, 90% of the patients experienced sedation or fatigue, 57% complained of dry mouth, 43% had faintness or dizziness, and 33% complained of irritability.

Comings, Comings, Tacket, and Li (1990) conducted an open trial of the transdermal patch on 270 patients
with Tourette syndrome, ADHD, or conduct disorder.
The results indicated that 62% showed some improvement, 40% had improvement in half or more of their
symptoms, and 12% had worsening symptoms. Some
patients demonstrated an excellent response to the patch
after experiencing no effect from the oral medication.
Comings et al. suggested that transdermal clonidine
should be the drug of first choice for Tourette syndrome.
In contrast to this recommendation, Singer et al. (1995)
compared the efficacy of clonidine to desipramine in
patients with Tourette syndrome and ADHD. A double-
blind placebo-controlled protocol was used, and
improvement with desipramine was superior to clonidine
in alleviating both ADHD symptoms and tic severity.

ADHD

Hunt, Minderaa, and Cohen (1985) reported results of
the first treatment study showing positive results for
ADHD in a trial of 10 children with IQs greater than
80 and with ages between 8 and 13 years. Seven of the
10 children improved significantly, according to ratings
made by parents and teachers. The dose of clonidine was
gradually increased to 4 to 5 µg/kg/day, or approximately 0.05 mg qid; it was administered for eight weeks. The
main side effect was sleepiness, which occurred for 30
to 60 minutes beginning 1 hour after the dose. The
sleepiness subsided after three weeks in all but 1 child.
Lowering the dose also helped to alleviate sleepiness.
The blood pressure decreased on average 10%, but this
did not cause any symptoms except for a rare case of
lightheadedness after exertion. An overall calming effect
with improved frustration tolerance was observed;
improvement occurred in hyperactivity, impulsivity, and
inattention. The children who responded best were
overactive and lacked inhibition, whereas a child who
had depression and another who had schizoid personality disorder responded poorly. This first study of clonidine use for children with ADHD is probably the most
frequently cited; however, the experimental design used
may have been problematic. Clonidine was given to
each child in eight-week blocks, whereas placebo was
given for two weeks before and two weeks after clonidine (to half of the subjects) or for four weeks after
clonidine (to half of the subjects). This is a potential
difficulty because drug and time may have been
confounded, and because anyone with a knowledge of
the design would have known that placebo necessarily

would have to be the last treatment condition (i.e.,
blindness may have been compromised).

Hunt et al. (1985) hypothesized that only some
subgroups of children with ADHD respond optimally to
clonidine; specifically, they suggested that improvement
is most marked for those either with an increased noradrenergic state or with an excessive activity of another
neurochemical system that is secondarily modulated by
norepinephrine. Clonidine has a modulating effect on
the firing of dopaminergic neurons under conditions of
stress (Antelman & Caggiula, 1977). Additionally,
clonidine has an indirect inhibition on serotonin
systems, causing a decrease in firing in the raphe nucle-
us and a decrease in serotonin turnover, both thought
to be mediated by decreased norepinephrine transmission from the locus coeruleus to the raphe (Svensson,
Bunney, & Aghajakian, 1975). The modulation effects
of clonidine on the dopamine system may be mediated
indirectly through the serotonergic raphe system
(Bunney & DeRiemers, 1982).

Anecdotal reports also suggest that clonidine is helpful for treating spontaneous or drug-induced sleep disturbances for children with ADHD (Wilens, Biederman, &
Spencer, 1994). A nightly dose often induces drowsiness
and subsequent sleep. If increased afternoon rebound
occurs while a child is taking stimulants, clonidine may
be substituted later in the day for the stimulant. In an
open trial, it was found that 96% of children with
ADHD and a comorbid tic disorder benefited from
clonidine, compared with 53% of children with ADHD
only (Steingard, Biederman, Spencer, Wilens, &
Gonzalez, 1993).

Schvehla, Mandoki, and Sumner (1994) reported
results of an open trial of clonidine with 18 prepubertal
boys who had a dual diagnosis of ADHD and conduct
disorder and who were unresponsive to conventional
therapy. The clonidine was initiated on an inpatient
basis, and follow-up occurred after one and two months
of outpatient treatment. Sixty-one percent (11 patients)
had significant improvement on clonidine alone and an
additional 4 patients (22%) did well when a stimulant
was added to the clonidine.

As was previously noted, Singer et al. (1995)
compared the efficacy of clonidine (0.05 mg four times
daily) and desipramine (25 mg four times daily) in treating 37 children with ADHD and Tourette syndrome and
found desipramine to be superior for alleviating hyperactivity, anxiety, and tic frequency. Desipramine appears
to be an effective alternative to clonidine, although four
cases of sudden death in children treated with desipramine
has led to cautious use and careful cardiovascular

follow-up (Singer et al., 1995). In summary, clonidine appears to be a useful medication for some patients with ADHD who also have associated chronic tic disorders, severely decreased appetite, sleep problems, or growth rate problems as a primary complaint or secondary to treatment with stimulants (Fox & Rieder, 1993; Golden, 1990; Hunt, 1987; Hunt et al., 1986).

In an open trial, guanfacine showed significant effects on hyperactivity, inattention, and immaturity in 13 children diagnosed with ADHD (Hunt, Arnsten, & Asbell, 1995). The authors found guanfacine to be better tolerated than clonidine because it has a longer half-life (18 hours) and is less sedating. They also cited unpublished data that show that some patients with ADHD may respond better to a combination of guanfacine and methylphenidate than to either medication alone.

The use of combined pharmacotherapy is relatively common because of the frequency of comorbid diagnoses, beneficial synergistic effects, and lowered adverse effects, particularly if lower doses of each medication are used (Wilens, Spencer, Biederman, Wozniak, & Connor, 1995). Clonidine has been combined with stimulants to treat children with ADHD, especially when stimulants alone have not had optimal benefit. Hunt et al. (1990) used a combination of methylphenidate and clonidine in treating those with ADHD and conduct disorder. Wilens et al. (1995) combined methylphenidate and clonidine in treating patients with aggressive ADHD and patients with oppositional defiant or conduct disorders and found greater efficacy than with either agent alone.

Other Disorders

Both serotonin and norepinephrine systems are implicated in aggressive behavior. On the one hand, serotonin has an inhibitory function in many neuronal systems; enhancement of serotonin inhibits aggressive behavior in response to an adverse stimulus (Coccaro, 1989). On the other hand, norepinephrine promotes impulsive aggressive behavior. Central norepinephrine systems regulate the level of arousal and responsiveness to stimuli (Coccaro et al., 1991).

Kemph, DeVane, Levin, Jarocke, and Miller (1993) hypothesized that clonidine would be helpful in controlling aggression. This hypothesis was based on two findings: (1) Clonidine stimulates release of gamma-aminobutyric acid (GABA) in specific regions of rat brains, including the frontal cortex (Pittaluga & Raiteri, 1988), and (2) GABA is the major inhibitory neurotransmitter of the

CNS and is involved in inhibiting aggression. For example, animal studies have shown that a GABA agonist or an inhibitor of GABA uptake decreases fighting in mice (Puglisi-Allegra & Mandel, 1980).

Kemph et al. (1993) tested their hypothesis in an open trial of clonidine. They treated 17 severely aggressive children, aged 5 to 15, who met diagnostic criteria for either conduct disorder or oppositional defiant disorder. The doses ranged from 0.15 mg to 0.40 mg/day for 1 to 18 months. The results indicated that aggression decreased in 15 of the 17 children. A follow-up with 6 children showed that 5 who responded positively to clonidine had significant increases in GABA and that the one who did not show clinical improvement also did not show an increase in GABA. Although this study is intriguing, no controls were utilized. Further study of the treatment of aggression and the role of GABA is warranted.

The cardiovascular effects of clonidine have led to a variety of uses. As was already noted, clonidine is most widely used as an antihypertensive agent for both children and adults. Because of its peripheral vasoconstriction effects, the transdermal patch has been used in treating menopausal hot flashes (Nagamani, Kelver, & Smith, 1987). It is also helpful in the differential diagnosis of primary hypertension from pheochromocytoma. Plasma concentrations of norepinephrine are markedly reduced after a single dose of clonidine in primary hypertension, but not so with pheochromocytoma. The lack of suppression of plasma norepinephrine to less than 500 pg/ml three hours after an oral dose of 0.3 mg clonidine suggests pheochromocytoma. Clonidine has also been used in endocrine studies. Two stimulation tests are required for the assessment of GH secretion and one such stimulus can employ clonidine in a dose of 4 μg/kg given orally. GH response is evaluated 60 to 120 minutes subsequently (Lewis, Underwood, & Jackson, 1992).

Clonidine may temporarily reduce the intensity of anxiety associated with panic disorder, but it is not effective for long-term treatment (Hunt et al., 1990; Uhde et al., 1989). Preliminary observations have also suggested that clonidine yields a partial response in people treated for post-traumatic stress and phobias (Hoehn-Saric, Merchant, Keyser, & Smith, 1981). Friedman (1988) has shown that clonidine reduces sympathetic hyperarousal, sleep problems, and anxiety associated with post-traumatic stress disorder in adults.

The efficacy of clonidine for mania has not been established. A randomized, double-blind study of clonidine with lithium treatments did not support the effectiveness of clonidine (Giannini, Pascarzi, Loiselle, Price,

& Giannini, 1986). However, an open trial of clonidine with 24 patients with acute mania (Hardy, Lecrubier, & Widloecher, 1986) suggested a significant improvement in 50% of the patients, especially for those who had a family history of mania or who did not respond favorably to neuroleptics. Much more research is needed to evaluate the effects of clonidine on mania.

Clonidine has been used to treat withdrawal symptoms from narcotics, alcohol, and tobacco (Bjorkqvist, 1975; Glassman et al., 1988; Jasinski, Johnson, & Kocher, 1985). It suppresses activity of the locus coeruleus at withdrawal, thereby decreasing adverse and excessive sympathetic activity. Drug craving is only modestly relieved, however. The investigators of an open trial with three patients concluded that clonidine was ineffective in alleviating withdrawal symptoms of benzodiazepines (Goodman, Charney, Price, Scott, & Herringer, 1986). In opiate withdrawal, effective reduction of autonomic symptoms including hypertension, tachycardia, sweating, lacrimation, and rhinorrhea were evident. Clonidine can be used alone or in combination with naltrexone. It may be more effective in the withdrawal of methadone than of other narcotics (Charney, Heninger, & Kleber, 1986; Riordan & Kleber, 1980; Sensy, Dovus, & Oldberg, 1977).

Recent preliminary observations suggest the possible role of clonidine in the treatment of apparent life threatening event (near-miss sudden infant death syndrome). Two male infants, aged 5 and 7 months, presented with recurrent severe episodes of apnea, cyanosis, and muscle flaccidity associated with oxygen desaturation. Their episodes were diagnosed as severe prolonged expiratory apnea that were refractory to atropine. Following treatment with clonidine (2-3 μg/kg/day in two divided doses), the episodes disappeared completely for one infant and decreased significantly for the other both in terms of the number and severity of episodes. Blood pressure remained stable. Treatment was discontinued at the age of 10 months for one infant, whereas the other was still on the drug at the time of this writing (E. Tirosh, personal communication, June 15, 1995). Further investigations are required before any conclusions can be made.

Issa (1992) reported results of the use of clonidine with 10 men with obstructive sleep apnea. Six improved with clonidine and two worsened. Clonidine suppressed REM sleep in general and affected the breathing mechanisms during sleep. In some cases, clonidine enhanced airway patency. Clonidine was observed to improve speech fluency in a stutterer;

however, further research is required to verify this possible effect (Vink, Althaus, Goorhuis-Brouwer, & Minderaa, 1992).

CLINICAL INDICATIONS IN MENTAL RETARDATION

Indications Based on Controlled Studies

Published reports on the use of clonidine for children with mental retardation are extremely limited. Only two double-blind crossover, placebo-controlled studies have been reported, and both concerned children with autism. Jaselskis, Cook, and Fletcher (1992) observed eight hyperactive children with autistic disorder; the mean IQ was 59. Clonidine in a daily dose of 4 to 10 μg/kg/day for six weeks significantly improved ratings of hyperactivity, irritability, stereotypy, and inappropriate speech. There was also a significant increase in drowsiness and decreased activity compared to placebo. Six of the eight children continued on clonidine after the study. However, four of the children had developed a tolerance to clonidine at long-term follow-up. The medication was discontinued because higher doses led to an intolerable increase in irritability and drowsiness (Jaselskis et al., 1992).

Fankhauser et al. (1992) observed nine male subjects with autism, aged 5 to 33 years. Transdermal clonidine in a dose of 5 μg/kg/day for four weeks was compared to placebo. Significant improvements were seen in hyperarousal behavior, self-stimulation, stereotypies, hyperactivity, and hypervigilance. Both parents and clinicians noted a calming effect in the majority of the participants, specifically noting improved attention, reduced repetitive behavior, and improved social interactions. The authors suggested that clonidine may reduce overactivity of the noradrenergic system. Lake, Ziegler, and Murphy (1977) found that higher plasma levels of norepinephrine and decreased plasma activity of dopamine-hydroxylase (which converts dopamine to norepinephrine) are associated with autism.

Indications Based on Clinical Observations

The fragile X syndrome is associated with hyperarousal and hyperactivity in people with mental retardation (Hagerman, 1996). This is the most common form of inherited mental retardation; the prevalence of female carriers is approximately 1 in 259 in the general population (Rousseau et al., 1995). Hyperactivity occurs in approximately 80% of men and 35% of women who are affected by the syndrome (Hagerman, 1996).

Clonidine has been reported anecdotally to be of benefit in boys with fragile X and hyperactivity (Hagerman, 1996; Leckman, 1987). It is often used successfully in conjunction with methylphenidate to treat the hyperactivity, which is usually severe in this disorder. Clonidine also may improve irritability and tantrum behavior. A dose in the evening appears to help with bedtime processing and sleep disturbances, which are common in fragile X syndrome. The sleepiness associated with clonidine's use appears to be helpful in the evenings. Hagerman, Riddle, Roberts, Brease, and Fulton (1995) interviewed the parents of 35 children with fragile X syndrome (mean age 8.5 years) who were prescribed clonidine. They found that 77% of the children were still taking clonidine (mean length of use 1.6 years). Overall, 11% of the parents felt that their children's behavior was worse on clonidine, 6% said clonidine had no effect, 20% said clonidine helped a little, and 60% said clonidine was very beneficial. Methylphenidate was also used for 49% of the patients because of a synergistic effect with clonidine to alleviate symptoms of ADHD. These results need to be replicated by controlled trials before conclusions can be drawn.

Zarkowska, Crawley, and Locke (1989) used clonidine to treat a girl who had both severe mental retardation and Tourette syndrome. Clonidine did not reduce her tic frequency, but pimozide did. It is premature to draw any conclusions, however. We have seen several patients who had both mental retardation and Tourette syndrome who improved on clonidine.

Cesena, Lee, Cebollero, and Steingard (1995) used clonidine to treat a 4-year-old boy who had both developmental delays and AIDS. Because of the encephalopathy associated with his HIV-1 infection, he developed hyperactivity, irritability, and a sleep disturbance. These three problems all responded well to clonidine.

Sovner (1995) used clonidine to treat adults with mental retardation who experienced withdrawal symptoms from a thioridazine taper. The symptoms included agitation, sleep disturbance, and anxiety. When these symptoms were successfully treated with clonidine, the thioridazine was tapered and discontinued.

CONCLUSION

Clonidine is a presynaptic alpha$_2$-adrenergic agonist that lowers the sympathetic output from the CNS and plasma norepinephrine levels and that indirectly affects both dopaminergic and serotonergic systems. Because of these properties, clonidine is an effective antihypertensive agent. But it has also been helpful in the treatment of some behavioral problems. Because of its general calming effect, it may alleviate hyperactivity, irritability, and inattention, improve concentration, and lessen tic frequency, particularly in people with Tourette syndrome.

Sedation is a very common side effect, but it is one that may be beneficial in nighttime dosing and in alleviating sleep disturbances. Sedation usually declines after the first two weeks and can also be lessened by lowering the dose. There have been reports of sudden death in children receiving clonidine in conjunction with other psychotropic drugs. Given the widespread use of this drug and the specific medical complications in the reported cases of sudden death, it is difficult to know whether clonidine played *any* role in these fatalities; however, prudence suggests a cautious approach. Recent reports of cardiac dysrhythmia also suggest that caution should be taken in using clonidine and that follow-up EKGs are needed, especially when it is used with other medications. Families should be warned to avoid overdose, which can be life threatening. However, clonidine generally is a safer medication than neuroleptics and should be tried initially in the treatment of tics and hyperactivity in Tourette syndrome. Sudden discontinuance of clonidine can cause hypertensive rebound and is to be avoided.

Although the use of clonidine to treat patients with mental retardation is new, preliminary data suggest potential benefits. The medication appears to reduce hyperarousal, anxiety, aggression, and hyperactivity. These are common problems in many patients with mental retardation who are seen for behavioral difficulties. Clonidine can be used by itself or in combined pharmacotherapy. It is the most widely used medication available for decreasing norepinephrine levels. As more knowledge is gained regarding the neurochemistry of various developmental disorders, the indications for clonidine may increase.

REFERENCES

Antelman, S.M., & Caggiula, A.R. (1977). Norepinephrine-dopamine interactions and behavior. *Science, 194,* 646–653.

Bjorkqvist, S.E. (1975). Clonidine in alcohol withdrawal. *Acta Psychiatrica Scandinavica, 52,* 256–263.

Borison, R., Arg, L., Hamilton, W., Diamond, B., & David, J. (1983). Treatment approaches in Gilles de la Tourette syndrome. *Brain Research Bulletin, 11,* 205–208.

Bunney, B.S., & DeRiemers, S. (1982). Effect of clonidine on dopaminergic neuron activity in the substantia nigra: Possible indirect mediation by noradrenergic regulation of the serotonergic raphe system. In A.J. Friedhoff & T.N. Chase (Eds.), *Gilles de la Tourette syndrome* (pp. 99–104). New York: Raven Press.

Cesena, M., Lee, D.O., Cebollero, A.M., & Steingard, R.J. (1995). Case study: Behavior symptoms of pediatric HIV-1 encephalopathy successfully treated with clonidine. *Journal of the American Academy of Child and Adolescent Psychiatry, 34,* 302–306.

Chandran, K.S.K. (1994). ECG and clonidine. *Journal of the American Academy of Child and Adolescent Psychiatry, 33,* 1351–1352.

Chapman, N.A. (1994). Safety of clonidine and nortriptyline. *Journal of the American Academy of Child and Adolescent Psychiatry, 33,* 142–143.

Charney, D.S., Heninger, G.R., & Kleber, H.D. (1986). The combined use of clonidine and naltrexone as a rapid, safe, and effective treatment of abrupt withdrawal from methadone. *American Journal of Psychiatry, 143,* 831–837.

Clementy, J., Castagné, D., Wicker, P., Dallocchio, M., & Bricaud, H. (1986). Study of the electrophysiologic properties of clonidine administered intravenously. *Journal of Cardiovascular Pharmacology, 8*(Suppl. 3), 24–29.

Coccaro, E.F. (1989). Central serotonin and impulsive aggression. *British Journal of Psychiatry, 155*(Suppl. 8), 52–62.

Coccaro, E.F., Lawrence, T., Trestman, R., Gabriel, S., Klar, H.M., & Siever, L.J. (1991). Growth hormone responses to intravenous clonidine challenge correlate with behavioral irritability in psychiatric patients and healthy volunteers. *Psychiatry Research, 39,* 129–139.

Cocco, G., & Ague, C. (1977). Interactions between cardioactive drugs and antidepressants. *European Journal of Clinical Pharmacology, 11,* 389–393.

Cohen, D.J., Riddle, M.A., & Leckman, J.F. (1992). Pharmacotherapy of Tourette's syndrome and associated disorders. *Psychiatric Clinics of North America, 15,* 109–129.

Cohen, D.J., Young, J.G., Nathanson, J.A., & Shaywitz, B.A. (1979). Clonidine in Tourette's syndrome. *Lancet, 2,* 551–553.

Cohen, D.L., Detlor, J., Young, G. & Shaywitz, B.A. (1980). Clonidine ameliorates Gilles de la Tourette. *Archives of General Psychiatry. 37,* 1350–1357.

Comings, D.E., Comings, B.F., Tacket, T., & Li, S. (1990). The clonidine patch and behavior problems. *Journal of the American Academy of Child and Adolescent Psychiatry, 29,* 667–668.

Conner, C.S., & Watanabe, A.S. (1979). Clonidine overdose: A review. *American Journal of Hospital Pharmacology, 36,* 906–911.

Dawson, P.M., VanderZanden, J.A., Werkman, S.L., Washington, R.L., & Tyma, T.A. (1989). Cardiac dysrhythmia with the use of clonidine in explosive disorder. *DICP, The Annals of Pharmacotherapy, 23,* 465–466.

Elliott, H.L., Whiting, B., & Reid, J.L. (1983). Assessment of the interaction between mianserin and overall acting antihypertensive drugs. *British Journal of Clinical Pharmacology, 15*(Suppl.), 323S–328S.

Fankhauser, M., Karumanchi, V., German, M., Yates, A., & Karumanchi, S. (1992). A double-blind, placebo-controlled study of the efficacy of transdermal clonidine in autism. *Journal of Clinical Psychiatry, 53,* 77–82.

Fenichel, R.R. (1995). Combining methylphenidate and clonidine: The role of postmarketing surveillance. *Journal of Child and Adolescent Psychopharmacology, 5,* 155–156.

Fender, L., Inserra, F., & Medina, F. (1987). Safety aspects of long-term antihypertensive therapy (10 years) with clonidine. *Journal of Cardiovascular Pharmacology, 10*(Suppl. 12), 104–108.

Fox, A.M., & Rieder, M.J. (1993). Child risks and benefits of drugs used in the management of the hyperactive child. *Drug Safety, 9,* 38–50.

Friedman, M.J. (1988). Toward rational pharmacotherapy for post-traumatic stress disorder: An interim report. *American Journal of Psychiatry, 145,* 281–285.

Giannini, A.J., Pascarzi, G.A., Loiselle, R.H., Price, W.A., & Giannini, M.C. (1986). Comparison of clonidine and lithium in the treatment of mania. *American Journal of Psychiatry, 143,* 1608–1609.

Gillon, J.Y., Quintin, L., Ghigone, M., & Pujol, J.F. (1987). Clonidine modulated the ventrolateral medullary catechol metabolic hyperactivity induced by hypotension. *Brain Research, 418,* 157–163.

Glassman, A.H., Stetner, F., Walsh, T., Raizman, P.S., Fleiss, J.L., Cooper, T.B., & Covey, L.S. (1988). Heavy smokers, smoking cessation and clonidine. *Journal of the American Medical Association, 259,* 2863–2866.

Goetz, C.G., Shannon, K.M., Carroll, V.S., Tanner, C.M., & Weingarten, R. (1987). The autonomic nervous system in Gilles de la Tourette's syndrome. *Movement Disorder, 2,* 99–102.

Goetz, C., Tanner, C., Wilson, R., Carroll, B.S., Connor, P., & Shannon, K. (1987). Clonidine and Gilles de la Tourette syndrome: Double-blind study using objective rating measures. *Annals of Neurology, 21,* 307–310.

Golden G.S. (1990). Tourette syndrome: Recent advances. *Neurological Clinics, 8,* 705–714.

Goodman, U.K., Charney, D.S., Price, L.J., Scott, W.W., & Herringer, G.R. (1986). Ineffectiveness of clonidine in the treatment of the benzodiazepine withdrawal syndrome. *American Journal of Psychiatry, 143,* 900–903.

Goodman, & Gilman, A.G. (1990) *The pharmacological basis of therapeutics* (8th ed., pp. 208–211). New York: Pergamon Press.

Hagerman, R.J. (1996). Medical follow-up and pharmacotherapy. In R.J. Hagerman & A. Cronister (Eds.), *Fragile X syndrome: Diagnosis, treatment and intervention.* 2nd edition, Baltimore, MD: Johns Hopkins University Press, p.p. 283–331.

Hagerman, R.J., Riddle, J.E., Roberts, L.S., Brease, K., & Fulton, M. (1995). A survey of the efficacy of clonidine in fragile X syndrome. *Developmental Brain Dysfunction. 8,* 336–344.

Hardy, M.C., Lecrubier, Y., & Widloecher, D. (1986). Efficacy of clonidine in 24 patients with acute mania. *American Journal of Psychiatry, 143,* 1450–1453.

Hedland, H., Dymbling, J.F., & Humbelt, B. (1972). The effect of insulin-induced hypoglycemia on plasma renin activity and urinary catecholamines before and following clonidine in man. *Acta Endocrinologica, 71,* 321.

Hewlett, W.A., Vinogradov, S., & Agras, W.S. (1992). Clomipramine, clonazepam and clonidine treatment of obsessive-compulsive disorder. *Journal of Clinical Psychopharmacology, 12,* 420–426.

Hoehn-Saric, R., Merchant, A.F., Keyser, M.L., & Smith, V.R. (1981). Effects of clonidine on anxiety disorders. *Archives of General Psychiatry, 38,* 1278–1282.

Huisjes, H.J., Hadders-Algra, M., & Touwen, B.C.L. (1986). Is clonidine a behavioral teratogen in the human? *Early Human Development, 14,* 43–48.

Huk, S.G. (1989). Transient exacerbation of tics in treatment of Tourette's syndrome with clonidine. *Journal of the American Academy of Child and Adolescent Psychiatry, 28,* 583–586.

Hunt, R.D. (1987). Treatment effects of oral and transdermal clonidine in relation to methylphenidate: An open pilot study. *Psychopharmacology Bulletin, 23,* 111–114.

Hunt, R.D., Arnsten, A.F.T., & Asbell, M.D. (1995). An open trial of guanfacine in the treatment of attention-deficit hyperactivity disorder. *Journal of the American*

Academy of Child and Adolescent Psychiatry, 34, 50–54.

Hunt, R.D., Capper, L., & O'Connell, P. (1990). Clonidine in child and adolescent psychiatry. Journal of Child and Adolescent Psychopharmacology, 1, 87–102.

Hunt, R.D., Minderaa, R.B., & Cohen, D.J. (1985). Clonidine benefits children with attention-deficit disorder and hyperactivity: Report of a double-blind placebo-crossover therapeutic trial. Journal of the American Academy of Child Psychiatry, 24, 617–629.

Hunt, R.D., Minderaa, R.B., & Cohen, D.J. (1986). The therapeutic effect of clonidine in attention-deficit disorder with hyperactivity: A comparison with placebo and methylphenidate. Psychological Bulletin, 22, 229–236.

Issa, F.G. (1992). Effect of clonidine in obstructive sleep apnea. American Review of Respiratory Disease, 145, 435–439.

Jaffe, R., Livshits, T., & Bursztyn, M. (1994). Adverse interaction between clonidine and verapamil. Annals of Pharmacotherapy, 28, 881–883.

Jaselskis, C.A., Cook, E.H. Jr., & Fletcher, K.E. (1992). Clonidine treatment of hyperactive and impulsive children with autistic disorder. Journal of Clinical Psychopharmacology, 12, 322–327.

Jasinski, D.R., Johnson, R.E., & Kocher, T.R. (1985). Clonidine in morphine withdrawal: Differential effects on signs and symptoms. Archives of General Psychiatry, 42, 1063–1066.

Kallio, A., Saraste, M., Scheinin, M., Hartiala, J., & Scheinin, H. (1990). Acute hemodynamic effects of medetomidine and clonidine in healthy volunteers: A noninvasive echocardiographic study. Journal of Cardiovascular Pharmacology, 16, 28–33.

Kemph, J.P., DeVane, C.L., Levin, G.M., Jarocke, R., & Miller, R.L. (1993). Treatment of aggressive children with clonidine: Results of an open pilot study. Journal of the American Academy of Child and Adolescent Psychiatry, 32, 577–581.

Kibler, L.E. and Gazes, P.C. (1977). Effects of clonidine on atriogen atrioventricular conduction. Journal of the American Medical Association, 238, 1930–1932.

Kugler, J., Seus, R., Krauskopf, R., Brecht, H.M., & Raschig, A. (1990). Differences in psychic performance with guanfacine and clonidine in normotensive subjects. British Journal of Clinical Pharmacology, 99, 803–809.

Kunchandy, J., & Kulkarni, S.K. (1986). Reversal by alpha-2 agonists of diazepam withdrawal hyperactivity in rats. Psychopharmacology, 90, 198–202.

Lake, C.R., Ziegler, M.G., & Murphy, D.L. (1977). Increased norepinephrine levels and decreased dopamine-hydroxylase activity in primary autism. Archives of General Psychiatry, 34, 533–536.

Leckman, J.F., Detlor, J., Harcherik, D.F., Ort, S., Shaywitz, B.A., & Cohen D.J. (1985). Short- and long-term treatment of Tourette's syndrome with clonidine: A clinical perspective. Neurology, 35, 347–351.

Leckman, J., Hardin, M., Riddle, M., Stevenson, J., Ort, S., & Cohen, D. (1991). Clonidine treatment of Gilles de la Tourette's syndrome. Archives of General Psychiatry, 48, 324–328.

Lewis, E., Underwood, L.E., & Van Wykis (1992). Normal and aberrant grown. In Wilson & Foster (eds) Textbook of Endocrinology, 8th edition. Philadelphia, W.B. Sounders. pp. 1079–1138.

Li, G., Regunathan, S., Barrow, C.J., Eshraghi, J., Cooper, R., & Reis, D.J. (1994). Agmatine: An endogenous clonidine-displacing substance in the brain. Science, 263, 966–969.

Max, J.E., & Rasmunsen, S.A. (1986). Clonidine in the treatment of Tourette's syndrome exacerbation due to haloperidol withdrawal. Journal of Nervous and Mental Disease, 174, 246–247.

Nagamani, M., Kelver, M.E., & Smith, E.R. (1987). Treatment of menopausal hot flashes with transdermal administration of clonidine. American Journal of Obstetrics and Gynecology, 156, 561–565.

Pittaluga, A., & Raiteri, M. (1988). Clonidine enhances the release of endogenous gamma aminobutyric acid through alpha-z and alpha-1 presynaptic adreno receptors differentially located in rat cerebral cortex sub-regions. Journal of Pharmacology and Experimental Therapeutics, 245, 682–686.

Popper, C.W. (1995). Combining methylphenidate and clonidine: Pharmacologic questions and new reports about sudden death. Journal of Child and Adolescent Psychopharmacology, 5, 157–166.

Puglisi-Allegra, S., & Mandel, P. (1980). Effects of sodium n-dipropylacetate, muscimaol hydrobromide and (R,S) nipecotic acid amide on isolation induced aggressive behavior in mice. Psychopharmacology, 70, 287–290.

Quintin, L., Ghigone, M., & Pujol, J.F. (1987). The ability of the alpha2-adrenergic agonist clonidine to suppress central noradrenergic hyperactivity secondary to hemodynamic or environmental stimuli. Journal of Cardiovascular Pharmacology, 10(Suppl. 12), 128–134.

Quintin, L., Gonon, F., Buda, M., Ghigone, M., Hilaire, G., & Pujol, J.F. (1986). Clonidine modulated locus coeruleus metabolic hyperactivity induced by stress in behaving rats. Brain Research, 362, 366–369.

Riordan, C.E., & Kleber, H.D. (1980). Rapid opiate detoxification with clonidine and naloxone. Lancet, 1, 1079–1080.

Rousseau, F., Rouillard, P., Morel, M.L., Khandijian, E.W., Morgan, K. (1995).

Prevalance of carriers of premutation-sized alleles of the FMRI gene and implications for the population genetics of the fragile X syndrome. American Journal of Human Genetics, 57, 1006–1018.

Schvehla, T.J., Mandoki, M.W., & Summer, G.S. (1994). Clonidine therapy for comorbid attention deficit hyperactivity disorder and conduct disorder: Preliminary findings in a children's inpatient unit. Southern Medical Journal, 87, 692–695.

Sensy, E.C., Dovus, W.S., & Oldberg, F. (1977). Withdrawal from methadone maintenance: Rate of withdrawal and expectation. Archives of General Psychiatry, 34, 361–367.

Singer, H.S., Brown, J., Quaskey, S., Rosenberg, L.A., Mellits, E.D., & Denekla, M.B. (1995). The treatment of attention-deficit hyperactivity disorder in Tourette syndrome: A double-blind placebo-controlled study with clonidine and desipramine. Pediatrics, 95, 74–81.

Sovner, R. (1995). Thioridazine withdrawal-induced behaviorl deterioration treated with clonidine. Mental Retardation, 33, 221–225.

Steingard, R., Biederman, J., Spencer, J., Wilens, T., & Gonzalez, A. (1993). Comparison of clonidine response in treatment of attention-deficit hyperactivity disorder with and without comorbid tic disorders. Journal of the American Academy of Child and Adolescent Psychiatry, 32, 350–353.

Svensson, T.H., Bunney, B.S., & Aghajakian, G.K. (1975). Inhibition of both noradrenergic and serotonergic neurons in brain by the adrenergic agonist clonidine. Brain Research, 92, 291–306.

Swanson, J.M., Flockhart, D., Udrea, D., Cantwell, D., Connor D., & Williams, L. (1995). Clonidine in the treatment of ADHD: Questions about safety and efficacy. Journal of Child and Adolescent Psychopharmacology, 5, 301–304.

Uhde, T.W., Stein, M.B., Vittone, B.J., Siever, L.J., Boulenger, J.P., Klein, E., & Mellman, T.A. (1989). Behavioral and physiologic effects of short-term and long-term administration of clonidine in panic disorder. Archives of General Psychiatry, 46, 170–177.

Uhlen, S., & Wikberg, J.E.S. (1991). Delineation of rat kidney alpha-2A- and alpha-2B-adrenoceptors with [3H] RX821002 radioligand binding: Computer modeling reveals that guanfacine is an alpha-2A-selective compound. European Journal of Pharmacology, 202, 235–243.

Vink, H.J.F., Althaus, A.M., Goorhuis-Brouwer, S.M., & Minderaa, R.B. (1992). Clonidine and stuttering. American Journal of Psychiatry, 149, 717–718.

Volta, C., Ghizzoni, L., Muto, G., Spaggiari, R., Virdis, R., & Bernasconi, S. (1991). Effectiveness of growth-promoting therapies: Comparisons among growth hormone, clonidine and levodopa. *American Journal of Diseases of Children, 145,* 168–171.

Wasserman, G.S. (1989). Clonidine intoxication. *Veterinarian Human Toxicology, 31,* 391.

Wedin, G.P., Richardson, S.L., & Wallace, G.H. (1990). Clonidine poisoning in children. *American Journal of Diseases of Children, 144,* 853–854.

Wilens, T.E., & Biederman, J. (1994). Reply to safety of clonidine and nortriptyline. *Journal of the American Academy of Child and Adolescent Psychiatry, 33,* 143.

Wilens, T.E., Biederman, J., & Spencer, T. (1994). Clonidine for sleep disturbances associated with attention-deficit hyperactivity disorder. *Journal of the American Academy of Child and Adolescent Psychiatry, 33,* 424–426.

Wilens, T.E., Spencer, T., Biederman, J., Wozniak, J., & Connor, D. (1995). Combined pharmacotherapy: An emerging trend in pediatric psychopharmacology. *Journal of the American Academy of Child and Adolescent Psychiatry, 34,* 110–112.

Wiley, J.F., Wiley, C.C., Torrey, S.B., & Henretig, F.M. (1990). Clonidine poisoning in young children. *Journal of Pediatrics, 116,* 654–658.

Zarkowska, E., Crawley, B., & Locke, J. (1989). A behavioral intervention for Gilles de la Tourette syndrome in a severely mentally handicapped girl. *Journal of Mental Deficiency Research, 33,* 245–253.

Beta-Adrenergic Blockers

W. I. Fraser[1], Stephen Ruedrich[2], Michael Kerr[3], and Andrew Levitas[4]

Beta-adrenergic blocking medications have a 40-year history of use in psychiatric disorders. The initial report concerned the treatment of anxiety (Granville-Grossman & Turner, 1966), but they also have been reported anecdotally to have benefits in psychosis, aggression, and in other conditions (Arnold & Aman, 1991; Coffey, 1990; Lader, 1988). Non-psychiatric uses include a variety of cardiovascular disorders, migraine headaches, and glaucoma. Despite widespread uses, beta-adrenergic blockers are among the least well-studied classes of medications in patients with psychiatric illness, with or without developmental disability.

DEFINITION, CLASSES, AND NAMES

Beta-adrenergic blocking medications are competitive inhibitors of the effects of catecholamines at beta-adrenergic nerve receptor sites. As inhibitors of catecholamine activity, they are also known as beta-adrenergic antagonists, because they oppose, or antagonize, the sympathetic nervous system. The sympathetic nervous system contains two types of receptors (termed *alpha* and *beta*), and at least two receptor subtypes have been identified for each (α_1 and α_2, β_1 and β_2) (Hoffman & Lefkowitz, 1996). Drugs that are ß blockers are classified based on whether they antagonize either the β_1 or β_2 receptor subtype, or both, or have some pro-sympathetic (agonist) activity (called Intrinsic Sympathetic Activity or ISA). A feature used in classification is whether or not the drug produces blockade (antagonism) of receptors (Prichard, 1978).

The largest class of ß blockers are called non-selective, in that they block catecholamine effects at both β_1 and β_2 receptors. These include: carteolol, labetolol, levobunolol, nadolol, oxprenolol, penbutolol, pindolol, propranolol, sotalol, and timolol. Most of these, with the exception of nadolol, propranolol, and timolol, also have some ISA, and most do not cause blockade. A second group produce only β_1 blockade, and are therefore called selective β_1 blockers. These would include: acebutolol, atenolol, betaxolol, bisoprolol, esmolol, and metoprolol. No currently available agent selectively blocks β_2 receptors (Hoffman & Lefkowitz, 1996). Generic and trade names, as well as ß receptor selectivity, can be found in Table 16-1.

PHARMACOLOGY

Pharmacodynamics

Beta blockers are competitive inhibitors of the effects of catecholamines at ß-adrenergic sites both in the nervous system and at locations in non-nerve tissue (Arnold & Aman, 1991). Alpha receptors found in vascular and other smooth muscle are mainly excitatory; most ß receptors, when activated, exert an inhibitory effect on their target organ, although ß receptors in the heart are excitatory (Hoffman & Lefkowitz, 1996). Alpha and ß receptors respond differentially to various sympathetic transmitters (or medications). The ß receptors in the nervous system are activated by catecholamines (primarily epinephrine and norepinephrine) released from adjacent nerve cells; ß receptors located in non-nerve tissue (found in the pancreas, liver, and kidney) are activated by catecholamines circulating in the vascular system. Beta receptors in the heart and brain are mostly β_1 (Conway, Greenwood, & Middlemiss, 1978; Palacios & Kuhar, 1980); those in the vascular system, lung bronchi, and gastrointestinal (GI) system are mostly β_2 (Hoffman & Lefkowitz, 1996).

1 Professor of Mental Handicap, University of Wales College of Medicine, South Glamorgan, Wales, United Kingdom
2 Associate Professor of Psychiatry, Case Western University, Cleveland, OH
3 Lecturer in Learning Disability, University of Wales College of Medicine, South Glamorgan, Wales, United Kingdom
4 Assistant Professor of Clinical Psychiatry, University of Medicine and Dentistry of New Jersey, Stratford, NJ

Table 16-1. Beta Blockers

NON-SELECTIVE ß BLOCKERS

Generic Name	Trade Name	ß₁ Blockade	ß₂ Blockade	ISA	Lipid Solubility
carteolol	Cartrol	Yes	Yes	Yes	Low
labetolol	Normodyne	Yes	Yes	Yes	High
levobunolol	Betagan	Yes	Yes	No	Low
nadolol	Corgard	Yes	Yes	No	Low
oxprenolol	Trasicor	Yes	Yes	Yes	?
penbutolol	Levatol	Yes	Yes	Yes	High
pindolol	Visken	Yes	Yes	Yes	Moderate
propranolol	Inderal	Yes	Yes	No	High
sotalol	Betapace	Yes	Yes	No	Low
timolol	Blocadren	Yes	Yes	No	Moderate

SELECTIVE ß BLOCKERS

Generic Name	Trade Name	ß₁ Blockade	ß₂ Blockade	ISA	Lipid Solubility
acebutolol	Sectral	Yes	No	Some	Moderate
atenolol	Tenormin	Yes	No	No	Low
betaxolol	Betoptic	Yes	No	No	Low
bisoprolol	Zebeta	Yes	No	No	Moderate
esmolol	Brevibloc	Yes	No	No	Moderate
metoprolol	Lopressor, Toprol	Yes	No	No	Moderate

Because β_1 receptors outside of the brain are mostly found in the heart, ß blockers which are selective for β_1 are sometimes referred to as cardioselective. It should be noted that such cardioselectivity is relative, and does not imply cardiospecificity, so that even cardioselective β_1 blockers can also exert effects on β_2 receptors found in the lung and vascular system (Lewis & Lofthouse, 1993).

Another important pharmacodynamic quality of some ß blockers is ISA. This refers to the property of some ß blockers to exert an agonist (pro-sympathetic) effect, even while blocking the ß receptor. Beta blockers with ISA, such as oxprenolol and pindolol, are less likely to cause bradycardia and coldness of the extremities than their non-ISA counterparts (Fitzgerald, 1993).

In addition to their effect on ß receptors, ß blockers may bind to (promote) (Hjorth & Carlsson, 1986) or antagonize serotonergic (5-HT) receptors (Hoyer, 1988; Weinstock & Weiss, 1980), and alter the uptake and release of serotonin from platelets (Bygdeman & Johnson, 1969; Weksler, Gillick, & Pink, 1977).

A majority of pharmacodynamic effects of ß blockers are mediated through their action on ß receptors. Other non-receptor actions include a membrane-stabilizing effect, which does not seem to have clinical significance at usual therapeutic doses, but may be important in an overdose (Hayes & Schulz, 1983; Hoffman & Lefkowitz, 1996).

It should be noted that the effects of ß blockers, particularly on cardiac function, are most evident under conditions of increased sympathetic activity (Hoffman & Lefkowitz, 1996). Beta receptor blockade has little effect on the function of the resting heart (when base-line stimulation of the ß receptor is low), but with increased sympathetic activity induced by stress, exercise, or sympathetic agonists, ß blockers exert a more profound blocking effect (Cruickshank & Prichard, 1987).

Pharmacokinetics

Probably the most important pharmacokinetic quality of ß blockers is their differing solubility in fat (lipid) versus water. Those that are highly soluble in the fat tissues of the body are called lipophilic (fat-liking), contrasted to others that are hydrophilic (water-liking). Lipophilicity affects two important pharmacokinetic properties. First, highly lipophilic medications are more rapidly and completely absorbed from the GI system after oral administration than are water soluble compounds. Second, lipophilic ß blockers are more heavily distributed into the lipid-containing tissues of the body (the brain and central nervous system [CNS]), while hydrophilic compounds do not easily cross the blood-brain barrier (BBB), and are largely excluded from the CNS (Hoffman & Lefkowitz, 1996). Some portions of the CNS, such as the pineal and periventricular nuclei, do not have a BBB, and can be affected by hydrophilic ß blockers (Arnold & Aman, 1991). In general, however, the hydrophilic ß blockers exert their effect primarily through action on ß receptors outside the CNS (peripheral NS), while lipophilic ß blockers can affect both central and peripheral ß receptors. This also means lipophilic ß blockers are more likely to cause side effects thought to be secondary to central CNS effects such as nightmares, insomnia, hallucinations, toxic psychosis (Conway et al., 1978), or fatigue and depression (Neppe, 1989).

Absorption and Bioavailability. Lipophilicity affects not only absorption and bioavailability, but also distribution and elimination. The lipid-soluble ß blockers are more quickly absorbed after oral administration and generally have a shorter half-life of action, requiring multiple daily dosing. They are more highly metabolized by the liver in their initial pass through the portal circulation, so that less medication reaches the systemic circulation (Wood et al., 1978). However, there are significant differences between individual patients in the hepatic first-pass clearance of lipid-soluble ß blockers, resulting in significant variability in plasma concentration in patients given the same dose of a lipophilic ß blocker (Hoffman & Lefkowitz, 1996). The effect of hepatic metabolism is also altered based on the particular dose of each lipophilic drug, with less inter-individual variability at higher oral doses. Some of the lipophilic ß blockers also have metabolites with ß receptor activity, which can complicate clinical trials comparing doses of the same drug, or one lipophilic compound to another (Fitzgerald & O'Donnell, 1971; Shand, 1975). Finally, the lipophilic ß blockers are more likely to be bound in the vascular system to plasma proteins, which can be of theoretical importance in low protein states, such as the nephrotic syndrome (Hoffman & Lefkowitz, 1996). Genetic polymorphism can lead to an inability to metabolize lipophilic ß blockers via P450 liver enzymes and can lead to higher-than-expected or toxic drug concentrations in some indi-

viduals (Benfield, Clissold, & Brogden, 1986).

The hydrophilic (water-soluble) ß blockers are incompletely absorbed from the GI system, and are excreted unchanged in the urine (little or no hepatic metabolism) (Hoffman & Lefkowitz, 1996). This makes them potentially safer for patients with impaired hepatic function, but perhaps more dangerous for patients with renal disease.

The majority of ß blockers are given orally, but two (esmolol and labetolol) are available in an intravenous form, and can be used for rapid (or emergency) ß blockade. Esmolol is very short acting; it has a half-life of 8 minutes after IV administration (Hoffman & Lefkowitz, 1996). Several others (timolol, betaxolol, levobunolol) are available in topical (eye drop) forms for the treatment of glaucoma (Brooks & Gillies, 1992). Although topical, most have systemic absorption through the eye, and can cause typical ß blocker side effects even when given topically.

Beta Blockers in the Elderly. Additional care must be exercised in treating elderly patients with ß blocking medications. Although absorption is relatively stable over the lifespan, the other determinants of pharmacokinetics (distribution, metabolism, and excretion) are all affected by aging (Spar & La Rue, 1990). Lipophilic ß blockers will be distributed into the relatively increased lipid volume of the elderly, resulting in lower plasma concentrations. Hydrophilic ß blocker levels will appear increased, based on a relatively lower volume of body water seen in older patients. Plasma proteins also decrease with aging, so that levels of unbound drug are higher, causing greater drug effect. Finally, hepatic and renal functions are decreased by aging. This effect appears to be more significant for the kidney, so that hydrophilic (water-soluble) compounds may be more likely to produce higher-than-expected plasma levels (and ß blockade) than lipophilic agents. The actual effect of the drug on the receptor may also change with aging, although this is less well-documented (Young & Meyers, 1991). The sum total of these changes should result in extra caution and additional monitoring of both response and side effects in elderly patients.

System/Physical Effects

The clinical effects of ß blockade depend on the receptor subtype and its location/action on each target organ. Beta$_1$ receptors are primarily found in the heart and brain; ß$_2$ receptors in the innervation of the peripheral vascular system, bronchial tree, and GI tract.

Cardiovascular Effects. Catecholamines acting on ß$_1$

receptors in the heart result in accelerated heart rate and contractility, so that blockade of these effects slows the heart rate and decreases cardiac output. These effects are minimal in resting states, but blockade of β_1 receptors can decrease heart rate by 35% and cardiac output by up to 25% during periods of exercise or stress (Cruickshank & Prichard, 1987). This probably accounts for the ß blocker efficacy in decreasing the cardiac acceleration seen in angina and performance anxiety (Brantigan, Brantigan, & Joseph, 1982). Beta blockers also function as antiarrhythmic agents, by reducing sinus rate, suppressing ectopic pacemakers in the heart, and slowing conduction. In these ways, they function both to slow the heart and prevent rapid (tachy) arrhythmias. Both of these cardiac effects, along with others, make ß blockers useful in preventing further cardiac damage after acute myocardial infarction (Frishman & Lazar, 1990).

The ß blockers also exert a significant effect in lowering peripheral blood pressure, and are widely used as antihypertensive agents. Generally, their blood pressure lowering effect is not significant in the absence of hypertension, causing modest decreases in patients without hypertension (Hoffman & Lefkowitz, 1996). The mechanism of their antihypertensive action is not completely understood, but may be related to blockade of renin in the kidney, the release of which can cause elevated blood pressure. They also seem to decrease peripheral vascular resistance, which, along with decreased cardiac output, also produces an antihypertensive benefit. Some ß blockers also function directly as peripheral vasodilators, through either blockade or ISA ß receptor agonism (Prichard, 1978). Non-selective ß blockers, however, can inhibit vasodilation and should be used cautiously in patients with epinephrine-secreting tumors (Hoffman & Lefkowitz, 1996). This may also account for their tendency to produce coldness in the extremities and to worsen the symptoms of peripheral vascular disease (Fitzgerald, 1993).

Respiratory Effects. Bronchial smooth muscle is innervated by β_2 receptors, which when stimulated dilate the bronchial tree. Non-selective ß blockers (affecting β_1 and β_2) thus cause bronchoconstriction, narrowing air passages and aggravating diseases such as asthma and chronic obstructive pulmonary disease. This effect can be life-threatening in patients with bronchoconstrictive disease but does not seem clinically problematic in patients with normal lung function (Hayes & Schulz, 1987). It should be noted that even cardioselective (β_1) blockers can cause some β_2 blockade and should be used with caution (or not at all) in patients with airway disease.

Autonomic/Metabolic Effects. Catecholamines promote the production and release of glucose; this effect is antagonized by ß blocking medications. This is particularly true for the metabolic response to hypoglycemia (low blood sugar); patients taking ß blockers may not be able to mobilize to increase glucose and can have a delayed recovery from insulin-induced hypoglycemia (Hoffman & Lefkowitz, 1996). Beta blockers can also prevent the tachycardia usually seen in hypoglycemic states so that individuals suffering low blood sugar may not have this warning sign. Both of these effects mean the ß blockers should be used with caution in patients with diabetes, particularly if blood sugar is labile.

Beta receptors are also involved in the activation of lipase, which leads to the release of fatty acids into the blood stream, producing energy for exercising muscle. Beta blockade blunts their release, but over time ß blockers modestly elevate plasma triglycerides and decrease high density lipoproteins, perhaps with negative effects on hypertension (Rabkin, 1993).

Beta agonists cause potassium to be taken into muscle, decreasing its level in the serum. Beta blockers oppose this effect and can cause a state of mildly elevated potassium called hyperkalemia (Hoffman & Lefkowitz, 1996).

Other Effects. Beta blockers can decrease tremor induced by catecholamines, lithium, and as part of Parkinsonism (Jefferson, 1974; Neppe, 1989). In all of the effects mentioned previously, cardioselectivity (predominance of β_1 blockade) and ISA are important. In general, ß blockers which are cardioselective or have ISA are less likely to produce the same magnitude of effect as that seen with non-selective blockers with no ISA. Decreases in heart rate and cardiac output, increased pulmonary bronchoconstriction, and glucose intolerance are all less severe with cardioselective or ISA compounds.

Side Effects/Toxic Effects

Nearly all of the adverse effects of ß blockers are a result of their primary action in blocking ß-adrenergic receptors, with infrequent adverse reactions related to non-receptor effects (Lewis & Lofthouse, 1993). Therefore, most adverse effects are pharmacologically predictable. Most are well tolerated, but several are dangerous and can be lethal; some of these can be difficult to monitor, such as the impaired glucose response to insulin-induced hypoglycemia.

The primary toxic effects are seen in the cardiovascular and pulmonary systems, in which a large number of ß receptors are found. In the heart, ß blockers, by decreasing heart rate and cardiac output, can produce or aggravate congestive heart failure. This is particularly problematic following recent myocardial infarction, in that ß blockers can help patients who have heart injury not complicated by heart failure. Other adverse cardiac effects can include bradyarrhythmias (slowed heart rate), which can be dangerous if patients are already taking medications which slow cardiac conduction. Finally, when used in patients with angina, ß blockers should not be abruptly discontinued, in that greater-than-usual ß agonist response (hypersensitivity) can ensue, and patients can have more frequent angina or even myocardial infarction. In these, and probably in all patients with any cardiac disease, ß blockers should be discontinued gradually, such as tapering dose over 2-3 weeks (Hoffman & Lefkowitz, 1996; Lewis & Lofthouse, 1993).

Based on the capacity of non-selective ß blockers to produce bronchoconstriction, they (and perhaps all ß blockers) should be avoided, or used with great caution, in patients with bronchoconstrictive disease (asthma, chronic obstructive pulmonary disease). Drugs which are cardio-selective or possess ISA may be slightly safer, but their use is also relatively contraindicated in these patients.

Based on their blunting of the glucose increase to insulin-induced hypoglycemia, ß blockers should be avoided in patients with labile diabetes or hypoglycemia. Glucose tolerance should be investigated before using ß blockers. Plasma triglycerides can also be increased by ß blockers (Hoffman & Lefkowitz, 1996).

Patients with hyperthyroidism are sometimes given ß blockers to address the tachycardia that may accompany this disease; patients should be screened for the presence of thyroid axis disease (causing either tachy- or brady-arrhythmias) before ß blockers are prescribed.

Because of their effect on limiting vasodilation, ß blockers can cause peripheral vasospasm, resulting in complaints of coldness of the extremities in many patients without peripheral vascular disease (Bai, Webb, & Hamilton, 1982). In patients with peripheral vascular disease, ß blockers have the potential to worsen symptoms of intermittent claudication (Lepauntalo, 1985) or produce Raynaud's phenomenon.

CNS Side Effects. Less predictable are the CNS side effects of the ß blockers, which are of considerable interest in persons with mental retardation. Beta blockers have been anecdotally reported to produce nightmares, insomnia, hallucinations, and even toxic psychosis (Conway et al., 1978; Lewis, Jackson, & Ramsay, 1984), presumably through a central β_1 blockade. Others have reported fatigue and depression (Neppe, 1989; Thiessen, Wallace,

Blackburn, Wilson, & Bergman, 1990). Presumably, CNS effects are likely to be more prevalent with agents which are lipophilic; however, this is not a consistent pattern (Drayer, 1987; Gengo, Hintoon, & McHugh, 1981; Gerber & Nies, 1985). Several authors have described difficulties in short-term memory, concentration, and alertness in normal subjects being treated with ß blockers for hypertension (Currie, Lewis, McDevitt, Nicholson, & Wright, 1988; Lichter, Richardson, & Wyke, 1986; Solomon et al., 1983), but in most studies, the methods used cannot unequivocally relate these side effects to ß blocker treatment.

Of significant interest in the area of CNS effects of ß blockers have been reports of their potential for causing depression (Lader, 1988). A number of studies have investigated this issue (Griffen & Friedman, 1986; Petrie, Maffucci, & Woosley, 1982); at this time available evidence does not demonstrate proof of a causal relationship between ß blockers and depression (Sorgi, Ratey, Knoedler, Arnold, & Cole, 1992; Yudofsky, 1992). This issue is clinically controversial, however, and it should be noted that some of the symptomatology of ß blocker toxicity (fatigue, insomnia, decreased physical activity) may be confused with depressive symptomatology. Such affective symptoms should not be confused with affective disorders.

Finally, ß blockers produce rare, but occasional allergic reactions, constipation, indigestion, and diarrhea (Hoffman & Lefkowitz, 1996). Sexual dysfunction can occur, but this effect is poorly understood. Most ß blockers are pregnancy category C, indicating that human studies of their effects on pregnant women are lacking, although animal studies reveal risk. Acebutolol, pindolol, and sotalol are risk category B (no evidence of risk in humans), and atenolol is category D (positive evidence of risk) (Widerhorn, Rubin, Frishman, & Elkayam, 1987).

Rare reported adverse reactions have included a psoriasis-like eruption (Gold, Holy, & Roenigk, 1988) and an unusual form of keratoconus (Wright, 1975). This may be important in patients with Down syndrome who have susceptibility to kerato-conjunctival infections. Additionally, there is one report of a pleural pulmonary Lupus syndrome (Burgess Record, 1981).

Drug Interactions

Pharmacokinetic interactions involve drugs that affect either the absorption of ß blockers or their metabolism by the liver. Lipophilic ß blockers are hepatically metabolized and are more likely to have significant interactions. Drugs that induce hepatic enzymes may decrease circulating levels of ß blockers. Drugs that decrease hepatic blood flow may decrease metabolism of ß blockers and increase the plasma levels of ß blockers. Similarly, ß blockers themselves may compete for hepatic metabolism with other drugs (e.g., chlorpromazine, theophylline, warfarin) and increase their levels if given concurrently (Hoffman & Lefkowitz, 1996; Lewis & Lofthouse, 1993; Lewis & McDevitt, 1986). A recent report describes two adolescents in whom the combination of propranolol and imipramine (a tricyclic antidepressant) produced near-toxic levels of imipramine within a few days after introduction of the second drug, presumably based on competitive hepatic metabolism (Gillette & Tannery, 1994).

Pharmacodynamic drug interactions occur when ß blockers are combined with other medications for an additive pharmacologic effect; examples include combinations of ß blockers and other antihypertensives for hypertension not responsive to either drug alone. Indomethacin and other non-steroidal anti-inflammatory drugs may oppose the antihypertensive effects of ß blockers (Hoffman & Lefkowitz, 1996).

CLINICAL INDICATIONS EXCLUSIVE OF MENTAL RETARDATION

Although initially developed for treatment of cardiovascular disorders, ß blockers also have been prescribed for a variety of psychiatric illnesses.

Anxiety Disorders

Granville-Grossman and Turner (1966) are generally given credit for being the first to demonstrate the efficacy of ß blocking drugs in the treatment of anxiety disorders. In a controlled trial versus placebo, they reported that propranolol 80 mg per day was superior in controlling the peripheral autonomic symptoms and signs of anxiety. More than 15 controlled studies have replicated this finding, in comparison to placebo or measured against benzodiazepine anxiolytics (Agras, 1990; Covelli, Antonacci, & Pagliarulo, 1983; Greenwood, 1990; Hayes & Schulz, 1983; Kathol et al., 1980; Matuzas & Jack, 1991; Meibach, Mullane, &

Binstok, 1987; Noyes, 1982, 1985; Peet & Ali, 1986; Saul, Jones, Edwards, & Tweed, 1985; Tanna, Penningroth, & Woolson, 1977; Tyrer, 1988). In addition to anxiety disorders, patients with acute stress-related anxiety such as performance anxiety may have hyperadenergic symptoms that respond to ß blockers (Brantigan et al., 1982; Drew, Barnes, & Evans, 1985; Fredrickson, Klein, & Ohman, 1990; James, Griffith, Pearson, & Newbury, 1977). Famularo, Kinscherff, and Fenton (1988) reported their efficacy for post-traumatic stress disorder symptomatology in children. When given adjunctively to patients receiving relaxation/biofeedback training for migraine headache, ß blockers produce improvement in migraine activity and decreased analgesic use (Holroyd et al., 1995; Mathew, 1981).

A number of general guidelines have emerged regarding the role and method of ß blocker use in anxiety disorders (Ananth, 1986; Arnold & Aman, 1991; Lader, 1988; Manchanda, 1988; Noyes, 1985; Tyrer, 1988). These guidelines include the following:

1. Beta blockers appear to be effective for the somatic, non-psychological symptoms of anxiety. These may occur in generalized anxiety disorder, acute stress reactions, adjustment disorder with anxiety, and social phobias. Patients with anxiety manifesting in bodily symptoms may be particularly responsive. In these patients, the response to ß blockers seems most related to a peripheral effect in decreasing autonomic symptoms, is generally rapid, and requires modest doses of medication. In patients taking ß blockers for acute situational stress or performance anxiety, relatively low doses may be useful, and PRN doses preceding anticipated stressful situations may be sufficient.
2. Panic disorder, in spite of its significant somatic component, is seen as relatively non-responsive to ß blockers (Gorman et al., 1983).
3. Specific phobias, including agoraphobia, are not responsive to ß blockers.
4. Beta blockers may be of particular value in patients with anxiety disorders or symptoms who have a history or predisposition to drug dependency involving other anxiolytics.

This anxiolytic effect of ß blockers is thought to be due to ß blockade, in that the dextro-isomer of propranolol, which has little ß blocking activity, also has little antianxiety effect (Bonn & Turner, 1971).

Psychotic Disorders

Since a report by Atsmon et al. (1971), a number of investigators have assessed the therapeutic effect of ß blockers in psychotic illness (Berlant, 1987; Eccleston, Fairbairn, Hassanyeh, McClelland, & Stephens, 1985; Lipinski, Keck, & McElroy, 1988; Manchanda & Hirsch, 1986; Myers, Campbell, & Cocks, 1981; Peet, Middlemiss, & Yates, 1981). Reports can be separated into those in which ß blockers are used adjunctively (or as "add-on") to pre-existing treatment with neuroleptics versus those in which they were used alone (monotherapy). Regarding the former, Yorkston et al. (1977) reported favorably on the addition of propranolol to phenothiazine therapy in 14 patients with chronic schizophrenia, and several additional studies have generally supported this view (Alpert et al., 1990; Myers et al., 1981; Yorkston, Zaki, Malik, Morrison, & Havard, 1974).

A number of different mechanisms have been postulated for the potential efficacy of adjunctive ß blocker therapy, in that ß blockers do not seem to block dopamine in the manner demonstrated by neuroleptic medication (Hanssen et al., 1980). Possible actions could include reduction in anxiety (Lader, 1988), serotonin blockade (Eccleston et al., 1985), membrane stabilization (Hayes & Schulz, 1983), elevation of serum neuroleptic levels (Alpert et al., 1990; Silver, Yudofsky, Kogan, & Katz, 1986), or reduction in neuroleptic-induced akathisia (Lipinski et al., 1988).

When used as monotherapy, Eccleston et al. (1985) reported that propranolol produced significant benefits in both positive and negative symptoms of schizophrenia in a double-blind comparison with thioridazine. However, Manchanda and Hirsch (1986), in a placebo-controlled trial of 36 patients with acute schizophrenia, reported no clinically significant benefit from propranolol.

Most reports on ß blockers given for psychosis have involved significantly higher doses than generally are given for either cardiovascular or other psychiatric disorders, with doses ranging from 500 to greater than 2000 mg per day of propranolol (Emrich et al., 1979; Lindstrom & Persson, 1980; Shepard, 1979; Yorkston et al., 1977). Such high doses are more likely to support the idea that ß blockers are acting centrally in producing benefit (Neppe, 1989).

Berlant (1987) and Lader (1988), reviewing the literature in this area, concluded that no good evidence existed to support ß blockers as monotherapy for psychoses and that their benefit as adjunctive therapy is questionable and potentially risky. *At this time, it cannot be advocated that ß blockers (alone or adjunctively) have a role in the management of psychoses.*

Aggression

Elliott (1977) was among the first to describe the use of ß blockers for aggressive behavior. Since then a number of individual case reports (Mattes, 1985; Polakoff, Sorgi, & Ratey, 1986; Ratey, Morrill, & Oxenkrug, 1983), small case series (Sorgi, Ratey, & Polakoff, 1986; Yudofsky, Williams, & Gorman, 1981), and larger retrospective reviews (Silver & Yudofsky, 1987; Williams, Mehl, Yudofsky, Adams, & Roseman, 1982) have supported the view that ß blockers are helpful in managing aggressive rage and self-injurious behavior in patients with a variety of psychiatric diagnoses. Besides aggression occurring in individuals with mental retardation, other diagnoses that have been studied include intermittent explosive disorder, "organic aggressive syndromes," schizophrenia, organic mental disorders following head injury, drug/alcohol abuse, and dementia (Eimer, 1989; Mattes, Rosenberg, & Mays, 1984; Volavka, 1988; Yudofsky, Stevens, Silver, Barsa, & Williams, 1984). Several methodologically sound studies have also reported efficacy for ß blockers in alleviating aggression in patients with dementia and other organic brain syndromes (Alpert et al., 1990; Greendyke, Berkner, Webster, & Gulya, 1989; Greendyke & Kanter, 1986; Greendyke, Kanter, Schuster, Verstreate, & Wootton, 1986; Mattes, 1990) and schizophrenia (Ratey et al., 1992). Although most authors have speculated that the most likely mechanism of action for ß blockers' anti-aggressive efficacy is CNS ß blockade (Neppe, 1989), others have reported benefit from nadolol, a hydrophilic ß blocker with little CNS effect (Alpert et al., 1990; Ratey et al., 1987a; Ratey et al., 1987b).

Whereas there are only a few relevant reports, and few prospective controlled methodologies, there does appear to be sufficient evidence to support ß blocker use for patients with serious recurrent aggressive behavior, particularly if based in head injury or other organic mental disease (Ayd, 1985; Brizer, 1988; Mattes, 1986; Smith & Perry, 1992). *There is some justification for the use of ß blockers in treatment of resistant aggressive patients with a variety of psychiatric disorders, particularly those involving head injury.*

Akathisia

Akathisia is a syndrome of motor restlessness which occurs in up to 45% (average 20%) of patients receiving neuroleptic medication (Braude, Barnes, & Gore,

1983; Lipinski et al., 1988). Beta blockers, notably propranolol, are widely used to treat this condition (Adler, Angrist, Peselow, Corwin, & Rotrosen, 1985; Lipinski, Zubenko, Cohen, & Barreira, 1984). A randomized controlled cross-over trial (Adler et al., 1986) indicated that propranolol was superior to placebo in 12 patients. The same group of investigators who had conducted this trial reported a subsequent study in which five days of treatment with propranolol 80 mg per day and benztropine 6 mg per day were equally effective versus placebo in 28 patients with neuroleptic-induced akathisia (Adler, Peselow, Rosenthal, & Angrist, 1993). The mechanism of action for ß blockers in decreasing akathisia remains unknown, but reports of nadolol's efficacy (suggesting a peripheral mechanism) suggest a possible reduction in general arousal through peripheral ß blockade. *There are sufficient data to support the use of β blockers in low doses to treat neuroleptic-induced akathisia.*

Other Disorders

Other psychiatric disorders in which ß blockers have been prescribed include substance withdrawal (Carlsson, 1976; Carlsson & Johansson, 1971), winter depression (Schlager, 1994), attention-deficit hyperactivity disorder (Buitelaar, van der Gaag, Swaab-Barneveld, & Kuipers, 1994; Ratey, Greenberg, & Lindem, 1991), and others (Neppe, 1989). *Presently, there are insufficient data to advocate routine use of β blockers in these other conditions.*

INDICATIONS IN MENTAL RETARDATION

Clinical practice involving the use of ß blockers with people with mental retardation and developmental disabilities is based on extrapolation of research findings from the general population of people who do not have a developmental disability. At this time, there are few methodologically sound studies of the use of ß blockers in patients with mental retardation, so that firm guidelines regarding their clinical utility or indications are difficult to determine. What information is available can be separated into indications that are established and data based, those that are unproven but about which some consensus exists, and those which are speculative. A summary of the available research appears in Table 16-2.

Established/Data Based Indications

Behavioral Effects. As previously noted, some data support the use of ß blockers for some anxiety disorders, anxiety problems, aggression in the context of head injury or organic brain syndromes, and neuroleptic-induced akathisia. Of these, the only area in which ß blockers have been specifically studied in persons with mental retardation and developmental disabilities is the area of aggression. At this time, there are almost no data regarding the efficacy of ß blockers in the treatment of anxiety disorders, psychosis, neuroleptic-induced akathisia, or other psychiatric disorders in persons who have mental retardation.

Nevertheless, some data reports provide preliminary support for the use of ß blockers in aggressive or self-injurious behavioral disorders in people with mental retardation and developmental disabilities. The initial reports were anecdotal. They were based on single patients or small case series and involved open-label, non-blind treatment with ß blockers, often in conjunction with other psychotropic medications. Most reports did not include placebo controls or objective measures of change (Connor, 1994; Jenkins & Maruta, 1987; Kastner, Burlingham, & Friedman, 1990; Kuperman & Stewart, 1987; Lang & Remington, 1994; Luchins & Dojka, 1989; Matthews-Ferrari & Karroum, 1992; Polakoff et al., 1986; Ratey et al., 1983; Ratey et al., 1986; Ratey et al., 1987a; Ratey et al., 1987b; Ratey et al., 1992; Ruedrich, Grush, & Wilson, 1990; Silver & Yudofsky, 1987; Sims & Galvin, 1990; Williams et al., 1982; Yudofsky et al., 1981). Many of these included psychiatric patients both with and without mental retardation (Jenkins & Maruta, 1987; Kuperman & Stewart, 1987; Ratey et al., 1983; Ratey et al., 1987a; Ratey et al., 1987b; Ratey et al., 1992; Silver & Yudofsky, 1987; Sims & Galvin, 1990; Williams et al., 1982; Yudofsky et al., 1981).

A few reports involved single subjects or groups in which ß blockers were used with blinded and placebo-controlled methodologies. Cohen, Tsiouris, and Pfadt (1991) described a significant reduction in aggression and stereotypy in a 32-year-old male with fragile X and pervasive developmental disorder, treated with propranolol 80-320 mg per day, in comparison to placebo, over a 24-week trial (cross-over design, double-blind). In the largest series reported thus far (14 adults with autism), Ratey and Lindem (1991) found that pindolol 10-40 mg per day produced a 40% decrease in the frequency of aggression and self-injurious behavior, in comparison to a 12% decrease seen in placebo-treated controls over 16 weeks of treatment. The same investigators (Ratey & Lindem, 1991) also reported that nadolol (40-120 mg per day, 16 weeks) produced a 33% decrease in aggression in 14 additional adults with autism in comparison to placebo-treated patients (6% decrease). Both studies utilized blind raters using the Modified Overt Aggression Scale ([MOAS]; Silver & Yudofsky, 1987).

The apparent efficacy of ß blockers in decreasing aggressive or self-injurious behavior has been hypothesized to occur as a result of peripheral ß blockade of over-aroused adrenergic activity (Polakoff et al., 1986), CNS ß blockade (Baumeister & Sevin, 1990), a combination of the two (Ratey & Lindem, 1991), or serotonin agonist activity (Coccaro, 1989). Another hypothesis holds that the key factor is membrane stabilization (Ratey & Lindem, 1991). Since most of the studies evaluating ß blockade for people with mental retardation involved the concurrent use of other psychotropic drugs, usually neuroleptics, the observed effects cannot be attributed to ß blockade (Silver et al., 1986; Lipinski et al., 1988). None of the studies involving the concurrent use of ß blockers and neuroleptics in persons with mental retardation controlled for the neuroleptic serum level or presence of neuroleptic-induced akathisia, although many of the reports indicated significant behavior improvement in the face of decreased or discontinued neuroleptic medication. This latter fact would seem to argue against a neuroleptic-associated action as the primary determinant of ß blocker efficacy in these reports.

Effects on Learning/Cognition

As previously noted, the ß blockers can produce a number of deleterious and other CNS effects (Conway et al., 1978; Neppe, 1989; Thiessen et al., 1990). Lichter et al. (1986) reported mild but consistent memory deficits in patients treated with atenolol. McAnish and Cruickshank (1990) reviewed 15 studies of the effects of ß blockers on memory (four with volunteers plus 11 clinical studies) and found that most showed no effect of propranolol or atenolol on memory. However, five demonstrated some memory dysfunction with propranolol treatment. The issue was addressed further by a number of other researchers (Blumenthal, Ekelund, & Emery, 1990; Bulpitt & Fletcher, 1992; Deary, Capewell, Hajducka, & Muir, 1991; Dietrich & Herrmann, 1989; Dimsdale, Newton, & Joist, 1989; Greenblatt, Scavone, Harmatz, Engelhardt, & Shader, 1993; Palac et al., 1990; Powell, Pickering, Wyke, & Goggin, 1993; Streufert, DePadova, McGlynn, Piasecki, & Pogash, 1989), some

of whom noted methodological problems in assessing neuropsychiatric effects of ß blocking drugs, particularly when dosage schedules are for antihypertensive effect.

Many studies evaluated the effects of ß blockers on memory in non-human subjects. The results of these studies indicated a detrimental effect of ß blockers on memory function as tested by learning rate and retention (Gallagher, 1985; McGaugh, Introini-Collison, & Nagahara, 1988).

Clinical Guidelines

Several recent reviewers outlined recommendations for the use of ß blockers in treating persons with mental retardation and developmental disabilities who are verbally or physically aggressive or self-injurious (Arnold & Aman, 1991; Connor, 1993; Haspel, 1995; Ruedrich, 1996). These guidelines include the following:

1. Evaluate proposed patients with history, physical examination, and laboratory examination to exclude individuals with significant cardiovascular disease (e.g., angina, congestive heart failure), bronchoconstrictive disease (e.g., asthma, chronic obstructive pulmonary disease), insulin-dependent diabetes, significant peripheral vascular disease, hyperthyroidism, renal pathology, or ß blocker allergy. This would generally include chemistry profile, CBC, thyroid functions, and EKG.

2. Beta blockers may be an initial treatment for persons with aggression, self-injurious behavior, or rage associated with known head injury or other organic etiology. They also may be prescribed for individuals who have not responded adequately to other interventions or medications. In these latter situations, the ß blocker can be added to existing psychotropic treatment, although care must be taken when adding ß blockers to neuroleptics, anticonvulsants, or antidepressants, in that ß blockers can significantly increase the levels of these drugs to the point of toxicity. Routine monitoring of serum levels of concurrent medications should be undertaken.

3. Choice of medication is generally made on the basis of receptor selectivity, ISA, lipophilicity, and practitioner comfort and experience. Most of the available literature has focused on the use of metoprolol, nadolol, pindolol, and propranolol. The available data do not favor one of these drugs over the others, although nadolol may be favored for

Table 16-2. Psychiatric Studies of ß Blockers with at Least One-third

Authors	No. of Subjects (MR/Total)	Age Range (Years)	Characterization of Subjects	Objective Measures[a]
Yudofsky et al., 1981	1/4	22	Female	N
Williams et al., 1982	13/30	7-35	Conduct disorder Intermittent explosive disorder Pervasive developmental disorder	N
Ratey et al., 1983	2/3	25-49	Major mental disorders	N
Polakoff et al., 1986[d]	1/1	36	Severe assaultive behaviors with impulsivity	N
Ratey et al., 1986[e]	19/19	22-49	Severely retarded patients who showed assaultive or self-injurious behaviors	Y[f]
Jenkins and Maruta, 1987	4/8	14-50	Intermittent explosive disorder	N
Kuperman and Stewart, 1987	8/16	4-24	Physically aggressive behavior that played significant role in behavior management or in the psychiatric diagnosis	N
Ratey et al., 1987a and 1987b[g]	5/8	25-50	Autistic adults with assaultive and/or self-injurious behavior	N Y[h]
Luchins and Dojka, 1989	6/6	25-45	Institutionalized adults with both aggressive and self-injurious behavior	Y
Calamari et al., 1990	1/1	23	Severely retarded, female, institutionalized	Y
Kastner et al., 1990	2/2	16-23	Severe mental retardation	N
Ruedrich et al., 1990	1/1	25	Organic personality disorder, explosive type, with major motor seizure disorder	Y[i]

of the Sample With Mental Retardation or Other Developmental Disorder

Mean Dose[b] (and range)	No. Positive Responses[c]	Results
510mg	4/4 1/1 (MR)	Reduced rage previously unresponsive to phenothiazines, lithium, and ECT.
161mg (50-960)	24/30 ?/13 (MR)	Reduced rage outbursts. IQ unrelated to outcome.
197mg (90-300)	3/3 2/2 (MR)	Reduced verbal/physical assaults, temper outbursts, unprovoked rage.
200mg nadolol 80[d]	1/1 1/1 (MR)	Reduced spitting, screaming, self-induced vomiting on others, urinating on others.
120mg (40- 240)	16/19 16/19 (MR)	11 patients regarded as substantially improved, 5 as moderately improved, 3 as unchanged. Prior psychotropic drugs often reduced or discontinued. 7 subjects developed hypotension and/or bradycardia and were unable to go above 100mg/day.
175mg (80-300)	5/8 3/4 (MR)	Reduced verbal and physical aggression in 5 of 8 subjects. Based on global impressions from medical records.
164mg (80-280)	10/16 6/8 (MR)	Physical aggression rated as moderately or much improved for 10 children. Possible predictors of response: (1) presence of mental retardation, (2) nonresponders showed more bradycardia to propranolol than responders.
214mg (100-420) nadolol 120[d]	8/8 5/5 (MR)	All subjects reported to have decreased ritualized behaviors and increased attention span. Six reported as having improved social skills and greater openness to human contact. (Not clear whether the latter had MR or not) All subjects reported to show moderate to marked improvement in aggression and self-injurious behavior. In most cases, improvements were gradual, over first 6 weeks of treatment.
287mg (90-410)	5/6 5/6 (MR)	Both aggression and self-injury decreased in 5 subjects. Aggression decreased by 28% and self-injury decreased by 58%, based on incomplete summary data.
30-400mg	1/1	Dramatic decrease in aggression; modest decrease in SIB.
metoprolol 200-250mg	2/2	Alprazolam and thioridazine discontinued.
120mg (30-160)	1/1 1/1 (MR)	Reported to show fewer aggressive acts, less impulsivity, greater frustration tolerance, less self-injury.

Authors	No. of Subjects (MR/Total)	Age Range (Years)	Characterization of Subjects	Objective Measures [a]
Sims and Galvin, 1990	3/7	5-14	Children with intermittent explosive disorder, oppositional disorder, organic personality disorder, conduct disorder, etc.	N
Cohen et al., 1991	1/1	32	Severely retarded male with fragile X and PDD	Y
Ratey and Lindem, 1991	14/14	18-55	Moderate to profound retardation	MOAS, [k] NOSIE, CGI, PPVT, VABS
Ratey and Lindem, 1991	14/14	18-55	Aggressive, self-injurious adults, all met DSM III-R criteria for Autism	MOAS, NOSIE, CGI, PPVT, VABS
Ratey et al., 1992	4/16	Adult Mean age 40	Chronic inpatients, mostly schizophrenic, schizoaffective	OAS, BPRS, CGI
Matthews-Ferrari and Karroum, 1992	1/1	11	IQ 91, impulsive, hyperactive, aggressive, short attention span	N
Connor, 1994	1/1	11	PPD and pica	CAPS, [l] ABC, SIB and pica counts
Lang and Remington, 1994	1/1	14	Severe retardation, DiGeorge syndrome, severe hearing loss	Y SIB counts systematically sampled

Note. In most studies, psychotropic medication was given in conjunction with ß blockers, usually one or more neuroleptics, except for one child taking phenytoin for epilepsy in Kuperman and Stewart (1987), methylphenidate in Matthews-Ferrari and Karroum (1992).

a Before- and after-medication count of aggressive acts provided.
b Daily dose of propranolol unless otherwise specified.
c Proportion of responders for whole sample/Proportion of responders with mental retardation (MR) or other developmental disabilities.
d Nadolol used as well as propranolol (daily dose so tagged is nadolol).
e This report includes the subject described in Polakoff et al., 1986.
f Numeric data reported for 12 of 19 subjects.
g Nadolol used to replace propranolol or instead of propranolol in 3 subjects, 2 of whom were mentally retarded. Same study, with autistic and aggressive behaviors discussed in separate publications.
h Numeric data reported for 3 of 8 subjects regarding aggression and SIB, but not for autistic behavior.
i Objective measures obtained but not reported.
j Includes one child with borderline IQ.
k BPRS - Brief Psychiatric Rating Scale   OAS - Overt Aggression Scale
   CGI - Clinical Global Impression   PPVT - Peabody Picture Vocabulary Test
   MOAS - Modified Overt Aggression Scale   VABS - Vineland Adaptive Behavior Scale
   NOSIE - Nurse's Observation Scale for Inpatient Evaluation
l CAPS - Child Attention Problems Scale
   ABC - Aberrant Behavior Checklist

Mean Dose[b] (and range)	No. Positive Responses[c]	Results
99mg	5/7 1/3 (MR)[j]	Improvements seen in physical aggression, destructiveness, unpredictable rage, agitation, and impulsivity.
320mg	1/1	Dose dependent decrease in stereotypy and non-dose depdendent decrease in aggression without medication.
pindolol 10-40mg	14/14	24-week study, 16 active Rx; MOAS decreased by 40%, compared to 12% (controls); communication skills improved 47%, compared to 8% (controls); social skills improved 61%, compared to 29% (controls). Only one subject took concurrent neuroleptic.
nadolol 40-120mg	14/14	24-week study, 16 weeks active Rx; MOAS decreased 33%, compared to 6% (controls).
nadolol 40-120mg	?/4	17-week study, 15 active Rx; nadolol significantly decreased OAS and BPRS, but not CGI, compared to controls; "hyperarousal" on BPRS significantly decreased.
metaprolol 75mg	1/1	Carbamazepine produced no benefit; methylphenidate improved ADHD, but not aggression. Metoprolol decreased aggresive outbursts to zero.
propranolol 80mg, then nadolol 80mg	1/1	Previously unsuccessful trials of diphenhydramine, imipramine pemoline, methylphenidate, haloperidol. Nadolol produced significant decrease in CAPS; propranolol little benefit; pica not affected.
300mg	1/1	Fluoxetine 12mg and thioridazine 60mg per day produced no benefit; average frequency counts of SIB/10 minutes decreased from 154 to 40-70; thioridazine decreased but not discontinued.

Adapted and extended by permission from Arnold L.E. & Aman, M.G. (1991). "Beta blockers in mental retardation and developmental disorders," *Journal of Child and Adolescent Psychopharmacology, 1,* 361–383.

peripheral blockade and propranolol or metoprolol for central blockade.

4. Attempts should be made to utilize a prospective behavioral monitoring system for a reasonable baseline before initiation of medication and during treatment (see Chapter 6 for a review of possible instruments.)

5. Treatment can begin with propranolol 10-40 mg per day in divided doses, increasing the dose by 10-30 mg twice per week until a therapeutic dose is reached. Larger dose increases are more easily tolerated by adults than by adolescents or children.

6. It is necessary to monitor vital signs throughout ß blocker treatment and particularly during dosage titration. This can be done daily with inpatients and on each visit with outpatients. Heart rate of less than 50 beats per minute (60 in children/adolescents) and blood pressure less than 90 systolic should result in withholding of doses, delay in dose increase, or even decreasing total daily dose (Coffey, 1990). It is believed that individuals with mental retardation or other developmental disabilities may be sensitive to lower doses of psychotropic medication, and that more caution should be exercised in dose titration and ultimate daily dose.

For adults with developmental disabilities, this total daily dose is generally between 200-240 mg per day of propranolol (with a range from 40-400 mg per day). This is lower than the doses that have sometimes been described for the treatment of rage occurring in patients without mental retardation, where doses above 1000 mg per day have been utilized. Generally the dose can be titrated upward until cardiovascular effects appear, improvement occurs, or the dose is in the 200-300 mg per day range. Improvement may rarely occur within days of initiation; more commonly there is gradual improvement over 2-4 months of adequate treatment. A trial should not be considered a failure until an adequate dose has been administered for at least two months.

7. On discontinuing ß blocker therapy, the dose should be tapered slowly over 2-3 weeks to prevent rebound tachycardia or hypertension.

8. Following a period of successful treatment with a ß blocker, consideration should be given to an attempt to lower the dose gradually, watching for evidence of deterioration. If symptoms recur, the medication can be increased to the previously effective dose.

Clinical Observations (Not Scientifically Proven)

Behavioral Effects. There are uses for ß blockers for persons with developmental disabilities that have not been scientifically validated but are supported by clinical considerations. The first is in the treatment of various forms of anxiety or anxiety disorders; the second in the treatment of neuroleptic-induced akathisia. Few current data exist to support the use of ß blockers directly for anxiety disorders or akathisia in this population (Gross, Hull, Lytton, Hill, & Piersel, 1993). Nevertheless, these indications are supported by sound research with persons without developmental disabilities. The use of ß blockers can be extrapolated from these data for similar indications in persons with mental retardation.

Some authorities say that anxiety disorders have been underdiagnosed in persons with developmental disabilities (Levine, 1985). However, there are persons whose generalized anxiety disorder or adjustment disorder with anxiety results in adrenergic symptoms of tachycardia, diaphoresis, hypertension, tremor, and agitation; in these persons a ß blocker trial is a reasonable approach and may be preferable to treatment with a neuroleptic or benzodiazepine anxiolytic (Fahs, 1989). Although the issue of benzodiazepine and anxiolytic dependence may be somewhat less problematic in persons with developmental disabilities, the possibility of benzodiazepines causing behavioral disinhibition in this population also suggests that ß blockers is a better choice (Fahs, 1989).

ß blockers have become the treatment of choice for neuroleptic-induced akathisia. They produced fewer side effects in controlled trials than did anticholinergic medications (Adler et al., 1993). Akathisia is an under-recognized side effect of neuroleptic medication, particularly in persons with mental retardation. Such patients may not be able to self-report the restlessness and motor tension produced by these medications (Ganesh, Rao, & Cowie, 1989; Stone, May, Alvarez, & Ellman, 1989). A trial of low-dose ß blocker therapy is indicated for persons with developmental disabilities who develop motor restlessness or non-specific agitation within several weeks after the initiation of neuroleptic treatment. It also is indicated for persons who continue to manifest these symptoms after extended treatment with neuroleptics. Systematic attempts should be made to assess the duration and intensity of restlessness before a drug trial by using standardized rating scales (Bodfish, Newell, Sprague, Harper, & Lewis, 1997; Gaultieri, 1993) or videotaping methods in which results are compared for baseline and post-treatment periods. A usual therapeutic dose of propranolol is 20-60 mg per day; a clinical response should be seen within 2-4 days if the restlessness is secondary to neuroleptic-induced akathisia (Adler et al., 1993; Blaisdell, 1994). Negative effects on learning and cognition should be minimal given the low doses of propranolol used to treat this condition. However, caution still must be taken regarding drug interactions between neuroleptics and ß blockers.

There does not appear to be any role for the use of ß blockers in persons with psychosis and mental retardation.

Other Therapies and Hypotheses

Several considerations suggest that ß blockers help persons with mental retardation *uncomplicated* by concurrent psychiatric or behavioral disorders. As previously noted, ß blockers provide relief in a variety of anxiety states, particularly those with prominent somatic symptomatology, acute stress-related anxiety, and performance anxiety. All three areas, but particularly the latter two, are not well studied in persons with developmental disabilities. Of special interest is the relationship between physiological arousal and subjective anxiety; when such arousal becomes excessive, it may interfere with the capacity of the individual to process information (Sands & Ratey, 1986). Whether persons with mental retardation benefit from ß blockers given in low doses to suppress anxious over-arousal is unclear. If utilized in this manner, it would seem prudent to treat those individuals who show prominent signs of physiologic arousal in novel or threatening circumstances, where the arousal is counter-productive and interferes with the individual's habilitation and learning. Since anxiety-producing situations can arise from many experiences (Levine, 1985), ß blocker therapy should be considered only for those for whom physiological anxiety is especially frequent. Beta blockers are preferable to trials of benzodiazepines or neuroleptics. If utilized in this manner, low doses of ß blockers, on the order of magnitude of those recommended for performance anxiety (propranolol 10-60 mg) should be utilized, and patients should undergo that same pre-treatment evaluation for safety of ß blockers and standardized assessment as recommended earlier.

Consideration should be given to efforts to use medications in combination with cognitive-behavior therapy. There is very strong evidence for the use of cognitive-behavior therapy in the treatment of anxiety disorders (McNally, 1994). (At the time this chapter was prepared, a large multi-site study comparing cognitive-

behavior therapy and drug therapy for the treatment of panic disorder was nearing completion.) Recently, cognitive-behavioral researchers have shown that anxiety sensitivity (Reiss, Peterson, Gursky, & McNally, 1986) is an early risk factor for spontaenous panic attacks (see Reiss, 1997; Schmidt, Lerew, & Jackson, 1997). Independent of the frequency or intensity of physiological arousal, the presence of anxiety sensitivity beliefs predict such attacks. Reports of panic disorder and certain other types of anxiety disorders in people with mental retardation are rare (Reiss, 1994).

Researchers have made considerable progress in developing psychological measures of specific components of anxiety (Reiss, 1997). For the most part, these measures have not been adapted for use with people with mental retardation. A fear survey schedule has been adapted for this population (King, Ollendick, Gullone, Cummins, & Josephs, 1990). Moreover, the new Reiss Profile of Fundamental Goals and Motivational Sensitivities (Reiss & Havercamp, 1997) includes an assessment of anxiety sensitivity. Much more research is indicated along these lines.

CONCLUSIONS

Beta-adrenergic blocking medications have a 40-year history of use in psychiatric disorders. With appropriate pre-treatment evaluation and adequate monitoring, they can be administered safely to persons with mental retardation. Available research does not support widespread use of ß blocking medications; however, at this time, three major indications seem justified.

Anxiety Disorder. The ß blockers seem indicated for the treatment of the somatic manifestations of anxiety disorders in generalized anxiety disorder and perhaps in performance anxiety. For these individuals, a trial of ß blockers seems justified and would be preferable to approaching these symptoms with benzodiazepines or neuroleptic medication. Cognitive-behavioral techniques are effective in the treatment of many anxiety disorders and should be adapted where this is practical.

Aggression and Self-Injurious Behavior. ß blocking medications may be indicated for the treatment of aggression or self-injurious behavior not attributable to a specific psychiatric disorder. Therapeutic trials of ß blockers appear warranted with strict adherence to prescribing guidelines, after exclusion of contraindications, and following failure of behavioral interventions. Studies utilizing newer objective measures of these behaviors, with appropriate methodology and controls, are needed. Future researchers should identify the types and forms of aggression or self-injury that is ß blocker responsive and determine whether or not the response is primary or a secondary to the attenuation of autonomic overarousal and motor agitation.

Akathisia. ß blockers are indicated for the sympto-matic relief of akathisia secondary to neuroleptic therapy in persons with mental retardation. This would seem particularly true given the less-than-adequate response of akathisia to standard anticholinergic therapy. Moreover, anticholinergic medications can lead to cognitive deterioration, which is a special concern when it is used with people with mental retardation.

REFERENCES

Adler, L., Angrist, B., Peselow, E., Corwin, J., Maslanski, R., & Rotrosen, J. (1986). A controlled assessment of propranolol in the treatment of neuroleptic-induced akathisia. *British Journal of Psychiatry, 149,* 42–45.

Adler, L., Angrist, B., Peselow, E., Corwin, J., & Rotrosen, J. (1985). Efficacy of propranolol in neuroleptic-induced akathisia. *Journal of Clinical Psychopharmacology, 5,* 164–166.

Adler, L.A., Peselow, E., Rosenthal, M., & Angrist, B. (1993). A controlled comparison of the effects of propranolol, benztropine, and placebo on akathisia: An interim analysis. *Psychopharmacology Bulletin, 29,* 283–286.

Agras, W.S. (1990). Treatment of social phobias. *Journal of Clinical Psychiatry, 51* (Suppl.), 52–55.

Alpert, M., Allas, E.R., Citrome, L., Laury, G., Sison, C., & Sudilovsky, A. (1990). A double-blind, placebo-controlled study of adjunctive nadolol in the management of violent psychiatric patients. *Psychopharmacology Bulletin, 26,* 367–371.

Ananth, J. (1986). Propranolol in psychiatry: Therapeutic uses and side effects. *Neuropsychobiology, 10,* 20–27.

Arnold, L.E., & Aman, M.G. (1991). Beta-blockers in mental retardation and developmental disorders. *Journal of Child and Adolescent Psychopharmacology, 1,* 361–373.

Atsmon, A., Blum, I., Wijsenbeek, H., Maoz, B., Steiner, M., & Ziegelman, G. (1971). The short term effects of adrenergic-blocking agents in a small group of psychiatric patients: Preliminary clinical observations. *Neurologie, Psihiatrie, Neurochirurgie, 74,* 251–258.

Ayd, F.J. (1985). Propranolol for aggression: Literature review and clinical guidelines. *International Drug Therapy Newsletter, 20,* 9–12.

Bai, T.R., Webb, D., & Hamilton, M. (1982). Treatment of hypertension with beta-adrenoreceptor blocking drugs. *Journal of the Royal College of Physicians of London, 16,* 239–241.

Baumeister, A.A., & Sevin, J.A. (1990). Pharmacologic control of aberrant behavior in the mentally retarded: Toward a more rational approach. *Neuroscience and Biobehavioral Reviews, 14,* 253–262.

Benfield, P., Clissold, S.P., & Brogden, R.N. (1986). Metoprolol. *Drugs, 31,* 376–429.

Berlant, J.L. (1987). One more look at propranolol for the treatment of refractory schizophrenia. *Schizophrenia Bulletin, 13,* 705–714.

Blaisdell, G.D. (1994). Akathisia: A comprehensive review and treatment summary. *Pharmacopsychiatry, 27,* 139–146.

Blumenthal, J.A., Ekelund, L.G., & Emery, C.F. (1990). Quality of life among hypertensive patients with a diuretic background who are taking atenolol and enalapril. *Clinical Pharmacology Therapy, 48,* 447–454.

Bodfish, J.W., Newell, K.M., Sprague, R.L., Harper, V.N., & Lewis, M.H. (1997). Akathisia in adults with mental retardation: Development of the Akathisia Ratings of Movement Scale (ARMS). *American Journal on Mental Retardation, 101,* 413–423.

Bonn, J., & Turner, P. (1971). Propranolol and anxiety. *Lancet, 1,* 1355–1356.

Brantigan, C.O., Brantigan, T.A., & Joseph, N. (1982). Effect of beta-blockade and beta-stimulation on stage fright. *American Journal of Medicine, 72,* 88–94.

Braude, W.M., Barnes, T.R., & Gore, S. (1983). Clinical investigation of akathisia: A systematic investigation of acute psychiatric inpatient admissions. *British Journal of Psychiatry, 143,* 139–150.

Brizer, D.A. (1988). Psychopharmacology and the management of violent patients. *Psychiatric Clinics of North America, 11,* 551–568.

Brooks, A.M., & Gillies, W.E. (1992). Ocular beta blockers in glaucoma management: Clinical pharmacological aspects. *Drugs and Aging, 22,* 208–221.

Buitelaar, J.K., van der Gaag, R.J., Swaab-Barneveld, H., & Kuipers, M. (1994). A placebo-controlled comparison of methylphenidate and pindolol in ADHD. *Scientific Proceedings of the American Society of Child and Adolescent Psychiatry, 10,* 43.

Bulpitt, C.J., & Fletcher, A.E. (1992). Cognitive function and angiotensin converting enzyme inhibitors in comparison with other antihypertensive drugs. *Journal of Cardiovascular Pharmacology, 32* (Suppl. 6), s100–s104.

Burgess Record, N. (1981). Acebutolol-induced pleuropulmonary lupus syndrome. *Annals of Internal Medicine, 95,* 326–327.

Bygdeman, S., & Johnson, O. (1969). Studies on the effect of adrenergic blocking drugs and catecholamine-induced platelet aggregation and uptake of noradrenaline and 5HT. *Acta Physiologica Scandinavica, 75,* 129.

Calamari, J.E., McNally, R.J., Benson, D.S., & Babington, C.M. (1990). Case Study: Use of propranolol to reduce aggressive behavior in a woman who is mentally retarded. *Behavioral Residential Treatment, 5,* 287–296.

Carlsson, C. (1976). Propranolol in the treatment of alcoholism: A review. *Postgraduate Medical Journal, 52,* 166–167.

Carlsson, C., & Johansson, T. (1971). The psychological effects of propranolol in the abstinence phase of chronic alcoholics. *British Journal of Psychiatry, 119,* 605–606.

Coccaro, E.F. (1989). Central serotonin and impulsive aggression. *British Journal of Psychiatry, 155* (Suppl. 8), 52–62.

Coffey, B.J. (1990). Anxiolytics for children and adolescents: Traditional and new drugs. *Journal of Child and Adolescent Psychopharmacology, 1,* 57–83.

Cohen, I.L., Tsiouris, J.A., & Pfadt, A. (1991). Effects of long-acting propranolol on agonistic and stereotyped behaviors in a man with pervasive developmental disorder and fragile X syndrome: A double-blind, placebo-controlled study. *Journal of Clinical Psychopharmacology, 11,* 398–399.

Connor, D.F. (1993). Beta blockers for aggression: A review of the pediatric experience. *Journal of Child and Adolescent Psychopharmacology, 3,* 99–114.

Connor, D.F. (1994). Nadolol for self-injury, overactivity, inattention, and aggression in a child with pervasive developmental disorder. *Journal of Child and Adolescent Psychopharmacology, 4,* 101–111.

Conway, J., Greenwood, D.T., & Middlemiss, C. (1978). Central nervous actions of beta-adrenoreceptor antagonist. *Clinical Science and Molecular Medicine, 54,* 119–124.

Covelli, V., Antonacci, F., & Pagliarulo, E. (1983). Propranolol: Further evidence of its anti-anxiety effect. *Acta Pharmaceutica, 9,* 367–373.

Cruickshank, J.M., & Prichard, B.N.C. (1987). *Beta-blockers in clinical practice.* Edinburgh: Churchill Livingstone.

Currie, D., Lewis, R.V., McDevitt, D.G., Nicholson, A.N., & Wright, N.A. (1988). Central effects of beta-adrenergic antagonists: 1. Performance and subjective assessment of mood. *British Journal of Clinical Pharmacology, 26*, 121–128.

Deary, I.J., Capewell, S., Hajducka, C., & Muir, A.G. (1991). The effects of captopril v atenolol on memory, information processing and mood: A double-blind crossover study. *British Journal of Clinical Pharmacology, 33*, 347–353.

Dietrich, B., & Herrmann, W.M. (1989). Influence of cilazapril on memory functions and sleep behavior in comparison with metoprolol and placebo in healthy subjects. *British Journal of Clinical Pharmacology, 27*, 249s–261s.

Dimsdale, J.E., Newton, R.P., & Joist, T. (1989). Neuropsychological side effects of beta blockers. *Archives of Internal Medicine, 149*, 514–525.

Drayer, D.E. (1987). Lipophilicity, hydrophilicity, and the central nervous system side effects of beta blockers. *Pharmacotherapy, 7*, 87–91.

Drew, P.J.T., Barnes, J.N., & Evans, S.J. (1985). The effect of acute beta-adrenergic blockade on examination performance. *British Journal of Clinical Pharmacology, 19*, 783–786.

Eccleston, D., Fairbairn, A.F., Hassanyeh, F., McClelland, H.A., & Stephens, D.A. (1985). The effect of propranolol and thioridazine on negative symptoms of schizophrenia. *British Journal of Psychiatry, 147*, 623–630.

Eimer, M. (1989). Management of the behavioral symptoms associated with dementia. *Primary Care, 16*, 431–450.

Elliott, F.A. (1977). Propranolol for the control of belligerent behavior following acute brain damage. *Annals of Neurology, 1*, 438–491.

Emrich, H.M., von Zerssen, D., Moller, H.J., Kissling, W., Cordig, C., Schietsch, J.H., & Riedel, E. (1979). Action of propranolol in mania: Comparison of effects of the d- and the 1-stereoisomer. *Pharmacopsychiatrie-Neuro-Psychopharmacologie, 12*, 295–304.

Fahs, J.J. (1989). Anxiety disorders. In T.B. Karasu (Ed.), *Treatments of psychiatric disorders: A task force report of the American Psychiatric Association* (pp. 14–19, 85–90). Washington, DC: American Psychiatric Association.

Famularo, R., Kinscherff, R., & Fenton, T. (1988). Propranolol treatment for childhood posttraumatic stress disorder, acute type: A pilot study. *American Journal of Diseases of Children, 142*, 1244–1247.

Fitzgerald, J.D. (1993). Do partial agonist ß blockers have unproved clinical utility? *Cardiovascular Drugs and Therapy, 7*, 303–310.

Fitzgerald, J.D., & O'Donnell, S.R. (1971). Pharmacology of 4-hydroxypropranolol, a metabolite of propranolol. *British Journal of Pharmacology, 43*, 222–235.

Fredrickson, M., Klein, K., & Ohman, A. (1990). Do instructions modify effects of beta-adrenergic blockade on anxiety? *Psychophysiology, 27*, 309–317.

Frishman, W.H., & Lazar, E.J. (1990). Reduction of mortality, sudden death and non-fatal reinfarction with ß-adrenergic blockers in survivors of acute myocardial infarction: A new hypothesis regarding the cardioprotective action of ß-adrenergic blockade. *American Journal of Cardiology, 6*, 66G–70G.

Gallagher, M. (1985). Reviewing modulation of learning and memory, in N.M. Weinberger, J.L. McGaugh, & G. Lynch (Eds.), *Memory systems in the brain: Animal and human cognitive processes* (pp. 311–334). New York: Guilford Press.

Ganesh, S., Rao, M., & Cowie, V.A. (1989). Akathisia in neuroleptic medicated mentally handicapped subjects. *Journal of Mental Deficiency Research, 33*, 323–329.

Gengo, F.M., Hintoon, L., & McHugh, W.B. (1981). Lipid-soluble and water-soluble ß blockers: Comparison of the central nervous system dependent effect. *Archives of Internal Medicine, 147*, 39–43.

Gerber, J.G., & Nies, A.S. (1985). *Beta-adrenergic blocking drugs*. Denver CO: University of Colorado Health Sciences Center.

Gillette, D.W., & Tannery, L.P. (1994). Beta blocker inhibits tricyclic metabolism. *Journal of the American Academy of Child and Adolescent Psychiatry, 33*, 223–224.

Gold, M.H., Holy, A.K., & Roenigk, H.H. (1988). Beta-blocking drugs and psoriasis. *Journal of the American Academy of Dermatology, 19*, 37–841.

Gorman, J.M., Levy, G.F., Liebowitz, M.R., McGrath, P., Appleby, I.L., Dillon, D.J., Davies, S.O., & Klein, D.F. (1983). Effect of acute beta-adrenergic blockade on lactate-induced panic. *Archives of General Psychiatry, 40*, 1079–1082.

Granville-Grossman, K.L., & Turner, P. (1966). The effect of propranolol on anxiety. *Lancet, 1*, 788–790.

Greenblatt, D.J., Scavone, J.M., Harmatz, J.S., Engelhardt, N., & Shader, R.I. (1993). Cognitive effects of beta-adrenergic antagonists after single doses: Pharmacokinetics, pharmacodynamics of propranolol, atenolol, lorazepam and placebo. *Clinical Pharmacology Therapy, 53*, 577–584.

Greendyke, R.M., Berkner, J.P., Webster, J.C., & Gulya, A. (1989). Treatment of behavioral problems with pindolol. *Psychosomatics, 30*, 161–165.

Greendyke, R.M., & Kanter, D.R. (1986a). Therapeutic effects of pindolol on behavioral disturbances associated with organic brain disease: A double-blind study. *Journal of Clinical Psychiatry, 47*, 423–426.

Greendyke, R.M, Kanter, D.R., Schuster, D.B., Verstreate, S., & Wootton, J. (1986b). Propranolol treatment of assaultive patients with organic brain disease. *Journal of Nervous and Mental Disease, 174*, 290–294.

Greenwood, D.T. (1990). Stress, catecholamines and beta-adrenoreceptor blockade. *Postgraduate Medical Journal, 66* (Suppl.), s36–s40.

Griffen, S.J., & Friedman, M.J. (1986). Depressive symptoms in propranolol users. *Journal of Clinical Psychiatry, 47*, 453–457.

Gross, E.J., Hull, H.G., Lytton, G.T., Hill, J.A., & Piersel, W.C. (1993). Case study of neuroleptic-induced akathisia: Important implications for individuals with mental retardation. *American Journal on Mental Retardation, 98* 156–164.

Gualtieri, C.T. (1993). The problem of tardive akathisia. *Brain and Cognition, 23*, 102–109.

Hanssen, T., Heyden, T., Sundberg, I., Alfredsson, G., Nyback, H., & Wetterberg, L. (1980). Propranolol in schizophrenia. *Archives of General Psychiatry, 37*, 685–690.

Haspel, T. (1995). Beta blockers and the treatment of aggression. *Harvard Review of Psychiatry, 2*, 274–281.

Hayes, P.E., & Schulz, S.C. (1983). The use of beta-adrenergic blocking agents in anxiety disorders and schizophrenia. *Pharmacotherapy, 3*, 101–117.

Hayes, P.E., & Schulz, S.C. (1987). Beta blockers in anxiety disorders. *Journal of Affective Disorders, 13*, 119–130.

Hjorth, S., & Carlsson, A. (1986). Is pindolol a mixed agonist/antagonist at central serotonin (5-HT) receptors? *European Journal of Pharmacology, 129*, 131–138.

Hoffman, B.B., & Lefkowitz, R.J. (1996). Catecholamines, sympathomimetic drugs, and adrenergic receptor antagonists, In J.G. Hardman, A.G. Gilman and L.E. Limbird (Eds.), *Goodman and Gilman's the pharmacological basis of therapeutics*, (9th ed., pp. 199–248). New York: McGraw Hill.

Holroyd, K.A., France, J.L., Cordingley, G.E., Rokicki, L.A., Kvaal, S.A., Lipchik, G.L., & McCool, H.R. (1995). Enhancing the effectiveness of relaxation-thermal biofeedback training with propranolol hydrochloride. *Journal of Consulting and Clinical Psychology, 63*, 327–330.

Hoyer, D. (1988). Functional correlates of serotonin 5-HT1 recognition sites. *Journal of Receptor Research, 8*, 59–81.

James, I.M., Griffith, D.N.W., Pearson, R.M., & Newbury, P. (1977). Effect of oxprenolol on stage fright in musicians. *Lancet, 2*, 952–954.

Jefferson, J.W. (1974). Beta-adrenergic blocking drugs in psychiatry. *Archives of General Psychiatry, 31*, 681–691.

Jenkins, S.C., & Maruta, T. (1987). Therapeutic use of propranolol for intermittent explosive disorder. *Mayo Clinic Proceedings, 62*, 204–214.

Kastner, T., Burlingham, K., & Friedman, D.L. (1990). Metoprolol for aggressive behavior in persons with mental retardation.

American Family Physician, 42, 1595–1588.

Kathol, R.G., Noyes, R., Slyman, D.J., Crowe, R.R., Clancy, J., & Kerber, R.E. (1980). Propranolol in chronic anxiety disorders. *Archives of General Psychiatry, 37,* 1361–1365.

King, N.J., Ollendick, T.H., Gullone, E., Cummins, R.A., Josephs, A. (1990). Fear and phobias in children and adolescents with intellectual disabilities: Assessment and intervention strategies. *Australia and New Zealand Journal of Devepmental Disablities, 16,* 97–108.

Kuperman, S., & Stewart, M.A. (1987). Use of propranolol to decrease aggressive outbursts in younger patients. *Psychosomatics, 28,* 315–319.

Lader, M. (1988). Beta adrenoceptor antagonists in neuropsychiatry: An update. *Journal of Clinical Psychiatry, 49,* 213–223.

Lang, C., & Remington, D. (1994). Treatment with propranolol of severe self-injurious behavior in a blind, deaf, retarded adolescent. *Journal of the American Academy of Child and Adolescent Psychiatry, 33,* 265–269.

Lepautalo, M. (1985). Chronic effects of labetolol, pindolol, and propranolol on calf blood flow in intermittent claudication. *Clinical Pharmacology and Therapeutics, 37,* 7–12.

Levine, H.G. (1985). Situational anxiety and everyday life experiences of mildly mentally retarded adults. *American Journal of Mental Deficiency, 90,* 27–33.

Lewis, R.V., Jackson, P.R., & Ramsay, L.E. (1984). Quantification of side effects of beta-adrenoreceptor blockers using visual analogue scales. *British Journal of Clinical Pharmacology, 18,* 325–330.

Lewis, R.V., & McDevitt, D.G. (1986). Adverse reactions and interactions with beta-adrenergic blocking drugs. *Medical Toxicology and Adverse Drug Experience, 1,* 343–361.

Lewis, R.V., & Lofthouse, C. (1993). Adverse reactions with beta-adrenergic blocking drugs. *Drug Safety, 9,* 272–279.

Lichter, I., Richardson, P.J., & Wyke, M.A. (1986). Differential effects of atenolol and enalapril on memory during treatment for essential hypertension. *British Journal of Clinical Pharmacology, 21,* 641–645.

Lindstrom, L.H., & Persson E. (1980). Propranolol in chronic schizophrenia: A controlled study of neuroleptic-treated patients. *British Journal of Psychiatry, 137,* 126–130.

Lipinski, J.F., Keck, P.E., & McElroy, S. (1988). Beta adrenergic antagonists in psychosis: Is improvement due to treatment of neuroleptic-induced akathisia? *Journal of Clinical Psychopharmacology, 8,* 409–416.

Lipinski, J.F., Zubenko, G.S., Cohen, B.M., & Barreira, P.J. (1984). Propranolol in the treatment of neuroleptic-induced akathisia. *British Journal of Psychiatry, 141,* 412–415.

Luchins, D.J., & Dojka, M.S. (1989). Lithium and propranolol in aggression and self-injurious behavior in the mentally retarded. *Psychopharmacology Bulletin, 25,* 372–375.

Manchanda, R. (1988). Propranolol: The wonder drug for psychiatric disorders? *British Journal of Hospital Medicine, 39,* 267–271.

Manchanda, R., & Hirsch, S. (1986). Does propranolol have an antipsychotic effect? A placebo-controlled study in acute schizophrenia. *British Journal of Psychiatry, 148,* 701–707.

Mathew, N.T. (1981). Prophylaxis of migraine and mixed headache: A randomized controlled study. *Headache, 21,* 105–109.

Mattes, J.A. (1985). Metroprolol for intermittent explosive disorder. *American Journal of Psychiatry, 142,* 1108–1109.

Mattes, J.A. (1986). Psychopharmacology of temper outbursts: A review. *Journal of Nervous and Mental Disease, 174,* 464–470.

Mattes, J.A. (1990). Comparative effectiveness of carbamazepine and propranolol for rage outbursts. *Journal of Neurophsychiatry, 2,* 159–164.

Mattes, J.A., Rosenberg, J., & Mays, D. (1984). Carbamazepine versus propranolol in patients with uncontrolled rage outbursts: A random assignment study. *Psychopharmacology Bulletin, 20,* 98–100.

Matthews-Ferrari, K., & Karroum, N. (1992). Metoprolol for aggression [Letter to the editor]. *Journal of the American Academy of Child and Adolescent Psychiatry, 31,* 994.

Matuzas, W., & Jack, E. (1991). The drug treatment of panic disorders. *Psychological Medicine, 9,* 213–215.

McAnish, J., & Cruickshank, J.M. (1990). Beta-blockers and central nervous system side effects. *Pharmacology and Therapeutics, 46,* 163–197.

McGaugh, J.L., Introini-Collison, I.B., & Nagahara, A.H. (1988). Memory-enhacing effects of post-training naloxone: Involvement of ß-noradrenergic influences in the amygdaloid complex. *Brain Research, 444,* 37–49.

McNally, R.J. (1994). *Panic disorder.* New York: Guilford Press.

Meibach, R.C., Mullane, J.F., & Binstok G. (1987). A placebo-controlled multi-center trial of propranolol and chlordiazepoxide in the treatment of anxiety. *Critical Therapy Research, 41,* 65–76.

Myers, D.H., Campbell, P.L., & Cocks, N.M. (1981). A trial of propranolol in chronic schizophrenia. *British Journal of Psychiatry, 139,* 105–111.

Neppe, V.M. (1989). *Innovative Psychopharmacotherapy.* New York: Raven Press.

Noyes, R., Jr. (1982). Beta-blocking drugs and anxiety. *Psychosomatics, 23,* 155–170.

Noyes, R., Jr. (1985). Beta-adrenergic blocking drugs in anxiety and stress. *Psychiatric Clinics of North America, 8,* 119–132.

Palac, D., Cornish, R.D., McDonald, W.J., Middaugh, D.A., Howieson, D., & Bagby, S.P. (1990). Cognitive functioning in hypertensives treated with atenolol or propranolol. *Journal of General Internal Medicine, 5,* 310–318.

Palacios, J.R., & Kuhar, M.J. (1980). Beta-adrenergic-receptor localization by light microscopic autoradiography. *Science, 208,* 1378–1380.

Peet, M., & Ali, S. (1986). Propranolol and atenolol in the treatment of anxiety. *International Journal of Psychopharmacology, 1,* 314–319.

Peet, M., Middlemiss, D.N., & Yates, R.A. (1981). Propranolol in schizophrenia: II. Clinical and biochemical aspects of combining propranolol with chlorpromazine. *British Journal of Psychiatry, 138,* 112–117.

Petrie, W.M., Maffucci, R.J., & Woosley, R.L. (1982). Propranolol and depression. *American Journal of Psychiatry, 139,* 92–93.

Polakoff, S.A., Sorgi, P.J., & Ratey, J.J. (1986). The treatment of impulsive and aggressive behavior with nadolol. *Journal of Clinical Psychopharmacology, 6,* 125–126.

Powell, J., Pickering, A., Wyke, M., & Goggin, T. (1993). The effects of antihypertensive medication on learning and memory. *British Journal of Clinical Pharmacology, 35,* 105–113.

Prichard, B.N.C. (1978). Beta-adrenergic receptor blockade in hypertension, past, present and future. *British Journal of Clinical Psychopharmacology, 5,* 379–399.

Rabkin, S.W. (1993). Mechanisms of action of adrenergic receptor blockers on lipids during antihypertensive drug treatment. *Journal of Clinical Pharmacology, 33,* 286–291.

Ratey, J.J., Bemporad, J., Sorgi, P., Polakoff, S., Bick, P., O'Driscoll, G., & Mikkelsen, E. (1987a). Brief report: Open trial effects of beta blockers on speech and social behaviors in 8 autistic adults. *Journal of Autism and Developmental Disorders, 17,* 439–446.

Ratey, J.J., Greenberg, M.S., & Lindem, K.J. (1991). Combination of treatment for attention deficit hyperactivity disorder in adults. *Journal of Nervous and Mental Disease, 179,* 699–701.

Ratey, J.J., & Lindem, K.J. (1991). Beta blockers as primary treatment for aggression and self-injury in the developmentally disabled. In J.J. Ratey (Ed.), *Mental Retardation: Developing pharmacotherapies* (pp. 51–82). Washington, DC: American Psychiatric Association.

Ratey, J.J., Mikkelsen, E.J., Smith, G.B., Upadhyaya, A., Zuckerman, H.S., Marello, D., Sorgi, P., Polakoff, S., & Bemporad, J. (1986). Beta blockers in the severely and profoundly mentally retarded. *Journal of Clinical Psychopharmacology, 6,* 103–107.

Ratey, J.J., Mikkelsen, E., Sorgi, P.,

Zuckerman, S., Polakoff, S., Bemporad, J., Bick, P., & Kaddish, W. (1987b). Autism: The treatment of aggressive behaviors. *Journal of Clinical Psychopharmacology, 7*, 35–41.

Ratey, J.J., Morrill, R., & Oxenkrug, G. (1983). Use of propranolol for provoked and unprovoked episodes of rage. *American Journal of Psychiatry, 140*, 1356–1357.

Ratey, J.J., Sorgi, P., O'Driscoll, G.A., Sands, S., Daehler, M.L., Fletcher, J.R., Kadish, W., Spruiell, G., Polakoff, S., Lindem, K.J., Bemporad, J.R. Richardson, L., & Rosenfeld, B. (1992). Nadolol to treat aggression and psychotic symptomatology in chronic psychiatric inpatients: A double-blind, placebo-controlled study. *Journal of Clinical Psychiatry, 53*, 41–46.

Reiss, S. (1997). Trait anxiety: It's not what you think it is. *Journal of Anxiety Disorders, 11*, 201–214.

Reiss, S. (1994). *Handbook of challenging behavior: Mental health aspects of mental retardation.* Worthington, OH: IDS Publishing.

Reiss, S., & Havercamp, S.M. (1997). *The development of a scale to measure aberrant motivation in persons with mental retardation.* Unpublished manuscript, The Ohio State University Nisonger Center.

Reiss, S., Peterson, R.A., Gursky, D.M., & McNally, R.J. (1986). Anxiety sensitivity, anxiety frequency, and the prediction of fearfulness. *Behaviour Research and Therapy, 24*, 1–8.

Ruedrich, S.L., Grush, L., & Wilson, J. (1990). Beta adrenergic blocking medications for aggressive or self-injurious mentally retarded persons. *American Journal on Mental Retardation 95*, 110–119.

Ruedrich, S.L. (1996) Beta adrenergic blocking medications for treatment of rage outbursts in mentally retarded persons. *Seminars in Clinical Neuropsychiatry, 1*, 115–121.

Sands, S., & Ratey, J.J. (1986). The concept of noise. *Psychiatry, 49*, 290–297.

Saul, P., Jones, B.P., Edwards, K.G., & Tweed, J.A. (1985). Randomized comparison of atenolol and placebo in the treatment of anxiety: A double-blind study. *European Journal of Clinical Pharmacology, 28*(Suppl.), 109–110.

Schlager, D. (1994). Early-morning administration of short-acting ß blockers for treatment of winter depression. *American Journal of Psychiatry, 151*, 1383–1385.

Schmidt, N.B., Lerew, D.R., & Jackson, R.L. (1997). The role of anxiety sensitivity in the pathogenesis of panic: Prospective evaluation of spontaneous panic attacks during acute stress. *Journal of Abnormal Psychology, 3*, 355–364.

Shand, D.G. (1975). Drug therapy: Propranolol. *New England Journal of Medicine, 293*, 280–284.

Shepard, G. (1979). High dose propranolol and schizophrenia. *British Journal of Psychiatry, 134*, 470–476.

Silver, J., & Yudofsky, S. (1987). Documentation of aggression in the assessment of the violent patient. *American Journal of Psychiatry, 143*, 1290–1292.

Silver, J.M., Yudofsky, S.C., Kogan, M., & Katz, B.L. (1986). Elevation of thioridazine plasma levels by propranolol. *American Journal of Psychiatry, 143*, 1290–1292.

Sims, J., & Galvin, M.R. (1990). Pediatric psychopharmacologic uses of propranolol. *Journal of Child and Adolescent Psychiatric Mental Health Nursing, 3*, 18–24.

Smith, D.A., & Perry, P.J. (1992). Non-neuroleptic treatment of disruptive behavior in organic mental syndromes. *The Annals of Pharmacotherapy, 26*, 1400–1408.

Solomon, S., Hutchkiss, E., Saravay, S.M., Bayer, C., Ramsey, P., & Blum, R.S. (1983). Impairment of memory function by antihypertensive medication. *Archives of General Psychiatry, 41*, 1109–1112.

Sorgi, P., Ratey, J.J., Knoedler, D., Arnold, W., & Cole, L. (1992). Depression during treatment with beta blockers: Results from a double-blind, placebo-controlled study. *Journal of Neuropsychiatry and Clinical Neurosciences, 4*, 187–189.

Sorgi, P.J., Ratey, J.J., & Polakoff, S. (1986). Beta-adrenergic blockers for the control of aggressive behavior in patients with chronic schizophrenia. *American Journal of Psychiatry, 143*, 775–776.

Spar, J.E., & La Rue, A. (1990). *Concise guide to geriatric psychiatry* (pp. 11–37). Washington, DC: American Psychiatric Association Press.

Stone, R.K., May, J.E., Alvarez, W.F., & Ellman, G. (1989). Prevalence of dyskinesia and related movement disorders in a developmentally disabled population. *Journal of Mental Deficiency Research, 33*, 41–53.

Streufert, S., DePadova, A., McGlynn, T., Piasecki, M., & Pogash, R. (1989). Effects of beta-blockade with metoprolol on simple and complex task performance. *Health Physiology, 8*(2), 143–158.

Tanna, V.T., Penningroth, R.P., & Woolson, R.F. (1977). Propranolol in the treatment of anxiety neurosis. *Comprehensive Psychiatry, 18*, 319–326.

Thiessen, B.Q., Wallace, S.M., Blackburn, J.L., Wilson, T.W., & Bergman, U. (1990). Increased prescribing of antidepressants subsequent to beta blocker therapy. *Archives of Internal Medicine, 150*, 2286–2290.

Tyrer, P. (1988). Current status of beta-blocking drugs in the treatment of anxiety disorders. *Drugs, 36*, 773–783.

Volavka, J. (1988). Can aggressive behavior in humans be modified by beta blockers? *Postgraduate Medicine,* (Special Number), 163–168.

Weksler, B.B., Gillick, M., & Pink, J. (1977). Effect of propranolol on platelet function. *Blood, 49*, 185.

Weinstock, M., & Weiss, C. (1980). Antagonism by propranolol of isolation-induced aggression in mice: Correlation with 5-hydroxytryptamine receptor blockade. *Neuropharmacology, 19*, 653–656.

Widerhorn, J., Rubin, J.N., Frishman, W.H., & Elkayam, V. (1987). Cardiovascular drugs in pregnancy. *Cardiology Clinics, 5*, 651–674.

Williams, D.T., Mehl, R., Yudofsky, S., Adams, D., & Roseman, B. (1982). The effect of propranolol on uncontrolled rage outbursts in children and adolescents with organic brain dysfunction. *Journal of the American Academy of Child Psychiatry, 21*, 129–135.

Wood, A.J.J., Carr, K., Vestal, R.E., Belcher, S., Wilkinson, G.R., & Shad, H.G. (1978). Direct measurement of propranolol bioavailability during accumulation to steady state. *British Journal of Clinical Pharmacology, 6*, 345–350.

Wright, P. (1975). Untoward effects associated with practolol administration: Oculomucocutaneous syndrome. *British Medical Journal, 1*, 595–598.

Yorkston, N.J., Gurzelier, J.H., Zaki, S.A., Hollander, D., Pitcher, D.R., & Sergeant, H.G. (1977). Propranolol as an adjunct to the treatment of schizophrenia. *Lancet, 2*, 575–578.

Yorkston, N.J., Zaki, S.A., Malik, M.K.U., Morrison, R.C., & Havard, C.W.H. (1974). Propranolol in the control of schizophrenic symptoms. *British Medical Journal, 4*, 633–635.

Young, R.C., & Myers, B.S. (1991). Psychopharmacology. In J. Sadavoy, L.W. Lazarus, & L.F. Jaruk (Eds.), *Comprehensive review of geriatric psychiatry,* (pp 435–468). Washington, DC: American Psychiatric Association Press.

Yudofsky, S.C. (1992). Beta blockers and depression: The clinician's dilemma. *Journal of the American Medical Association, 267*, 1826–1827.

Yudofsky, S.C., Stevens, L., Silver, J., Barsa, J., & Williams, D. (1984). Propranolol in the treatment of rage and violent behavior associated with Korsakoff's psychosis. *American Journal of Psychiatry, 141*, 114–115.

Yudofsky, S.C., Williams, D., & Gorman, J. (1981). Propranolol in the treatment of rage and violent behavior in patients with chronic brain syndrome. *American Journal of Psychiatry, 138*, 218–230.

Opiate Blockers

Curt A. Sandman[1], Travis Thompson[2], Rowland P. Barrett[3],
Willem M.A. Verhoeven[4], James A. McCubbin[5], Stephen R. Schroeder[6], and William P. Hetrick[7]

Opioid blockers are a class of compounds that antagonize endogenous opioid receptors. The first clinically useful opiate blocker—nalorphine—was described in the early 1900s and was used in the treatment of opioid toxicity (Archer, 1980). Nalorphine was not a pure opioid antagonist but rather a partial kappa agonist that possessed significant dysphoric effects. The search for pure antagonists led to the synthesis in the 1960s of naloxone hydrochloride (Narcan) and naltrexone hydrochloride (ReVia, formerly called Trexan). Naloxone and naltrexone reversibly block the mu-opioid receptor, have few effects in the absence of exogenously administered or endogenously released (i.e., during physical stress) opioids, and are currently the most commonly administered drugs in this class. Naltrexone is structurally and functionally similar to naloxone; the primary differences are that naltrexone is administered orally, is more potent, and has a longer duration of bioactivity. Throughout this chapter, the terms *opioid blocker* and *opioid antagonist* will be used interchangeably.

The primary therapeutic use of opioid antagonists is for the treatment of acute opiate overdose. Recently, naltrexone was labeled for use in the treatment of alcohol dependency and also has been used as an adjunctive treatment for narcotic dependence. Naltrexone was designated an orphan drug by the U. S. Food and Drug Administration for use with people with mental retardation or with developmental delay and may be administered to children and adults at the physician's discretion.

Opioid antagonists are among the newest psychoactive drugs used to treat self-injurious behavior (SIB) and symptoms of autism. Researchers have proposed three noteworthy hypotheses for treating SIB with opioid antagonists (Barron & Sandman, 1985; Deutsch, 1986; Sandman, 1990/1991; Sandman & Hetrick, 1995). As discussed later in this chapter, these hypotheses suggest that opioid antagonists may eliminate the motivation for SIB, lower pain sensory thresholds so that SIB is experienced as painful in individuals who otherwise do not experience much pain, and restore regulation of the stress system. The rationale for treating autistic symptoms is that the drugs antagonize the excessive brain opioid activity that is hypothesized to underlie social, communicative, and attentional disturbances (Panksepp, 1979). The first reports of the effects of opiate antagonists on autistic features were published in the early 1980s and described the suppression of SIB with acute naloxone treatment. The majority of subsequent published studies were focused on the efficacy of naltrexone, which has a therapeutic advantage over naloxone. For this reason, this chapter focuses on naltrexone.

PHARMACODYNAMICS AND PHARMACOKINETICS

Both naloxone and naltrexone are pure opioid antagonists with primary affinity for mu-receptors and have few, if any, agonist effects (Martin, 1983). Both drugs reversibly block the effects of opioids by competitive binding at mu-receptors primarily, but also at kappa- and sigma-opioid receptors (McEvoy, Litvak, & Welsh, 1995). These drugs block the subjective and addictive effects of intravenously administered opioids and are known to antagonize the effects of endogenously-mediated opioid activity (Jaffe & Martin, 1991). On a weight basis, naltrexone's antagonist activity is reportedly 2 to 9 times more than that of naloxone. Naltrexone's primary metabolite, $6\text{-}\beta\text{-naltrexol}$, has weaker opioid antagonist effects on a weight basis than naltrexone, but its concentrations in plasma are 2 to 4 times greater and its duration of action longer. The drug's antagonistic effects are linearly related to dose and

1 Professor-in-Residence, Department of Psychobiology, Department of Psychiatry and Human Behavior, University of California, Irvine, CA
2 Professor of Psychology and Director of John F. Kennedy Center, Vanderbilt University, Nashville, TN
3 Associate Professor of Psychiatry, Brown University, Providence, RI
4 Director of Residency Training, Vincent Van Gogh Institute of Psychiatry, Vanray, The Netherlands
5 Professor and Chairman, Department of Psychology, Clemson University, Clemson, SC
6 Director of Schiefelbusch Institute for Life Span Studies, University of Kansas
7 Department of Psychology, Ohio State University, Columbus, OH

systemic availability (Meyer, Straughn, Lo, Schary, & Whitney, 1984; Verebey, Volavka, Mule, & Resnick, 1976). Single doses block the pharmacologic effects of intravenously administered heroin for up to 24 hours at 50 mg, 48 hours at 100 mg, and 72 hours at 150 mg (see Gonzalez & Brogden, 1988).

Naltrexone is orally administered and is absorbed (about 95%) by the gastrointestinal tract (McEvoy et al., 1995). The drug is 80% to 95% metabolized during the first pass through the liver, primarily to 6-β-naltrexol (Meyer et al., 1984). The onset of opioid antagonism is 15 to 30 minutes after ingestion, and plasma levels of naltrexone and 6-β-naltrexol peak between 1 and 2 hours after administration (Verebey et al., 1976). Naltrexone and β-naltrexol decline in a triphasic manner (through alpha, beta, and gamma stages) in plasma (McEvoy et al., 1995). The beta half-lives of naltrexone and β-naltrexol are about 4 and 12 hours, whereas the gamma (terminal) phases are about 18 and 96 hours, respectively (Meyer et al., 1984; Verebey et al., 1976). Receptor binding data indicate that the half-life of mu-receptor blockade in the brain by 50 mg of naltrexone is between 72 and 108 hours in humans (Lee et al., 1988). The percentage of receptor blockade at 48, 72, 120, and 168 hours after 50 mg of naltrexone was 91%, 80%, 46%, and 30%, respectively, demonstrating the extended duration of action produced with a small dose of naltrexone.

Daily administration of naltrexone increases plasma 6-β-naltrexol concentrations by about 40% (McEvoy et al., 1995), and a steady-state equilibrium of the drug and its major metabolite is achieved within 24 hours, that is, after the second dose (Verebey et al., 1976). Because elevated plasma concentrations of 6-β-naltrexol are strongly associated with increased pharmacodynamic effects (Verebey et al., 1976), the increased potency of naltrexone resulting from chronic dosing must be considered carefully when extrapolating from data that were based on single-administration protocols.

SYSTEM AND PHYSICAL EFFECTS

The opioid antagonists appear to be well tolerated in humans. Even at high doses of naltrexone, subjective effects are rarely reported (Gonzalez & Brogden, 1988). Naltrexone has few, if any, intrinsic actions in humans besides the opioid-blocking properties. Some reports suggest that it can produce pupillary constriction, miosis,

increased blood pressure, increased sensory-evoked potential amplitude, decreased EEG alpha and beta frequency, decreased respiratory rate, or decreased body temperature (Gonzalez & Brogden, 1988; McEvoy et al., 1995). Naltrexone may possess appetite suppressant qualities but no persistent, clinically significant effects on human obesity have been observed (Atkinson, 1987; Mitchell et al., 1987; Spiegel et al., 1987). In people with autism, acute naltrexone treatment does not significantly influence body weight (Campbell et al., 1989, 1993; Gonzalez et al., 1994).

Naltrexone's endocrine effects in humans are not well understood, but an increase in plasma LH has been observed (Veldhuis, Rogol, & Johnson, 1983). Naloxone has been shown to increase plasma epinephrine, ACTH, cortisol, and beta-endorphin-like immunoreactivity in some subjects (McCubbin, Surwit, Williams, Nemeroff, & McNeilly, 1989). Preliminary data from studies of people with autism (Ernst et al., 1993) or with mental retardation (Sandman, Hetrick, Chicz-DeMet, & Taylor, 1995) indicated that plasma beta-endorphin concentrations were not systematically affected by naltrexone treatment. Subjective and physical effects have been reported in a few individuals and primarily at doses exceeding commonly used therapeutic levels (0.5 to 2.0 mg/kg per day).

SIDE EFFECTS

Naltrexone appears to be a safe drug without serious side effects. Treatment studies of people with developmental disabilities generally support this opinion (e.g., Barrett, Feinstein, & Hole, 1989; Campbell et al., 1989, 1993; Herman, Hammock, Arthur-Smith, Kuehl, & Appelgate, 1989; Kolmen, Feldman, Handen, & Janosky, 1995; Sandman et al., 1993; Thompson, Hackenberg, Cerutti, Baker, and Axtell, 1994). Sandman (1995) evaluated side effects of naltrexone treatment in 10 individuals with mental retardation who exhibited SIB. Based on ratings on the Naltrexone Side Effects Scale, no significant side effects were observed at the end of six months of treatment for any individual in the study. (See Figure 17-1.)

About 10% of people treated with naltrexone develop one or more of the following symptoms: difficulty sleeping, transient anxiety, nervousness, abdominal pain or cramps, nausea, low energy, joint and muscle pain, and headache. In a study of naltrexone treatment for alcoholism, Volpicelli, Alterman, Hayashida, and O'Brien (1992) reported that two patients developed nausea and one showed increased pain from arthritis. There were no mood or psychiatric changes associated with the treatment. In another study of alcohol dependency, the majority of the subjects tolerated well 50 mg/day naltrexone but some nausea, dizzi-

ness, and weight loss were reported (O'Malley et al., 1992). Kenny (1994) found that naltrexone was effective (but glucocorticoids were not) in reducing self-mutilation in three of five zoo animals. No adverse effects were noted and two successfully treated male animals eventually sired healthy offspring. Some concern has been raised about cardiovascular changes

Figure 17-1. Naltrexone Side Effects Scale
D.V. Taylor, C.A. Sandman, & W.P. Hetrick
University of California Irvine & Fairview Developmental Center
Costa Mesa, CA 92626

Client: _____   Date of Evaluation: _____

Evaluator: _____   Shift (circle one): AM / PM / NOCs

Notes: _____

Please evaluate the client for signs or complaints of the following side effects using the scale below. Circle the appropriate number.

1 = No symptoms observed or reported.
2 = Symptoms almost never seen.
3 = Symptoms seldom seen.
4 = Symptoms observed frequently.
5 = Symptoms are a constant characteristic of client's condition.

#	Item	Response				
1.	Yawning or apparent drowsiness	1	2	3	4	5
2.	Loss of energy	1	2	3	4	5
3.	Sleeps more than usual	1	2	3	4	5
4.	Sleeps less than usual	1	2	3	4	5
5.	Anxiety and nervousness	1	2	3	4	5
6.	Abdominal discomfort	1	2	3	4	5
7.	Vomiting	1	2	3	4	5
8.	Loss of appetite	1	2	3	4	5
9.	Excessive runny nose or mucosal discharge	1	2	3	4	5
10.	Skin rash or irritation	1	2	3	4	5
11.	Blurred vision	1	2	3	4	5
12.	Chills or shivering	1	2	3	4	5
13.	Increased thirst	1	2	3	4	5

(e.g., increased blood pressure and tachycardia) caused by naltrexone; however, careful studies among individuals with SIB generally showed there are no effects on heart rate or blood pressure outside the normal range (Thompson et al., 1994). In young children with autism, naltrexone did not significantly change pulse, blood pressure, respiration, or weight (Campbell et al., 1989; Herman et al., 1989; Kolmen et al., 1995). Campbell et al. (1993) found that overall ratings of adverse effects were equivalent for naltrexone and a placebo condition, although a few children taking naltrexone developed sedation, vomiting, and decreased appetite.

Withdrawal Effects

Discontinuation of naltrexone after prolonged administration does not precipitate a withdrawal syndrome. Discontinuation of other opioid antagonists, such as cyclaozine and nalorphine, can produce effects similar to, but not as intense as those of morphine withdrawal (Jaffe & Martin, 1991). There is no evidence that naltrexone produces drug craving or physical dependence; moreover, people with opiate addictions who are treated with naltrexone do not view the effects as pleasurable.

Naloxone and naltrexone can precipitate withdrawal symptoms in opiate-dependent individuals, but chronic administration of either drug does not appear to result in psychological or physical dependence. However, data from animal studies suggest that chronic treatment (8 days) with naltrexone increases the density of opiate receptors in the CNS and produces opioid sensitivity (Yoburn, Duttaroy, Shah, & Davis, 1994; Yoburn, Luke, Pasternak, & Inturisi, 1988). Marley et al. (1995) found that repeated administration of naltrexone in rats may result in both decreased mu-receptor binding in the midbrain and increased mu-receptor binding in the hindbrain. Naltrexone increased delta-receptors in both mid- and hindbrain. No effects were observed in the cortex. The authors reported moderately increased behavioral sensitivity for the drug. These effects may modify the efficacy of long-term naltrexone treatment and explain the durable, apparent carry-over effects (i.e., reduced SIB) that are occasionally observed following termination of naltrexone (Barrett et al., 1989; Crews, Bonaventura, Rowe, & Bonsie, 1993; Panksepp & Lensing, 1993; Walters, Barrett, Feinstein, Mercurio, & Hole, 1990).

Hepatotoxicity

Concern has been expressed about the use of naltrexone for individuals with elevated liver enzymes (Medical Economics Data, 1996). However, researchers have found no effect of naltrexone on liver functioning in both adults and children with mental retardation and developmental disabilities (Barrett et al., 1989; Bernstein, Hughes, Mitchell, & Thompson, 1987; Campbell et al., 1989; Herman et al., 1989; Kolmen et al., 1995; Leboyer et al., 1992). Liver toxicity has been reported with high doses (300 mg/day) and for obese subjects (Mitchell et al., 1987), but not under other conditions.

The effects of prolonged naltrexone treatment on serum concentrations of liver enzymes were studied for one patient with developmental delay, SIB, and persistent viral hepatitis (Hetrick et al., 1993). The client was treated with 25 mg/day for 5 months. Serial blood samples were collected over a six-year period, preceding and including the treatment period. At dosage levels necessary for the treatment of SIB, naltrexone did not exacerbate hepatocellular damage (serum glutamate oxaloacetic transaminase [SGOT], serum glutamate pyruvate transaminase [SGPT], alkaline phosphatase [ALP], lactate dehydrogenase [LDH], albumin, and bilirubin).

Sandman (1995) studied the hepatotoxic effects of six-months treatment with naltrexone for 10 people with mental retardation and developmental disabilities. Serial assessments of ALP, LDH, SGOT, and SGPT were made. During drug treatment none of the subjects had enzyme levels above the normal range. These results are consistent with previous findings that SGOT and SGPT were not elevated in eight individuals receiving acute treatment of naltrexone for one week (Thompson et al., 1994).

Recently, naltrexone was used to treat dyskinesia associated with Huntington's disease in a group of 10 patients (Sax, Kornetsky, & Kim, 1994). Doses of 50 to 300 mg/day were administered for 10-36 months. For one subject, initiation of naltrexone treatment resulted in dose-related increases in SGOT and SGPT, and another subject had increases in SGPT. However, these elevations decreased to normal levels with continued treatment, and no changes in hepatic function were observed in the other subjects. In persons with heroin addictions, long-term treatment with naltrexone did not significantly change hepatic enzyme levels (Braden, Capone, & Capone, 1988; Pini, Ferretti, Trenti, Ferrari, & Sternieri, 1991).

Other Side Effects

Barrett et al. (1989) reported visual impairment in a patient with SIB after a treatment combination of naltrexone and chlorpromazine. The patient, a positive responder to naltrexone, experienced an abrupt loss of vision in both eyes during downward titration from chlorpromazine while receiving naltrexone. Treatment with corticosteriods partially restored vision. However, this and other adverse reactions were not found for two adults with developmental disabilities and SIB who continuously received chlorpromazine during an acute, double-blind, multiple-dose naltrexone treatment study (Sandman et al., 1993). Although visual impairment is not associated with the use of naltrexone alone, the interaction between naltrexone treatment and titration from chlorpromazine may constitute a risk.

In a study of 24 volunteers, one person with post-traumatic stress disorder exhibited unusual hypervigilance and anger outbursts after a single, double-blind dose of 50 mg of naltrexone (Ibarra et al., 1994). The symptoms were distorted vision, paranoid behavior, and increased cardiovascular responses. Increased aggression was reported for another patient who showed decreased SIB under naltrexone treatment (Taylor et al., 1991) and some panic symptoms were observed in two patients with autism (Panksepp & Lensing, 1991). Anecdotal reports in recent studies suggest that a minority of individuals with SIB who are treated with naltrexone show increased agitation (Sandman, 1995). Several investigators have found that up to about 10% of patients may show increased SIB after changes in dose of naltrexone (Barrett, 1992; Sandman, 1995). For the most part, adverse effects are rarely observed with naltrexone treatment in the therapeutic dose range of 0.5 to 2.0 mg/kg.

CLINICAL INDICATIONS EXCLUSIVE OF MENTAL RETARDATION

The initial and primary use of opioid antagonists was for the treatment of opioid poisoning. However, researchers have found additional clinical applications. Two separate, double-blind studies of 97 (O'Malley et al., 1992) and 70 (Volpicelli et al., 1992) people with alcoholism showed that naltrexone improved abstention rates and reduced relapse in drinking-related problems. Both groups of researchers concluded that naltrexone may be an effective adjunctive therapy for alcohol-dependent subjects.

Opioid antagonists may prevent some stress-related overeating and suppress appetite, although these effects are not clinically significant (Atkinson, 1987; Mitchell et al., 1987; Spiegel et al., 1987). One case study indicated that naltrexone was effective in the treatment of bulimia nervosa; naltrexone decreased the urge to binge and increased plasma beta-endorphin levels (Chatoor, Herfman, & Harzler, 1994). Two studies with patients with Tourette syndrome yielded inconsistent results. One double-blind clinical trial with 10 patients with Tourette syndrome showed that naltrexone reduced self-reported frequency of tics but not tic severity, attentional ability, or obsessive-compulsive symptoms (Kurlan et al., 1991). However, these effects were not found consistently in a second study of 10 Tourette patients (Muller, Putz, & Straube, 1994). In a study of Rett syndrome, 4 of 10 patients deteriorated one or more clinical stages after naltrexone, compared to none of the patients tested with placebo (Percy et al., 1994). This deleterious effect cautions against the use of naltrexone in this population.

Opiate antagonists improve both learning acquisition and retention in animals (Aigner & Mishkin, 1988; Flood, Cherkin, & Morley, 1987; Gallagher & Kapp, 1978; Gallagher, King, & Young, 1983). They increase the arousal necessary for learning by removing the tonic inhibitory influences of opioids on adrenergic and dopaminergic tone (Izquierdo & Dias, 1980; Izquierdo & Gradients, 1980; McGaugh, Ines, & Nagahara, 1988) and by decreasing inhibitory effects of opiate peptides on acetylcholinergic neurons (Botticelli & Wurtman, 1981, 1982). Memory-enhancing effects do not appear to be pronounced in healthy people (Cohen, Cohen, Weingartner, & Murphy, 1983; Morley et al., 1980). Treatment with naltrexone, however, has resulted in improved memory consolidation for Alzheimer's patients (Reisberg, Ferris, & Anand, 1983) and in enhanced event-related potentials and normalized reaction times in a young woman with a mental illness (Sandman, Barron, Crinella, & Donnelly, 1987). For people with mental retardation and developmental disabilities, improved paired associate learning was reported for an adolescent boy (Taylor et al., 1991) and improvement on several parameters of learning, including independence and compliance, was reported for adults (Sandman et al., 1993). However, one study showed no effect of naltrexone on discrimination learning in children with autism (Campbell et al., 1993).

INDICATIONS IN MENTAL RETARDATION

Indications Based on Established Data

In a review of pre-1991 studies on naloxone, Sandman (1990/1991) found eight published studies in which injectable naloxone was tested in a total of 10 individuals with SIB. A decrease in SIB was reported for 7 individuals. Sandman (1990/1991) also summarized 12 published studies of naltrexone treatment, most of which were case studies or studies with very small samples. Of 45 people with mental retardation and developmental disabilities who had been treated with naltrexone, 38 had positive responses of various degrees, including 24 of 28 people with SIB. A review of 13 studies (including several in the Sandman 1990/1991 review) concluded that about one-third of the patients treated with naltrexone experienced decreased SIB (Verhoeven & Tuinier, in press). Several studies in this second review included juvenile patients under the age of 8 (Campbell et al., 1993) and patients with primary behavioral problems related to aggression and agitation (Zingarelli et al., 1992). These two groups should be considered separately because immature nervous systems may respond to naltrexone differently than do mature nervous systems and because aggression and agitation are not etiologically or phenomenologically similar to SIB. Aman (1993) also reviewed much of this literature. He concluded that a suppression of SIB occurred in 11 of 22 studies; for the remaining 11 studies, the results were equivocal in 7 and negative in 4. Aman observed that uncontrolled case reports generally were more positive than were controlled studies and concluded that there was a need for more outcome research before firm conclusions can be drawn.

The results of three recent placebo-controlled studies of the effects of naltrexone on SIB have been reported. Sandman et al. (1993) found that, in a double-blind, placebo-controlled, dose-finding study, 18 of 21 individuals with SIB responded favorably to at least one of the doses, which ranged from 0.5 mg/kg to 2.0 mg/kg. In this study, each individual was observed directly for 1,200 minutes. Acute treatment, defined as one week at each of three doses of naltrexone, reduced the frequency of SIB without producing major side effects. Rated behavior, activity, stereotypy, involuntary movement, and neurological status were not influenced by naltrexone. The researchers found that the highest dose (2 mg/kg) was the most effective for reducing SIB, confirm-

ing earlier results obtained for this population (Sandman, Barron, Chicz-DeMet, & DeMet, 1990). Of 8 patients who responded best at the highest dose, 7 also responded favorably to the 1.0 mg/kg dose; and 6 responded at the 0.5 mg/kg dose. Eleven subjects responded positively to both the 1.0 and 2.0 mg/kg doses. Another noteworthy finding was that subjects with the most frequent SIB were the most positive responders to higher doses of naltrexone (between 1 and 2 mg/kg), consistent with previous findings of this dosage range (Herman et al., 1987; Sandman et al., 1990). A small minority of subjects responded most favorably to lower doses.

Thompson et al. (1994) reported results of a double-blind, placebo-controlled, fixed-dose study of eight adults with severe to profound retardation. They concluded that treatment with naltrexone reduced head hitting, head banging, and self-biting. The eight individuals evaluated displayed 18 forms of SIB. Improvement was observed in 77% of the head-hitting and head-banging episodes and in 100% of the self-biting forms. Episodes of high-frequency SIB also were sensitive to treatment with naltrexone. The 100 mg dose was more effective than the 50 mg dose in reducing SIB. For several individuals, some forms of SIB (e.g., head hitting and self-biting) decreased after naltrexone treatment was started, but other forms (e.g., throat poking) did not change. Four of the subjects in this trial received concomitant treatment with clonidine, but no effects on SIB or interactions with naltrexone were observed. These findings suggested that naltrexone may be effective for treating some forms of SIB but ineffective for other forms of SIB.

In contrast to these results, Willemsen-Swinkels, Buitelaar, Nijhof, and van Engeland (1995) reported results of a double-blind, placebo-controlled study of 35 adults with autism, 11 of whom had SIB. Outcomes were assessed by means of direct observation ($\underline{n}$=11) and on the basis of scores on standardized rating scales. This was a two-phase study including a single acute dose (100 mg) phase and a long-term phase in which individuals received either fixed doses of 50 mg or 150 mg. For both the acute and long-term phases, observations of SIB were based on only 40 minutes for each individual. The reported results were unfavorable. Naltrexone treatment was not observed to have therapeutic effects on SIB and autism. The investigators noted some evidence that drug treatment was associated with a worsening of behavioral conditions. The investigators questioned the effectiveness of naltrexone, asserting that all previous reports of benefits were obtained in methodologically flawed studies. However, methodological limitations in this study may have accounted for the negative finding. The results were based on many fewer minutes (40 versus 1200) of observations than in Sandman et al. (1993), the ratings of behavior were global, and only 11 subjects had SIB. The results may be subject to reinterpretation; they are largely consistent with the hypothesis that naltrexone does not improve the complex symptoms of autism, but rather has specific effects on SIB.

Most published reports of long-term effects of naltrexone on SIB are case studies. In the first, a total of 24 days of naltrexone treatment resulted in the elimination of SIB in a 12-year-old girl that persisted for at least 22 months (Barrett et al., 1989). A similar finding was reported after one year of continuous treatment with naltrexone in a 28-year-old woman with severe SIB. Not only did treatment eliminate SIB, but also the near-zero rate persisted through placebo and no-drug phases (> 6 months) of the study (Crews et al., 1993). A one-year trial of naltrexone reduced SIB and stereotypic motor behaviors and increased social behavior in two women with developmental disabilities (Smith, Gupta, & Smith, 1995). These positive effects ceased when naltrexone was withdrawn, but were restored with subsequent treatment. Additionally, positive long-term effects were reported in three of four people with severe mental retardation and autism treated for as long as a year with open-labeled naltrexone (Panksepp & Lensing, 1991).

In a recent clinical trial to test the long-term effectiveness of naltrexone in 25 individuals with SIB and developmental delay, 18 responded positively during an acute dose-finding phase (Sandman, 1995). Seven of the individuals continued to improve during long-term treatment; 4 had positive responses during an initial six-month treatment phase, continuing through a two-month drug holiday. However, their SIB increased *after* the drug holiday period was over when the previously effective dose of naltrexone was resumed. For two individuals, SIB was controlled by increasing the dose by 0.5 mg/kg. Three others showed significant decreases in one type of SIB but not in other forms of SIB. In one case, naltrexone eliminated life-threatening head-banging behavior, but did not influence less severe, frequent behaviors such as head slapping.

The effects of naltrexone on behavioral symptoms in young children with autism have, for the most part, been modest. Improvements in ratings of hyperactivity and restlessness have been the only consistent findings across studies with sample sizes of 10 or more, but these observations may have been related to observed sedative effects (Campbell et al., 1989, 1993; Kolmen et al., 1995). A careful, placebo-controlled study of 13 children with autism between the ages of 3 and 8 showed that 8 children improved on several criteria (Kolmen et al., 1995). Of these 8, 4 showed increased communication initiation in an interaction with an adult and decreased actometer or disruptive behavior ratings. These results are consistent with those that have suggested that naltrexone may increase social behavior (e.g., verbal production and eye contact) and decrease SIB and stereotypies for children with autism (Barrett et al., 1989; Campbell et al., 1989; Lensing et al., 1992; Panksepp & Lensing, 1991).

Indications Based on Clinical Observations

The primary, perhaps sole, application of opioid antagonists in mental retardation and developmental disabilities is for SIB. The *symptom* of self-injury appears to be selectively influenced by naltrexone, although the effect may occur only for some people and only for certain types of SIB. Treatment benefits seem most likely with adolescents and adults and less likely with children prior to puberty. Treatment with naltrexone has had some benefit in about half of the patients examined. High-frequency SIB, SIB directed at the head, and self-biting appear especially sensitive to treatment. Daily and every-other-day dosing has been reported, although our experience favors every-other-day dosing. Doses between 1.0 and 2.0 mg/kg or a fixed dose between 50 and 100 mg (depending on the size of the patient) are the most effective for reducing SIB. The most effective dose for a given individual must be tailored by a careful dose-finding protocol.

An analysis of the risk:benefit ratio may support a trial of naltrexone in many cases of SIB because naltrexone appears to be a safe drug without major or contraindicating side effects and alternative treatments have limited effectiveness. Most individuals who had entered into naltrexone trials had exhibited severe SIB for which other forms of treatment had been ineffective. They had not responded to electric shock, protective shielding for the body, physical restraint, other medications, and sedation. Often the SIB had potentially life-threatening consequences and prevented enjoyment of a less restrictive environment. In this context, the possible benefits of a significant reduction in some form of SIB by treatment with naltrexone outweighed the risks of possible adverse side effects. As far as we could determine, there have been no serious side effects attributable solely to the administration of naltrexone for people with mental retardation and developmental disabilities.

A careful study by Campbell et al. (1993) showed that naltrexone was ineffective in reducing core autistic symptoms, including SIB, in children under 8 years old. This conclusion is at variance with Campbell's earlier studies and the study of Kolmen et al. (1995). The application of naltrexone treatment to young children requires additional study. Treatment of SIB with naltrexone should be applied to individuals with a mature (post-pubescent) nervous system.

Treatment with naltrexone should be avoided during pregnancy. Naloxone administered to pregnant women during the late third trimester reduced fetal distress (Goodlin, 1981); however, it resulted in increased pain during childbirth for the mother. Kenny (1994) reported that two zoo animals successfully treated for self-mutilation sired healthy offspring. Naltrexone also should be avoided when patients are known to be in pain requiring narcotic analgesics, for example, for post surgical patients or those with bone fractures. Furthermore, alternate plans for treatment of severe, acute pain should be maintained for patients receiving naltrexone. Non-steroidal anti-inflammatory drugs may be used for this purpose. Figure 17-2 provides guidelines for managing pain in patients maintained on opiate antagonists.

HYPOTHESES OF THE ROLE OF OPIATES IN SELF-INJURY

Three hypotheses have emerged to explain why endogenous opiates may be responsible for maintaining SIB. Whether or not any of these hypotheses is valid is not known at this time; however, research findings on naltrexone are compatible with each hypothesis. One hypothesis is that individuals who self-injure may have elevated sensory thresholds for pain. Most people with SIB do not exhibit the usual signs of experiencing pain when they cut or hurt themselves. Perhaps SIB is related to both insensitivity to pain and a general sensory depression induced either by elevated endogenous opiates or by super-sensitive opiate receptors (Cataldo & Harris, 1982; Deutsch, 1986; Sandman, 1988; Sandman et al., 1983). These possibilities are supported by findings that opiate receptor blockers (a) reverse congenital insensitivity to pain (Dehen, Willer, Boureau, & Cambier, 1977), (b) reverse hypothalamic-peptide dysfunction coexisting with elevated pain threshold (Dunger, Leonard, Wolff, & Preece, 1980), and (c) increase brain responses to sensory information (Arnsten et al., 1983). These observations are consistent with extensive research

Figure 17-2. Sample Protocol for Inducing Non-opioid Analgesia
Prepared by V.P. Martinazzi, Pharm.D.
Fairview Developmental Center
Costa Mesa, CA 92626

FIRST

If clinically appropriate, use an orally administered non-steroidal anti-inflammatory drug (NSAID) up to a maximum dose (e.g., ibuprofen, 3.2 g/day; naproxen, 1.25 g/day). Terminate naltrexone treatment.

OR

If clinically warranted, analgesia *may* be achieved more rapidly with the injectable NSAID agent ketorolac (the only NSAID currently available for pain in injectable form). Administer 60 mg of ketorolac intra-muscularly (IM) as a loading dose followed by 30 mg every six hours. For individuals weighing 50 kg or less, the loading dose should be 30 mg IM followed by a maintenance dose of 15 mg every six hours. Treatment should be limited to no longer than 5 days.

Ketorolac has compared favorably to meperidine and morphine in the short-term treatment of moderate to severe postoperative pain. The onset of analgesia can be ten minutes, but peak analgesic effects may take 1 to 2 hours. Adverse effects and contraindications must be considered on a case-by-case basis.

SECOND

Opioid agonists (narcotics) are not recommended for treatment of pain experienced by individuals treated with naltrexone. However, in an emergency situation, cautious use of a rapidly-acting narcotic may be necessary with the understanding that higher-than-normal doses may be required. Adverse effects of narcotics must be carefully considered.

on animals indicating that opioid antagonists lower the pain threshold (e.g., Sandman et al., 1979). Taken together, these findings support a pain hypothesis that implies that self-injurious individuals do not feel pain because they have chronically elevated endogenous opiates or opiate receptor disregulation.

Another hypothesis is that the addictive properties of opiates may be responsible for maintaining SIB. If painful SIB results in the release of opiates, then perhaps individuals commit self-inflicted harm to receive the euphoric effects of increased opiates. From this perspective, SIB constitutes an addiction to the endogenous opiate system. The addictive properties of beta-endorphins have been indicated by studies showing development of tolerance (Lal, 1975; Madden, Akil, Patrick, & Barchas, 1977), physical dependence (Wei & Loh, 1976), and euphoric effects after repeated administration (Belluzzi & Stein, 1977). The repetitive, often compulsive and ritualistic patterns of SIB (e.g., injury to one area of the head or body, stereotyped patterns of behavior, catastrophic responses if the environment is slightly changed) are similar to rituals and compulsive patterns often associated with addictive behaviors. The addiction hypothesis maintains that individuals with SIB may endure the pain to enjoy the pleasure it produces, as well as to avoid a withdrawal effect.

A third hypothesis is that some people may use SIB to modulate stress. The opiate system is a component of the general stress response of the hypothalamic-pituitary-adrenal (HPA) axis. For instance, beta-endorphin is co-released from the anterior pituitary with ACTH in response to a variety of stressors. Both of these peptides are contained in the pre-protein molecule, proopiomelanocortin, and both are controlled by the hypothalamic peptide corticotropin-releasing hormone. It is unknown if stress uncouples the HPA system and SIB is an attempt to regulate the system, or if SIB is the event that deregulates the HPA axis (Verhoeven & Tuinier, 1995). Because SIB appears to elevate beta-endorphin (Sandman & Hetrick, 1995; Tuinier & Verhoeven, 1995a, 1995b), it may disregulate the HPA arousal system (Verhoeven & Tuinier, in press). Naltrexone, therefore, may be effective because it regulates this arousal system. This hypothesis predicts that naltrexone should be most effective in the early stages of development of aberrant behaviors such as SIB and stereotypy.

Some informal reports indicated that naltrexone may be an effective treatment for SIB for periods of months, after which SIB may reappear. One clinical observation linked the reappearance of SIB after effective control with naltrexone to a painful accident that the patient experienced. This interesting possibility may relate to hyperalgesia after naltrexone and is worthy of systematic investigation.

CONCLUSION

Naltrexone may be an important pharmacological agent for the treatment of SIB. The available data suggest that at least some people with SIB experience significant short-term improvement, although long-term benefits require additional study. The rate of positive response in studies that directly observed behavior was between 35% and 70% for the individuals tested. One recent study showed no positive responders (Willemsen-Swinkels et al., 1995), although the failure to find benefit may have been a consequence of inadequate observation. The individuals who may be most likely to respond positively to naltrexone are those with frequent SIB involving their heads and those who bite themselves. Three hypotheses have been advanced to explain the effects of naltrexone in reducing SIB, but much additional research is needed to test the validity of these hypotheses. Some recent reports have suggested that a reduction in SIB may be predicted by an increase in beta-endorphins after an SIB episode. Additional controlled research is needed to evaluate in more detail the nature of the effects of this medication.

A risk:benefit analysis will support the use of naltrexone in many cases, especially when alternative treatments have been found to be ineffective and the SIB poses health risks. Many of the people treated with naltrexone have had severe and frequent SIB and have been intractable to all other treatments. Naltrexone is a relatively safe drug with minor side effects, although caution should be exercised if it is used with chlorpromazine, if chlorpromazine is withdrawn during treatment with naltrexone, for people with liver disease or elevated liver enzymes, and for pregnant women.

REFERENCES

Aigner, T.G., & Mishkin, M. (1988). Improved recognition memory in monkeys following naloxone administration. *Psychopharmacology, 94*, 21–23.

Aman, M.G. (1993). Efficacy of psychotropic drugs for reducing self-injurious behavior in the developmental disabilities. *Annals of Clinical Psychiatry, 5*, 171–188.

Archer, S. (1980). Historical perspective on the chemistry and development of naltrexone. In R.E. Willette & G. Barnett (Eds.), *NIDA research monograph 28. Narcotic antagonists: Naltrexone pharmacochemistry and sustained-release preparations* (pp. 3–9). Rockville, MD: National Institute on Drug Abuse.

Arnsten, A.F., Segal, D.S., Neville, H.B., Hillyard, S.A., Janowsky, D.S., Judd, L.L., & Bloom, F.S. (1983). Naloxone augments electrophysiological signs of selective attention in man. *Nature, 304*, 725–727.

Atkinson, R.L. (1987). Opioid regulation of food intake and body weight in humans. *Federal Proceedings, 46*, 178–182.

Barrett, R.P. (1992, December). *Advances in the treatment of self-injurious behavior in children and adolescents with autism and mental retardation: The opiate antagonists.* East Providence, RI: Brown University, School of Medicine, Department of Psychiatry and Human Behavior.

Barrett, R.P., Feinstein, C., & Hole, W.T. (1989). Effects of naloxone and naltrexone on self-injury: A double-blind, placebo-controlled analysis. *American Journal on Mental Retardation, 93*, 644–651.

Barron, J.L., & Sandman, C.A. (1985). Paradoxical excitement to sedative-hypnotics in mentally retarded clients. *American Journal of Mental Deficiency, 2*, 124–129.

Belluzzi J.D., & Stein, L. (1977). Enkephalin may mediate euphoria and drive-reduction reward. *Nature, 266*, 556–558.

Bernstein, G.A., Hughes, R.J., Mitchell, J.E., & Thompson, T. (1987). Effects of narcotic antagonists in self-injurious behavior: A single case study. *Journal of the American Academy of Child and Adolescent Psychiatry, 26*, 886–889.

Botticelli, L.J., & Wurtman, R.J. (1981). Choline reverses naloxone-induced decreases in hippocampal acetylcholine content and suppresses escape behavior in opiate-dependent rats. *Brain Research, 210*, 479–484.

Botticelli, L.J., & Wurtman, R.J. (1982). Septohippocampal cholinergic neurons are regulated trans-synaptically by endorphin and corticotropin neuropeptides. *Journal of Neuroscience, 2*, 1316–1321.

Braden, L.S., Capone, T.J., & Capone, D.M. (1988). Naltrexone: Lack of effect on hepatic enzymes. *Journal of Clinical Pharmacology, 28*, 64–70.

Campbell, M., Anderson, L.T., Small, A.M., Adams, P., Gonzalez, N.M., & Ernst, M. (1993). Naltrexone in autistic children: Behavioral symptoms and attentional learning. *Journal of the American Academy of Child and Adolescent Psychiatry, 32*, 1283–1291.

Campbell, M., Overall, J.E., Small, A.M., Sokol, M.S., Spencer, E.K., Adams, P., Foltz, R.L., Monti, K.M., Perry, R., Nobler, M., & Roberts, E. (1989). Naltrexone in autistic children: An acute open dose tolerance trial. *Journal of the American Academy of Child and Adolescent Psychiatry, 28*, 200–206.

Cataldo, M.F., & Harris, J. (1982). The biological basis for self-injury in the mentally retarded. *Analysis of the Intervention of Developmental Disabilities, 2*, 21–39.

Chatoor, I., Herfman, B.H., & Harzler, J. (1994). Effects of opiate antagonist, naltrexone, on binging antecedents and plasma beta-endorphin concentrations. *Journal of the American Academy of Child and Adolescent Psychiatry, 33*, 748–752.

Cohen, R.M., Cohen, M.R., Weingartner, H., & Murphy, D. (1983). High dose naloxone affects task performance in normal human subjects. *Psychiatric Research, 8*, 127–136.

Crews, W.D., Jr., Bonaventura, S., Rowe, F.B., & Bonsie, D. (1993). Cessation of long-term naltrexone therapy and self-injury: A case study. *Research in Developmental Disabilities, 14*, 331–340.

Dehen, H., Willer, J.C., Boureau, F., & Cambier, J. (1977). Congenital insensitivity to pain, and endogenous morphine-like substances. *Lancet, 2*, 293–294.

Deutsch, S.I. (1986). Rationale for the administration of opiate antagonists in treating infantile autism. *American Journal on Mental Retardation, 90*, 631–635.

Dunger, D.B., Leonard, J.V., Wolff, O.H., & Preece, A. (1980). Effect of naloxone in a previously undescribed hypothalamic syndrome. *Lancet, 2*, 1277–1281.

Ernst, M., Devi, L., Silva, R.R., Gonzalez, N.M., Small, A.M., Malone, R.P., & Campbell, M. (1993). Plasma beta-endorphin levels, naltrexone, and Haloperidol in autistic children. *Psychopharmacology Bulletin, 29*, 221–227.

Flood, J.F., Cherkin, A., & Morley, J.E. (1987). Antagonism of endogenous opioids modulates memory processing. *Brain Research, 422*, 218–234.

Gallagher, M., & Kapp, B. S. (1978). Manipulation of opiate activity in the amygdala alters memory processes. *Life Sciences, 23*, 1973–1978.

Gallagher, M., King, R. A., & Young, N. B. (1983). Opiate antagonists improve spatial memory. *Science, 221*, 975–976.

Gonzalez, J.P., & Brogden, R.N. (1988). Naltrexone: A review of its pharmacodynamic and pharmacokinetic properties and therapeutic efficacy in the management of opioid dependence. *Drugs, 35*, 192–213.

Gonzalez, N.M., Campbell, M., Small, A.M., Shay, J., Bluhm, L.D., Adams, P.B., & Frotz, R.L. (1994). Naltrexone plasma levels, clinical response and effect on weight in autistic children. *Psychopharmacology Bulletin, 30*, 203–208.

Herman, B.H., Hammock, M.K., Arthur-Smith, A., Egan, J., Chatoor, I., Werner, A., & Zelnik, N. (1987). Naltrexone decreases self-injurious behavior. *Annals of Neurology, 22*, 550–552.

Herman, B.H., Hammock, M.K., Arthur-Smith, A., Kuehl, K., & Applegate, K. (1989). Effects of acute administration of naltrexone on cardiovascular function, body temperature, body weight, and serum concentrations of liver enzymes in autistic children. *Developmental Pharmacology Therapeutics, 12*, 118–127.

Hetrick, W.P., Rusu, L., Krutzik, M., Taylor, D., Martinazzi, V., & Sandman, C.A. (1993). Naltrexone has no hepatoxic effects in a self-injurious patient with chronic hepatitis. *Journal of Clinical Psychopharmacology, 13*, 46.

Ibarra, P., Bruehl, S.P., McCubbin, J.A., Carlson, C.R., Wilson, J.F., Norton, J.A., & Montgomery, T.B. (1994). An unusual reaction to opioid blockade with naltrexone in a case of post-traumatic stress disorder. *Journal of Traumatic Stress, 7*, 303–309.

Izquierdo, I., & Dias, R.D. (1980). Effect of ACTH, epinephrine, beta-endorphin, naloxone, and the combination of naloxone and beta-endorphin with ACTH or epinephrine on memory consolidation. *Psychoneuroendocrinology, 8*, 81–87.

Izquierdo, I., & Gradients, M. (1980). Memory facilitation by naloxone is due to release of dopaminergic and beta-adrenergic systems from tonic inhibition. *Psychopharmacology, 67*, 265–268.

Jaffe, J.H., & Martin, W.R. (1991). Opioid analgesics and antagonists. In A.G. Goodman, T.W. Rall, A.S. Neis, & P.Taylor (Eds.), *Goodman and Gilman's the pharmacological basis of therapeutics* (pp. 485–521). Elmsford, NY: Pergamon Press.

Kenny, D.E. (1994). Use of naltrexone for treatment of psychogenically induced dermatoses in five zoo animals. *Journal of the American Veterinary Medical Association, 205*, 1021–1023.

Kolmen, B.K., Feldman, H.M., Handen, B.L., & Janosky, J.E. (1995). Naltrexone in young autistic children: A double-blind, placebo-controlled crossover study. *Journal of the American Academy of Child and Adolescent Psychiatry, 34*, 223–231.

Kurlan, R., Majamar, L., Deeley, C., Mudholkar, G.S., Plumb, S., & Como, P.G. (1991). A controlled trial of propoxphene and naltrexone with Tourette's syndrome. *Annals of Neurology, 30*, 19–23.

Lal, H. (1975). Narcotic dependence, narcotic action and dopamine receptors. *Life Sciences, 17*, 483–495.

Leboyer, M., Bouvard, M.P., Launay, J.M., Tabuteau, F., Waller, D., Dugas, M., Kerdelhue, B., Lensing, P., & Panksepp, J. (1992). Brief report: A double-blind study of naltrexone in infantile autism. *Journal of Autism and Developmental Disorders, 22*, 309–319.

Lee, M.C., Wagner, H.N., Jr., Tanada, S., Frost, J.J., Bice, A.N., & Dannals, R.F. (1988).

Duration of occupancy of opiate receptors by naltrexone. *The Journal of Nuclear Medicine, 29,* 1207–1211.

Lensing, P., Klinger, D., Lampl, C., Leboyer, M., Bouvard, M., Plumet., M.H., & Panksepp, J. (1992). Naltrexone open trial with a 5-year-old-boy: A social rebound reaction. *Acta Paedopsychiatrica, 55,* 169–173.

Madden, J.I., Akil, H., Patrick, R.L., & Barchas, J.D. (1977). Stress-induced parallel changes in central opioid levels and pain responsiveness in the rat. *Nature, 265,* 358–360.

Marley, R.J., Shimosato, K., Gewiss, M., Thorndike, E., Goldberg, S.R., & Schindler, C.W. (1995). Long-term sensitization to the behavioral effects of naltrexone is associated with regionally specific changes in the number of mu and delta opioid receptors in rat brain. *Life Sciences, 56,* 767–774.

Martin, W.R. (1983). Pharmacology of opioids. *Pharmacological Review, 35,* 283–323.

McCubbin, J., Surwit, R., Williams, R., Nemeroff, C., & McNeilly, M. (1989). Altered pituitary hormone response to naltrexone in hypertension development. *Hypertension, 7,* 808–811.

McEvoy, G.K., Litvak, K., & Welsh, O.H. (Eds.). (1995). *AHFS drug information.* Bethesda, MD: American Society of Health-System Pharmacists.

McGaugh, J.L., Ines, B.I.C., & Nagahara, A. (1988). Memory-enhancing effects of post-training naloxone: Involvement of beta-noradrenergic influences in the amygdaloid complex. *Brain Research, 446,* 37–49.

Medical Economics Data. (1996). *Physicians' desk reference* (50th ed.). Montvale, NJ: Author.

Meyer, M.C., Straughn, A.B., Lo, M., Schary, W., & Whitney, C.C. (1984). Bioequivalence, dose-proportionality, and pharmacokinetics of naltrexone after oral administration. *Journal of Clinical Psychiatry, 45,* 15–19.

Mitchell, J.E., Morley, J.E., Levine, A.S., Hatsukami, D., Gannon, M., & Pfohl, D. (1987). High-dose naltrexone therapy and dietary counseling for obesity. *Biological Psychiatry, 22,* 35–42.

Morley, J. E., Barenetsky, H. G., Wengert, T. D., Hershman, H. E., Melmed, J. M., Levin, S. R., Jamison, K., Weitzman, R., Chang, J., & Vaner, A. A. (1980). Endocrine effects of naloxone-induced opiate receptor blockade. *Journal of Clinical Endocrinology and Metabolism, 50,* 251–257.

Muller, N., Putz, A., & Straube, A. (1994). The opiate system in Gilles de la Tourette syndrome: Diverse effects of naltrexone treatment. *European Psychiatry, 9,* 39–44.

O'Malley, S.S., Jaffe, A.J., Change, G., Schottenfeld, R.S., Meyer, R.E., & Roundsaville, B. (1992). Naltrexone and coping skills therapy for alcohol dependence: A controlled study. *Archives of General Psychiatry, 49,* 881–887.

Panksepp, J. (1979). A neurochemical theory of autism. *Trends in Neuroscience, 2,* 174–177.

Panksepp, J., & Lensing, P. (1991). Brief report: A synopsis of an open-trial of naltrexone treatment of autism with four children. *Journal of Autism and Developmental Disorders, 21,* 243–249.

Percy, A.K., Glaze, D.G., Schultz, R.J., Zoghbi, H.Y., Williamson, D., Frost, J.D., Jr., Jankovic, J.J., del Juco, D., Skender, M., & Waring, S. (1994). Rett syndrome: Controlled study of an oral opiate antagonist, naltrexone. *Annals of Neurology, 35,* 466–470.

Pini, L.A., Ferretti, C., Trenti, T., Ferrari, A., & Sternieri, E. (1991). Effects of long-term treatment with naltrexone on hepatic enzyme activity. *Drug Metabolism and Drug Interactions, 9,* 161–174.

Reisberg, B., Ferris, S. H., & Anand, R. (1983). Effects of naloxone in senile dementia: A double-blind trial. *New England Journal of Medicine, 308,* 721–722.

Reisine, T., & Pasternak, G. (1996). Opioid analgesics and antagonists. In J.G. Hardman, L.E. Limbird, P.B. Molinoff, R.W. Ruddon, & A.G. Gilman (Eds.), *The pharmacological basis of therapeutics* (pp. 521–556). New York: McGraw-Hill.

Sandman, C.A. (1988). Beta-endorphin disregulation in autistic and self-injurious behavior: A neurodevelopmental hypothesis. *Synapse, 2,* 193–199.

Sandman, C.A. (1990/1991). The opiate hypothesis in autism and self-injury. *Journal of Child Adolescent Psychopharmacology, 1,* 235–246.

Sandman, C.A., Barron, J.L., Chicz-DeMet, A., & DeMet, E. (1990). Plasma beta-endorphin levels in patients with self-injurious behavior and stereotypy. *American Journal on Mental Retardation, 95,* 84–92.

Sandman, C.A. (1995). *Efficacy of naltrexone in self-injurious behavior: Final report.* Washington, DC: U.S. Food and Drug Administration.

Sandman, C. A., Barron, J. L., Crinella, F. M., & Donnelly, J. (1987). The influence of naloxone on the brain and behavior of a self-injurious woman. *Biological Psychiatry, 22,* 899–906.

Sandman, C.A., Datta, P.C., Barron-Quinn, J., Hoehler, F.K., Williams, C., & Swanson, J.M. (1983). Naloxone attenuates self-abusive behavior in developmentally disabled clients. *Applied Research in Mental Retardation, 4,* 5–11.

Sandman, C.A., & Hetrick, W.P. (1995). Opiate and non-opiate mechanisms in self-injury. *Mental Retardation and Developmental Disabilities Research Reviews, 1,* 1–7.

Sandman, C.A., Hetrick, W.P., Chicz-DeMet, A., & Taylor, D.V. (1995). [Effects of naltrexone on beta-endorphin, ACTH, CRH, and cortisol]. Unpublished data.

Sandman, C.A., Hetrick, W.P., Taylor, D.V., Barron, J.L., Touchette, P., Lott, I., Crinella, F., & Martinazzi, V. (1993). Naltrexone reduces self-injury and improves learning. *Experimental and Clinical Psychopharmacology, 1,* 242–258.

Sandman, C.A., McGivern, R.F., Berka, C., Walker, J.M., Coy, D.H., & Kastin, A.J. (1979). Neonatal administration of beta-endorphin produces "chronic" insensitivity to thermal stimuli. *Life Sciences, 25,* 1755–1760.

Sax, D.S., Kornetsky, C., & Kim, A. (1994). Lack of hepatoxicity with naltrexone treatment. *Journal of Clinical Pharmacology, 34,* 898–901.

Smith, S.G., Gupta, K.K., & Smith, S.H. (1995). Effects of naltrexone on self injury, stereotypy, and social behavior of adults with developmental disabilities. *Journal of Developmental and Physical Disabilities, 35,* 283–323.

Spiegel, T.A., Stunkard, A.J., Shrager, E.E., O'Brien, C.P., Morrison, M.F., & Stellar, E. (1987). Effect of naltrexone on food intake, hunger, and satiety in obese men. *Physiology and Behavior, 40,* 135–141.

Taylor, D.V., Hetrick, W.P., Neri, C.L., Touchette, P., Barron, J.L., & Sandman, C.A. (1991). Effect of naltrexone upon self-injurious behavior, learning and activity: A case study. *Pharmacology, Biochemistry and Behavior, 40,* 79–82.

Thompson, T., Hackenberg, T., Cerutti, D., Baker, D., & Axtell, S. (1994). Opioid antagonist effects on self-injury in adults with mental retardation: Response form and location as determinants of mediation effects. *American Journal on Mental Retardation, 99,* 85–102.

Tuinier, S. & Verhoeven, W.M.A. (1995a). Dimensional classification and behavioral pharmacology of personality disorders: A review and hypothesis. *European Neuropsychopharmacology, 5,* 135–146.

Tuinier, S., & Verhoeven W.M.A. (1995b). Stress and stereotypy: Reflections about its relationship and neurobiological substrate. In R.J. Fletcher, D. McNelis, & L. Fusaro (eds.), *Proceedings of the International Congress II on the Dually Diagnosed* (pp. 57–61). Kingston, NY: National Association for the Dually Diagnosed.

Veldhuis, J.D., Rogol, A.D., & Johnson, M.L. (1983). Endogenous opiates modulate the pulsatile secretion of biologically active luteinizing hormone in man. *Journal of Clinical Investigation, 72,* 2031–2040.

Verebey, K., Volavka, J., Mule, S.J., & Resnick, R.B. (1976). Naltrexone: Disposition, metabolism, and effects after acute and chronic dosing. *Clinical Pharmacology and Therapeutics, 20,* 315–328.

Verhoeven, W.M.A., & Tuinier, S. (in press) *Pharmacotherapy in aggressive and auto-aggressive behavior.* Washington, D.C.: American Psychiatric Press.

Volpicelli, J.R., Alterman, A.I., Hayashida, M. & O'Brien, C.P. (1992). Naltrexone in the treatment of alcohol dependence. *Archives of General Psychiatry, 49,* 876–880.

Walters, A.S., Barrett, R.P., Feinstein, A.M.,

Mercurio, A.K, & Hole, W.T. (1990). A case report of naltrexone treatment of self-injury and social withdrawal in Autism. *Journal of Autism and Developmental Disorders, 20,* 169–176.

Wei, E., & Loh, H. (1976). Physical dependence of opiate-like peptides. *Science, 193,* 1262–1263.

Yoburn, B.C., Duttaroy, A., Shah, S., & Davis, T. (1994). Opioid antagonist-induced receptor upregulation: Effects of concurrent agonist administration. *Brain Research Bulletin, 33,* 237–240.

Yoburn, B.C., Luke, M.C., Pasternak, G.W., & Inturisi, C.E. (1988). Upregulation of opioid receptor subtypes correlates with

pregnancy changes of morphine and DADLE. *Life Sciences, 43,* 1319–1324.

Zingarelli, G., Ellman, G., Hom, A., Wymore, M., Heidorn, S., & Chicz-DeMet, A. (1992). Clinical effects of naltrexone on autistic behavior. *American Journal on Mental Retardation, 97,* 57–63.

Fenfluramine

Christopher Gillberg[1], Michael G. Aman[2], and Alan Reiss[3]

Fenfluramine was introduced in the late 1960s and marketed under various trade names, most commonly Pondimin, Ponderax, and Ponderal. The U.S. Food and Drug Administration (FDA) had approved the drug for short-term use in the treatment of exogenous obesity. The drug has been used "off-label" with people with autism, and to a lesser extent, people with mental retardation. Because of concerns about significant adverse effects, the drug was recalled on September 15, 1997 after about 30 years' of use (see editor's note on page 310). In part because there is a significant possibility that the drug will be found safe and remarketed—and in part because the drug had been given in the recent past to many people with developmental disabilities—this chapter remains relevant in our field.

In doses of approximately 1.5 mg/kg per day, fenfluramine lowered whole blood serotonin by about 50% in one study of children (Ekman, Miranda-Linne, Gillberg, Garle, & Wetterberg, 1989). (It also has potent effects on brain serotonin in animals.) Since autism is associated with high whole blood serotonin in an important minority of cases (Cook, 1990), Geller, Ritvo, Freeman, and Yuwiler (1982) hypothesized that fenfluramine might decrease autistic symptoms by lowering levels of serotonin. This hypothesis has stimulated some interesting research on fenfluramine and autism. Because many people with mental retardation also have high whole blood serotonin levels (even if they do not have autism), researchers have also conducted clinical trials with this population. We now have an interesting literature on the effects of fenfluramine on people with various kinds of developmental disabilities and behavior disorders associated with mental retardation.

PHARMACODYNAMICS AND PHARMACOKINETICS

Fenfluramine is a substituted phenylethylamine with a trifluoromethyl group at the 3-position on the phenyl ring, a methyl substitute on the alpha-carbon, and an ethyl sub-

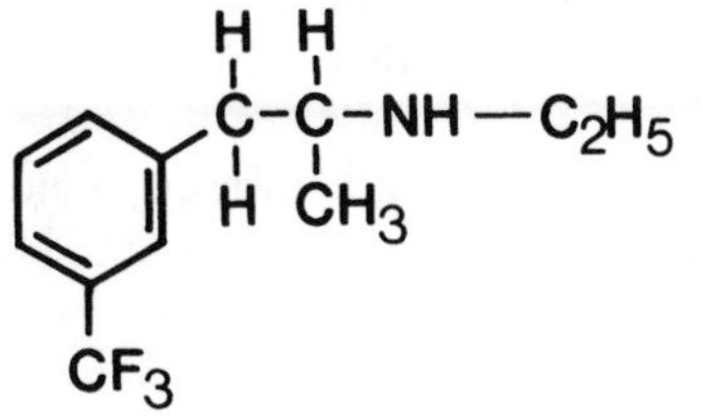

$C_{11}H_{16}F_3N_1$ Mw; 219.3 (free base)

Figure 18-1. Chemical structure of fenfluramine.

stitute on the amine terminal (see Figure 18-1). Following oral administration, it is well absorbed from the gastrointestinal tract. The absorption half-life is about 1.2 hours in adults (Pinder, Brogden, Sawyer, Speight, & Avery, 1975). Plasma half-life in adults is approximately 20 hours, and steady-state levels are reached after three to four days. The drug seems to have considerable inter-subject variation in steady state level. In one study on young children with autism, the blood level varied between 4 and 260 μ/ml with a standard dose of 1.5 mg/kg per day divided into two daily doses (Ekman et al., 1989).

After absorption into the bloodstream, fenfluramine rapidly distributes to various tissues, most notably brain, fat, and muscle.

Fenfluramine is metabolized in the liver. The major metabolite (through de-ethylation) is norfenfluramine. Animal studies suggest that this metabolite has effects similar to those of fenfluramine (Pinder et al., 1975). Some dealkylation may occur in the intestine. It may undergo further metabolism to 3-trifluoromethylbenzoic acid before excretion, which is mostly via the kidneys.

The main effect of fenfluramine appears to be serotoninolytic. Fenfluramine decreases blood serotonin (Pinder et al., 1975). It also produces release of neuronal

1 Professor of Child and Adolescent Psychiatry, University of Goteborg, Goteborg, Sweden
2 Professor of Psychology and Psychiatry, Ohio State University Nisonger Center, Columbus, OH
3 Associate Professor of Psychiatry and Pediatrics, Behavior Genetics and Neuroimaging Research Center, Kennedy Kreiger Institute, Baltimore, MD

serotonin, and it inhibits the uptake of serotonin by its nerve terminals (Garattini, Jori, Buczko, & Samanin, 1975). Brain serotonin effects are observed at low doses of fenfluramine, whereas brain norepinephrine effects are also observed at high doses (Costa, Groppetti, & Revuelta, 1971). Blood serotonin has been reduced in fenfluramine studies of children with autism. However, whether or not the brain and cerebral spinal fluid (CSF) levels of serotonin or its metabolites are also affected by fenfluramine is not known for children with autism or mental retardation.

One study showed a trend toward lowering abnormally high CSF-beta-endorphin levels in nine children with autism. The children were treated with fenfluramine for almost four months (Ross, Klykylo, & Hitzemann, 1987). Fenfluramine has also been shown to block dopamine receptors and increase striatal homovanillic acid (HVA) in animals (Garattini et al., 1975). Fenfluramine is a relatively potent serotonin depletor, and blood serotonin is reduced by about 50% even after short-term treatment. Brain serotonin returns to pre-treatment levels in animals soon after drug discontinuation (Duhault & Boulanger, 1977).

Some investigators have reported that serotonin nerve terminals in the brains of some animal species, including rhesus monkeys, may be destroyed by fenfluramine (Schuster, Lewis, & Seiden, 1986). It is not known whether or not these findings generalize to humans. Fenfluramine increases glucose uptake in muscles, reducing blood glucose levels (Pinder et al., 1975). Reduced levels of cholesterol in plasma have been reported, but these may be secondary to reduced food consumption following anorexia.

SYSTEM EFFECTS AND PHYSICAL EFFECTS

The effects of fenfluramine on the central nervous system include a sedative-type effect on EEGs, reductions in REM sleep, increases in number of arousals, changes in slow-wave sleep, and poorer quality of sleep (Pinder et al., 1975). Three studies showed no effects of fenfluramine on cortical and brain stem average evoked responses (August et al., 1984; Pritchard, Raz, & August, 1987; Raz, Pritchard, & August, 1987). However, Raz et al. (1987) found a decrease in alpha and an increase in theta activity, a pattern characteristic of neuroleptic drugs. In spite of (or perhaps because of) its stimulant-like effects, fenfluramine effectively reduced the rate of

seizures in one of four children with epilepsy among a total of eight children with autistic features (Gastaut, Zifkin, & Rufo, 1987). The behavioral effects of fenfluramine in humans are variable (Campbell, 1988), and in adults they are dose-dependent. The unpredictability of individual responses could be related to the large variability of plasma concentrations of the drug, even with standard dosage (Ekman et al., 1989; Innes et al., 1977).

The effects of fenfluramine on heart rate and blood pressure require further study. On the one hand, some studies showed such effects. For pre-adolescent hyperactive children with mental retardation, a fenfluramine dose of 1.5 mg/kg per day decreased both heart rate and blood pressure, although by less than 10% (Aman, Kern, McGhee, & Arnold, 1993a). The blood pressure findings were replicated in a second study (Aman et al., in press). On the other hand, blood pressure, EKG, pulse, heart, and respiration rates were unaffected in other studies involving children with autistic disorder (Campbell, Deutsch, Perry, Wolsky, & Palij, 1986; Campbell et al., 1987; Realmuto et al., 1986).

In terms of gastrointestinal effects, fenfluramine reduces some degree of anorexia in many cases treated with common doses and, indeed, this is the drug's only FDA approved use.

SIDE EFFECTS AND DRUG INTERACTIONS

Probably the most common side effect is weight loss, which is usually mild to moderate and transient. One group of researchers found that pre-adolescent children lost approximately 1.8 pounds (.82 kg) over a four-week period (Aman et al., 1993a), which was more loss than they found for either placebo or methylphenidate. The weight loss may be caused by anorexia, which is a common side effect of fenfluramine. Another side effect is mild or moderate stomachaches; fenfluramine *may* even have been associated with the development of gastric ulcer in one case (Piggott, Gdowski, & Villaneuva, 1987).

Drowsiness and sedation are frequent side effects (Raich, Rickels, & Raab, 1966), but some people show instead irritability (Kohler, Shortland, & Rolles, 1987) or agitation, especially when the dosage is above the therapeutic range. Insomnia, other sleep problems, and underactivity have been observed. There is some limited evidence that fenfluramine can produce movement disorder. Spontaneous and involuntary teeth grinding in sleep (Ekman et al., 1989; Lewis, Oswald, & Dunleavy, 1971), oral dyskinetic movements (Brandon, 1969), and acute dystonic reactions (Sananman, 1974) are possible effects. Dizziness was observed by one group of researchers (Realmuto et al., 1986), but in another study (Ekman et al., 1989) dizziness was noted only in the placebo condition. Headache improved when fenfluramine was discontinued for one patient (Ross et al., 1987).

Fenfluramine is controversial. In addition to recent findings of possible adverse cardiovascular effects (see page 310), some researchers found evidence of irreversible neurochemical changes when large doses were given to laboratory animals (e.g., Schuster et al., 1986). Long-lasting depletion of serotonin was found in the brains of rats, guinea pigs, and rhesus monkeys after doses of fenfluramine ranging from 12.5 mg/kg per day to 100 mg/kg per day. These doses are much larger than those used in humans, and thus may not be relevant to the clinical context. Additionally, the effects on animals may not hold for people. The drug has been available since the late 1960s, and there are no data indicating long-lasting neurological effects in people given doses in therapeutic ranges. Fenfluramine is well tolerated, although the issue of possible neurotoxicity is unresolved (Aman & Kern, 1989).

Fenfluramine interacts with the following medications, according to a review of the literature by Pinder et al. (1975): (a) standard antihypertensive drugs (e.g., guanethidine, methyldopa, and reserpine) used for patients with hypertension; (b) drugs with a sedative or depressant action; and (c) tricyclic antidepressants in regard to their antidepressant effect (by increasing plasma levels). Fenfluramine appears to antagonize the action of many stimulant drugs. Fenfluramine should not be given in conjunction with traditional monoamine oxidase inhibitors (MAOIs); the MAOIs prevent metabolism of the parent drug and its primary metabolite, norfenfluramine. Pinder et al. (1975) noted one instance in which a toxic confusional state was reported, resulting from the concurrent use of fenfluramine and phenelzine.

CLINICAL INDICATIONS IN MENTAL RETARDATION

Five possible clinical indications of fenfluramine are obesity, bulimia nervosa, autism, mental retardation associated with nonautistic behavior problems, and Prader-Willi syndrome. Uses for obesity and bulimia nervosa in the general population are beyond the scope of this chapter. This review focuses on indications for people with autism, people with both hyperactivity and mental retardation, and people with Prader-Willi syndrome.

Autism

Geller et al. (1982) conducted a case study in which fenfluramine (40 mg/day) was administered to two preschool boys with autism under double-blind and placebo-controlled conditions. They found substantial increases in IQ and marked improvements in several dimensions of behavior. Much of the behavioral improvement was temporary; it was not evident at retesting three months after discontinuation of treatment. No untoward effects were observed. This preliminary study stimulated a substantial amount of subsequent research.

The very marked improvements in IQ reported in the first study did not replicate in larger-scale, placebo-controlled studies. At least 30 studies of fenfluramine treatment for autism, most involving fewer than 10 participants, were reported (for recent reviews, see Aman & Kern, 1989; Aman et al., 1993a). The majority of studies were negative or equivocal in terms of the effect of fenfluramine on the core symptoms of autism. Usually, fenfluramine did not improve speech, language, and IQ. However, several studies showed that the hyperactivity and inattention of children with autism were improved. The evidence concerning an improvement in social behavior is less convincing because different research groups reported conflicting results. Some researchers reported improved social behavior, as measured by the social subscale of the Real Life Rating Scale for Autism (see Aman & Kern, 1989); others found little or no improvement in social behavior, as measured by the Griffiths Personal-Social subscale (Ekman et al., 1989). A few studies found improvement on the sensory motor subscale of the Real Life Rating Scale for Autism, indicating decreases in stereotypic behavior. However, other studies reported *increases* in stereotypies (Barthelemy et al., 1990; Piggott et al., 1987), so that the evidence must be regarded as equivocal in this respect.

Some methodological problems with several of the early fenfluramine studies are noteworthy. Some studies were unbalanced, in that fenfluramine was given for longer periods of time than placebo and usually as the second of three conditions. Also, it is not clear that double-blind conditions were maintained, as adult patients and their physicians were able to identify correctly the type of medication 70% of the time in at least one study of this drug (Brownell & Stunkard, 1982). Furthermore, the same design was used in many of the early studies, so that personnel working on a given protocol may have inadvertently learned the medication sequence from reading about other studies (Aman & Kern, 1989).

In most studies on autism, the dose of fenfluramine was about 1.5 mg/kg per day. In two studies in which higher doses were used (2.0 and 1.9 mg/kg per day) no improvement whatsoever was found, and agitation occurred in some patients (see Aman & Kern, 1989). It is unclear whether doses under 1.5 mg/kg per day might produce positive effects in some individuals.

There have been a number of attempts to predict response to fenfluramine. In most studies on autism, there was no correlation between whole blood serotonin concentrations and therapeutic responses. Beeghly, Kuperman, Perry, Wright, and Tsai (1987) found that the combined level of fenfluramine and its metabolite, norfenfluramine, was more than twice as high for two children with autism who were good responders to fenfluramine than the average levels in those who did not respond as well. However, this finding was not confirmed by Ekman et al. (1989). Ekman et al. used a double-blind placebo-controlled crossover study of fenfluramine in 20 3- to 12-year-old children with autism. CSF-beta-endorphin levels dropped after fenfluramine treatment, although not significantly. Three children improved with regard to behavior, but the behavioral improvement was not correlated with the change in CSF-beta-endorphin levels for all children. In one study, urinary HVA rose markedly in a group of children with autism who responded favorably to fenfluramine treatment (Barthelemy et al., 1990).

It appears that fenfluramine may lead to some improvement in both hyperactivity and inattention in autism, particularly if treatment with methylphenidate or d-amphetamine has been disappointing. However, the drug is unlikely to do much, if anything, to the core symptoms of autism.

Mostly inconsistent results have been reported regarding the effects of fenfluramine on cognitive-performance tasks. In one balanced study, significant gains on the Hearing and Speech subscale of the Griffiths scale were only seen when fenfluramine was given before placebo and not when the order was reversed (Ekman et al., 1989). This indicates that the improvements could have been due to chance or linked to a particular medication sequence but were not a *general* effect of the drug. Stern et al. (1990) reported significant improvements in the

language quotients of 19 children who were treated with fenfluramine. Two studies by Campbell's group suggested that fenfluramine may have an adverse effect on discrimination learning, even though the finding did not reach statistical significance in the second of these studies (Campbell et al., 1987). However, Groden et al. (1987) did not find any effect of fenfluramine on performance, using a test of stimulus overselectivity. All of these studies involved only participants with autism or severe degrees of autistic behavior. Given lack of consistent results, it is difficult to attribute any cognitive effects to fenfluramine at this time.

Hyperactivity and Attention-Deficit Hyperactivity Disorder (ADHD)

In a controlled case study of a severely hyperactive 4-year-old boy with moderate mental retardation, Gadow and Pomeroy (1990) found dramatic improvement with fenfluramine treatment. In a more extensive evaluation, Aman et al. (1993a) studied 28 children with ADHD and mental retardation treated with placebo, methylphenidate (0.4 mg/kg per day), and fenfluramine (gradually increased to 1.5 mg/kg per day) for four weeks each in a double-blind crossover design. Teachers found methylphenidate to be much better than placebo, but only marginally superior to fenfluramine, for producing improvements in conduct, hyperactivity, inattention, and irritability. Parents, however, found fenfluramine to be superior in respect to reducing irritability, inappropriate speech, and hyperactivity.

Aman et al. (1997a) compared three doses of fenfluramine (1.0, 1.5, and 2.0 mg/day) with methylphenidate (0.4 mg/day) and placebo in children with mental retardation or borderline intelligence and ADHD. Each child received all drug conditions for two weeks each in a double-blind crossover design. Of the 30 participants, 24 (80%) were regarded as positive responders to one or more doses of fenfluramine, whereas 12 participants (40%) were regarded as methylphenidate responders. However, 6 participants could not tolerate the medium or high doses of fenfluramine. When each child's optimal fenfluramine dose condition was compared with methylphenidate and placebo, the parents rated their children as significantly improved on several subscales assessing hyperactivity and conduct problems, but the children were also rated as somewhat more lethargic. Teachers also rated the children as less hyperactive and irritable with fenfluramine than with placebo, but these changes were less impressive than those from the parents' ratings. Significant methylphenidate improvements were confined to 2 of 11 subscales completed by teachers. Most of the significant dosage effects favored the high dose (2.0 mg/day) over the low dose (1.0 mg/day) as rated by parents, but there was also evidence of greater side effects and poorer learning performance with the high dose. Aman et al. (in press) recommended that practitioners strive for a dose of 1.5 mg/kg per day or less, given in divided doses and reached over two to three weeks for most children.

In a study of children with mental retardation and ADHD, Aman, Kern, McGhee, and Arnold (1993b) found some indications that fenfluramine enhanced memory performance and slowed response tempo. The finding of slower response times was subsequently replicated in a similar group of children with ADHD (Aman et al., 1997b). In these studies, computer tests were used to record response time, and the automated procedures in place may have allowed for a more precise measure of response tempo than was possible in studies of subjects with autism. Aman et al. (1997b) regarded fenfluramine's slowing of response time to be its most robust and repeatable cognitive effect. In both studies, laboratory examiners who were blind to type of treatment perceived the children as being more attentive (Aman et al., 1993b, 1997a). Those perceptions were not confirmed by the children's scores on the Continuous Performance Task in the first study (Aman et al., 1993b), but there were significantly fewer omission errors on this task with each child's optimal dose of fenfluramine than with placebo in the second investigation (Aman et al., 1997b). All participants had presented with pervasive and severe hyperactivity. The depressant effect of fenfluramine on agitation and hyperarousal in these children may have had beneficial effects on cognition. (This would not be the effect of *any* depressant drug, however. For instance, thioridazine, a drug with clear depressant effects on some hyperactive children, had no positive effects on cognition in the Aman et al. [1991] study.)

Donnelly et al. (1989) assessed the effects of fenfluramine on children with ADHD and *normal* intelligence and found no improvements in terms of teachers' ratings, vigilance, or motor activity. It is unclear why IQ or developmental level should determine responsiveness to fenfluramine, but the available data, although very limited, are consistent with this hypothesis.

Some preliminary recommendations are warranted at this time, although much more research is needed. Fenfluramine appears to be at least as effective in reducing hyperactivity in children with mental retardation (and no autism) as it is in children with both autism and mental retardation and, also, in children with autism

alone (no mental retardation). If it can be shown to be safe, fenfluramine might be worth considering in such individuals when trials with traditional psychostimulants and tricyclic antidepressants are not successful.

Prader-Willi Syndrome

Fifteen research participants with Prader-Willi syndrome and a mean age of 14 (ranging from 5 to 27) received fenfluramine alternating with placebo, each for a period of six weeks, in a double-blind fashion (Selikowitz, Sunman, Pendergast, & Wright, 1990). Children aged 5 to 7 years received 10 mg of fenfluramine three times a day; those aged 8 to 15 received 20 mg three times a day (after a week of 10 mg x 3); and those aged 16 and above received 40 mg three times a day (after a first week of 20 mg x 3). Significant weight loss, improved food-related behavior, and reduced aggression toward others were observed. No improvement in self-aggression and no side effects were observed. The findings suggested that short-term treatment with fenfluramine may be beneficial in the management of some patients with Prader-Willi syndrome. The medication may be used during periods when exposure to large amounts of food cannot be avoided and when aggressive behavior is anticipated. The investigators suggested further that fenfluramine may be useful for people with Prader-Willi syndrome whose lives are threatened by complications of obesity. However, it should be noted that the number of patients included in the study was small (13 to 14 for some analyses) and that no clear description was provided of how well the patients' conditions met accepted diagnostic (including genetic) criteria. Therefore, the recommendations should be regarded as only preliminary.

In the Selikowitz et al. (1990) study of fenfluramine in subjects with Prader-Willi syndrome, no untoward effects on learning were noted. However, because the study did not include a specific measure of effects on cognition, additional research is needed.

INDICATIONS BASED ON CLINICAL OBSERVATIONS

Sherman, Factor, Swinson, and Darjes (1989) observed 15 children aged 7 to 16 with a mean IQ of 31 and found that when treated with fenfluramine they showed marginally more destructive behavior than when treated with placebo. Similar observations were made with two children in the Ekman et al. (1989) study, although the finding was not published because it was not statistically significant. M. Aman and R. Kern have observed marked reductions in stereotypic behavior and self-injury with fenfluramine treatment.

C. Gillberg has observed that the effects of fenfluramine on learning and cognition may vary considerably from one person to another: Some people with both autism and mild to moderate mental retardation appear to show considerable improvement in attention as measured by on-task behavior, whereas non-hyperactive children with autism and at least near average intelligence may show impaired attention.

INDICATIONS FOR WHICH FURTHER RESEARCH IS NEEDED

To our knowledge, fenfluramine has not been systematically tried with adults with mental retardation and behavior disorders (without autism included). Reiss, Egel, Feinstein, Goldsmith, and Borengasser-Caruso (1988) included two adults in their study, but neither improved. Similarly, adolescents with autism and ADHD have only seldom been included in the fenfluramine studies. Both adolescents and adults should be given priority in future research on fenfluramine, because medication is often requested throughout the age span.

Although Donnelly et al. (1989) failed to find any significant behavioral improvement in children with ADHD and no mental retardation who were treated with fenfluramine (some individuals even showed signs of excessive sedation), more research is needed in this population. It is likely that fenfluramine has not hitherto been tried more often, because safe and effective treatment is usually available in the form of conventional psychostimulants; and fear may exist that there may be neural toxicity with fenfluramine. Fenfluramine research may also be indicated for obsessive-compulsive disorder, because this disorder involves serotonergic dysfunction. In one open study, six of seven patients with obsessive-compulsive disorder improved with the addition of fenfluramine to various other serotonin reuptake inhibitors (Goodman, McDougle, & Price, 1992).

CONCLUSION

Fenfluramine has been recalled from the marketplace because of concerns about adverse effects (see page 310). However, experience with this drug since the early 1980s suggests that it may reduce hyperactivity in autism, but it has little or no effect on most other symptoms. A few researchers have reported some gains in reducing stereotypic or ritualistic behavior, but most have found no improvement in the basic social deficits. Serotonin in whole blood is consistently reduced with doses of fenfluramine of about 1.5 mg/kg per day, but therapeutic effects are not correlated with changes in serotonin. Untoward effects are usually mild to moderate, with excessive sedation, increased irritability, and transient weight loss being the most common. Although some research with animals has shown neurotoxic effects of fenfluramine, data suggestive of neuropsychological or other damage have not emerged from the studies of humans. Fenfluramine has shown some promise in the treatment of hyperactivity and inattention in children with mental retardation in a limited number of studies.

REFERENCES

Aman, M.G., & Kern, R.A. (1989). Review of fenfluramine in the treatment of developmental disabilities. *Journal of the American Academy of Child and Adolescent Psychiatry, 28,* 549–565.

Aman, M.G., Kern, R.A., McGhee, D.E., & Arnold, L.E. (1993a). Fenfluramine and methylphenidate in children with mental retardation and ADHD: Clinical and side effects. *Journal of the American Academy of Child and Adolescent Psychiatry, 32,* 851–859.

Aman, M.G., Kern R.A., McGhee, D.E., & Arnold, L.E. (1993b). Fenfluramine and methylphenidate in children with mental retardation and attention deficit hyperactivity disorder: Laboratory effects. *Journal of Autism and Developmental Disorders, 23,* 491–506.

Aman, M.G., Kern, R.A., Osborne, P., Tumuluru, R., Rojahn, J., & Del Medico, V. (1997a). Fenfluramine and methylphenidate in children with mental retardation and borderline intelligence: Clinical effects. *American Journal on Mental Retardation, 101,* 521–534.

Aman, M.G., Kern, R.A., Osborne, P., Tumuluru, R., Rojahn, J., & Del Medico, V. (1997b). *Fenfluramine and methylphenidate in children with mental retardation and borderline intelligence: Cognitive effects.* Manuscript submitted for publication, Ohio State University.

Aman, M.G., Marks, R.E., Turbott, S.H., Wilsher, C.P., & Merry, S.N. (1991). Methylphenidate and thioridazine in the treatment of intellectually subaverage children: Effects on cognitive-motor performance. *Journal of the American Academy of Child and Adolescent Psychiatry, 30,* 816–824.

August, G.J., Raz, N., Papanicolaou, A.C., Baird, T.D., Hirsch, S.L., & Hsu, L.L. (1984). Fenfluramine treatment in infantile autism. *Journal of Nervous and Mental Disease, 172,* 604–612.

Barthelemy, C., Bruneau, N., Jouve, J., Martineau, J., Muh, J.P., & LeLord, G. (1990). Urinary dopamine metabolites as indicators of the responsiveness to fenfluramine treatment in children with autistic behavior. *Journal of Autism and Developmental Disorders, 19,* 241–254.

Beeghly, J.H., Kuperman, S., Perry, P.J., Wright, G.J., & Tsai, L.Y. (1987). Fenfluramine treatment of autism: Relationship of treatment response to blood levels of fenfluramine and norfenfluramine. *Journal of Autism and Developmental Disorders, 17,* 541–548.

Brandon, S. (1969). Unusual effects of fenfluramine. *British Medical Journal, 682,* 557–558.

Brownell, K.D., & Stunkard, R.J. (1982). The double-blind in danger: Untoward consequences of informed consent. *American Journal of Psychiatry, 139,* 1487–1489.

Campbell, M. (1988). Fenfluramine treatment of autism. *Journal of Child Psychology and Psychiatry and Allied Disciplines, 29,* 1–10.

Campbell, M., Deutsch, S.I., Perry, R., Wolsky, B.B., & Palij, M. (1986). Short-term efficacy and safety of fenfluramine in hospitalized preschool-age autistic children. *Psychopharmacology Bulletin, 22,* 141–147.

Campbell, M., Small, A.M., Palij, M., Perry, R., Polonsky, B.B., Lukashock, D., & Anderson, L.T. (1987). The efficacy and safety of fenfluramine in autistic children: Preliminary analysis of a double-blind study. *Psychopharmacology Bulletin, 23,* 123–127.

Cook, E.H. (1990). Autism: Review of neurochemical investigation. *Synapse, 6,* 292–308.

Costa, E., Groppetti, A., & Revuelta, A. (1971). Action of fenfluramine on monoamine stores of rat tissues. *British Journal of Pharmacology, 41,* 57–64.

Donnelly, M., Rapoport, J.L., Potter, W.Z., Oliver, J., Keysor, C.S., & Murphy, D.L. (1989). Fenfluramine and dextroamphetamine treatment of childhood hyperactivity. *Archives of General Psychiatry, 46,* 205–212.

Duhault, J., & Boulanger, M. (1977). Fenfluramine long-term administration and brain serotonin. *European Journal of Pharmacology, 43,* 203–205.

Ekman, G., Miranda-Linne, F., Gillberg, C., Garle, M., & Wetterberg, L. (1989).

Fenfluramine treatment of twenty children with autism. *Journal of Autism and Developmental Disorders, 19,* 511–532.

Gadow, K.D., & Pomeroy, J.C. (1990). A controlled case study of methylphenidate and fenfluramine in a young mentally retarded, hyperactive child. *Australia and New Zealand Journal of Developmental Disabilities, 16,* 323–334.

Garattini, S., Jori, Q., Buczko, W., & Samanin, R. (1975). The mechanism of action of fenfluramine. *Postgraduate Medical Journal, 51* (Suppl. 1), 27–35.

Gastaut, H., Zifkin, B., & Rufo, M. (1987). Compulsive respiratory stereotypies in children with autistic features: Polygraphic recording and treatment with fenfluramine. *New England Journal of Medicine, 17,* 391–407.

Geller, E., Ritvo, E.R., Freeman, B.J., & Yuwiler, A. (1982). Preliminary observations on the effect of fenfluramine on blood serotonin and symptoms in three autistic boys. *New England Journal of Medicine, 307,* 165–169.

Goodman, W.K., McDougle, C.J., & Price, L.H. (1992). Pharmacotherapy of obsessive compulsive disorder. *Journal of Clinical Psychiatry, 53* (Suppl.), 29–37.

Groden, G., Groden, J., Dondey, M., Zane, T., Pueschel, S.M., & Veliceur, W. (1987). Effects of fenfluramine on the behavior of autistic individuals. *Applied Research in Mental Retardation, 8,* 203–211.

Innes, J.A., Watson, M.L., Ford, M.J., Munro, J. F., Stoddart, M.E., & Campbell, D.B. (1977). Plasma fenfluramine levels, weight loss, and side effects. *British Medical Journal, 2,* 1322–1325.

Kohler, J.A., Shortland, G., & Rolles, C.J. (1987). Effect of fenfluramine on autistic symptoms. *British Medical Journal, 295,* 885.

Lewis, S.A., Oswald, I., & Dunleavy, D.L. (1971). Chronic fenfluramine administration: Some cerebral effects. *British Medical Journal, 3,* 67–70.

Piggott, L.R., Gdowski, C.L., & Villaneuva, D. (1987). Side effects of fenfluramine in autistic children. *Journal of the American Academy of Child and Adolescent Psychiatry, 25,* 287–289.

Pinder, R.M., Brogden, R.N., Sawyer, P.R., Speight, T.M., & Avery, G.S. (1975). Fenfluramine: A review of its pharmaco-

logical properties and therapeutic efficacy in obesity. *Drugs, 10,* 241–238.

Pritchard, W.S., Raz, N., & August, G.J. (1987). No effects of chronic fenfluramine on the P300 component of the event-related potential. *International Journal of Neurosciences, 35,* 105–110.

Raich, W.A., Rickels, K., & Raab, E. (1966). A double-blind evaluation of fenfluramine in anxious somatizing neurotic medical clinic patients. *Current Therapeutic Research and Clinical Experiment, 8,* 31–33.

Raz, N., Pritchard, W.S., & August, G.J. (1987). Effects of fenfluramine on EEG and brainstem average evoked response in infantile autism. *Neuropsychobiology, 18,* 105–109.

Realmuto, G.M., Jensen, J., Klykylo, W., Piggott, L., Stubbs, G., Yuwiler, A., Geller, E., Freeman, B.J., & Ritvo, E. (1986). Untoward effects of fenfluramine in autistic children. *Journal of Clinical Psychopharmacology, 6,* 350–355.

Reiss, A.L., Egel, A.L., Feinstein, C., Goldsmith, B., & Borengasser-Caruso, M.A. (1988). Effects of fenfluramine on social behavior in autistic children. *Journal of Autism and Developmental Disorders, 18,* 617–625.

Ross, D.L., Klykylo, W.M., & Hitzemann, R. (1987). Reduction of elevated CSF-beta-endorphin by fenfluramine in infantile autism. *Pediatric Neurology, 3,* 83–86.

Sananman, M.L. (1974). Dyskinesia after fenfluramine. *New England Journal of Medicine, 291,* 422.

Schuster, C.R., Lewis, M., & Seiden, L.S. (1986). Fenfluramine: Neurotoxicity. *Psychopharmacology Bulletin, 22,* 148–151.

Selikowitz, M., Sunman, J., Pendergast, A., & Wright, S. (1990). Fenfluramine in Prader-Willi syndrome: A double-blind, placebo-controlled trial. *Archives of Diseases in Childhood, 65,* 112–114.

Sherman, J., Factor, D.C., Swinson, R., & Darjes, R.W. (1989). The effects of fenfluramine (hydrochloride) on the behaviors of fifteen autistic children. *Journal of Autism and Developmental Disorders, 19,* 533–543.

Stern, L.M., Walker, M.K., Sawyer, M.G., Oades, R.D., Badcock, N.R., & Spence, J.G. (1990). A controlled crossover trial of fenfluramine in autism. *Journal of Child Psychology and Psychiatry, 31,* 569–585.

Editor's Note:
RECALL OF FENFLURAMINE

On September 15, 1997 Wyeth-Ayerst Laboratories voluntarily withdrew its two diet medications, fenfluramine (Pondimin) and dexfenfluramine (Redux). This followed a report from the Mayo Clinic of 24 women who had taken a combination of fenfluramine and phentermine (colloquially called "fen-phen") for weight reduction (Connolly et al., 1997). All of the patients presented with cardiovascular symptoms or a heart murmur. All were women who had valvular heart disease, and eight also had newly-diagnosed pulmonary hypertension, an often fatal disease. Other case reports of valvular disease associated with fenfluramine, dexfenfluramine, or either in combination with phentermine appeared in the same issue (Mark, Patalas, Chang, Evans, & Kessler, 1997; Graham & Green, 1997); one patient died of sudden cardiac arrest 8 months after taking fen-phen for 23 days.

Subsequently a notice on the World Wide Web posted by the FDA[a] described 101 cases with valvular disorders; 85 patients had taken fenfluramine plus phentermine (fen-phen), 3 fenfluramine, 9 dexfenfluramine, and 4 had taken fen-phen and dexfenfluramine at different times. A subset of 46 cases had adequate detail on valvular leakage (valvular regurgitation) to enable a determination of pathology. Some 38 of these (83%) had evidence of pathology: aortic involvement in 28 of the 38 positive cases (74%), mitral valve involvement in 27 (71%), and both aortic and mitral involvement in 18 (47%).

Elsewhere in this notice[a] data were reported on 291 asymptomatic patients from six clinical settings. Of 271 patients taking fen-phen, 32% had valvular regurgitation. Some 30% of those taking dexfenfluramine had valvulopathy.

Fenfluramine, fen-phen, and dexfenfluramine have been widely prescribed to overweight patients in the U.S. One report cited a figure of 18 million prescriptions for fenfluramine in 1996 (Connolly et al., 1997). Fenfluramine has been on the market for nearly 30 years, and one naturally wonders why this side effect was not detected sooner if indeed it is a side effect. Another FDA notice[b] reports that this type of valvular disease is a highly unusual type of drug reaction and that it is not normally screened in clinical trials, even those seeking an FDA indication. The notice observed that the number of patients reported with valvular disease is very small as compared with the number that have received fen-phen, fenfluramine, or dexfenfluramine. However, it also is of interest that there was a serious outbreak of primary pulmonary hypertension between 1967 and 1972 in Western Europe following the introduction of another anorectic agent, aminorex (Menocil), which on post mortem was found to cause lesions in the pulmonary arteries (Curfman, 1997).

Wyeth-Ayerst Laboratories is funding a study to look at the presence of valvular disease in 400 patients who took dexfenfluramine, 400 who took fen-phen, and 400 who took neither (Johannes & Langreth, 1997). One article commented that it has not been proved that fenfluramine or dexfenfluramine caused valvulopathy in these patients and that valvulopathy may somehow be related to their obesity. Depending on the outcome of the Wyeth-Ayerst investigation (and other studies underway) fenfluramine and dexfenfluramine may be back on the market in the future.

---

a FDA analysis of cardiac valvular dysfunction with use of appetite suppressants. http://www.fda.gov/cder/news/slides/index.htm

b Questions and Answers about withdrawal of fenfluramine (Pondimin) and dexfenfluramine (Redux). http:www.fda.gov/cder/news/fenphenqa2.htm

REFERENCES

Connolly, H.M., Crary, J.L., McGoon, M.D., Hunsrud, D.D., Edwards, B.S., Edwards, W.D., & Hartzell, V.S. (1997). Valvular heart disease associated with fenfluramine-phentermine. New England Journal of Medicine, 337, 581–588.

Curfman, G.D. (1997). Diet Pills Redux. New England Journal of Medicine, 337, 629–630.

Graham, D.J., & Green, L (1997). Further cases of valvular heart disease associated with fenfluramine-phentermine. New England Journal of Medicine, 337, 635.

Johannes, L. & Langreth, R. (September 18, 1997). Diet drugs' side effects are still a mystery. The Wall Street Journal, pp. B1, B5.

Mark, E.J., Patalas, E.D., Chang, H.T., Evans, R.J., & Kessler, S.C. (1997). Fatal pulmonary hypertension associated with short-term use of fenfluramine and phentermine. New England Journal of Medicine, 337, 602–606.

Vitamin, Mineral, and Dietary Treatments

Nirbhay N. Singh[1], Cynthia R. Ellis[2], James A. Mulick[3], and Alan Poling[4]

Beginning in the late 1970s, nutritional approaches to producing behavioral, emotional, and cognitive changes in individuals with developmental disabilities flourished for about a dozen years. Although an occasional paper is still published, there has been little serious research activity in this field in recent years. Given that a psychotropic drug can be defined as "any substance administered for the purpose of producing behavioral, emotional, or cognitive changes" (Aman & Singh, 1988a, p. 1), nutritional substances, such as vitamins and minerals that are used for this purpose, can be considered as psychotropic drugs. Furthermore, the research methodologies appropriate for evaluating the effects of nutritional approaches to treatment are nearly identical to those for assessing the effects of standard psychotropic drugs (Aman & Singh, 1988c).

In this chapter, we review research on the effects of various nutritional approaches to treating individuals with developmental disabilities. Our interest is in nutritional approaches that are intended to enhance cognitive ability or to treat behavior problems; therefore, we will not review the literature on the nutritional status of individuals with developmental disabilities. We recognize that these individuals have a number of problems that may compromise their nutritional well-being and therefore require nutritional interventions. For example, individuals with developmental disabilities may have folic acid, calcium, and vitamin D deficiencies as a result of taking anticonvulsant medication for a seizure disorder. If untreated, these deficiencies may lead to megaloblastic anemia and disturbances in bone marrow. Those with chewing and swallowing difficulties may have a vitamin deficiency because their food is softened, pureed, or overcooked, thereby depleting vitamins. Furthermore, some individuals with developmental disabilities have metabolic disorders (e.g., maple syrup urine disease, phenylketonuria, and galactosemia) that may require treatment with specific nutrients or diets. The treatments for these disorders are also not discussed in this chapter.

HISTORICAL OVERVIEW

Individuals with developmental disabilities have experienced treatment with a large variety of nutrients, with some substances being suggested to be highly effective in producing marked behavioral and IQ gains. The early literature included descriptions of treatments using vitamins (e.g., thiamine [B1], vitamin E), glutamic acid, celastrus paniculata, sicca cell therapy, thyroid therapy, and pituitary extracts. As often happens with new therapies, there was an initial enthusiasm for them, with several reports of their effectiveness—typically anecdotal in nature—but the enthusiasm waned with the introduction of rigorous experimental evaluation that showed little or no effect. Indeed, all of the proponents of nutrients touted in the early literature on this topic made exaggerated claims for their efficacy. Yet none of these were proven to be effective in producing beneficial behavioral, emotional, or cognitive changes in individuals with developmental disabilities (Louttit, 1965; Share, 1976).

"U" SERIES TREATMENT

The "U" series of nutrients for the treatment of individuals with Down syndrome was introduced by Turkel (1961, 1975), who claimed that such individuals can be brought to near-normality in intellectual functioning by altering inborn structural anomalies. The treatment consists of 48 vitamins, minerals, enzymes, and common drugs that are given in specific quantities depending on the individual's age and weight. The following is an example of the claims made by Turkel for the effectiveness of this treatment: "Mongoloids and

1 Professor of Psychiatry, Medical College of Virginia, Richmond, VA
2 Assistant Professor of Pediatrics and Psychiatry, Medical College of Virginia, Richmond, VA
3 Professor of Pediatric Psychology, Ohio State University, Columbus, OH
4 Professor of Psychology, Western Michigan University, Kalamazoo, MI

other types of physically and mentally retarded individuals can be brought to near-normalcy by the "U" series of drugs in a treatment which the physician can manage from his office while the patient remains at home" (cited in Bumbalo, Morelewicz, & Berens, 1964, p. 361).

The "U" series is an example of a treatment that failed to meet expectations when scientifically tested for efficacy. The initial data supporting Turkel's claims consisted of case histories. For example, Turkel presented a case report of a five-year-old girl whose pretreatment IQ of 44 increased to 85 following three years on the "U" series (Turkel, Nusbaum, & Baker, 1984). However, when the "U" series was independently evaluated, with Turkel providing the "U" series as well as placebo, no improvement was found for experimental subjects compared to control subjects (Bumbalo et al., 1964). The "U" series was never approved by the Food and Drug Administration for use in the United States, but according to Turkel et al. (1984), it is used extensively in other countries, such as Japan and Norway.

HARRELL VITAMIN SUPPLEMENTATION

Dramatic gains in IQ and collateral improvements in the growth, appearance, and behavior of a diagnostically mixed group of children with mental retardation were reported in a study by Harrell, Capp, Davis, Peerless, and Ravitz (1981). Harrell et al. used a megavitamin and mineral formula manufactured by Bronson Pharmaceuticals; their hypothesis was that some of the children had genotypic diseases in which they inherited a need for an augumented supply of various nutrients. At the end of the first part of the study, the children in the treatment group showed a statistically significant 5-point gain in IQ as compared to those in the control group. In the second part of the study, Harrell et al. continued to give the megavitamins to the treatment group and initiated the same treatment for the control group. This part of the study was uncontrolled. At the end of this part, the control group children showed average IQ gains of 16 points, and the children in the original treatment group showed an average gain of 14 points during the entire study. It was further observed that there was a significant gain in height and improved general appearance in three children with Down syndrome.

Such dramatic results caused a great deal of excite-

ment in the lay press as well as in academic journals, and the race to replicate the study began immediately. At least seven studies were published within the next five years (Bennett, McClelland, Kriegsmann, Andrus, & Sells, 1983; Chanowitz, Ellman, Silverstein, Zingarelli, & Ganger, 1985; Coburn, Schaltenbrand, Mahuren, Clausman, & Townsend, 1983; Ellis & Tomporowski, 1983; Ellman, Silverstein, Zingarelli, Schafer, & Silverstein, 1984; Smith, Spiker, Peterson, Cicchetti, & Justine, 1984; Weathers, 1983). All of these studies were well designed, incorporating double-blind, placebo-controlled, between-groups designs, and all included larger samples than those used by Harrell et al. (1981). These studies also included a wide array of dependent variables that were related to the IQ and cognitive development, behavioral adjustment, motor proficiency, growth and development, and general health status of the children. However, the spectacular increases in IQ reported by Harrell et al. were not replicated in any of these studies. A difference between these studies and the original one was that, with the exception of Chanowitz et al., researchers did not combine the thyroid supplements with the megavitamin supplements. However, in the study in which thyroid supplementation was controlled (Chanowitz et al., 1985), the results were no different from the others. Furthermore, thyroid supplementation was probably not critical to the treatment, because the two children in the Harrell et al. study who were not on the thyroid supplement also showed an increase of 13 IQ points. Thus, the dramatic results claimed by Harrell et al. were not supported by independent, well controlled research.

Since the publication of these studies, an additional attempt has been made to replicate the Harrell et al. (1981) study. Menolascino et al. (1989) replicated the Harrell et al. procedures with 24 children with mental retardation, aged 5 to 15 years, in a double-blind study for eight months. The children were divided into five experimental groups. During the first four months, the different groups of children received the following combination of nutrients: active-vitamin, active-thyroid (Group 1); active-vitamin, placebo-thyroid (Group 2); placebo-vitamin, active-thyroid (Group 3); and placebo-vitamin, placebo-thyroid (Groups 4 & 5). During the second four months of the trial, the first four groups received active-vitamin, active-thyroid supplements and the last group remained on placebo (control group). The Menolascino et al. study replicated the Harrell et al. methodology except that it "was larger in size, maintained its double-blind conditions, utilized a rationale for decreased amounts of desiccated thyroid, utilized a vitamin and mineral supplement which contained slight variations in biotin and calcium phosphate contents, and employed a control group in both phases of the study" (Menolascino et al., 1989, p. 185).

At the end of the first four months, some statistically significant differences between the different groups were found on six outcome measures. On the Nebraska Neuropsychological Exam (Golden, 1985), (a) the vitamin-only group performed significantly worse than the placebo group on the Purposeful Movement test, (b) the thyroid-only group performed significantly worse than the placebo group on the Drawing test, (c) the vitamin-only group performed significantly better than the placebo group on the Visual-Spatial and General Intelligence tests, and (d) the vitamin and thyroid group performed significantly worse than the placebo group on the Reading Recognition test. On the Vineland Social Maturity Scale (Doll, 1965), the vitamin-only group had a significantly higher Social Quotient than the placebo group. However, all of these significant differences disappeared at the end of the second four months of the trial. Other effects included general calming in the behavior of 5 of the 24 children, with the best improvement noted in an 11-year-old girl from the control (placebo) group. This study provided a definitive replication of the procedures used by Harrell et al. (1981), but did not replicate the dramatic findings of the earlier study.

Regardless of the outcome of the Harrell et al. (1981) replication studies, parents have continued to demand high-dosage vitamin-mineral supplements for their children with mental retardation. For example, Bidder, Gray, Newcombe, Evans, and Hughes (1989) used a double-blind, placebo-controlled, crossover design to evaluate the effects of multivitamins and minerals on 19 children with Down syndrome. The results showed that the developmental quotient of most children increased more during placebo than during treatment with multivitamins and mineral supplements. Observations showed no difference in the behavior of the children under placebo and active treatment conditions. Adverse effects of the treatment included problems with appetite and concentration, flushing, tightness of skin, and vomiting. However, regardless of these adverse effects and a clear lack of benefits from the vitamin-mineral supplements, many parents of the children were not only willing to continue with the treatment but also recommended it to other parents. This is a serious problem, because megadoses of vitamins and minerals may have adverse side effects..

FOLIC ACID AND VITAMIN B$_6$ TREATMENTS

During the 1980s, the vitamin folic acid received considerable attention following a report by Lejeune (1982) that suggested that it reduced psychotic-like behavior in some individuals with fragile X syndrome, a genetically-determined subtype of mental retardation. At least 15 studies have been published in which the effects of folic acid on individuals with fragile X were assessed, and several excellent summaries of this literature are available. For example, in a critical review, Aman and Kern (1990/1991) concluded, "folic acid cannot be considered to have established efficacy for managing behavior problems or enhancing adaptive functioning in children or adolescents with fragile X syndrome" (p. 285). There is some indication that folic acid may be somewhat useful with adults who have this disorder, but the evidence is very limited (Hagerman, 1987). These conclusions echo the report of the Third International Workshop on fragile X and X-Linked Mental Retardation: "folic acid treatment ... cannot any longer be regarded as adequate therapy for fragile X patients" (Neri et al., 1988, p. 7).

In the 1980s, there was also some research interest in the possibility that vitamin B$_6$ (pyridoxine) may be of some therapeutic value for children with Down syndrome and autism. Children with Down syndrome have a vitamin B$_6$ deficiency and probably a smaller body pool of B$_6$ as compared to control subjects (Coleman et al., 1985). Further, 5-hydroxytryptamine (serotonin) concentrations in the peripheral blood of children with Down syndrome are lower than in control subjects (Pueschel, Reed, Cronk, & Goldstein, 1980). Both Coleman et al. and Pueschel et al. have hypothesized that the administration of vitamin B$_6$ may increase serotonin levels in children with Down syndrome because pyridoxine, as pyridoxal phosphate, is a coenzyme that participates in the decarboxylation of 5-hydroxytryptophan to 5-hydroxytryptamine. Three studies were undertaken to test this hypothesis, but the data were equivocal and not in support of this hypothesis (Coleman et al., 1985; Frager, Barnet, Weiss, & Coleman, 1985; Pueschel et al., 1980).

Rimland's (1973) survey showed that parents used vitamins extensively with their children who had a variety of mental disorders. He also reported the results of an uncontrolled study in which 59% of children with autism showed a definite improvement on vitamin B$_6$. This study provided the impetus for further investigation of the effects of vitamin B$_6$ on children with autism

(Barthelemy et al., 1981; Callaway, 1977; Gualtieri, Van Bourgondien, Hartz, Schopler, & Marcus, 1981; Lelord et al., 1981; Martineau, Barthelemy, Garreau, & Lelord, 1985; Martineau, Barthelemy, & Lelord, 1986; Martineau, Garreau, Barthelemy, Callaway, & Lelord, 1981). Aman and Singh (1988c) reviewed these studies and found that (a) all studies reported improvements in the subjects given vitamin B_6, (b) all studies had serious methodological problems, and (c) there is no good rationale for using vitamin B_6 with this population.

Two additional studies have been reported since the Aman and Singh (1988c) review. Martineau, Barthelemy, Cheliakine, and Lelord (1988) assessed the effects of vitamin B_6 combined with magnesium in an eight-week open trial. Clinical, biochemical, and electrophysiological measures were obtained for 11 vitamin B_6-responsive children with autism who had participated in an earlier study (Martineau et al., 1985). The authors reported improvement and no significant side effects of the vitamin B_6-magnesium combination. In the other study, researchers examined evoked potential conditioning in children whose behavior improved following treatment with combined vitamin B_6 and magnesium (Martineau, Bartelemy, Roux, Garreau, & Lelord, 1989). Again, this was an open trial with a very small sample of children. The methodological problems encountered in the earlier studies were evident in these two studies as well. Taken in their best light, these studies suggested that some children with autism may benefit from a course of vitamin B_6 therapy. However, the studies have methodological problems, and there is no good rationale for using this nutrient as a psychotropic medication.

MINERAL TREATMENTS

Humans need only minute quantities of minerals, such as chromium, cobalt, copper, fluorine, iron, iodide, magnesium, manganese, molybdenum, selenium, and zinc (Canadian Pediatric Society, 1990). Typically, the level of minerals needed by humans can be obtained through a balanced diet. In the absence of an underlying disease or disorder, supplementation is rarely warranted. However, deficiencies in minerals may have behavioral and cognitive effects. For example, iron deficiency may result in fatigue, irritability, and short attention span and may impair children's performance on laboratory tasks and simple memory tests (Pollitt, Leibel, & Greenfield, 1983). Also, excess mineral intake leads to toxic effects (O'Dell, 1984) and with some minerals, such as zinc,

excessive intake may lead to reduced absorption of others, such as copper and iron (O'Dell, 1989).

A recent study has indicated that the typical North American diet may be marginally deficient in zinc (Moser-Veillon, 1990). Zinc deficiency may result in behavior deficits, such as irritability, mood disturbance, and tremor, and it has been suggested that it may be responsible for attention-deficit hyperactivity disorder ([ADHD]; Colquhoun & Bunday, 1981). Zinc has also been suggested as an etiological factor in the expression of pica in individuals with developmental disabilities (Bhalla, Khanna, Srivastava, Sur, & Bhalla, 1983). Bhalla et al. hypothesized that zinc deficiency results in pica because individuals are driven to seek zinc from sources other than their regular diets. Indeed, when they treated a group of zinc-deficient children with oral zinc sulphate, their pica was eliminated within three to four weeks.

Lofts, Schroeder, and Maier (1990) surveyed 806 residents of an institution for individuals with mental retardation and found that 15.8% (n = 128) of them engaged in pica. Of the 128 residents who engaged in pica, 54% had serum zinc levels below normal range as compared to 7% in a control sample. Sixty-nine zinc-deficient individuals with mental retardation were given a supplement of 100 mg of chelated zinc for two weeks and then reassessed for pica. All except three responded to the zinc supplement and showed reduced rates of pica. The effects of zinc supplementation were further tested with a 51-year-old woman with profound mental retardation who had low zinc levels and engaged in high rates of pica. The effectiveness of zinc supplementation was demonstrated with a reversal design. This study suggests that a trace mineral evaluation should be conducted with individuals with mental retardation who engage in pica because some of their behavioral difficulties may be due to a mineral deficiency.

MELATONIN TREATMENT

Melatonin is a hormone produced by the pineal gland, a pea-sized gland located in the base of the brain. In a multistep process that is synchronized with the sensory perception of light and darkness by the retina, tryptophan, an essential amino acid, is metabolized into the neurotransmitter serotonin which is subsequently converted into melatonin. Melatonin is typically secreted in a diurnal pattern, with the highest levels of the hormone produced during the night and the lowest levels during the day. A number of studies have shown that the administration of exogenous melatonin may be useful in regulating sleep in individuals with abnormal sleep patterns resulting from conditions such as chronic insomnia (MacFarlane, Cleghorn, Brown, & Streiner, 1991), jet lag (Arendt et al., 1987), and shift work (Weitzman et al., 1981). Furthermore, melatonin has also been used to improve the disruptive sleep patterns of several blind adults (Folkard, Arendt, Aldhous, & Kennett, 1990; Miles, Raynal, & Wilson, 1977; Sack, Lewy, Blood, Stevenson, & Keith, 1991).

There have been two reports indicating that individuals with autism may have dysfunctional melatonin production. In the first study, Ritvo et al. (1993) measured melatonin concentrations in the overnight and first-morning urine samples of 9 adolescents with autism and 1 adolescent with autism and mental retardation, 25 of their relatives (parents, grandparents, and siblings) and 10 healthy, unrelated volunteers. Although the groups did not differ in their overnight melatonin concentrations, there was a significant increase in first-morning melatonin concentrations in the urine of the individuals with autism and mental retardation and some of their relatives when compared to the unrelated control subjects. Urinary melatonin concentrations reflect serum melatonin levels; therefore, the increased first-morning urine melatonin concentrations indicated an abnormal persistence of melatonin production into daylight hours. Zapella (1993) reported data on two sets of twins with autism and hypomelanosis of Ito (a neurocutaneous syndrome characterized by hypopigmented streaks and patches of skin on the trunk and limbs that occur frequently in children with developmental delay and brain damage). One of the twins, a 15-year-old boy who had mental retardation and a severe sleep disturbance, had abnormally high daytime levels of melatonin.

The association between autism and dysfunctional melatonin production has prompted the use of melatonin in a small number of children with developmental disabilities. In the first case report, Palm, Blennow, and Wetterberg (1991) normalized the sleep pattern of a 9-year-old boy with mental retardation and a visual impairment with melatonin (0.5 mg) given daily at bedtime. Using a double-blind, placebo-controlled, crossover design, Jan, Espezel, and Appleton (1994) examined the effects of melatonin on 15 children with severe sleep disturbances that had been previously unresponsive to conventional management. The children ranged in age from 6 months to 14 years; 10 children had multiple developmental disabilities (7 with visual impairments), 2 had visual impairments only, 2 had ADHD, and 2 had congenital sleep disorders of unde-

termined etiologies. All of the children showed at least some improvement within several days of initiating melatonin treatment, with the most benefit seen in the children with neurologic abnormalities. The duration of response was variable, and some children were still receiving melatonin one year later with a beneficial response. There were no adverse side effects associated with the melatonin treatment. Although the scientific evidence supporting the use of melatonin to treat some sleep disorders in individuals with developmental disabilities is limited, further clinical trials are indicated.

TREATMENTS FOR EFFECTS OF DIETARY SUBSTANCES

Many studies evaluated hypotheses about the effects of various foods on the behavior of children. Investigators assessed the effects of such dietary substances as milk, wheat, oats, rye, eggs, cocoa, and corn. However, most of this literature has been concerned with children with either ADHD or learning disabilities rather than with individuals with developmental disabilities. We briefly summarize the studies with individuals with developmental disabilities.

Bird, Russo, and Cataldo (1977) investigated the effects of a food allergy on the behavior of a 9-year-old boy with moderate mental retardation who was purportedly allergic to wheat gluten. The effects of the wheat gluten were tested in a single-subject design, and it was found that the wheat gluten did not contribute to the boy's behavior problems. However, his behavior problems were subsequently well controlled with a behavioral intervention implemented by his mother. This study demonstrated that a suspected food allergy can be easily and accurately tested with a single subject design.

Much has been written about Feingold's (1975) suggestion that food additives, such as artificial flavors and colors, and foods containing natural salicylates (e.g., almonds and apples) and preservatives are linked to hyperactivity and other behavior problems (Conners, 1980, 1990). Feingold maintained that some foods have a toxic effect on some children, which results in a behavioral rather than a physical reaction (e.g., impulsivity or short attention span rather than asthma or nasal stuffiness). He developed the Kaiser-Permanente (K-P) diet for children affected by food additives. However, extensive research on the effects of the K-P diet shows that it generally is ineffective in treating the problems of children with hyperactivity and that probably only 1%

to 5% of children respond favorably to it (Conners, 1980, 1990; Wender, 1986).

Three studies have yielded data on the effects of the K-P diet on the behavior of individuals with developmental disabilities. In a double-blind crossover study with 30 institutionalized children and young adults, Harner and Foiles (1980) evaluated the effects of the K-P diet and a control diet, each in effect for 6 weeks. There were no statistically significant differences between children on the two diets with respect to measures of excitability, attention span, and general activity level. In a double-blind challenge design with 10 children with moderate mental retardation, Thorley (1984) evaluated the behavioral and cognitive effects of the K-P and a challenge of artificial color or placebo, each given for 14 days. There were no statistically significant differences between the challenge and the placebo conditions on behavior rating scales, psychometric tests, and measures of motor activity. In the final study, the effects of the K-P diet combined with anticonvulsant medication were assessed on the seizure frequency and hyperactivity of a young boy with mental retardation (Haavik, Altman, & Woelk, 1979). In an open trial using a repeated reversal design, the boy's family diet was alternated with the K-P diet while the anticonvulsant medication was unchanged. The results showed that the boy's seizures were reduced when he was on the K-P diet as compared to when he was on the family diet. However, the K-P diet did not have any effect on the boy's hyperactivity.

There has been a great deal of controversy about the hypothesized effects of sugar on the behavior of children, particularly those with hyperactivity and learning disabilities (Milich, Wolraich, & Lindgren, 1986). Well controlled studies with children with ADHD (Milich & Pelham, 1986; Wolraich, Milich, Stumbo, & Schultz, 1985) and learning disabilities (Behar, Rapoport, Adams, Berg, & Cornblath, 1984) have failed to provide empirical support for the hypothesis that sugar intake leads to behavioral problems. Despite these findings, many parents and physicians continue to implicate sugar in the behavior problems of children. The anecdotal evidence on which they base their opinions can be explained in terms of the expectancy effects of the mothers: Those who believe in behavioral sugar effects in their children tend to act toward their children in a manner congruent with their expectancy (Hoover & Milich, 1994). Although Gschwend, Ryan, Atchison, Arslanian, and Becker (1995) recently found that hyperglycemia following sugar ingestion caused no adverse behavioral symptoms, they did report that hypoglycemia

can result in transient decrements in the cognitive functioning of children. Furthermore, Jones et al. (1995) reported that the fall in plasma glucose levels seen after sugar ingestion can precipitate an exaggerated epinephrine response in healthy children compared to adults, resulting in increased symptoms of sympathetic nervous system stimulation (e.g., feeling shaky and sweaty) as well as decreased cognitive performance. The authors hypothesized that it was this enhanced adrenomedullary responsiveness to the induced hypoglycemia, rather than the reactive hypoglycemia itself, that produced the behavioral and cognitive effects they observed. Given these findings, we are unable as yet to resolve the controversy regarding the association of sugar and behavior and attention.

The effects of sugar on children with developmental disabilities were tested in two studies. In an uncontrolled study, sugar was implicated in the hyperactive and disruptive behavior of an 8-year-old boy with autism (O'Banion, Armstrong, Cummings, & Stange, 1978). However, other foods (e.g., wheat, corn, tomatoes, mushrooms, and dairy products) were also correlated with the boy's increased disruptive behavior. In a study using a single-subject withdrawal design, Kanabay (1984) assessed the effects of sugar on the disruptive behavior and attention of a young boy with autism. The data showed that increased sugar consumption was correlated with increased levels of disruptive behavior but not with attention. Given conflicting findings from just two children, no conclusions can be drawn about the effects of sugar on the behavior of individuals with developmental disabilities.

It has been hypothesized that caffeine and sugar may have additive effects in the development or exacerbation of behavior problems in children as well as contribute to the symptomatology of children with hyperactivity and learning disorders (Powers, 1973). Caffeine is a CNS stimulant that is present in coffee, tea, chocolate, and cola drinks. Although there is only limited research on the effects of caffeine, there does not appear to be any empirical data from well controlled studies to show that caffeine either produces or exacerbates the behavior problems of children. Only one study evaluated the effects of caffeine on the behavior of individuals with mental retardation (Podboy & Mallory, 1977). When compared to whole coffee, decaffeinated coffee significantly reduced the aggressive behavior of the young men with mental retardation. However, this was an uncontrolled study, and the findings need to be replicated in a controlled trial before any firm conclusions can be drawn.

SEROTONIN-ENHANCING DIETS

Some natural foods have been used as treatment for behavior problems because of their effect on the production of brain neurotransmitters. Tryptophan, which is converted to serotonin, is sometimes hypothesized to have calming or anti-anxiety properties. Some psychiatric and developmental conditions are associated with lowered levels of serotonin, including Down syndrome, PKU, and Tourette syndrome. A dysfunction of the serotonergic system has also been associated with the self-injurious behavior (SIB) seen in Lesch-Nyhan syndrome, and although it has not been a consistent finding in all studies, SIB in some of these individuals has been reduced by treatment with tryptophan (a serotonin precurser) or tryptophan in conjunction with carbidopa or imipramine (Castells et al., 1979; Mizuno & Yugari, 1975; Nyhan, Johnson, Kaufman, & Jones, 1980). Research on the use of serotonin-enhancing diets began in the 1970s (e.g., Coleman, 1973; Wurtman & Fernstrom, 1974), and several subsequent studies have indicated that diets high in carbohydrates cause an increase in brain tryptophan, which may lead to an increase in brain serotonin content (Blum et al., 1992; Fernstrom, 1986; Prinz & Riddle, 1986; Steglink, 1987; Wurtman, 1987; Wurtman & Wurtman, 1988).

Five studies have been reported in which dietary modifications were used to enhance the serotonin levels of adults with mental retardation in an effort to control their SIB or aggressive behaviors. In the first, the diet of a 26-year-old woman with Down syndrome and profound mental retardation was modified to increase central serotonin (Gedye, 1990). The modified diet provided a low protein/high carbohydrate ratio, enrichment with serotonin-containing foods and foods high in potassium, and elimination of caffeine and chocolate, which lower endogenous serotonin production. Her SIB was reduced by 90% and maintained at follow-up six months later. In the second study, the same dietary modifications were combined with trazodone to treat aggression in a 58-year-old man with Down syndrome (Gedye, 1991b). The effects of the serotonin-enhancing diet and the medication were not independently assessed, but the combined treatment approach resulted in a 96% decrease in his aggression. In the third study, the dietary modification combined with buspirone was compared to the use of buspirone alone in the treatment of aggression of a 39-year-old woman with moderate mental retardation (Gedye, 1991a). The combined treatment was more effective than medication alone. In another study, the same serotonin-enhancing

diet (Gedye, 1990) was used alone and in combination with trazodone to treat aggression and SIB in a 34-year-old woman with profound mental retardation, PKU, and depression (Barrera, Selmeci, Donovan, Murray, & Goldberg, 1993). Although a reduction in the aggression was noted with the serotonin-enhancing diet alone, a clinically significant improvement was observed with the concurrent use of the serotonergic diet and trazodone. In a fifth study, an ABCD design was used to determine the effects of a serotonergic diet alone and in combination with paroxetine and sertraline on the SIB of a 6-year-old boy with mental retardation and Lesch-Nyhan syndrome (Kirkpatrick-Sanchez, Williams, Gualtieri, & Raichman, 1994). The serotonergic diet alone and the diet plus paroxetine decreased SIB, but the most effective treatment was the diet in combination with sertraline, which resulted in a 57% decrease in the boy's SIB. These case reports suggested that augmenting a serotonin medication with a diet designed to enhance serotonin levels should be considered in the treatment of SIB and aggression in individuals with mental retardation. However, all of these studies are based on single cases, and blood and cerebrospinal fluid serotonin levels were not measured directly in any of these studies. Furthermore, it can be argued that the concurrent medication was responsible for any changes reported in some of these studies. Therefore, additional evaluations using larger samples are needed before the clinical use of serotonin-enhancing diets can be justified.

CONCLUSION

Some individuals with developmental disabilities are at risk for nutritional deficiencies because of their unique problems, such as swallowing and feeding difficulties, and may require specific nutritional supplements. For other individuals who have genetically transmitted metabolic disorders, specialized dietary treatments are also indicated. However, there is little in the literature to support the use of nutrients and other dietary treatments as psychotropic medications for individuals with developmental disabilities.

Numerous claims have been made regarding the effects of food additives and special diets on the behavior of children with ADHD and learning disabilities. A number of specific dietary regimens, such as vitamin-thyroid supplements and the "U" series of vitamins and minerals, were advocated for individuals with developmental disabilities. However, virtually none of these claims have been substantially based on controlled investigations. There is little evidence for the efficacy of megavitamins, folic acid, vitamin B$_6$, or other dietary treatments with individuals with developmental disabilities.

Two remarkable aspects of the literature on the behavioral effects of nutrient and dietary treatments should be noted. First, the research is overwhelmingly anecdotal and poorly controlled (Aman & Singh, 1988b). The behavioral effects of nutrients and other dietary treatments are subtle and require methodologies and assessment instruments that are sensitive to subtle changes. The experimental protocols and methodologies that are useful for psychopharmacological research in the developmental disabilities (Aman & Singh, 1980; Sprague & Werry, 1971) can be used in this area of research as well. Furthermore, Schwab and Conners (1986) have presented a series of guidelines for research on the behavioral effects of nutrients in children that can provide the basis for similar research with individuals with developmental disabilities. Although it may be difficult to conduct methodologically sound evaluations of the effects of dietary variables in this population, such work is possible and should be conducted.

REFERENCES

Aman, M.G., & Kern, R.A. (1990/91). The efficacy of folic acid in fragile X syndrome and other developmental disabilities. *Journal of Child and Adolescent Psychopharmacology, 1,* 285–295.

Aman, M.G., & Singh, N.N. (1980). The usefulness of thioridazine for treating childhood disorders: Fact or folklore? *American Journal of Mental Deficiency, 84,* 331–338.

Aman, M.G., & Singh, N.N. (1988a). Patterns of drug use: Methodological considerations, measurement techniques, and future trends. In M.G. Aman & N.N. Singh (Eds.), *Psychopharmacology of the developmental disabilities* (pp. 1–28). New York: Springer-Verlag.

Aman, M.G., & Singh, N.N. (1988b). *Psychopharmacology of the developmental disabilities.* New York: Springer-Verlag.

Aman, M.G., & Singh, N.N. (1988c). Vitamin, mineral, and dietary treatments. In M.G. Aman & N.N. Singh (Eds.), *Psychopharmacology of the developmental disabilities* (pp. 168–196). New York: Springer-Verlag.

Arendt, J., Aldhous, M., English, J., Marks, V., Arendt, J.H., Marks, M., & Folkard, S. (1987). Some effects of jet-lag and their alleviation by melatonin. *Ergonomics, 30,* 1379–1393.

Barrera, F.J., Selmeci, T., Donovan, C., Murray, A., & Goldberg, B. (1993, March). *Serotonergic diet effects on aggression and self-injury.* Paper presented at the meeting of the Ontario Association of Developmental Disabilities, Kitchener, Ontario, Canada.

Barthelemy, C., Garreau, B., Leddet, I., Ernouf, D., Muh, J.R., & Lelord, G. (1981). Behavioral and biological effects of oral magnesium, vitamin B$_6$ and combined magnesium-vitamin B$_6$ administration in autistic children. *Magnesium Bulletin, 2,* 150–153.

Behar, D., Rapoport, J.L., Adams, A.J., Berg, C.J., & Cornblath, M. (1984). Sugar challenge testing with children considered behaviorally "sugar reactive." *Nutrition and Behavior, 1,* 277–288.

Bennett, F.C., McClelland, S., Kriegsmann, E.A., Andrus, L.B., & Sells, C.J. (1983). Vitamin and mineral supplementation in Down's syndrome. *Pediatrics, 72,* 707–713.

Bhalla, J.N., Khanna, P.K., Srivastava, J.R., Sur, B.K., & Bhalla, M. (1983). Serum zinc levels and pica. *Indian Pediatrics, 20,* 667–670.

Bidder, R.T., Gray, P., Newcombe, R.G., Evans, B.K., & Hughes, M. (1989). The effects of multivitamins and minerals on children with Down's syndrome. *Developmental Medicine and Child Neurology, 31,* 532–537.

Bird, B.L., Russo, D.C., & Cataldo, M.F. (1977). Considerations in the analysis and treatment of dietary effects on behavior disorders. *Journal of Autism and Childhood Schizophrenia, 7,* 373–382.

Blum, I., Vered, Y., Graff, E., Grosskopf, Y., Don, R., Harsat, A., & Raz, O. (1992). The influence of meal composition on plasma serotonin and norepinephrine concentrations. *Metabolism, 41,* 137–140.

Bumbalo, T.S., Morelewicz, H.V., & Berens, D.L. (1964). Treatment of Down's syndrome with the "U" series of drugs. *Journal of the American Medical Association, 187,* 361.

Callaway, E. (1977). Response of infantile autism to large doses of B$_6$. *Psychopharmacology Bulletin, 13,* 57–58.

Canadian Pediatric Society, Nutrition Committee. (1990). Mega-vitamin and mega-mineral therapy in childhood. *Canadian Medical Association Journal, 143,* 1009–1013.

Castells, S., Chakrabarti, C., Winsberg, B.G., Hurwic, M., Perel, J.M., & Nyhan, W.L. (1979). Effects of L-5-hydroxytryptophan on monoamine and amino acids turnover in the Lesch-Nyhan syndrome. *Journal of Autism and Developmental Disorders, 9,* 95–103.

Chanowitz, J., Ellman, G., Silverstein, C.I., Zingarelli, G., & Ganger, E. (1985). Thyroid and vitamin-mineral supplement fail to improve IQ of mentally retarded adults. *American Journal of Mental Deficiency, 90,* 217–219.

Coburn, S.P., Schaltenbrand, W.E., Mahuren, J.D., Clausman, R.J., & Townsend, D. (1983). Effect of megavitamin treatment on mental performance and plasma vitamin B$_6$ concentrations in mentally retarded young adults. *American Journal of Clinical Nutrition, 38,* 352–355.

Coleman, M. (1973). *Serotonin in Down's syndrome.* New York: American Elsevier.

Coleman, M., Sobel, S., Bhagavan, H.N., Coursin, D., Marquardt, A., Guay, M., & Hunt, C. (1985). A double-blind study of vitamin B$_6$ in Down's syndrome infants: Part 1. Clinical and biochemical results. *Journal of Mental Deficiency Research, 29,* 233–240.

Colquhoun, I., & Bunday, S. (1981). A lack of essential fatty acids as a possible cause of hyperactivity in children. *Medical Hypotheses, 7,* 673–679.

Conners, C.K. (1980). *Food additives and hyperactive children.* New York: Plenum Press.

Conners, C.K. (1990). *Feeding the brain: How foods affect children.* New York: Plenum Press.

Doll, E.A. (1965). *Vineland Social Maturity Scale.* Circle Pines, MN: American Guidance Service.

Ellis, N.R., & Tomporowski, P.D. (1983). Vitamin/mineral supplements and intelligence of institutionalized mentally retarded adults. *American Journal of Mental Deficiency, 88,* 211–214.

Ellman, G., Silverstein, C.I., Zingarelli, G., Schafer, E.W.P., & Silverstein, L. (1984). Vitamin-mineral supplement fails to improve IQ of mentally retarded young adults. *American Journal of Mental Deficiency, 88,* 688–691.

Feingold, B.F. (1975). *Why your child is hyperactive.* New York: Random House.

Fernstrom, J.D. (1986). Acute and chronic effects of protein and carbohydrate ingestion on brain tryptophan levels and serotonin synthesis. *Nutrition Reviews, 44* (Suppl.), 25–36.

Folkard, S., Arendt, T., Aldhous, M., & Kennett, H. (1990). Melatonin stabilises sleep onset time in a blind man without entrainment of cortisol or temperature rhythms. *Neuroscience Letters, 113,* 193–198.

Frager, J., Barnet, A., Weiss, I., & Coleman, M. (1985). A double-blind study of vitamin B$_6$ in Down's syndrome infants: Part 2. Cortical auditory evoked potentials. *Journal of Mental Deficiency Research, 29,* 241–246.

Gedye, A. (1990). Dietary increase in serotonin reduces self-injurious behavior in a Down's syndrome adult. *Journal of Mental Deficiency Research, 34,* 195–203.

Gedye, A. (1991a). Buspirone alone or with serotonergic diet reduced aggression in a developmentally delayed adult. *Biological Psychiatry, 30,* 88–91.

Gedye, A. (1991b). Serotonergic treatment for aggression in a Down's syndrome adult showing signs of Alzheimer's disease. *Journal of Mental Deficiency Research, 35,* 247–258.

Golden, C.J. (1985). *Nebraska Neuropsychological Exam: Manual.* Los Angeles, CA: Western Psychology Services.

Gschwend, S., Ryan, C., Atchison, J., Arslanian, S., & Becker, D. (1995). Effects of acute hyperglycemia on mental efficiency and counterregulatory hormones in adolescents with insulin-dependent diabetes mellitus. *Journal of Pediatrics, 126,* 178–184.

Gualtieri, C.T., Van Bourgondien, M.E., Hartz, C., Schopler, E., & Marcus, L. (1981). *A pilot study of pyridoxine treatment in autistic children.* Paper presented at the meeting of the American Psychiatric Association, New Orleans, LA.

Haavik, S., Altman, K., & Woelk, C. (1979). Effects of the Feingold diet on seizures and hyperactivity: A single-subject analysis. *Journal of Behavioral Medicine, 2,* 365–374.

Hagerman, R.J. (1987). Fragile X syndrome. *Current Problems in Pediatrics, 17,* 621–674.

Harner, I.C., & Foiles, R.A.L. (1980). Effect of Feingold's K-P diet on a residential, mentally handicapped population. *Journal of the American Dietetic Association, 76,* 575–580.

Harrell, R.F., Capp, R.H., Davis, D.R., Peerless, J., & Ravitz, L.R. (1981). Can nutritional supplements help mentally retarded children? An exploratory study. *Proceedings of the National Academy of Science, 78,* 574–578.

Hoover, D.W., & Milich, R. (1994). Effects of sugar ingestion expectancies on mother-child interactions. *Journal of Abnormal Child Psychology, 22,* 501–515.

Jan, J.E., Espezel, H., & Appleton, R.E. (1994). The treatment of sleep disorders with melatonin. *Developmental Medicine and Child Neurology, 36,* 97–107.

Jones, T.W., Borg, W.P., Boulward, S.D., McCarthy, G., Sherwin, R.S., & Tamborlane, W.V. (1995). Enhanced adrenomedullary response and increased susceptibility to neuroglycopenia: Mechanisms underlying the adverse effects of sugar ingestion in healthy children. *Journal of Pediatrics, 126,* 171–177.

Kanabay, G.P. (1984). The effects of sugar upon the behavior of an autistic child within a structured work situation. *Dissertation Abstracts International, 45,* (2B).

Kirkpatrick-Sanchez, S., Williams, D.E., Gualtieri, C.T., & Raichman, J. (1994, May). *The use of serotonergic diet and antidepressants in the treatment of self-injury in Lesch-Nyhan syndrome.* Paper presented at the meeting of the Association for Behavior Analysis, Atlanta, GA.

Lejeune, J. (1982). Is the fragile X syndrome amendable to treatment? *Lancet, 1,* 273–274.

Lelord, G., Muh, J.P., Barthelemy, C., Martineau, J., Garreau, B., & Callaway, E. (1981). Effects of pyridoxine and magnesium on autistic symptoms: Initial observations. *Journal of Autism and Developmental Disorders, 11,* 219–230.

Lofts, R.H., Schroeder, S.R., & Maier, R.H. (1990). Effects of serum zinc supplementation on pica behavior of persons with mental retardation. *American Journal of Mental Retardation, 95,* 103–109.

Louttit, R. (1965). Chemical facilitation of intelligence among the mentally retarded. *American Journal of Mental Deficiency, 69,* 495–501.

MacFarlane, J.G., Cleghorn, J.M., Brown, G.M., & Streiner, D.L. (1991). The effects of exogenous melatonin on the total sleep time and daylight alertness of chronic insomniacs: A preliminary study. *Biological Psychiatry, 30,* 371–376.

Martineau, J., Barthelemy, C., Cheliakine, C., & Lelord, G. (1988). Brief report: An open middle-term study of combined vitamin B$_6$-magnesium in a subgroup of autistic children selected on their sensitivity to this treatment. *Journal of Autism and Developmental Disorder, 18,* 435–447.

Martineau, J., Barthelemy, C., Garreau, B., & Lelord, G. (1985). Vitamin B$_6$, magnesium, and combined B$_6$-Mg: Therapeutic effects in childhood autism. *Biological Psychiatry, 20,* 467–478.

Martineau, J., Barthelemy, C., & Lelord, G. (1986). Long-term effects of combined vitamin B$_6$-magnesium administration in an autistic child. *Biological Psychiatry, 21,* 511–518.

Martineau, J., Barthelemy, C., Roux, S., Garreau, B., & Lelord, G. (1989). Electrophysiological effects of fenfluramine or combined vitamin B$_6$ and magnesium on children with autistic behavior. *Developmental Medicine and Child Neurology, 31,* 721–727.

Martineau, J., Garreau, B., Barthelemy, C., Callaway, E., & Lelord, G. (1981). Effects of vitamin B$_6$ on averaged evoked potentials in infantile autism. *Biological Psychiatry, 16,* 627–641.

Menolascino, F.J., Donaldson, J.Y., Gallagher, T.F., Golden, C.J., Wilson, J.E., Huth, J.A., Ludvigsen, C.W., & Gillette, D.W. (1989). Vitamin supplements and purported learning enhancement in mentally retarded children. *Journal of Nutritional Science and Vitaminology, 35,* 181–192.

Miles, L.E.M., Raynal, D.M., & Wilson, M.A. (1977). Blind man living in normal society has circadian rhythms of 24.9 hours. *Science, 198,* 421–423.

Milich, R., & Pelham, W.E. (1986). Effects of sugar ingestion on the classroom and playground behavior of attention deficit disordered boys. *Journal of Consulting and Clinical Psychology, 54,* 714–718.

Milich, R., Wolraich, M., & Lindgren, S. (1986). Sugar and hyperactivity: A critical review of empirical findings. *Clinical Psychology Review, 6,* 493–513.

Mizuno, T., & Yugari, Y. (1975). Prophylactic effect of L-5-hydroxytryptophan on self-mutilation in the Lesch-Nyhan syndrome. *Neuropaediatrie, 6,* 13–23.

Moser-Veillon, P.B. (1990). Zinc: Consumption patterns and dietary recommendations. *Journal of the American Dietetic Association, 90,* 1089–1093.

Neri, G., Opitz, J.M., Mikkelsen, M., Jacobs, P.A., Davies, K., & Turner, G. (1988). Conference report: Third international workshop on the fragile X and X-linked mental retardation. *American Journal of Medical Genetics, 30,* 1–29.

Nyhan, W.L., Johnson, H.G., Kaufman, I.A., & Jones, K.l. (1980). Serotonergic approaches to the modification of behavior in the Lesch-Nyhan syndrome. *Applied Research in Mental Retardation, 1,* 25–40.

O'Banion, D., Armstrong, B., Cummings, R.A., & Stange, J. (1978). Disruptive behavior: A dietary approach. *Journal of Autism and Childhood Schizophrenia, 8,* 325–337.

O'Dell, B.L. (1984). Bioavailability of trace elements. *Nutrition, 42,* 301–308.

O'Dell, B.L. (1989). Mineral interactions relevant to nutrient requirements. *Journal of Nutrition, 119* (Suppl.), 1832–1845.

Palm, L., Blennow, G., & Wetterberg, L. (1991). Correction of non-24-hour sleep/wake cycle by melatonin in a blind retarded boy. *Annals of Neurology, 29,* 336–339.

Podboy, J.W., & Mallory, W.A. (1977). Caffeine reduction and behavior change in the severely retarded. *Mental Retardation, 15*, 40.

Pollitt, E., Leibel, R.L., Greenfield, D.B. (1983). Iron deficiency and cognitive test performance in preschool children. *Nutrition and Behavior, 1*, 137–146.

Powers, H.W.S. (1973). Dietary measures to improve behavior and achievement. *Academic Therapy, 9*, 203–214.

Prinz, R.J., & Riddle, D.B. (1986). Association between nutrition and behavior in five-year-old children. *Nutrition Reviews, 44*, 151.

Pueschel, S.M., Reed, R.B., Cronk, C.E., & Goldstein, B.I. (1980). 5-hydroxytryptophan and pyridoxine: Their effects in young children with Down's syndrome. *American Journal of Diseases of Childhood, 134*, 838–844.

Rimland, B. (1973). High-dosage levels of certain vitamins in the treatment of children with severe mental disorders. In D. Hawkins & L. Pauling (Eds.), *Orthomolecular psychiatry* (pp. 513–539). New York: Freeman.

Ritvo, E.R., Ritvo, R., Yuwiler, A., Brothers, A., Freeman, B.J., & Plotkin, S. (1993). Elevated daytime melatonin concentrations in autism: A pilot study. *European Child and Adolescent Psychiatry, 2*, 75–78.

Sack, R.L., Lewy, A.J., Blood, M.L., Stevenson, J., & Keith, L.D. (1991). Melatonin administration to blind people: Phase advances and entrainment. *Journal of Biological Rhythms, 6*, 249–261.

Schwab, E.K., & Conners, C.K. (1986). Nutrient-behavior research with children: Methods, considerations, and evaluation. *Journal of the American Dietetic Association, 86*, 319–324.

Share, J.B. (1976). Review of drug treatment for Down's syndrome persons. *American Journal of Mental Deficiency, 80*, 388–393.

Smith, G.F., Spiker, D., Peterson, C.P., Cicchetti, D., & Justine, P. (1984). Use of megadoses of vitamins with minerals in Down's syndrome. *Journal of Pediatrics, 105*, 228–234.

Sprague, R.L., & Werry, J.S. (1971). Methodology of psychopharmacological studies with the retarded. *International Review of Research in Mental Retardation, 5*, 147–219.

Stegink, L.D. (1987). The aspartame story: A model for the clinical testing of a food additive. *American Journal of Clinical Nutrition, 46*, 204–215.

Thorley, G. (1984). Pilot study to assess behavioural and cognitive effects of artificial food colours in a group of retarded children. *Developmental Medicine and Child Neurology, 26*, 56–61.

Turkel, H. (1961). Medical treatment of mongolism. In S. Otto (Ed.), *Organic bases and biochemical aspects of imbecility*. New York: S. Karger.

Turkel, H. (1975). Medical amelioration of Down's syndrome incorporating the orthomolecular approach. *Journal of Orthomolecular Psychiatry, 4*, 102.

Turkel, H., Nusbaum, I., & Baker, S. (1984). Intellectual improvement of a retarded patient treated with the "U" series. *Journal of Orthomolecular Psychiatry, 13*, 272–281.

Weathers, C. (1983). Effects of nutritional supplementation on IQ and certain other variables associated with Down syndrome. *American Journal of Mental Deficiency, 88*, 214–217.

Weitzman, E.D., Czeisler, C.A., Coleman, R.M., Spielman, A.J., Zimmerman, J.C., & Dement, W.C. (1981). Delayed sleep phase syndrome, a chronobiological disorder with sleep-onset insomnia. *Archives of General Psychiatry, 38*, 77–346.

Wender, E.H. (1986). The food additive-free diet in the treatment of behavior disorders: A review. *Journal of Developmental and Behavioral Pediatrics, 7*, 35–42.

Wolraich, M., Milich, R., Stumbo, P., & Schultz, F. (1985). Effects of sucrose ingestion on the behavior of hyperactive boys. *Journal of Pediatrics, 106*, 675–682.

Wurtman, J. (1987). Recent evidence from human studies linking central serotonergic function with carbohydrate intake. *Appetite, 8*, 211–213.

Wurtman, R.J., & Fernstrom, J.D. (1974). Effects of diet on brain neurotransmitters. *Nutrition Reviews, 32*, 193–200.

Wurtman, R.J., & Wurtman, J.J. (1988). Do carbohydrates affect food intake via neurotransmitter activity? *Appetite, 11* (Suppl.), 42–47.

Zappella, M. (1993). Autism and hypomelanosis of Ito in twins. *Developmental Medicine and Child Neurology, 35*, 826–832.

ABOUT THE EDITORS

Steven Reiss, Ph.D., is Professor of Psychology and Psychiatry and Director, Nisonger Center for Mental Retardation and Developmental Disabilities, The Ohio State University. He received an A.B. degree from Dartmouth College and a Ph.D. degree from Yale University. In the 1970s, he found that extrinsic rewards do not undermine intrinsic motivation, except when used in inappropriate ways. In the 1980s, he led a group that developed the concept, measure, and theory of anxiety sensitivity. Anxiety sensitivity has since been found to be a significant cognitive risk factor of Panic Disorder, a type of mental illness that affects about 5 million Americans. This work has been translated into 12 languages. Also in the 1980s, Reiss published articles on the co-occurrence of mental illness and mental retardation, helping to identify for public policy purposes a population of about one million Americans. This work was cited as part of the justification for the creation of hundreds of new specialty clinics and service programs. Recognitions include the Distinguished Research Award (The Arc of the United States), Distinguished Services Award (American Association on Mental Retardation), and Frank J. Menolascino Award (National Association on Dual Diagnosis). Media coverage includes an American Psychological Association national press conference, N.Y. Times, Today Show, Associated Press, Cable Network News, and CBS national radio. Recently, Reiss led the development of a new sensitivity (value-based) theory of human motivation.

Michael G. Aman, Ph.D., is Professor of Psychology and Psychiatry and Director of the Behavior Program at the Nisonger Center for Mental Retardation and Developmental Disabilities of The Ohio State University. He received an M.A. degree from the University of Illinois and a Ph.D. degree from the University of Auckland in New Zealand. He has published more than 125 scientific articles on the effects of psychiatric medications in children and adults with mental retardation, autism, and other developmental disabilities and on rating instruments. This work has produced scholarly reviews on most major classes of medication and related topics. Recognitions include peer-reviewed awards from the National Institute of Mental Health and from private sources. Since the mid-1980s, he co-developed a number of widely-used behavior rating instruments designed to strengthen scientific evaluations of the effects of psychotropic medications. He is the author of an influential NIMH-funded report on psychometric instruments and dual diagnosis. He also is co-editor of influential books, including a book on pediatric psychopharmacology.

AUTHORS

Norberto Alvarez, M.D., *Assistant Director of Neurology,* Harvard University Medical School, Boston, MA

Michael G. Aman, Ph.D., *Professor of Psychology and Psychiatry,* Nisonger Center, The Ohio State University, Columbus, OH

L. Eugene Arnold, M.D., *Special Expert,* Child and Adolescent Disorders Research Branch, National Institute of Mental Health. Now Emeritus Professor of Psychiatry, Ohio State University, Columbus, OH

Francisco J. Barrera, Ph.D., *Program Director,* Southwestern (Ontario) Regional Center, Blenheim, Ontario, Canada

Rowland P. Barrett, Ph.D., *Associate Professor of Psychiatry,* Brown University, Providence, RI

Alan A. Baumeister, Ph.D., *Assistant Professor of Psychiatry,* Louisiana State University, Baton Rouge, LA

William H. Benefield, Jr., Pharm.D., *Clinical Pharmacologist,* San Antonio State School, San Antonio, TX

John P. Board, Jr., M.D., *Chief of Medical Services,* Michigan Department of Mental Health, Lansing, MI

Nick Bouras, M.D., *Senior Lecturer in Psychiatry,* Guy's Hospital-London Bridge, London, England, United Kingdom

Joel D. Bregman, M.D., *Associate Professor of Psychiatry,* Emory Autism Research Center, Emory University School of Medicine, Atlanta, GA

Nancy Cain, M.D., *Clinical Assistant Professor of Psychiatry,* University of Rochester School of Medicine and Dentistry, Rochester, NY

Dennis P. Cantwell, M.D., *Joseph Campbell Professor of Child Psychiatry,* University of California at Los Angeles, Los Angeles, CA

David J. Clarke, M.D., *Senior Lecturer in Developmental Psychiatry,* University of Birmingham, Birmingham, England, United Kingdom

Edwin H. Cook, Jr., M.D., *Director,* Laboratory of Developmental Neurochemistry, University of Chicago, Chicago, IL

John A. Corbett, M.D., *Professor of Developmental Psychiatry,* University of Birmingham, Birmingham, England, United Kingdom

David L. Coulter, M.D., *Associate Professor of Pediatrics and Neurology,* Boston University School of Medicine, Boston, MA

Judy L. Curtis, Pharm.D., *Assistant Professor of Pharmacy Practice and Science,* University of Maryland at Baltimore, Baltimore, MD

Sharon Davis, Ph.D., *Director,* Department of Research and Program Services, The Arc of the United States, Arlington, TX

Howard Demb, M.D., *Assistant Professor of Psychiatry,* Albert Einstein College of Medicine, Bronx, NY

Anton Dosen, M.D., *President,* European Association on Dual Diagnosis, Venray, The Netherlands

Stuart Einfeld, M.D., *Lecturer in Child Psychiatry,* University of Sydney, Sydney, Australia

Cynthia R. Ellis, M.D., *Assistant Professor of Pediatrics and Psychiatry,* Medical College of Virginia, Richmond, VA

Sherman Fox, M.D., *Adjunct Professor of Psychiatry,* Dartmouth College Medical School, Hanover, NH

W.I. Fraser, M.D., *Professor of Mental Handicap,* University of Wales College of Medicine, South Glamorgan, Wales, United Kingdom

Kenneth D. Gadow, Ph.D., *Professor of Child and Adolescent Psychiatry,* State University of New York at Stony Brook, Stony Brook, NY

Angela Gedye, Ph.D., private practice, Vancouver, British Columbia, Canada

Christopher Gillberg, M.D., *Professor of Child and Adolescent Psychiatry,* University of Goteborg, Goteborg, Sweden

Benjamin Goldberg, M.D., *Emeritus Professor of Developmental Neuropsychiatry,* University of Western Ontario, London, Ontario, Canada

Randi J. Hagerman, M.D., *Professor of Pediatrics,* University of Colorado Health Science Center, Child Development Unit, The Children's Hospital, Denver, CO

William P. Hetrick, Department of Psychology, Ohio State University, Columbus, OH

Hans R. Huessy, M.D., *Professor Emeritus of Psychiatry,* University of Vermont College of Medicine, Burlington, VT

Anne DesNoyers Hurley, Ph.D., *Director of Clinical Services,* Bay Cove Human Services, MR/DD Divisions and *Assistant Professor of Psychiatry,* Tufts University School of Medicine, Boston, MA

Matti Iivanainen, M.D., Ph.D., *Professor of Child Neurology,* University of Helsinki Medical School, Helsinki, Finland

David H. James, M.D., *Consultant in Psychiatry of Developmental Disabilities,* Budock Hospital, Toro, England, United Kingdom

John E. Kalachnik, M.Ed., Minnesota Department of Human Services, St. Paul, MN

Theodore A. Kastner, M.D., *Associate Professor of Clinical Pediatrics,* Columbia University, and DDC Medical Director, Morristown Memorial Hospital, Morristown, NJ

Richard A. Kern, M.D., *Medical Director,* Ohio State University Nisonger Center, Columbus, OH

Michael Kerr, M.D., *Lecturer in Learning Disability,* University of Wales College of Medicine, South Glamorgan, Wales, United Kingdom

Bryan King, M.D., *Assistant Professor of Psychiatry,* University of California at Los Angeles, Los Angeles, CA

Margaret G. Klitzke, D.O. Associate Medical Director for DD Unit, Emma Pendleton Bradley Hospital, East Providence, RI

Bennett L. Leventhal, M.D., *Professor of Psychiatry and Pediatrics,* University of Chicago, Chicago, IL

Andrew Levitas, M.D., Assistant Professor of Clinical Psychiatry, University of Medicine and Dentistry of New Jersey, Stratford, NJ

Earl Loschen, M.D., *Chief, Department of Psychiatry,* Southern Illinois University, Springfield, IL

Rex S. Lott, Pharm.D., *Associate Professor,* Idaho State University, College of Pharmacy, Pocatello, ID

Fran Maher, *volunteer,* The Arc of New Jersey, North Brunswick, NJ

James A. McCubbin, Ph.D., *Professor and Chairman,* Department of Psychology, Clemson University, Clemson, SC

James A. Mulick, Ph.D., *Professor of Pediatric Psychology,* Ohio State University, Columbus, OH

Robert J. Pary, M.D., *Associate Professor of Psychiatry,* Southern Illinois University, Springfield, IL

Deborah A. Pearson, Ph.D., *Associate Professor of Psychiatry and Behavioral Science,* University of Texas Medical School, Houston, TX

Alice T. Plummer, M.D., Christian Health Care Center, Wyckoff, NJ

Ann R. Poindexter, M.D., *Consultant Physician,* Conway, AR

Alan Poling, Ph.D., *Professor of Psychology,* Western Michigan University, Kalamazoo, MI

Andrew H. Reid, M.D., *Consultant Psychiatrist,* Royal Dundee Liff Hospital, Dundee, Scotland (UK)

Allan L. Reiss, M.D., *Professor of Psychiatry and Pediatrics,* Behavior Genetics and Neuroimaging Research Center, Kennedy Krieger Institute, Baltimore, MD

Steven Reiss, Ph.D., *Professor of Psychology and Psychiatry and Director,* Nisonger Center, The Ohio State University, Columbus, OH

Christine Rinck, Ph.D., *Director of Research, Institute for Human Development,* University of Missouri at Kansas City, Kansas City, MO

Beverly Roberts, *Project Director,* The Arc of New Jersey, North Brunswick, NJ

Stephen Ruedrich, M.D., *Associate Professor of Psychiatry,* Case Western Reserve, Cleveland, OH

Judith Saklad, Pharm.D., *Clinical Assistant Professor of Pharmacy,* The University of Texas Health Sciences Center at Houston, Houston, TX

Luis Salvador-Carulla, M.D., Ph.D., *Associate Professor of Medical Psychology,* Universidad de Cardiz, Spain

Curt A. Sandman, Ph.D., *Professor-in-Residence,* Department of Psychobiology, Department of Psychiatry and Human Behavior, University of California, Irvine, CA

Stephen R. Schroeder, Ph.D., *Director of Schiefelbusch Institute for Life Span Studies,* University of Kansas, Lawrence, KS

Jay A. Sevin, Ph.D., *Psychologist,* Developmental Neuropsychiatric Unit, Southeast Louisiana Hospital, Mandeville, LA

Nirbhay N. Singh, Ph.D., *Professor of Psychiatry,* Medical College of Virginia, Richmond, VA

Roger W. Sommi, Pharm.D., *Associate Professor of Pharmacy Practice and Psychiatry,* University of Missouri at Kansas City, Kansas City, MO

Robert Sovner, M.D., *Associate Professor of Psychiatry,* Tufts University, Medford, MA

Ludwik S. Szymanski, M.D., *Director of Psychiatry,* Developmental Evaluation Center, Children's Hospital, Boston, MA

Travis Thompson, Ph.D., *Professor of Psychology and Director of John F. Kennedy Center,* Vanderbilt University, Nashville, TN

Emanuel Tirosh, M.D., *Pediatrician,* Hannah Khoushi Child Development Center, Haifa Medical Center, Haifa, Israel

Bruce Tonge, M.D., *Professor of Developmental Psychiatry,* Monash University, Clayton, Victoria, Australia

Luke Tsai, M.D., *Professor and Director, Developmental Disorders Clinic,* University of Michigan, Ann Arbor, MI

Christopher K. Varley, M.D., *Associate Professor of Psychiatry,* University of Washington, Seattle, WA

Willem M.A. Verhoeven, M.D., Ph.D., *Director of Residency Training,* Vincent Van Gogh Institute of Psychiatry, Vanray, The Netherlands

Kevin Walsh, Ph.D., *Director of Research,* Center for Human Development, Morristown Memorial Hospital, Morristown, NJ

Michael L. Wehmeyer, Ph.D., *Assistant Director, Department of Research and Program Services,* The Arc of the United States, Arlington, TX

Steven A. Weisblatt, M.D., *Assistant Professor of Clinical Psychiatry,* Albert Einstein College of Medicine, Bronx, NY

John S. Werry, M.D., *Emeritus Professor of Psychiatry,* University of Auckland, New Zealand

Jacquelyn Gardner Wilson, Pharm.D., *Clincal Assistant (Clinical) of Pharmacy Practice and Psychiatry,* Wayne State University, Detroit, MI

James Wilson, Pharm.D., *Clinical Pharmacologist,* San Antonio State School, San Antonio, TX

Henry Wisniewski, M.D., Ph.D., *Professor and Director,* NYS Institute for Basic Research in Developmental Disabilities, Staten Island, NY

INTERNATIONAL CONSENSUS PANEL: INVITED MEMBERS

Martin Agran, Ph.D., *Associate Professor of Special Education,* Utah State University, USA

Fredrik Almqvist, M.D., *Professor of Child Psychiatry,* University of Helsinki, FINLAND

Norberto Alvarez, M.D., *Assistant Professor of Neurology,* Harvard University Medical School, USA

Michael Aman, Ph.D., *Professor of Psychology & Psychiatry,* The Ohio State University, USA

L. Eugene Arnold, M.Ed., M.D., *Special Expert,* National Institute of Mental Health, USA

Francisco J. Barrera, Ph.D., *Director of Specialized Behavior Clinic,* Southwestern Regional Center, CANADA

Rowland P. Barrett, Ph.D., *Associate Professor of Psychiatry,* Brown University School of Medicine, USA

Alan A. Baumeister, Ph.D., *Professor of Psychology,* Louisiana State University, USA

William H. Benefield, Jr., Pharm.D., *Clinical Pharmacologist,* San Antonio State School, USA

John P. Board, Jr., M.D., *Chief of Medical Services,* Michigan Department of Mental Health, USA

Nick Bouras, M.D., Ph.D., *Senior Lecturer in Psychiatry,* Guy's Hospital, UNITED KINGDOM

Joel D. Bregman, M.D., *Associate Professor of Psychiatry,* Emory University School of Medicine, USA

Bruce A. Buehler, M.D., *Scottish Rite Distinguished Professor of Child Health; Director, Meyer Rehabilitation Institute,* University of Nebraska, & *President,* American Association of University Affiliated Programs, USA

Nancy N. Cain, M.D., *Clinical Associate Professor of Psychiatry,* University of Rochester School of Medicine and Dentistry, USA

Magda Campbell, M.D., *Professor of Psychiatry,* New York University, USA

Dennis P. Cantwell, M.D., *Joseph Campbell Professor of Child Psychiatry,* University of California at Los Angeles, USA

David J. Clarke, M.D., *Senior Lecturer in Developmental Psychiatry,* University of Birmingham, UNITED KINGDOM

Edwin H. Cook, Jr., M.D., *Director, Laboratory of Developmental Neurochemistry,* University of Chicago, USA

John A. Corbett, M.D., *Professor of Developmental Psychiatry,* University of Birmingham, UNITED KINGDOM

David L. Coulter, M.D., *Associate Professor of Pediatrics and Neurology,* Boston University School of Medicine, USA

Henry Crabbe, Ph.D., M.D., *Consultant Psychiatrist,* Psychiatric Medicine Center, USA

Judy L. Curtis, Pharm.D., *Assistant Professor of Pharmacy Practice and Science,* University of Maryland at Baltimore, USA

Philip W. Davidson, Ph.D., *Professor of Pediatrics and Psychiatry & Director,* Strong Center, University of Rochester, USA

Sharon Davis, Ph.D., *Director of Research & Program Services,* The Arc of the United States, USA

Kenneth A. Day, M.D., *Medical Director,* Northgate Hospital, UNITED KINGDOM

Howard B. Demb, M.D., *Assistant Professor,* Department of Psychiatry, Albert Einstein College of Medicine, USA

Anton Dosen, M.D., Ph.D., *President,* European Association on Dual Diagnosis, THE NETHERLANDS

Stuart L. Einfeld, M.D., *Lecturer in Child & Adolescent Psychiatry,* University of Sydney, AUSTRALIA

Cynthia R. Ellis, M.D., *Assistant Professor of Pediatrics & Psychiatry,* Medical College of Virginia, USA

Jeffrey J. Fahs, M.D., *Consulting Psychiatrist,* Department of Human Resources of North Carolina, USA

Carl B. Feinstein, M.D., *Associate Professor of Psychiatry and Pediatrics,* Brown University, USA

Celia Fisher, Ph.D., *Professor & Director,* Applied Developmental Psychology, Fordham University, USA

Sherman Fox, M.D., West Central Community Support Services of Claremont, N.H., USA

W.I. Fraser, M.D., *Professor of Mental Handicap,* University of Wales College of Medicine & *Editor, Journal of Intellectual Disability Research,* UNITED KINGDOM

Kenneth D. Gadow, Ph.D., *Professor of Psychiatry,* State University of New York at Stony Brook, USA

Angela Gedye, Ph.D., R.Psych., Private practice, Vancouver, CANADA

Christopher Gillberg, M.D., *Professor of Child & Adolescent Psychiatry,* University of Goteborg, SWEDEN

Benjamin Goldberg, M.D., *Professor of Developmental Neuropsychiatry,* University of Western Ontario, CANADA

C. Thomas Gualtieri, M.D., Private practice, Charlotte, North Carolina, USA

Randi J. Hagerman, M.D., *Associate Professor of Pediatrics,* University of Colorado Health Sciences Center, USA

Ruth Hamilton, Ph.D., *Research Assistant Professor,* University of Vermont, USA

Benjamin L. Handen, Ph.D., *Associate Professor of Psychiatry,* John Merck Outpatient Program, Western Psychiatric Institute and Clinic, Pittsburgh, USA

James R. Hillard, M.D., *Professor and Chairman of Psychiatry,* College of Medicine, University of Cincinnati, USA

Robert H. Horner, Ph.D., *Professor & Director of Specialized Training Program*, University of Oregon, USA
Hans R. Huessy, M.D., *Professor Emeritus of Psychiatry*, University of Vermont College of Medicine, USA
Anne D. Hurley, Ph.D., *Assistant Professor of Psychiatry*, Tufts University School of Medicine & *Co-editor, The Habilitative Mental Healthcare Newsletter*, USA
Matti Iivanainen, M.D., Ph.D., *Professor of Child Neurology*, University of Helsinki Medical School, FINLAND
David H. James, M.D., *Consultant in Psychiatry of Developmental Disabilities*, Budock Hospital, UNITED KINGDOM
John E. Kalachnik, M.Ed., *Planner*, Minnesota Department of Human Services, USA
Theodore A. Kastner, M.D., *Associate Professor of Clinical Pediatrics*, Columbia University, USA
Richard A. Kern, M.D., *Medical Director, Nisonger Center*, The Ohio State University, USA
Michael Kerr, M.D., *Lecturer in Learning Disability*, University of Wales College of Medicine, Cardiff, UNITED KINGDOM
Bryan H. King, M.D., *Assistant Professor of Psychiatry*, University of California at Los Angeles, USA
Margaret G. Klitzke, D.O., *Associate Medical Director for DD Unit*, Emma Pendleton Bradley Hospital, USA
A. Langa, M.D., *Acting Consultant Psychiatrist*, Lynebank Hospital, SCOTLAND
John Lantis, Ph.D., Department of Pediatrics, LaRabida Hospital, USA
Bennett L. Leventhal, M.D., *Professor of Psychiatry & Pediatrics*, The University of Chicago, USA
Michael J. Levine, M.D., *Medical Director*, Developmental Disabilities Services, Louisiana Healthcare Authority, USA
Andrew Levitas, M.D., *Assistant Professor of Clinical Psychiatry*, University of Medicine and Dentistry of New Jersey, USA
Earl C. Loschen, M.D., *Chief, Department of Psychiatry*, Southern Illinois University, USA
Rex S. Lott, Pharm.D., *Director of Pharmacy*, Fircrest School, State of Washington Department of Social and Human Services, USA
Fran Maher, *Volunteer*, The Arc of New Jersey, USA
Savita Malhotra, M.D., Ph.D., Postgraduate Institute of Medical Education & Research, INDIA
Gerhard E. Martin, M.D., *Professor Emeritus of Neurology*, The Ohio State University, USA
Mauri J. Mattila, M.D., *Professor of Pharmacology*, University of Helsinki, FINLAND
James A. McCubbin, Ph.D. University of Kentucky College of Medicine, Lexington, USA
James A. Mulick, Ph.D., *Professor of Pediatric Psychology*, The Ohio State University, USA
Walter J. Mysiw, M.D., *Associate Professor of Physical Medicine*, The Ohio State University, USA
Christine M. Nezu, Ph.D., *Associate Professor*, Medical College of Pennsylvania and Hahnemann University, Philadelphia, USA
Stephen C. Olson, M.D., *Associate Professor of Psychiatry*, The Ohio State University, USA
Edward Page-El, M.D., *Director of Diagnostic & Assessment Clinic*, Illinois UAP, University of Illinois at Chicago, USA
Robert J. Pary, M.D., *Associate Professor of Psychiatry*, Southern Illinois University, USA
Deborah A. Pearson, Ph.D., *Assistant Professor of Psychiatry & Behavioral Science*, University of Texas at Houston Mental Sciences Institute, USA
Alice T. Plummer, M.D., Christian Health Care Center, USA
Ann R. Poindexter, M.D., *Consultant Physician*, Conway, Arkansas, USA
Alan Poling, Ph.D., *Professor of Psychology*, Western Michigan University, USA
Andrew H. Reid, M.D., *Consultant Psychiatrist*, Dundee Psychiatric Service, SCOTLAND
Alan L. Reiss, M.D., *Associate Professor of Psychiatry & Pediatrics*, Johns Hopkins University, USA
Steven Reiss, Ph.D., *Professor of Psychology & Psychiatry*, The Ohio State University, USA
Christine Rinck, Ph.D., *Director of Research*, Institute for Human Development, University of Missouri at Kansas City, USA
Beverly Roberts, *Volunteer*, The Arc of New Jersey, USA
Brian T. Rogers, M.D., *Assistant Professor of Pediatrics and Neurology*, SUNY at Buffalo, USA
Stephen Ruedrich, M.D., *Associate Professor of Psychiatry*, Case Western Reserve University, Cleveland, USA
B. I. Sacks, M.D., University of London, UNITED KINGDOM
Judith J. Saklad, Pharm.D., *Clinical Assistant Professor of Pharmacology*, The University of Texas Health Sciences Center at Houston, USA

Luis Salvador-Carulla, M.D., Ph.D., *Associate Professor of Medical Psychology*, Universidad de Cadiz, SPAIN

Curt Sandman, Ph.D., *Professor-in-Residence*, Department of Psychobiology, Department of Psychiatry & Human Behavior, University of California at Irvine, USA

Stephen R. Schroeder, Ph.D., *Director of Schiefelbusch Institute for Life Span Studies*, University of Kansas & *Editor, American Journal on Mental Retardation*, USA

Jay A. Sevin, Ph.D., *Psychologist*, Southeastern Louisiana Hospital, USA

Nirbhay N. Singh, Ph.D., *Professor of Psychiatry*, Medical College of Virginia, USA

Roger W. Sommi, Pharm.D., *Assistant Professor of Pharmacy Practice & Psychiatry*, University of Missouri at Kansas City, USA

Robert Sovner, M.D., *Associate Professor of Psychiatry*, Tufts University & *Co-editor, The Habilitative Mental Healthcare Newsletter*, USA

Robert L. Sprague, Ph.D., *Professor*, Institute for Research on Human Development, University of Illinois at Champaign-Urbana, USA

Henry J. Svec, Ph.D., *Psychologist*, Southwestern Regional Center, CANADA

James M. Swanson, Ph.D., *Professor of Psychology*, University of California at Irvine, Newport, USA

Ludwik S. Szymanski, M.D., *Director of Psychiatry*, Developmental Evaluation Center, Children's Hospital, & *Chairperson, Mental Retardation Committee*, American Psychiatric Association, USA

Joseph Szyszko, M.A., *Acting Program Director*, University of Illinois at Chicago, USA

Akihiko Takahashia, M.D., *Associate Professor*, Japan College for Social Work & *Director*, Kisen Center for Developmental Disabilities, JAPAN

Travis Thompson, Ph.D., *Professor of Psychology & Director of John F. Kennedy Center*, Vanderbilt University, & *Liaison to Nisonger-The Arc International Psychopharmacology Conference*, American Psychological Association, USA

Emanuel Tirosh, M.D., *Pediatrician*, Ben Zion Medical Center, ISRAEL

Bruce J. Tonge, M.D., *Professor and Head*, Monash University Faculty of Medicine Center for Developmental Psychiatry, AUSTRALIA

Luke Y. Tsai, M.D., *Professor and Director*, Developmental Disorders Clinic, University of Michigan, USA

Rameshwari V. Tumuluru, M.D., *Assistant Professor of Child & Adolescent Psychiatry*, University of Pittsburgh, USA

Alina Vales, M.D., M.P.H., *Director*, Mental Retardation Program, Departmento de Salud, Puerto Rico, USA

Christopher K. Varley, M.D., *Associate Professor of Psychiatry*, University of Washington School of Medicine, USA

Willem M.A. Verhoeven, M.D., Ph.D., *Chief*, Department of Biological Psychiatry, Vincent Van Gogh Instituut, THE NETHERLAND

Peter M. Vietze, Ph.D., *Associate Director*, Institute for Basic Research in Developmental Disabilities, USA

Mary K. Walker, Ph.D., R.N., *Associate Professor of Nursing*, University of Kentucky Chandler Medical Center, USA

Kevin Walsh, Ph.D., *Director of Research*, Center for Human Development, Morristown Memorial Hospital, USA

Michael L. Wehmeyer, Ph.D., The Arc of the United States, USA

Steven A. Weisblatt, M.D., *Assistant Professor of Clinical Psychiatry*, Albert Einstein College of Medicine, USA

John S. Werry, M.D., *Emeritus Professor of Psychiatry*, University of Auckland, NEW ZEALAND

Jacquelyn Gardner Wilson, Pharm. D., *Clinical Assistant Professor*, University of Maryland, USA

James Wilson, Pharm.D., *Associate Professor of Pharmacy and Medicine*, University of Nebraska Medical Center, USA

Henry Wisniewski, M.D., Ph.D., *Professor and Director*, NYS Institute for Basic Research in Developmental Disabilities, & SUNY Health Science Center at Brooklyn, USA

1995 PSYCHOPHARMACOLOGY CONFERENCE PARTICIPANTS

Pasquale Accardo, M.D.

Mohammed Alam

William Bach, M.D.

Kenneth W. Beroza, M.D.

Sarah W. Bisconer, Ph.D.

Cheryll Bowers-Stephens, M.D.

Patricia E. Brierly-Bowers, Ed.D.

Richard Lee Burns, M.D.

Eddythe G. Carr, Ph.D.

Philip E. Devers, M.S., N.C.C.

Kelly Dobrin, M.A.

Flora Ewing, M.D.

Allen Fannin, Ph.D.

Kim Knox Faulkner, Ph.D.

David Fedders, M.D.

Jerome H. Feldstein, Ph.D.

Elizabeth Moran Fitzgerald, Ed.D., R.N., C.S.

Arturo Fogata, M.D.

Sue A. Gant

Russell Gardner, Jr., M.D.

Zev Goldberg, Ph.D.

Kate Haller, M.D.

Peter P. Heinbecker, M.D., J.D.

Jessica A. Hellings, M.D.

Patrick Holden, M.D.

Kay C. Hunter, Psy.D.

Susan L. Hyman, M.D.

Joanne M. Icovino, M.D.

Charlotte M. Kimmel, Ph.D.

William R. LeVine, M.D.

Stanley E. Lunde, Ph.D.

Lyle MacDonald, M.A.

Edmon L. Mann, Ph.D.

Joyce Elizabeth Mauk, M.D.

Philip May, Jr., M.D.

Robin R. Michaels, M.D.

Mary Kay Moore, R.N., M.A.

Jamshed R. Nuggud, M.D.

Benjamin K. Oko, M.D.

Stephen C. Olson, M.D.

Susan Pearlson, M.D.

Deborah Pearson, Ph.D.

David Pyles, Ph.D.

Rebecca Randall, R.N., B.S.N., M.A.

Joseph N. Ricciardi, Psy.D.

Robert W. Ricketts, M.S.

Donald R. Rochon, Ph.D.

Michael J. Romanelli, Ed.D.

Donald L Rynier, M.D.

Stephan A. Schwartz, Ph.D.

Susan N. Sherwood, Ph.D.

William E. Skuban, M.A.

Brenda H. Spence, Ph.D., L.L.P.

Richard M. Stevko, M.D.

Scott R. Stiefel, M.D.

Ruth C. Sullivan, Ph.D.

Kishore Sunkara, M.D.

John A. Tsiouris, M.D.

Craig Van Tuinen, M.D.

Rebecca S. Valla, M.D.

Robert S. White, M.D.

Joseph K. Yau, M.D.

CREDITS

SPONSORS: These organizations are the formal sponsors of this project.

Nisonger Center for Mental Retardation and Developmental Disabilities, A University-Affiliated Program

The Arc of the United States

LEADERS: This activity was supported by persons and organizations representing a diversity of interests, disciplines, and organizations. The following persons donated significant time and effort to help develop united support for this project.

Alan Abeson, Ed.D., Executive Director, Arc of the United States

Elizabeth Boggs, Ph.D., Arc of the United States

M. Doreen Croser, Executive Director, American Association on Mental Retardation

Sharon Davis, Ph.D., Director of Research and Program Services, The Arc of the United States

Robert Sovner, M.D., Associate Professor of Psychiatry, Tufts University

Ludwik S. Szymanski, M.D., Director of Psychiatry, Developmental Evaluation Clinic, Children's Hospital of Boston

Benedetto Vitiello, M.D., Child & Adolescent Disorders Research Branch, National Institute of Mental Health

Edward Zigler, Ph.D., Sterling Professor of Psychology, Yale University

FINANCIAL ASSISTANCE: The publication of this book is the culmination of a 6-year project costing approximately $350,000. The following individuals and organizations provided gifts to help support this activity or "The Nisonger—The Arc International Consensus Conference on Psychopharmacology" held June 15 and 16, 1995, at The Ohio State University. The provision of financial assistance for some or all of the activities that led to the development and publication of this book does not imply agreement or disagreement with any of the specific statements in the text.

Cincinnati Center for Developmental Disorders (CCDD) donated staff led by **Yvonne Bullock Fryberger** to organize and assist with local arrangements for the 1995 conference.

Robert Dilenschneider donated efforts of his New York publicity company, called **The Dilenschneider Group**, to help publicize the needs of the population.

Dr. Friedrich Christian Flick provided financial support for printing this book.

National Institute of Mental Health provided partial support for the 1995 conference.

Nisonger Center of Ohio State University provided funding plus in-kind resources to support all aspects of this project.

The **Office of Health Sciences** of The Ohio State University provided financial support for the 1995 international conference.

Simson First Foundation, Columbus, Ohio

EDITORIAL ASSISTANTS: The committees of the International Consensus Panel submitted 21 reports that needed to be organized into this book, verified for accuracy of fact and citation, made consistent with one another in terms of style and terminology, and proofread. The following individuals assisted the editors in accomplishing these tasks, which represented 2 years' effort.

Deanna D'Enrico, copyeditor

Susan M. Havercamp, M.A., assistant proofreading

Richard A. Kern, M.D., medical proofreading

Kathleen Kraft, secretarial support

Kate Matusak, secretarial support

Mary Ellen Milos, Ph.D., proofreader

Maggi Reiss, M.S., assistant proofreading

Jeanne Thomas, assistant proofreading

James Wiltz, assistant proofreading

BOOK MANUFACTURER: This book was developed and produced under the leadership of The Nisonger Center of The Ohio State University, which is the exclusive owner of the copyright. These companies provided contractual services to produce this book.

Braun-Brumfield, Inc., Ann Arbor, MI, printing & binding

Computer Publishing Services, Inc., Palos Heights, IL, typesetting & design

CONFERENCE CO-SPONSORS: 10 national organizations issued formal letters of co-sponsorship of the 1995 international conference for the purpose of alerting its membership on the importance of the population and issues addressed and also to recognize Nisonger Center leadership. Co-sponsorship of the conference does not imply agreement or disagreement with any of the statements made at that conference or with any of the specific statements that appear in this book. Co-sponsorship of the conference does not imply co-sponsorship of the activities preceding and following the conference.

American Academy of Child & Adolescent Psychiatry

American Association on Mental Retardation

American Association of University Affiliated Programs

American Psychiatric Association

American Psychological Association

Arc of the United States

European Association on Dual Diagnosis

National Association on Dual Diagnosis

President's Committee on Mental Retardation

U.S. Administration on Developmental Disabilities

U.S. Maternal & Child Health

CONFERENCE ASSISTANTS: These individuals assisted with arrangements for the 1995 conference.

Malcolm S. Baroway, University Communications

Antoinette L. Eaton, M.D., CME credit

Tom Gannon, volunteer

Pat Gardner, University Conferences

Susan M. Havercamp, M.A., organized student volunteers

Rebecca D. Jackson, M.D., CME credits

Kelly Kershner, University Communications

Alan G. Kraut, Ph.D., APS publicity

Yona Lunsky, organized student volunteers

Walter J. Mysiw, CME credits

Sarah A. Sieling, University Conferences

Marc J. Tasse, Ph.D., substantial technical assistance

Shawna Ryan, volunteer

Mark Shannon, volunteer

Benedetto Vitiello, M.D., NIMH support

Elizabeth B. Weller, M.D., CME credits

David Wilkerson, volunteer

Barry Zvolenski, substantial secretarial support

Ludwik Szymanski, M.D., APA co-sponsorship

1993 AAMR PRECONFERENCE: Steven Reiss and Michael Aman organized a preconference on psychopharmacology for the 1993 national meeting of the American Association on Mental Retardation held in Washington, D.C. The purpose of the preconference was to stimulate interest in the international consensus process. The following individual organized the arrangements for the preconference.

Marsha Aman, Columbus, Ohio

<u>Invitation</u>

The Nisonger - The Arc

INTERNATIONAL CONSENSUS CONFERENCE ON PSYCHOPHARMACOLOGY

June 15 and 16, 1995

The Ohio State University
Columbus, Ohio

<u>Organizing Committee</u>

Michael Aman, Ph.D., Co-chair
Sharon Davis, Ph.D., Co-chair
Yvonne Bullock Fryberger, M.S.
Richard Kern, M.D.
Steven Reiss, Ph.D., Chairperson
Ludwik S. Szymanski, M.D.
Marc J. Tasse, Ph.D.

Conference Aims and Purposes: A large percentage of people with mental retardation also have a mental illness or behavior disorder. These people are said to have a "dual diagnosis." Many physicians are trained either in mental retardation or mental illness, but not both. Because there is almost no cross-training, doctors make a relatively high number of mistakes in caring for people with a "dual diagnosis." These mistakes cost taxpayers billions of dollars and are very frustrating for families. They lead to unnecessary hospitalizations and to overmedication. Too many psychoactive drugs are given. The drugs may be given indefinitely, with no endpoint in treatment identified. They may lead to significant side effects. Particularly in children, they may interfere with learning, making acquisition of basic skills and knowledge even more difficult.

The conference represents a grass-roots, international initiative of hundreds of professors and physicians from eleven nations. The primary aim is to develop clinical information about the effects, side effects, and best practices regarding the use of psychoactive drugs in people with mental retardation. The conference will publish a handbook on psychopharmacology based on the common experiences of a large group of doctors, families, and health professionals. The book should reduce the number of mistakes made by physicians in working with people with a dual diagnosis. The book also should reduce unusual practices, alert caregivers to possible side effects, and reduce overmedication.

The conference will begin a national discussion on the need for public policies regarding training and research. In 1994 the nation's network of University-Affiliated Programs provided long-term training to only 32 psychiatrists in the entire country. The conference will consider a call to create 150 new ADD/MCH traineeships in psychiatry and behavior pediatrics to improve services and save billions of tax dollars.

In 1994 very little research was being conducted to develop new medicines or to evaluate clinical effects of commonly used medicines. The conference will consider a call for the pharmaceutical industry to fund two new MR research centers and to provide funds to create MR laboratories.

Sponsors: The Nisonger Center UAP and The Arc of the United States initiated this activity. The National Institute of Mental Health has helped fund the conference.

CME Credits: The Ohio State University Center for Continuing Medical Education is accredited by the Accreditation Council for Continuing Medical Education to sponsor medical education for physicians. This office certified that this program meets the criteria for 14.5 hours in Category I of the Physician's Recognition Award of the American Medical Association.

CEU Credits: Available for Psychology (Ohio Psychological Association), Social Work and Counseling (Ohio Department of Mental Health), Nursing, Adult Services and Case Management (Ohio Department of Mental Retardation.)

Local Arrangements: Yvonne Bullock Fryburger, Tom Gannon, Shawna Ryan, Mark Shannon, David Wilkerson, all UACCDD. Pat Gardner and Sarah A. Sieling, OSU Office of Continuing Education.

Assistance: Dr. Marc J. Tasse assisted with the scientific program and Barry Zvolenski provided general assistance. David Barlow, Antoinette L. Eaton, Gail E. Evans, Gary W. Goldstein, Dorothy W. Jackson, Rebecca D. Jackson, Christopher Keys, Susan Mineka, Walter J. Mysiw, Martin Seligman, Robert L. Sprague, Ludwik S. Szymanski, Benedetto Vitiello, Elizabeth B. Weller, Roger Weissberg, and Edward Zigler assisted with arrangements for co-sponsorships. Alan G. Kraut and Marilyn Brewer arranged for publicity with the American Psychological Society *Observer*.

Administrative Support: Administrative support for the conference was provided by E. Gordon Gee (President, The Ohio State University), Ronald St. Pierre (Associate Vice President for Health Services and Academic Affairs), and John R. Kleberg (Office of Business and Administration). Assistance regarding publicity was provided by Malcom S. Baroway (Director, University Communications), Earle M. Holland, Kelly Kershner, and The Dilenschneider Group of New York City.

PRESENTATIONS

COMMITTEE	PRESENTER	FACILITATOR
Antiepileptics	Alvarez, Kern	Coury
Antidepressants/MAOIs	Sovner	Silka
Anxiolytics	Werry	McNally
Beta Blockers	Fraser	McNally
Diagnostic Categories	Szymanski	Peterson
Ethical Issues	Davidson	Lottman
Interaction Effects	Sommi	St. Pierre
Mood Stabilizers	Poindexter	Silka
Neuroleptics	Sevin	McNally
Opiate Blockers	Sandman	McNally
Research Forum		
Past Research	Schroeder	
Reseach Methods	Swanson	
Instruments	Hurley	
Review Panels	Davis	Fish
Selected Drugs		
Clonidine	Hagerman	
Fenfluramine	Gillberg	
Vitamins	Singh	
Side Effects	Tsai	Aman
Standards of Care	Leventhal, Kalachnik	Peterson
Stimulants	Arnold	Coury

Note: The Epidemiology Committee, chaired by Christine Rinck, Ph.D., will present its report as part of the opening plenary session.

Facilitators

Michael Aman, Ph.D., Professor of Psychology and Psychiatry, The Ohio State University
Daniel L. Coury, M.D., Associate Professor of Clinical Pediatrics, The Ohio State University
Thomas Fish, M.S.W., Associate Director, Nisonger Center, The Ohio State University
Thomas Lottman, Adult Medical Services Program, UACCDD, University of Cincinnati
Richard J. McNally, Ph.D., Associate Professor of Psychology, Harvard University
Rolf A. Peterson, Ph.D., Professor of Psychology, George Washington University
Ronald St. Pierre, Ph.D., Associate Vice President for Health Services, The Ohio State University
Van R. Silka, M.D., Consultant Psychiatrist

Plenary Session, Thursday morning, June 15, 1995, Sullivant Hall

8:00 - 8:10   *Welcome to Ohio.*   **Jerome G. Manuel,** Director, Ohio Department of Mental Retardation and Developmental Disabilities
8:10 - 8:20   *Welcome to The Ohio State University.*   **Manuel Tzagournis, M.D.,** Vice-President for Health Sciences, The Ohio State University

NATIONAL PUBLIC HEALTH PERSPECTIVES
ON PSYCHOACTIVE DRUGS AND MENTAL RETARDATION

Moderator: **Stephen G. Pleasnick,** Franklin County Board of Mental Retardation and Developmental Disabilities

8:20 - 8:45   *Quantity and Quality of Use of Psychoactive Medications in Persons with Mental Retardation,* **Christine Rinck, Ph.D.,** Director of Research, Institute for Human Development, University of Missouri
8:45 - 9:15   *General Status of Research on Psychoactive Medications in Persons with Mental Retardation,* **Michael Aman, Ph.D.,** Professor of Psychology and Psychiatry, Nisonger Center, The Ohio State University
9:15 - 10:00   *A Public Health Perspective on Psychoactive Medications and Mental Retardation: National Need for Information, Training, and Research,* **Steven Reiss, Ph.D.,** Professor of Psychology and Psychiatry, The Ohio State University
10:00 - 10:15   *Discussant*: **Alan Abeson, Ed.D.,** Executive Director, The Arc of the United States

Nisonger Center UAP Awards Ceremony, Thursday evening, June 15, 1995, OSU Golf Clubhouse

Moderator: **Sharon Davis, Ph.D.,** Director of Research and Program Services, The Arc of the United States

7:40 - 7:50   **Elsie Helsel, Ph.D.,** *Herschel Nisonger Award and naming of the Elsie Helsel Toy and Technology Library.* Presented by: Steven Reiss, Ph.D., Director, Nisonger Center UAP
7:50 - 8:00   **Joseph Szyszko, M.A.,** *Simpson First Prize for Career Service Contributions to People with a Dual Diagnosis.* Award and $1,000 check presented by M. Doreen Croser, Executive Director, American Association on Mental Retardation.

Plenary Session, Thursday evening, June 15, 1995, OSU Golf Clubhouse

PUBLIC POLICY ISSUES

Moderator: **Senator Karen Gillmor,** Ohio Senate

8:00 - 8:20   *Role of Psychiatry at UAPs,* **Ludwik S. Szymanski, M.D.,** Harvard University
8:20 - 8:50   *National Institute of Mental Health: Current Activities and Future Directions,* **Benjamin Vitiello, M.D.,** Child and Adolescent Disorders Research Branch
8:50 - 9:10   *The Cochrane Initiative in Scotland,* **A. Lagna, M.D.,** Lynebank Hospital
9:10 - 9:30   *Discussants*: **Senator Grace Drake,** Chairperson, Health Committee, Ohio Senate and **Elizabeth Boggs, Ph.D.**

INTERNATIONAL CONSENSUS CONFERENCE ON PSYCHOPHARMACOLOGY

SCHEDULE OF ACTIVITIES

TIME	SULLIVANT HALL	WEXNER FILM LIBRARY	HAGERTY HALL
THURSDAY, 15 JUNE 1995			
7:00 am - ...	*REGISTRATION*		
8:00 am - 10:15 am	Plenary Session: Public Health Perspectives (SULLIVANT HALL)		
10:15 am - 10:45 am	*Break*		
10:45 am - 12:00 pm	Anxiolytics Werry/McNally	Standards of Care Leventhal & Kalachnik/Peterson	Stimulants Arnold/Coury
12:00 pm - 1:30 pm	*Lunch on your own*		
1:30 pm - 2:45 pm	Diagnostic Categories Szymanski/Peterson	Review Panels Davis/Fish	Research Committees Schroeder, Swanson, & Hurley
2:45 pm - 3:15 pm	*Break*		
3:15 pm - 4:30 pm	Neuroleptics Sevin/McNally	Antidepressants Sovner/Silka	Interaction Effects Sommi/St-Pierre
7:00 pm - 9:30 pm	*Dinner and Session - Ticket Required* Awards and NIMH Presentation (O.S.U. GOLF CLUBHOUSE)		
FRIDAY, 16 JUNE 1995			
8:45 am - 10:00 am	Opiate Blockers Sandman/McNally	Mood Stabilizers Poindexter/Silka	Ethical Issues Davidson/Lottman
10:00 am - 10:30 am	*Break*		
10:30 am - 11:45 am	Beta Blockers Fraser/McNally	Side Effects Tsai/Aman	
11:45 am - 1:00 pm	*Lunch on your own*		
1:00 pm - 2:15 pm	Antiepileptics Alvarez & Kern/Coury	Selected Drugs Gillberg, Hagerman, & Singh	
2:15 pm - 2:30 pm	*Break*		
2:30 pm - 3:15 pm	Keynote Address: David L. Hobson (R-Ohio, U.S. Congress) (FACULTY CLUB)		

\SCHEDUL7.WPD

FORMAT FOR CONCURRENT (BREAKOUT) SESSIONS

1. Volunteers will distribute a copy of the draft committee report to persons attending the session. **These reports should be regarded as works in progress** -- they will undergo additional revisions prior to publication. They are being developed as chapters in a forthcoming field-test version of a handbook to be published six to nine months after the conference. Due to costs, it will not be possible to give a copy of the draft report to persons not attending the session.

2. The facilitator will introduce the speaker(s), who will give a formal presentation based on the committee report. The facilitator will alert the last speaker when 5 and 0 minutes are left to the presentation.

3. After his/her presentation, the speaker will leave the podium and return to the speakers' table. The facilitator will go to the podium.

4. The facilitator will encourage audience comment on the committee report. The facilitator may use probe questions, which will be distributed at the conference. Examples of such questions are "Do you have experiences that are similar to, or different from, those summarized in the presentation?" "In what ways can the report be made more useful to you prior to publication?" Anyone in the audience may participate in the conversation, including persons who are on the International Panel but not members of the subcommittee giving the presentation.

5. The facilitator's job is to help the audience provide specific, factually oriented information. For example, if someone comments, "Our experience with medications has been negative," the facilitator might ask if the person can identify the specific medicine, the reason it was given, the length of time it was given, and any noticeable effects. If another person comments, "I've found that this drug helped in a case with a child with severe mental retardation," the facilitator might ask, "Can you tell us the behavioral condition that was being treated, the dosage level, the length of time of treatment, and how you evaluated the effects?"

6. Once the formal committee presentations are completed, the role of the speaker(s) is to take notes on the information provided by the audience. Speakers are asked not to comment on the discussion, not to ask or answer any questions during the discussion unless specfically requested to do so by the facilitator, and not to initiate any comments. The reason for these rules is that, on balance, they may encourage free and open conversation on the part of the audience. There will be a tape recorder in each room for backup purposes.

7. All comments and questions will be directed to the facilitator, who will direct them back to the audience. For example, if a member of the audience asks if the committee feels that xanax can be used to treat phobias, the facilitator will ask the audience what they think of this point.

8. At the end of the session, the speaker(s) should thank the audience for their comments and invite interested persons to submit additional written commentaries to Barry Zvolenski at Nisonger Center, who will distribute them to the appropriate committee chairpersons. Every comment will be considered by the committee, although that does not mean that the comment necessarily will be included in the final committee report.

9. Speakers are encouraged to invite members of the audience to talk with them privately during the conference if they have further questions or comments.

CO-SPONSORS

American Academy of Child & Adolescent Psychiatry (AACAP)[1]
American Association on Mental Retardation (AAMR)[2]
American Association of University Affiliated Programs (AAUAP)[3]
American Psychiatric Association (APA)[4]
American Psychological Association (APA)[5]
Arc of Ohio[6]
Cincinnati Center for Developmental Disorders (CCDD)[7]
European Association on Dual Diagnosis (EADD)[8]
National Institute of Mental Health (NIMH)[9]
National Association on Dual Diagnosis (NADD)[10]
Nisonger Center UAP[11]
Ohio Psychiatric Association[12]
President's Committee on Mental Retardation (PCMR)[13]
The Arc of the United States[14]
The Ohio State University[15]
U. S. Administration on Developmental Disabilities (ADD)[16]
U. S. Maternal & Child Health (MCH)[17]

[1] Virginia Q. Anthony, Executive Director
[2] Doreen Croser, Executive Director
[3] William Jones, Ph.D., Executive Director
[4] Melvin Sabshin, M.D., Executive Director
[5] Raymond G. Fowler, Ph.D., Executive Director
[6] Ray Ferguson, Executive Director
[7] Jack H. Rubenstein, M.D., Director
[8] Anton Dosen, M.D., President
[9] Peter Jensen, M.D., Chief, Child & Adolescent Disorders Research
[10] Robert Fletcher, D.S.W., Executive Director
[11] Steven Reiss, Ph.D., Director
[12] Phil Workman, M.D., Executive Director
[13] Gary H. Blumenthal, Executive Director
[14] Alan Abeson, Ph.D., Executive Director
[15] E. Gordon Gee, Ph.D., President
[16] Bob Williams, Commissioner
[17] Audrey H. Nora, M.D., M.P.H., Assistant Surgeon General

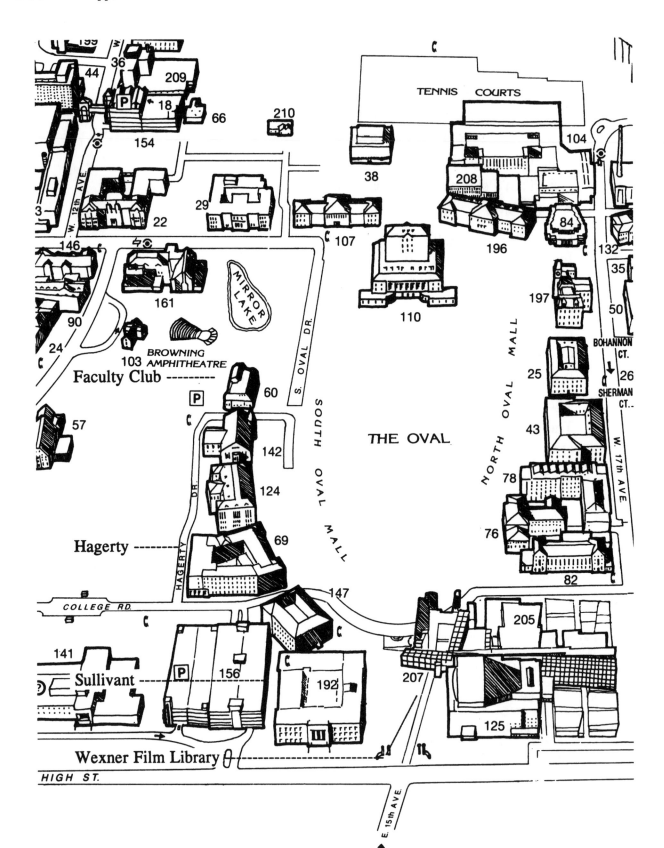

TENNIS   COURTS

MIRROR LAKE

BROWNING
103 AMPHITHEATRE

Faculty Club ----------

THE OVAL

NORTH OVAL MALL

SOUTH OVAL MALL

S. OVAL DR.

HAGERTY DR.

W. 12th AVE.

W. 17th AVE.

BOHANNON CT.

SHERMAN CT.

Hagerty --------

COLLEGE RD.

Sullivant ----------

Wexner Film Library

HIGH ST.

E. 15th AVE.

44   36   209   18   66   154   210   38   208   196   104   132   35   50   84   197   25   26   43   78   76   82   22   29   107   110   146   161   90   24   57   60   142   124   69   147   205   207   125   141   156   192   199

GLOSSARY OF MEDICINES

Note: Many drugs have more than one function and more than one brand name. The same drug may have different brand names in different countries. Some drugs have more than one scientific name. Some of the drugs mentioned in this book are still in a research phase and have not been approved for clinical use, at least not in the United States. Some of the medicines mentioned in this book are historical terms no longer in use. See subject index to find where in the text a medicine is mentioned. Some of the drug terms that are used in the text do not appear in this glossary because they refer to classes of drugs and are not names of a specific drug. In this glossary, only one function is listed and the brand name listed is the most common.

generic names are in lower case
first letters of brand names are in upper case

Names	Functional Categories	Comment
acebutolol	cardiovascular	brand name is Sectral
acetazolimide	antiepileptic	brand name is Diamox
acetophenazine	antipsychotic	brand name is Tindal
Achromycin	antibiotic	generic name is tetracycline hydrochloride
Adderall	stimulant	generic name is dextroamphetamine
Advil	analgesic	generic name is ibuprofen
Akineton	anti-Parkinson	generic name is biperiden hydrochloride
Aldomet	cardiovascular	generic name is methyldopa
alprazolam	anxiolytic	brand name is Xanax
Alurate	sedative	generic name is aprobarbital
amantadine	anti-Parkinson	brand name is Symmetrel
amiloride	diuretic	brand name is Midamor
Aminophyllin	antiasthmatic	generic name is aminophylline
aminophylline	antiasthmatic	brand name is Aminophyllin
amitriptyline	antidepressant	brand name is Elavil
amobarbital	sedative	brand name is Tuinal
amoxapine	antidepressant	brand name is Asendin
amphetamine	stimulant	brand name is Adderall
Amytal	sedative	generic name is amobarbital
Anafranil	antidepressant	generic name is clomipramine hydrochloride
Anaprox	analgesic	generic name is naproxen sodium
Anectine	autonomic	generic name is succinylcholine chloride
Antabuse	alcoholism	generic name is disulfiram
antipyrine	analgesic	brand name is Auralgan
aprobarbital	sedative	brand name is Alurate
Aquachloral	sedative	generic name is chloral hydrate
Artane	anti-Parkinson	generic name is trihexyphenidyl hydrochloride
Asendin	antidepressant	generic name is amoxapine
astemizole	antihistamine	brand name is Hismanal
Atarax	antihistamine	generic name is hydroxyzine hydrochloride
atenolol	cardiovascular	brand name is Tenormin
Ativan	anxiolytic	generic name is lorazepam
Auralgan	analgesic	generic name is antipyrine
Aventyl	antidepressant	generic name is nortriptyline hydrochloride
Benadryl	antihistamine	generic name is diphenhydramine hydrochloride
Benemid	antiarthritics	generic name is probenecid
Benzedrine	stimulant	generic name is amphetamine

Names	Functional Categories	Comment
benztropine	anti-Parkinson	brand name is Cogentin
Betagan	cardiovascular	generic name is levobunolol hydrochloride
Betapace	cardiovascular	generic name is sotalol hydrochloride
betaxolol hydrochloride	cardiovascular	brand name is Betoptic
bethanechol chloride	cholinergic agonist	brand name is Urecholine
Betoptic	cardiovascular	generic name is betaxolol hydrochloride
Biaxin	antibiotic	generic name is clarithromycin
biperiden hydrochloride	anti-Parkinson	brand name is Akineton
bisoprolol fumarate	cardiovascular	brand name is Zebeta
Blocadren	cardiovascular	generic name is timolol maleate
Brevibloc	cardiovascular	generic name is esmolol hydrochloride
bromocriptine mesylate	anti-Parkinson	brand name is Parlodel
bumetanide	diuretic	brand name is Bumex
Bumex	diuretic	generic name is bumetanide
bupropion hydrochloride	antidepressant	brand name is Wellbutrin
BuSpar	anxiolytic	generic name is buspirone hydrochloride
buspirone hydrochloride	anxiolytic	brand name is BuSpar
Butazolidin	analgesic	generic name is phenylbutazone
Calan	cardiovascular	generic name is verapamil hydrochloride
Capoten	cardiovascular	generic name is captopril
captopril	cardiovascular	brand name is Capoten
Carafate	treat ulcer	generic name is sucralfate
carbamazepine	antiepileptic	brand name is Tegretol
Cardizem	cardiovascular	generic name is diltiazem hydrochloride
carteolol hydrochloride	cardiovascular	brand name is Cartrol
Cartrol	cardiovascular	generic name is carteolol hydrochloride
Catapres	cardiovascular	generic name is clonidine hydrochloride
Celontin	antiepileptic	generic name is methsuximide
Centrax	anxiolytic	generic name is prazepam
chloral hydrate	sedative	brand name is Aquachloral
chlordiazepoxide	hydrochlorideanxiolytic	brand name is Librium
chlorpromazine	hydrochlorideantipsychotic	brand name is Thorazine
chlorpropamide	treat diabetes	brand name is Diabinese
chlorprothixene	antipsychotic	brand name is Taractan
Cibalith-S	antimanic	generic name is lithium citrate
cimetidine	treat ulcer	brand name is Tagamet
Cipro	antibiotic	generic name is ciprofloxacin hydrochloride
ciprofloxacin hydrochloride	antibiotic	brand name is Cipro
cisapride monohydrate	treat ulcer	brand name is Propulsid
clarithromycin	antibiotic	brand name is Biaxin
Clinoril	analgesic	generic name is sulindac
clomipramine hydrochloride	antidepressant	brand name is Anafranil
clonazepam	antiepileptic	brand name is Klonopin
clonidine hydrochloride	cardiovascular	brand name is Catapres
clorazepate dipotassium	anxiolytic	brand name is Tranxene
clorgyline	antidepressant	not available
clozapine	antipsychotic	brand name is Clozaril
Clozaril	antipsychotic	generic name is clozapine
Cogentin	anti-Parkinson	generic name is benztropine
Cognex	anticholinergic	generic name is tacrine hydrochloride

Names	Functional Categories	Comment
Compazine	antipsychotic	generic name is prochlorperazine
Corgard	cardiovascular	generic name is nadolol
Coumadin	anticoagulant	generic name is warfarin sodium
cyclosporine	immunosuppressant	brand name is Sandimmune
Cylert	stimulant	generic name is pemoline
cyproheptadine hydrochloride	antihistamine	brand name is Periactin
Dalmane	anxiolytic	generic name is flurazepam hydrochloride
Dantrium	neuromuscular	generic name is dantrolene sodium
dantrolene sodium	neuromuscular	brand name is Dantrium
Darvon	analgesic	generic name is propoxyphene hydrochloride
Deltasone	anti-inflammatory	generic name is prednisone
Depakene	antiepileptic	generic name is valproic acid
Depakote	antiepileptic	generic name is valproic acid
desipramine hydrochlorate	antidepressant	brand name is Norpramin
Desoxyn	stimulant	generic name is methamphetamine hydrochloride
Desyrel	antidepressant	generic name is trazodone hydrochloride
Dexedrine	stimulant	generic name is dextroamphetamine sulfate
dexfenfluramine	treat obesity	brand name is Redux
dextroamphetamine sulfate	stimulant	brand name is Dexedrine
Diabinese	treat diabetes	generic name is chlorpropamide
Diamox	antiepileptic	generic name is acetazolimide
diazepam	anxiolytic	brand name is Valium
diazoxide	cardiovascular	brand name is Hyperstat
diclofenac	analgesic	brand name is Voltaren
Diflucan	antibiotic	generic name is fluconazole
Dilantin	antiepileptic	generic name is phenytoin
diltiazem hydrochloride	cardiovascular	brand name is Cardizem
diphenhydramine hydrochloride	antihistamine	brand name is Benadryl
disulfiram	treat alcoholism	brand name is Antabuse
Dolophine	opiate agonist	generic name is methadone hydrochloride
Doral	anxiolytic	generic name is quazepam
Doxepin	antidepressant	generic name is doxepin hydrochloride
doxepin hydrochloride	antidepressant	brand name is Sinequan
Effexor	antidepressant	generic name is venlafaxine hydrochloride
Elavil	antidepressant	generic name is amitriptyline
Eldepryl	anti-Parkinson	generic name is selegiline hydrochloride
Elixophyllin	antiasthmatic	generic name is theophylline
Epilim	antiepileptic	generic name is valproic acid
Equanil	anxiolytic	generic name is meprobamate
Eskalith	antimanic	generic name is lithium carbonate
esmolol hydrochloride	cardiovascular	brand name is Brevibloc
estazolam	anxiolytic	brand name is ProSom
ethosuximide	antiepileptic	brand name is Zarontin
ethotoin	antiepileptic	brand name is Peganone
Euhypnos	anxiolytic	generic name is temazepam
felbamate	antiepileptic	brand name is Felbatol
Felbatol	antiepileptic	generic name is felbamate
Feldene	analgesic	generic name is piroxicam
fenfluramine hydrochlorate	treat obesity	brand name is Pondimin
Flagyl	antibiotic	generic name is metronidazole

Names	Functional Categories	Comment
fluconazole	antibiotic	brand name is Diflucan
fluoxetine hydrochloride	antidepressant	brand name is Prozac
fluphenazine decanoate	antipsychotic	brand name is Prolixin Decanoate
flurazepam hydrochloride	anxiolytic	brand name is Dalmane
furosemide	diuretic	brand name is Lasix
fluvoxamine	antidepressant	brand name is Luvox
gabapentin	antiepileptic	brand name is Neurontin
Grisactin	antibiotic	generic name is griseofulvine
griseofulvine	antibiotic	brand name is Grisactin
guanethidine monosulfate	cardiovascular	brand name is Ismelin
guanfacine hydrochloride	cardiovascular	brand name is Tenex
halazepam	anxiolytic	brand name is Paxipam
Halcion	anxiolytic	generic name is triazolam
Haldol	antipsychotic	generic name is haloperidol
haloperidol	antipsychotic	brand name is Haldol
Hismanal	antihistamine	generic name is astemizole
hydroxyzine hydrochloride	antihistamine	brand name is Atarax
hydroxyzine pamoate	antihistamine	brand name is Vistaril
Hyperstat	cardiovascular	generic name is diazoxide
ibuprofen	analgesic	brand name is Motrin
imipramine hydrochloride	antidepressant	brand name is Tofranil
Imovane	sedative	generic name is zopiclone
Inderal	anxiolytic	generic name is propranolol hydrochloride
Indocin	analgesic	generic name is indomethacin
indomethacin	analgesic	brand name is Indocin
INH	antibiotic	generic name is isoniazid
Ismelin	cardiovascular	generic name is guanethidine monosulfate
isocarboxazid	antidepressant	brand name is Marplan
isoniazid	antibiotic	brand name is INH
Isopto Eserine	anticholinergic	generic name is physostigmine salicylate
Isoptin	cardiovascular	generic name is verapamil hydrochloride
Kemadrin	anticholinergic agent	generic name procyclidine hydrochloride
ketoconazole	antibiotic	brand name is Nizoral
ketoprofen	analgesic	brand name is Orudis
Klonopin	antiepileptic	generic name is clonazepam
labetolol hydrochloride	cardiovascular	brand name is Normodyne
Lamictal	antiepileptic	generic name is lamotrigine
lamotrigine	antiepileptic	brand name is Lamictal
Larodopa	anti-Parkinson	generic name is levodopa
Lasix	diuretic	generic name is furosemide
Levatol	cardiovascular	generic name is penbutolol sulfate
levobunolol hydrochloride	cardiovascular	brand name is Betagan
levodopa	anti-Parkinson	brand name is Larodopa
Levoprome	sedative	generic name is methotrimeprazine
levothyroxine sodium	synthetic thyroid hormone	brand name is Synthroid
Librium	anxiolytic	generic name is chlordiazepoxide hydrochloride
lidocaine hydrochloride	anesthesia	brand name is Xylocaine Injectable
lisinopril	cardiovascular	brand name is Zestril
Lithane	antimanic	generic name is lithium carbonate
lithium carbonate	antimanic	brand name is Eskalith

Names	Functional Categories	Comment
lithium citrate	antimanic	brand name is Cibalith-S
Lithobid	antimanic	generic name is lithium carbonate
Lopressor	cardiovascular	generic name is metoprolol tartrate
lorazepam	anxiolytic	brand name is Ativan
loxapine succinate	antipsychotic	brand name is Loxitane
Loxitane	antipsychotic	generic name is loxapine succinate
Ludiomil	antidepressant	generic name is maprotiline hydrochloride
Luminal Sodium	antiepileptic	generic name is phenobarbital
Luvox	antidepressant	generic name is fluvoxamine
mannitol	diuretic	brand name is Osmitrol
maprotiline hydrochloride	antidepressant	brand name is Ludiomil
Marplan	antidepressant	generic name is isocarboxazid
Mebaral	antiepileptic	generic name is mephobarbital
Mellaril	antipsychotic	generic name is thioridazine hydrochloride
Mepergan	analgesic	generic name is meperidine hydrochloride
meperidine hydrochloride	analgesic	brand name is Mepergan
mephenytoin	antiepileptic	brand name is Mesantoin
mephobarbital	antiepileptic	brand name is Mebaral
meprobamate	anxiolytic	brand name is Miltown
Mesantoin	antiepileptic	generic name is mephenytoin
mesoridazine besylate	antipsychotic	brand name is Serentil
methadone hydrochloride	opiate agonist	brand name is Dolophine
methamphetamine hydrochloride	stimulant	brand name is Desoxyn
methenamine mandelate	antibiotic	brand name is Uroqid-Acid No. 2
methotrimeprazine	sedative	brand name is Levoprome
methsuximide	antiepileptic	brand name is Celontin
methyldopa	cardiovascular	brand name is Aldomet
methylphenidate hydrochloride	stimulant	brand name is Ritalin
metoclopramide hydrochloride	gastrointestinal	brand name is Reglan
metoprolol succinate	cardiovascular	brand name is Toprol XL
metoprolol tartrate	cardiovascular	brand name is Lopressor
metronidazole	antibiotic	brand names are Flagyl and Protostat
miconazole nitrate	antibiotic	brand name is Monistat
Midamor	diuretic	generic name is amiloride
midazolam hydrochloride	anxiolytic	brand name is Versed
Milontin	antiepileptic	generic name is phensuximide
Miltown	anxiolytic	generic name is meprobamate
Moban	antipsychotic	generic name is molindone hydrochloride
moclobemide	antidepressant	not available in U.S.
Moduretic	diuretic	generic name is amiloride
Mogadan	anxiolytic	generic name is nitrazepam
molindone hydrochloride	antipsychotic	brand name is Moban
Monistat	antibiotic	generic name is miconazole nitrate
Motrin	analgesic	generic name is ibuprofen
Mysoline	antiepileptic	brand name is primidone
nadolol	cardiovascular	brand name is Corgard
naloxone hydrochloride	opiate antagonist	brand name is Narcan
naltrexone hydrochloride	opiate antagonist	brand name is Trexan
Naprosyn	analgesic	generic name is naproxen
naproxen	analgesic	brand name is Naprosyn

Names	Functional Categories	Comment
naproxen sodium	analgesic	brand name is Anaprox
Narcan	opiate antagonist	generic name is naloxone hydrochloride
Nardil	antidepressant	generic name is phenelzine sulfate
Navane	antipsychotic	generic name is thiothixene
nefazodone	antidepressant	brand name is Serzone
Nembutal	antiepileptic	generic name is pentobarbital sodium
Neo-Synephrine	treat allergy	generic name is phenylephrine hydrochloride
Neurontin	antiepileptic	generic name is gabapentin
nialamide	antidepressant	brand name is Niamid
Niamid	antidepressant	generic name is nialamide
Nicoderm	smoking cessation	generic name is nicotine
nicotine	smoking cessation	brand name is Nicoderm
nifedipine	cardiovascular	brand name is Procardia
nimodipine	cardiovascular	brand name is Nimotop
Nimotop	cardiovascular	generic name is nimodipine
nitrazepam	anxiolytic	brand name is Mogadan
Nizoral	antibiotic	generic name is ketoconazole
Noctec	sedative	generic name is chloral hydrate
Norflex	anti-Parkinson	generic name is orphenadrine citrate
Normodyne	cardiovascular	generic name is labetolol hydrochloride
Norpramin	antidepressant	generic name is desipramine hydrochlorate
nortriptyline hydrochloride	antidepressant	brand name is Pamelor
olanzapine	antipsychotic	brand name is Zyprexa
omeprazole	treat ulcer	brand name is Prilosec
Orap	antipsychotic	generic name is pimozide
Orinase	antipsychotic	generic name is tolbutamide
orphenadrine citrate	anti-Parkinson	brand name is Norflex
Orudis	analgesic	generic name is ketoprofen
Osmitrol	diuretic	generic name is mannitol
oxazepam	anxiolytic	brand name is Serax
oxcarbazepine	antiepileptic	brand name is Trileptal
oxprenolol hydrochloride	cardiovascular	brand name is Trasicor
Pamelor	antidepressant	generic name is nortriptyline hydrochloride
Paradione	antiepileptic	generic name is paramethadione
Paral	antiepileptic	generic name is paraldehyde
paraldehyde	antiepileptic	brand name is Paral
paramethadione	antiepileptic	brand name is Paradione
Parlodel	anti-Parkinson	generic name is bromocriptine mesylate
Parnate	antidepressant	generic name is tranylcypromine sulfate
paroxetine hydrochloride	antidepressant	brand name is Paxil
Paxil	antidepressant	generic name is paroxetine hydrochloride
Paxipam	anxiolytic	generic name is halazepam
Peganone	antiepileptic	generic name is ethotoin
pemoline	stimulant	brand name is Cylert
penbutolol sulfate	cardiovascular	brand name is Levatol
pentobarbital sodium	antiepileptic	brand name is Nembutal
Periactin	antihistamine	generic name is cyproheptadine hydrochloride
perphenazine	antipsychotic	brand name is Trilafon
phenacemide	antiepileptic	brand name is Phenurone
phendimetrazine tartrate	stimulant	brand name is Plegine

Names	Functional Categories	Comment
phenelzine sulfate	antidepressant	brand name is Nardil
Phenergan	antihistamine	generic name is promethazine hydrochloride
phenobarbital	antiepileptic	brand name is Luminal Sodium
phensuximide	antiepileptic	brand name is Milontin
phentolamine mesylate	cardiovascular	brand name is Regitine
Phenurone	antiepileptic	generic name is phenacemide
phenylbutazone	analgesic	brand name is Butazolidin
phenylephrine hydrochloride	treat allergy	brand name is Neo-Synephrine
phenylpropanolamine	treat allergy	brand name is Propan
phenytoin	antiepileptic	brand name is Dilantin
physostigmine salicylate	anticholinergic	brand name is Isopto Eserine
pimozide	antipsychotic	brand name is Orap
pindolol	cardiovascular	brand name is Visken
piroxicam	analgesic	brand name is Feldene
Plegine	stimulant	generic name is phendimetrazine tartrate
Ponderal	treat obesity	generic name is fenfluramine hydrochloride
Ponderax	treat obesity	generic name is fenfluramine hydrochloride
Pondimin	treat obesity	generic name is fenfluramine hydrochloride
prazepam	anxiolytic	brand name is Centrax
prednisone	anti-inflammatory	brand name is Deltasone
Prilosec	treat ulcer	generic name is omeprazole
primidone	antiepileptic	brand name is Mysoline
Prinivil	cardiovascular	generic name is lisinopril
Priscoline	cardiovascular	generic name is tolazoline hydrochloride
probenecid	anti-arthritics	brand name is Benemid
Procardia	cardiovascular	generic name is nifedipine
prochlorperazine	antipsychotic	brand name is Compazine
procyclidine hydrochloride	anticholinergic agent	brand name is Kemadrin
Prolixin Decanoate	antipsychotic	generic name is fluphenazine decanoate
promazine hydrochloride	antipsychotic	brand name is Sparine
promethazine hydrochloride	antihistamine	brand name is Phenergan
propafenone hydrochloride	cardiovascular	brand name is Rythmol
Propan	treat allergy	generic name is phenylpropanolamine
propoxyphene hydrochloride	analgesic	brand name is Darvon
propranolol hydrochloride	anxiolytic	brand name is Inderal
Propulsid	treat ulcer	generic name is cisapride monohydrate
ProSom	anxiolytic	generic name is estazolam
Protostat	antibiotic	generic name is metronidazole
protriptyline hydrochloride	antidepressant	brand name is Vivactil
Prozac	antidepressant	generic name is fluoxetine hydrochloride
quazepam	anxiolytic	brand name is Doral
quinidine sulfate	cardiovascular	brand name is Quinidex
Quinidex	cardiovascular	generic name is quinidine sulfate
Redux	treat obesity	generic name is dexfenfluramine
Reglan	gastrointestinal	generic name is metoclopramide hydrochloride
Regitine	cardiovascular	generic name is phentolamine mesylate
reserpine	antipsychotic	brand name is Serpasil
Restoril	anxiolytic	generic name is temazepam
Rifadin	antibiotic	generic name is rifampin
rifampin	antibiotic	brand name is Rifadin

Names	Functional Categories	Comment
Rimactane	antibiotic	generic name is rifampin
Risperdal	antipsychotic	generic name is risperidone
risperidone	antipsychotic	brand name is Risperdal
Ritalin	stimulant	generic name is methylphenidate hydrochloride
Rufen	analgesic	generic name is ibuprofen
Rythmol	cardiovascular	generic name is propafenone hydrochloride
Sabril	antiepileptic	generic name is vigabatrin
Sandimmune	immunosuppressant	generic name is cyclosporine
scopolamine	anticholinergic	brand name is Transderm Scop
secobarbital	sedative	brand name is Seconal
Seconal	sedative	generic name is secobarbital
Sectral	cardiovascular	generic name is acebutolol
Seldane	antihistamine	generic name is terfenadine
selegiline hydrochloride	anti-Parkinson	brand name is Eldepryl
Serapax	anxiolytic	generic name is oxazepam
Serax	anxiolytic	generic name is oxazepam
Serentil	antipsychotic	generic name is mesoridazine besylate
Serpasil	antipsychotic	generic name is reserpine
sertindole	antipsychotic	not available at time of publication
sertraline hydrochloride	antidepressant	brand name is Zoloft
Serzone	antidepressant	generic name is nefazodone
Sinequan	antidepressant	generic name is doxepin hydrochloride
Sodium Sulamyd	antibiotic	generic name is sulfaphenazole
sotalol hydrochloride	cardiovascular	brand name is Betapace
Sparine	antipsychotic	generic name is promazine hydrochloride
spectinomycin hydrochloride	antibiotic	brand name is Trobicin
Stelazine	antipsychotic	generic name is trifluoperazine hydrochloride
succinylcholine chloride	autonomic	brand name is Anectine
sucralfate	treat ulcer	brand name is Carafate
sulfaphenazole	antibiotic	brand name is Sodium Sulamyd
sulindac	analgesic	brand name is Clinoril
sulpiride	D2 blocker	not available in U.S.
Surmontil	antidepressant	generic name is trimipramine maleate
Symmetrel	anti-Parkinson	generic name is amantadine
Synthroid	synthetic thyroid hormone	generic name is levothyroxine sodium
tacrine hydrochloride	anticholinergic	brand name is Cognex
Tagamet	treat ulcer	generic name is cimetidine
Taractan	antipsychotic	generic name is chlorprothixene
Tegretol	antiepileptic	generic name is carbamazepine
Temaril	antihistamine	generic name is trimeprazine tartrate
temazepam	anxiolytic	brand name is Restoril
Tenex	cardiovascular	generic name is guanfacine hydrochloride
Tenormin	cardiovascular	generic name is atenolol
terfenadine	antihistamine	brand name is Seldane
tetrabenazine	anti-Parkinson	brand name in U.K. is Nitoman
tetracycline hydrochloride	antibiotic	brand name is Achromycin
theophylline	antiasthmatic	brand name is Elixophyllin
thioridazine hydrochloride	antipsychotic	brand name is Mellaril
thiothixene	antipsychotic	brand name is Navane
Thorazine	antipsychotic	generic name is chlorpromazine hydrochloride

Names	Functional Categories	Comment
timolol maleate	cardiovascular	brand name is Timoptic
Timoptic	opthalmic	generic name is timolol maleate
Tindal	antipsychotic	generic name is acetophenazine
Tofranil	antidepressant	generic name is imipramine hydrochloride
tolazoline hydrochloride	cardiovascular	brand name is Priscoline
tolbutamide	antipsychotic	brand name is Orinase
Topamax	antiepileptic	generic name is topiramate
topiramate	antiepileptic	brand name is Topamax
Toprol XL	cardiovascular	generic name is metoprolol succinate
Transderm Scop	anticholinergic	generic name is scopolamine
Tranxene	anxiolytic	generic name is clorazepate dipotassium
tranylcypromine sulfate	antidepressant	brand name is Parnate
Trasicor	cardiovascular	generic name is oxprenolol hydrochloride
trazodone hydrochloride	antidepressant	brand name is Desyrel
Trexan	opiate antagonist	generic name is naltrexone hydrochloride
triazolam	anxiolytic	brand name is Halcion
Tridione	antiepileptic	generic name is trimethadione
trifluoperazine hydrochloride	antipsychotic	brand name is Stelazine
triflupromazine	antipsychotic	brand name is Vesprin
trihexyphenidyl hydrochloride	anti-Parkinson	brand name is Artane
Trilafon	antipsychotic	generic name is perphenazine
Trileptal	antiepileptic	generic name is oxcarbazepine
trimeprazine tartrate	antihistamine	brand name is Temaril
trimethadione	antiepileptic	brand name is Tridione
trimipramine maleate	antidepressant	brand name is Surmontil
Trobicin	antibiotic	generic name is spectinomycin hydrochloride
Tuinal	sedative	generic name is amobarbital
Urecholine	cholinergic agonist	generic name is bethanechol chloride
Uroqid-Acid No. 2	antibiotic	generic name is methenamine mandelate
Valium	anxiolytic	generic name is diazepam
Vallergan	antihistamine	generic name is trimeprazine tartrate
valproic acid	antiepileptic	brand name is Depakene
venlafaxine hydrochloride	antidepressant	brand name is Effexor
verapamil hydrochloride	cardiovascular	brand name is Calan
Versed	anxiolytic	generic name is midazolam hydrochloride
Vesprin	antipsychotic	generic name is triflupromazine
vigabatrin	antiepileptic	brand name is Sabril
Visken	cardiovascular	generic name is pindolol
Vistaril	antihistamine	generic name is hydroxyzine pamoate
Vivactil	antidepressant	generic name is protriptyline hydrochloride
Voltaren	analgesic	generic name is diclofenac
warfarin sodium	anticoagulant	brand name is Coumadin
Wellbutrin	antidepressant	generic name is bupropion hydrochloride
Xanax	anxiolytic	generic name is alprazolam
Xylocaine Injectable	anesthesia	generic name is lidocaine hydrochloride
Zarontin	antiepileptic	generic name is ethosuximide
Zebeta	cardiovascular	generic name is bisoprolol fumarate
Zestril	cardiovascular	generic name is lisinopril
Zoloft	antidepressant	generic name is sertraline hydrochloride
zopiclone	sedative	brand name is Imovane
Zyprexa	antipsychotic	generic name is olanzapine

SUBJECT INDEX

AAMR, see American Association on Mental Retardation

Aberrant Behavior Checklist (ABC), 6, 85, 86, 89, 90, 92, 186, 187, 192, 282

Abnormal Involuntary Movement Scale (AIMS), 59, 60, 110

absorption, 116

Accreditation Council for Facilities for the Mentally Retarded (ACMR), 47

Accreditation Council for Facilities for the Mentally Retarded and Other Developmentally Disabled Persons (ACMRDD), 47, 48, 53, 54, 59, 73

Accreditation Council on Services for People with Developmental Disabilities (ACDD), 47, 49, 53, 54, 57, 63

Accreditation Council on Services for People with Disabilities (ACD), 47, 49, 53, 58

acebutolol, 217, 272, 275

ACE inhibitors, 127

acetaldehyde, 204

acetaminophen, 119, 162

acetazolimide, 121, 127, 152, 219

acetylcholine, 135, 179, 180, 181, 209, 229, 295

acetylsalicylic acid, 163

ACTH, 292, 299

Adaptive Behavior Scale (ABS), 90, 92, 249

adaptive functioning, 5, 137, 138, 147

Adderall, 229

adjustment disorder, 15, 205, 208, 276, 284

adrenergic receptors, 123, 184, 211

adverse drug reactions (also see specific drugs), 48, 58, 60, 67, 95-111
   behavioral, 96-98
   cardiovascular, 98-99
   convulsive, 108
   endocrine & metabolic, 99-100
   hematologic, 101-102
   hepatic, 103-104
   immunologic & GI, 102-103
   masking by MR, 95
   monitoring guidelines, 108-109
   neuromuscular, 105-108
   rating scales, 109-111
   renal, 104-105
   sexual, 100-101

Adverse Drug Reaction Scale, 60, 110

African-Americans, 217

age, 35-36, 42, 80, 118, 311

aggressive behavior, 4, 8, 11, 12, 15, 21, 24, 25, 26-27, 32, 34, 35, 63, 95, 97, 124, 139, 143, 144, 145, 146, 155, 159, 172, 190, 179, 186, 191, 192, 193, 197, 204, 206, 207, 208, 211, 212, 219, 220, 221, 222, 223, 224, 225, 236, 238, 246, 247, 248, 249, 255, 264, 271, 277, 278, 279, 280, 281, 282, 283, 285, 286, 295, 296, 307, 316, 317

agmatine, 259

agoraphobia, see panic disorder

agranulocytosis 101, 102, 139, 157, 159

AIDS, 266

akathisia, 15, 32, 95, 96, 106, 138, 139, 140, 182, 205, 206, 208, 212, 213, 277-278, 279, 284, 285, 286

akinesia, 32, 96, 136, 138

albumin, 152, 153

alcohol, 24, 46, 115, 126, 140, 163, 186, 201, 203, 204, 262, 265, 291, 293

alcoholism, see substance abuse

Aldomet, see methyldopa

allergies, 210, 275, 315

aliphatic, 37

alopecia, 218

alprazolam, 39, 97, 119, 120, 125, 183, 201, 203, 206, 207, 281

Alzheimer's disease, 96, 193

amantadine, 32, 92, 104, 106

American Academy of Pediatrics, 167

American Association on Mental Deficiency, see American Association on Mental Retardation

American Association on Mental Retardation (AAMR), 4, 47

American Medical Association, 144

American Psychiatric Association (APA), 3, 4, 5, 8, 47, 58, 60, 66, 138, 142, 184, 189, 204

amiloride 100

amino acid, 152

aminophylline, 219

amitriptyline, 97, 100, 101, 123, 124, 139, 179, 180, 181, 182, 185, 189, 194, 224

ammonium chloride, 121

amnesia, 14, 97

amoxapine, 60, 97, 107, 108, 124, 180, 181, 182, 188

amphetamine, 14, 21, 23, 46, 97, 98, 124, 140, 229, 233, 234, 236, 237, 238, 244, 303

Anafranil, see clomipramine

analgesics, 201, 298

Anectine, 140

anemia, 101, 156, 157, 158, 159, 311

anesthesias, 261

anger, 295

dexamethasone, 119
Dexedrine, see dextroamphetamine
dextroamphetamine, 124, 126, 185, 229, 230, 231, 233, 236, 237, 244, 248, 250, 251, 252, 306
dextromethorphan, 125
diabetes, 158
diagnosis, see psychiatric diagnosis
Diagnostic Assessment of the Severely Handicapped (DASH), 89, 91
diagnostic overshadowing, 26, 86
Diamox, see acetazolimide
diarrhea, 103
diazepam, 24, 33, 37, 51, 102, 119, 125, 126, 151, 152, 170, 183, 201, 203, 206, 209
diazoxide, 99, 140
dibenzodiazepines, 32, 155
dibenzoxazepines, 32
dicarbamate, 152
diclofenac, 119, 121, 218
dicumarol, 163
diet, 26, 311-318
DiGeorge syndrome, 282
digitalis, 262
digoxin, 162, 183, 261
dihydroindolones, 32
Dilantin, see diphenylhydantoin 116
diltiazem, 119, 120, 129, 218
diphenhydramine, 23, 95, 105, 106, 138, 182, 209, 210, 283
diphenylbutylpiperidines, 32, 134
diphenylhydantoin, 23, 116, 117, 120, 163
disease entity, 3
disopyramide, 119
distractible, 12
disulfiram, 120, 204
diuretics, 218, 225, 262
divalproex sodium, 152
Doe v. Hudspeth, 58, 65, 66
dopamine, 59, 67, 106, 107, 123, 124, 135, 179, 180, 182, 229, 234, 263, 265, 266, 277, 295
dosage (see also specific medication)
    frequent changes, 63
    optimal, 62, 63-64, 67
    neuroleptics (antipsychotics), 66
    team monitoring, 80, 81
Dosage Record and Treatment Emergent Symptom Scale (DOTES), 60, 110
Down syndrome, 10, 96, 187, 190, 192, 193, 239, 275, 311, 312, 313, 317
doxepin, 96, 97, 124, 180, 181
doxycyline, 162

droperidol, 144
drug holiday, 36, 48, 62, 63, 80, 138, 297
DSM, see psychiatric diagnosis
dual diagnosis, 5, 26, 88, 142
dysarthria, 59, 217
dyskinesia, 96, 156, 158, 294, 305
Dyskinesia Identification System Condensed User Scale (DISCUS), 59, 60, 111, 139
dysphagia, 102
dysphasia, 86, 96, 102
dysthymic disorder, 10, 186, 196
dystonias, 32, 105, 106, 110, 138, 170, 305
E max, 122
eating disorder (also see anorexia), 179
ECT, see electroconvulsive shock
edema, 218
EEG, see electroencephalograpy
Effexor, see venlafaxine
EKG, see electrocardiogram
Elavil, see amitriptyline
Eldepryl, see selegiline
elderly, 124, 273
electrocardiogram (EKG), 136, 156, 185, 217, 261, 266, 279
electroconvulsive shock (ECT), 21, 22, 133, 141, 281, 297
electroencephalograpy (EEG), 157, 168, 217, 220, 233, 251, 292, 304, 314
emergencies, 50, 79, 209, 273
Emotional Problems Scales, see Behavior Rating Scales
enalapril, 127
enuresis, 7, 15, 104, 185, 197, 253
enzymes, 118, 119, 120-121, 123, 125, 136, 139, 153, 154, 155, 161, 182, 183, 184, 260, 273, 294, 299, 311, 313
eosinophilia, 101
ephedrine, 124
epilepsy, 20, 31, 32, 34, 51, 67, 86, 98, 108, 115, 122, 136, 139, 151-173, 193, 215, 220, 221, 222, 224, 233, 234, 250, 261,263, 304, 311
epinephrine, 140, 271, 292, 316
Equanil, see meprobamate
erythromycin, 119, 120, 122, 125, 163
Eskalith, see lithium
esmolol, 271, 272, 273
estrogen, 119, 137
ethanol, see alcohol
ethics, 24, 50
ethosuximide, 151, 152, 153, 156, 161, 162, 166, 167, 170
ethotoin, 152